AF734634

CANNABIS

Therapeutic Potential, Secondary Metabolites, Toxicity, and Regulations

Editors

Mahendra Rai

Department of Biotechnology
SGB Amravati University
Amravati, Maharashtra, India

Chistiane M. Feitosa

Laboratory of Research in Medicinal Plants and Experimental Neurochemistry
Federal University of Piauí
Teresina, PI, Brazil

CRC Press
Taylor & Francis Group
Boca Raton London New York

CRC Press is an imprint of the
Taylor & Francis Group, an **informa** business
A SCIENCE PUBLISHERS BOOK

First edition published 2027
by CRC Press
2385 NW Executive Center Drive, Suite 320, Boca Raton FL 33431

and by CRC Press
4 Park Square, Milton Park, Abingdon, Oxon, OX14 4RN

© 2027 Mahendra Rai and Chistiane M. Feitosa

CRC Press is an imprint of Taylor & Francis Group, LLC

Reasonable efforts have been made to publish reliable data and information, but the author and publisher cannot assume responsibility for the validity of all materials or the consequences of their use. The authors and publishers have attempted to trace the copyright holders of all material reproduced in this publication and apologize to copyright holders if permission to publish in this form has not been obtained. If any copyright material has not been acknowledged please write and let us know so we may rectify in any future reprint.

Except as permitted under U.S. Copyright Law, no part of this book may be reprinted, reproduced, transmitted, or utilized in any form by any electronic, mechanical, or other means, now known or hereafter invented, including photocopying, microfilming, and recording, or in any information storage or retrieval system, without written permission from the publishers.

For permission to photocopy or use material electronically from this work, access www.copyright.com or contact the Copyright Clearance Center, Inc. (CCC), 222 Rosewood Drive, Danvers, MA 01923, 978-750-8400. For works that are not available on CCC please contact mpkbookspermissions@tandf.co.uk

For Product Safety Concerns and Information please contact our EU representative GPSR@taylorandfrancis.com. Taylor & Francis Verlag GmbH, Kaufingerstraße 24, 80331 München, Germany.

Trademark notice: Product or corporate names may be trademarks or registered trademarks and are used only for identification and explanation without intent to infringe.

Library of Congress Cataloging-in-Publication Data (applied for)

ISBN: 978-1-041-08635-2 (hbk)
ISBN: 978-1-041-13130-4 (pbk)
ISBN: 978-1-003-66819-0 (ebk)

DOI: 10.1201/9781003668190

Typeset in Times New Roman
by Prime Publishing Services

Foreword

It gives me great pleasure to write the foreword for this important and timely volume, *Cannabis: Therapeutic Potential, Secondary Metabolites, Toxicity, and Regulations*, edited by Professors Mahendra Rai and Chistiane M. Feitosa. This book addresses a subject of growing global relevance at the intersection of science, health, and policy.

Cannabis has, for centuries, been both celebrated and stigmatized. In recent decades, however, advances in medical and pharmaceutical sciences have revealed its significant therapeutic potential, supported by an ever-growing body of evidence on its bioactive compounds. At the same time, questions regarding toxicity, safety, and regulation continue to generate robust debate among researchers, policymakers, and society at large. This book seeks to provide balanced insights into these complex issues.

What makes this volume particularly valuable is its interdisciplinary scope. By exploring the diverse secondary metabolites of cannabis, their pharmacological applications, potential adverse effects, and the regulatory frameworks governing their use, the editors and contributing authors offer a comprehensive resource for scientists, clinicians, students, and decision-makers alike. Such holistic treatment of the subject is essential in the context of One Health, where human health, plant science, and societal well-being are interconnected.

The Federal University of Piauí (UFPI) takes pride in supporting academic endeavors that bridge knowledge across borders and disciplines. This book not only enriches the scientific literature but also contributes to informed discussions on a topic that has social, economic, and ethical dimensions. I congratulate the editors and contributors for their dedication and vision in producing this volume, which I am confident will serve as a reference for future research and policy development in this field.

NADIR DO NASCIMENTO NOGUEIRA:18257135372

Assinado de forma digital por NADIR DO NASCIMENTO NOGUEIRA:18257135372
Dados: 2025.09.30 15:59:48 -03'00'

Prof. Dr. Nadir do Nascimento Nogueira
Rector

Federal University of Piauí (UFPI)
Teresina, Piauí – Brazil

Preface

Cannabis is native to South Asia and has been used for centuries in traditional medicine, particularly for the treatment of pain, insomnia, and gastrointestinal diseases. The plant has played a significant role in Asian and Egyptian cultures and has long been employed in China, India, and Egypt for managing a variety of diseases. In recent decades, however, its psychotropic activities and potential health risks have sparked considerable debate. Owing to rapid scientific advances and developing global regulations, cannabis has drawn the attention of scientists, medical professionals, policymakers, and society at large due to higher dose responsible for cardiovascular risks, brain disorders. It remains a subject of both scientific inquiry and public interest.

This book is organized into four sections: **Section 1** provides a general overview, discusses the current state of cannabis in the Asia-Pacific region, and examines its cultivation practices; **Section 2** explores the role of secondary metabolites produced by *Cannabis sativa* and their therapeutic potential. Topics include non-cannabinoid metabolites in therapy, the impact of cannabinoids on sleep, clinical trials and medical applications, the modulation of oxidative stress and inflammation by bioactive compounds, chemical and biological insights into *Cannabis sativa* roots, and the therapeutic potential of cannabis in metabolic disorders such as obesity, diabetes, dyslipidemia, and hypertension; **Section 3** addresses critical issues related to toxicity and risk assessment, including the risks and benefits of cannabis and cannabinoids in psychiatry, the association between cannabis use and psychosis or schizophrenia, and the implications of cannabis use during pregnancy; **Section 4** focuses on regulatory and socioeconomic perspectives, including global cannabis policies and regulatory frameworks.

This volume brings together diverse expertise to present a comprehensive and balanced perspective on *Cannabis sativa*. The book is highly interdisciplinary, with contributions from experts in medicine, pharmacology, agriculture, toxicology, and law. It serves as a valuable resource for researchers in botany, pharmacology, medicine, agriculture, and law; for policymakers; and for all readers interested in understanding cannabis and its applications.

We hope this volume will serve as an important resource for understanding the origin, cultivation, bioactive compounds, therapeutic applications, cultural significance, and regulatory landscape of cannabis.

We sincerely thank all contributors for their cooperation and research-based chapters.

Mahendra Rai

Chistiane M. Feitosa

Contents

Section 1
General Overview and Cultivation

Chapter 1

Introduction to Cannabis

History and Global Usage

Rishabh Agade, Ujban Hussain, Aditya Wadalkar, Divya Zambre, Veena S. Belgamwar and *Prashant Puranik*

1. Introduction

Cannabis is an adaptable and old plant of the Cannabis genus, which mainly comprises three species: *Cannabis sativa*, *Cannabis indica*, and *Cannabis ruderalis*. They have more than 100 cannabinoids, among which THC and CBD are the most researched. THC is the reason for the psychotropic effects of the plant, whereas CBD has captured international attention for its medicinal properties without causing intoxication (Schluttenhofer and Yuan 2017). Cannabis has played a variety of roles throughout history across civilizations, ritual, medicinal, recreational, and industrial. It was held sacred by ancient civilizations, whereas doctors in Asia and the Middle East utilized it for pain, inflammation, and mental illnesses (Zuardi 2006). Industrial hemp, a low-THC form of *Cannabis sativa*, on the other hand, was extensively employed for fabric, rope, and paper. Cannabis is a staple of both controversy and novelty today, standing at the nexus of law, medicine, commerce, and culture. To truly understand its multifaceted place in contemporary global society, it is necessary to understand its historical and botanical context (Russo 2005).

Cannabis possesses a deep and well-documented history in some of the world's most influential ancient cultures. Its first known reference is found in ancient China, where it was held in esteem for its medicinal and practical qualities. As early as 2700 BCE, cannabis was recorded in the Shennong Ben Cao Jing (The Divine Farmer's Materia Medica), one of the earliest books of Chinese herbal medicine. This ancient pharmacopoeia attributed healing properties to the plant, employing it in the treatment of conditions such as rheumatism, gout, malaria, and forgetfulness (Brand and Zhao 2017). In addition to medicine, hemp, originating from *Cannabis sativa*, was widely farmed for its fiber, playing a role in the manufacturing of clothing, ropes, fishing nets, and even early versions of paper. The Chinese also noted differences in the plant based on gender, with male and female varieties, demonstrating a surprisingly sophisticated understanding of botany for the time (Vasantha Rupasinghe et al. 2020).

In ancient India, cannabis was integrated into both religious and medicinal practices. Mentioned in the Atharva Veda (1500 BCE) as one of the five sacred plants, it was thought to be a divine gift.

Department of Pharmaceutical Sciences, Rashtrasant Tukadoji Maharaj Nagpur University, Nagpur-440033, Maharashtra, India.

* Corresponding author: vbelgamwar@gmail.com

DOI: 10.1201/9781003668190-2

Table 1: Historical timeline of cannabis usage across ancient civilizations.

Civilization	Approximate Period	Form of Use	Purpose	Key References
China	2700 BCE	Medicinal and Industrial (hemp)	Pain relief, malaria, fiber, and textiles	(Brand and Zhao 2017)
India	1500 BCE	Bhang (oral), Ayurvedic preparations	Rituals, digestion, sleep, and pain	(Jaiswal and Williams 2016)
Assyria/ Persia	1000 BCE	Incense and oral use	Religious rites, analgesia, and spiritual visions	(Crocq 2020)
Egypt	1500 BCE	Topical and inhaled remedies	Inflammation, hemorrhoids, and embalming rituals	(Metwaly et al. 2021)
Greece/Rome	1st century CE	Oil and edible cakes	Pain relief and digestive aid	(Totelin 2015)

In Ayurveda, cannabis was employed as a component in some preparations to stimulate appetite, ease pain, bring on sleep, and facilitate digestion. Perhaps most notably, the plant gained acceptance in religious festivals and ceremonies, particularly in bhang, the cannabis-infused milk beverage, and remains at the heart of celebrations such as that for Holi. It was believed to foster spiritual awareness, piety, and mystical visions, especially among Shaivite communities, where the deity Shiva is said to prefer the plant (Bapat 2016).

The Middle East also bears early witness to cannabis use, especially in Assyrian and Persian accounts from around the first millennium BCE. The Assyrians called cannabis "qunubu," a name some researchers think may have actually given rise to the current term cannabis. Assyrian writings speak of its use in religious incense, implying psychoactive uses in temple ceremonies. Persian medical authors and Zoroastrian literature speak of cannabis as an analgesic and a cause of spiritual awareness, pointing to its uses in both healing and mystical use.

In ancient Egypt, both archaeological and written evidence indicate that cannabis was used for medical and ritual purposes. Cannabis pollen has been identified in pharaonic tombs, including that of Ramses II, indicating its potential application in embalming practices or ritual ceremonies. Furthermore, medical treatises such as the Ebers Papyrus (c. 1550 BCE) document cannabis-based formulations for the treatment of inflammation and hemorrhoids, underscoring its early pharmacological relevance (Abdel-Salam et al. 2017). Classical civilizations like Greece and Rome also utilized cannabis in their medical practices. Greek physician Dioscorides, in his 1st-century work *De Materia Medica*, described cannabis as an effective treatment for earaches and for reducing sexual desire. Roman doctor Galen confirmed its pain-reducing property and its quality to make someone laugh when used in cakes. Table 1 shows timeline of cannabis usage across ancient civilization. While the use of the plant for recreational purposes was known, it was principally presented in terms of its health benefits and carefully prescribed.

Collectively, these varied civilizations illustrate the multifaceted use of cannabis—appreciated not just as a fiber and food crop but also as a sacred, medicinal, and psychoactive plant. Its incorporation into early medicine, spirituality, and society highlights the long-standing human connection with cannabis, laying the groundwork for its subsequent global spread and controversy (Charitos et al. 2020).

2. Cannabis and Colonial Economies

In the colonial period, cannabis, specifically in the guise of industrial hemp, became an important economic and strategic asset throughout European empires. Hemp, a low-THC form of *Cannabis sativa*, was crucial to naval powers such as Britain, France, and Spain because it was useful for making rope, sailcloth, and rigging necessary for maritime exploration and warfare (Vasantha Rupasinghe et al. 2020). The 17th and 18th-century European naval supremacy was primarily based on hemp fiber, which was extensively planted throughout Europe and its colonies. Colonial governments, such as the British Crown, issued mandates to colonial farmers in North America to cultivate hemp, recognizing its strategic potential for military and commercial expansion (Hyam 1993).

The introduction of cannabis to the Americas was facilitated by European powers, notably Spain and Britain, who brought both industrial hemp and psychoactive cannabis strains across the Atlantic. The Spanish introduced hemp to South America in the 16th century for fiber production, while the British colonial authorities promoted hemp cultivation in regions such as Virginia and Kentucky to support naval supplies. With time, psychoactive cannabis also migrated to the Americas through enslaved Africans and labour migrations, and caused varied patterns of medicinal as well as recreational use (Adebisi and Olaoye 2022).

Cannabis in Africa already had traditional roots in healing systems and spiritualities before European colonization. It was employed in rituals, medicinally for diseases such as malaria and dysentery, and even in childbirth as a sedative. With increasing colonial domination, the consumption of cannabis has at times been presented by colonial powers as undermining, especially if it was equated with resisting movements, mysticism, or worker solidarity by indigenous and enslaved peoples (Balthazar et al. 2022). Under plantation economies, hemp has traditionally been grown among other cash crops, thereby enhancing exploitative labour systems. The labor-intensive character of cannabis cultivation—be it for fiber or resin—made it wedded to colonial systems of coercive labor and helped entrench the economics of slavery, especially in the Americas and Caribbean (Višković et al. 2023).

3. Criminalization and the War on Drugs (1900–2000)

The 20th century marked a dramatic shift in global cannabis policy, transitioning from widespread traditional use and agricultural value to intense criminalization. This transformation was driven not purely by public health concerns, but also by political, racial, and economic motivations. The early decades saw the rise of prohibition campaigns, particularly in the United States, where cannabis began to be associated with marginalized groups, including Mexican immigrants and African Americans. This stigmatization laid the groundwork for legislative actions that would criminalize the plant for much of the century (Ransing et al. 2022).

A pivotal moment came in 1937 with the passage of the Marihuana Tax Act in the United States. Spearheaded by Harry Anslinger, the first commissioner of the Federal Bureau of Narcotics, the act effectively criminalized cannabis by imposing heavy taxes and bureaucratic restrictions on its sale and possession. Anslinger's campaign was rooted in sensationalist propaganda that linked cannabis use to crime, insanity, and moral decay. His rhetoric was steeped in racism, frequently targeting Black jazz musicians and Mexican laborers, and portraying them as dangerous users of "marihuana," a term deliberately chosen to emphasize foreignness and elicit fear.

The internationalization of cannabis prohibition followed shortly thereafter. Under pressure from the U.S., cannabis was included in several United Nations drug control conventions, including the 1961 Single Convention on Narcotic Drugs, which categorized cannabis alongside heroin and cocaine as a Schedule I substance. This classification required member nations to implement strict domestic controls, effectively globalizing the criminalization of cannabis. The 1971 Convention on Psychotropic Substances and the 1988 Convention Against Illicit Traffic in Narcotic Drugs further entrenched punitive policies, encouraging militarized enforcement and zero-tolerance approaches (Mills 2016).

Behind the legal architecture lay powerful racist and xenophobic propaganda that shaped public perception and policy. Films like *Reefer Madness* (1936) exaggerated the dangers of cannabis, claiming it caused madness, violence, and moral collapse. These narratives were often deployed to justify increased surveillance and policing of Black, Latino, and immigrant communities. The stigmatization of cannabis users as criminals, deviants, or threats to social order provided the political rationale for expanding state control, incarceration, and law enforcement budgets.

Table 2: Evolution of global cannabis control laws (1900–2000).

Year	Event	Description	References
1906	Pure Food and Drug Act (USA)	Required labeling of cannabis and other substances marked one of the earliest forms of federal regulation.	(Schroeder 2009)
1925	International Opium Convention (Geneva)	First international agreement to control cannabis; permitted export only for medical and scientific purposes.	(Riboulet-Zemouli 2025)
1937	Marihuana Tax Act (USA)	Effectively criminalized cannabis through taxation; launched the era of U.S.-led prohibition.	(Pacula and Smart 2017)
1961	UN Single Convention on Narcotic Drugs	Categorized cannabis as a Schedule I drug; signatory countries are mandated to restrict production and usage.	(Mills 2016)
1970	Controlled Substances Act (USA)	Officially placed cannabis in Schedule I, with no accepted medical use and high potential for abuse despite scientific opposition.	(Clark et al. 2011)
1971	UN Convention on Psychotropic Substances	Further restricted cannabis-related compounds and increased international compliance mechanisms.	(Lester et al. 2015)
1972	Shafer Commission Report (USA)	Recommended decriminalization; ignored by the Nixon administration.	(Nahas and Greenwood 1974)
1988	UN Convention Against Illicit Traffic in Narcotic Drugs	Strengthened global enforcement and criminal penalties; required national laws to criminalize possession and trafficking.	(Lines et al. 2017)
1996	California's Proposition 215	First U.S. state to legalize medical cannabis, signaling a shift in domestic and global perspectives.	(Satterlund et al. 2015)

The 1970s escalation under President Richard Nixon marked the onset of the formal "War on Drugs." Nixon's Controlled Substances Act of 1970 classified cannabis as a Schedule I drug, affirming its high abuse potential and supposed lack of medical use. Despite opposition from scientists and health professionals, the administration deliberately ignored recommendations from its own Shafer Commission, which advocated for decriminalization. Instead, Nixon used drug policy as a tool to target political adversaries. As later revealed by his domestic policy advisor, the strategy aimed to disrupt anti-war and Black civil rights movements by associating them with cannabis and heroin use, enabling their surveillance and mass arrest (Jackson 2024). Table 2 sumarizes evolution of gobal cannabies control laws in time period of 1990 to 2000

This period also saw a profound suppression of scientific research into cannabis. Federal grants for medical cannabis studies were withdrawn, and researchers faced bureaucratic obstacles in obtaining study materials. The decades-long chilling effect delayed advances in medical understanding and reinforced stigma. The Nixon-era policies cast a long shadow, influencing international drug policy, justifying mass incarceration, and distorting public discourse on cannabis for generations (National Academies of Sciences et al. 2017).

4. The Global Medical Cannabis Movement

After decades of strict prohibition, the late 20th century marked the re-emergence of medical cannabis as a legitimate area of clinical and policy interest. The shift was driven by both patient advocacy and renewed scientific exploration into the plant's therapeutic potential. By the 1970s and 1980s, clinical and anecdotal reports started to refute the myth that cannabis was just a dangerous drug of abuse, particularly as sick patients described symptom relief when mainstream treatments were not working (Hossain and Chae 2024). Table 3 illustrates examples of medical conditions in which cannabies showed possitive therapeutic effects.

Israel was one of the most significant centers of early research, with Professor Raphael Mechoulam and his colleagues conducting pioneering work in the field of cannabinoid science. In

Table 3: Summary of conditions supported by clinical evidence for cannabis treatment.

Medical Condition	Cannabinoid(s) Involved	Evidence Level	Therapeutic Effects	References
Chronic Neuropathic Pain	THC, THC:CBD combinations	Moderate to High	Pain reduction and improved sleep quality	(Mücke et al. 2018)
Epilepsy (e.g., Dravet Syndrome and LGS)	CBD	High (FDA-approved drug)	Seizure frequency reduction	(Kühne et al. 2023)
Multiple Sclerosis Spasticity	THC:CBD (e.g., Sativex)	Moderate	Muscle relaxation and reduced spasticity	(Russo et al. 2015)
Chemotherapy-Induced Nausea/Vomiting	THC (Dronabinol and Nabilone)	High	Anti-emetic effect and appetite stimulation	(Ware et al. 2008)
HIV/AIDS-related Cachexia	THC	Moderate	Appetite enhancement and weight gain	(Simon et al. 2021)
Post-Traumatic Stress Disorder (PTSD)	THC and CBD	Emerging	Reduction in nightmares, anxiety, and insomnia	(Sznitman et al. 2022)
Sleep Disorders	THC and CBD	Low to Moderate	Improved sleep latency and continuity	(Kaul et al. 2021)
Anxiety Disorders (Generalized and Social)	CBD	Low to Moderate	Anxiolytic effects without intoxication	(Smith et al. 2025)
Parkinson's Disease Symptoms	CBD	Preliminary	Improved quality of life and reduced tremors (limited evidence)	(Del-Bel et al. 2024)
Inflammatory Bowel Disease (IBD)	THC and CBD	Emerging	Reduced inflammation and pain (further research needed)	(Ahmed and Katz 2016)

the 1960s, they were able to isolate and synthesize THC and subsequently cannabidiol (CBD) and determine the psychoactive and non-psychoactive composition of the marijuana plant. Mechoulam's research also laid the groundwork for the identification of the endocannabinoid system, a human body system comprised of receptors that are key to mood control, appetite regulation, memory processes, and pain management. It was these advances that provided the scientific basis of contemporary cannabis medicines (Crippa et al. 2023).

America saw its first major policy change with California's Proposition 215, popularly referred to as the Compassionate Use Act of 1996. This historic bill enabled patients with specific medical ailments, such as cancer, AIDS, and chronic pain, to use cannabis, with a doctor's referral. The law followed grassroots movements by AIDS activists and cancer patients who found cannabis effective in treating nausea, pain, and appetite. Proposition 215 paved the way for other U.S. states and nations to reassess their medical cannabis legislation (Satterlund et al. 2015).

The clinical evidence base for medical cannabis has expanded considerably over the past few decades. Controlled trials and meta-analyses have shown its efficacy in treating a variety of conditions, such as chronic neuropathic pain, epilepsy (particularly treatment-resistant manifestations like Dravet syndrome), post-traumatic stress disorder (PTSD), spasticity in multiple sclerosis, chemotherapy-induced nausea and vomiting, and loss of appetite in HIV/AIDS. CBD, in fact, has been licensed by regulatory agencies such as the U.S. FDA in the form of Epidiolex, an agent for rare epilepsy (Hossain and Chae 2024).

In 2018, the World Health Organization (WHO) carried out a critical evaluation of cannabis and its derivatives. The WHO Expert Committee on Drug Dependence concluded that CBD is safe, non-addictive, and of therapeutic value, and advised that it be deleted from international drug control lists (Schlag et al. 2021). In addition, the committee advised that cannabis and related compounds be rescheduled to reflect better emerging evidence and minimize obstacles to research and medical use. These suggestions resulted in a landmark vote by the United Nations Commission on Narcotic

Drugs in December 2020, which rescheduled cannabis and recognized its medicinal utility, although nations still had the right to make their own laws (Nayak et al. 2023).

5. Legalization and Regulation Trends (2000–2025)

The early 21st century has witnessed a revolutionary change in the regulation and attitudes of countries towards cannabis. Increased awareness of its medicinal potential, coupled with the shortcomings of prohibitionist strategies, has resulted in the legalization and regulation of cannabis for medicinal and recreational purposes across various jurisdictions. This international shift has not only impacted health policy but also transformed global trade, human rights agendas, and pharmaceutical development (Smart and Pacula 2019).

Uruguay pioneered the full legalization of cannabis by adopting a law in 2013 permitting the cultivation and distribution of government-controlled cannabis. Intended to combat drug crime and control consumption, Uruguay's model was innovative, as it defied international narcotics conventions to place public health and safety above enforcement (Queirolo et al. 2019).

Canada subsequently enacted the Cannabis Act of 2018, the first G7 country to legalize recreational cannabis across the country. Canada's model features licensed commercial cultivation, adult-use retail sales, home growing, and robust public education efforts. Canada also allows medical cannabis by prescription and has emerged as a global leader in cannabis research and export (McDonald et al. 2025).

Medical cannabis was legalized in Germany in 2017, and in 2024, the nation legalized private use, home cultivation, and possession while opening pilot projects to legalize commercial sale under a controlled regime. Thailand followed a divergent approach and legalized medical cannabis in 2018 and decriminalized personal use in 2022, the first nation in Asia to make substantial inroads toward legalization (Manthey et al. 2024). South Africa's Constitutional Court legalized private cannabis use in 2018 on the grounds of constitutional privacy rights. Mexico's Supreme Court, on the other hand, ruled cannabis prohibition unconstitutional in 2018, and while complete regulation has been delayed, personal cultivation and consumption are now decriminalized (Riboulet-Zemouli and Clarke 2025).

In the U.S., despite federal prohibition, cannabis has been legalized for adult use in 24 states and Washington, D.C., as of 2025. Colorado, California, and New York are among the states that have established robust regulatory systems encompassing cultivation, distribution, taxation, and harm reduction. At the federal level, cannabis is still a Schedule I drug, posing intricate legal contradictions and hindering research (Orenstein and Glantz 2020).

Globally, these reforms have necessitated changes in the roles of the UN and regional agreements. In 2020, the United Nations Commission on Narcotic Drugs downgraded cannabis, taking it out of Schedule IV of the 1961 Single Convention, the most restrictive category for the most hazardous substances. Although still under Schedule I, the downgrade recognized the medical potential of cannabis, creating avenues for worldwide research and control (Mills 2016).

With these changes in the law comes an explosion of global market trends and pharma interest. The legalized cannabis market, valued at over $50 billion in 2024, encompasses a range of sectors, including wellness, cosmetics, food and beverage, and pharmaceutical markets (Baldwin et al. 2024). Firms are making investments in cannabinoid-derived drug development, such as synthetic THC analogs, purified CBD products, and nascent research into lesser-known cannabinoids such as CBG and CBN. International investment, patenting, and biotech entrepreneurship are transforming cannabis from an illicit drug into a science-based, regulated commodity of considerable economic and medicinal potential (Bonn-Miller et al. 2018).

Fully Legal (Dark green, Figure 1)

These countries have legalized both recreational and medical cannabis use for adults, often with regulated markets for cultivation, sale, and consumption:

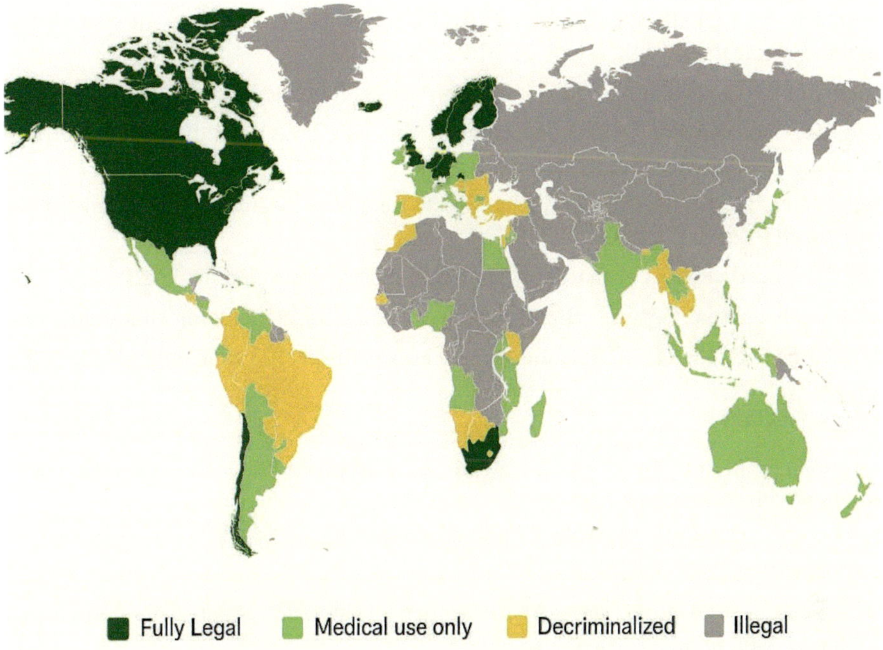

Figure 1: World Map of Cannabis Legal Status (2025).

- Canada: Legalized federally in 2018; includes licensed producers, storefronts, and home cultivation.
- Uruguay: First country to fully legalize cannabis (2013); state-monitored system with pharmacies and clubs.
- Germany: Legal for adult possession and home cultivation (2024); pilot retail projects under development.
- South Africa: Private personal use and cultivation legalized via court ruling (2018).
- Thailand: Cannabis decriminalized in 2022 with open access; pending stricter regulation.
- U.S.A (selected states): Recreational cannabis is legal in over half the states, though still federally prohibited.
- Malta and Luxembourg: Personal adult use and limited cultivation are allowed; sales are tightly regulated or in the planning stages.

Decriminalized (Yellow, Figure 1)

Cannabis possession and use are no longer criminal offenses, but are not legally authorized for commercial sale. Instead, administrative penalties like fines or warnings apply:

- Portugal: All drugs decriminalized since 2001; possession seen as a health issue.
- Spain: Private use decriminalized; cannabis clubs operate in legal gray zones.
- Jamaica: Decriminalized for small amounts and recognized for religious use (Rastafarian faith).
- Argentina, Colombia, and Chile: Personal use permitted, but sale and distribution remain illegal.
- India: Bhang (a cannabis preparation) is legally consumed in some states, especially during religious festivals.

Medical Use Only (Light green, Figure 1)

These countries have legalized cannabis strictly for medicinal use, often with specific qualifying conditions and medical oversight:

- Australia and New Zealand: Medical cannabis access regulated through federal programs.
- Brazil, Mexico, and Peru: CBD and medical cannabis laws passed; import and prescription regulated.
- Italy, Poland, the Netherlands, and the Czech Republic: Access to medicinal cannabis with prescription; local or imported.
- Israel: Advanced medical cannabis research and tightly controlled medical access.
- Thailand (also partially green): Broad access to medical care, including community cultivation.
- South Korea and Japan (CBD): Limited legal access to specific cannabinoids like CBD.

Illegal (Gray, Figure 1)

Cannabis remains fully prohibited in these countries. Possession, sale, and cultivation are criminal offenses, often with severe penalties:

- Asia: China, Indonesia, Malaysia, Singapore, and Japan maintain zero-tolerance policies, accompanied by harsh penalties.
- Middle East: Saudi Arabia, Iran, UAE, and others prohibit all cannabis activity; violations may carry long prison terms or worse.
- Africa: Most countries still consider cannabis illegal, though enforcement varies. Exceptions include Lesotho and Zimbabwe (medical cultivation).
- Russia and former Soviet states: Highly punitive cannabis laws with no legal pathways for use.

6. Cultural and Spiritual Uses in the Modern Era

In the contemporary world, cannabis remains a deep cultural and spiritual force in many societies, going beyond consumption to represent identity, resistance, and expression. Perhaps the most widely known spiritual connection with cannabis is in Rastafarianism, a religious and cultural movement that developed in Jamaica in the 1930s. Rastafarians see cannabis, called Ganja, as a sacred sacrament, being consumed in rituals and discussion periods to encourage self-reflection, spiritual enlightenment, and social bonding (Pretorius 2006). In part influenced by old Ethiopian culture and the Biblical text mentioning "herb," Rastafarians see cannabis as a gift of God that helps in the union with Jah. Although highly stigmatized in colonial and post-colonial times, cannabis is at the heart of their religious practice and opposition to Western materialism and oppression.

In South Asia, cannabis consumption is firmly embedded in Hindu spiritual practice, especially in India and Nepal. The plant is linked with Lord Shiva, who is frequently portrayed as consuming bhang, a cannabis-based drink. At festivals such as Maha Shivaratri and Holi, bhang is ritually consumed as a way of worship, purification, and transcendence. Sadhus, or Hindu ascetics, traditionally use cannabis to facilitate meditation and attain detachment from worldly troubles. In Nepal, particularly among Pashupatinath Temple precincts, cannabis use has traditionally been condoned as an element of religious practice, albeit against modern-day legal prohibitions (Shakya et al. 2021).

Cannabis has also had a lasting influence on artistic and musical movements, often as a symbol of rebellion, creativity, and non-conformity. In the jazz culture of the 1920s to 1940s, African American musicians used cannabis both as a stimulant for musical improvisation and as a subtle act of resistance against systemic racism. Subsequently, reggae music, made famous by artists such as Bob Marley, transmitted both the religious message of Rastafarianism and political messages that framed cannabis as a means of liberation. In hip-hop, especially from the 1990s onwards, cannabis was a powerful cultural symbol of authenticity, rebellion, and urban identity, although it also served to fuel stereotypes and law enforcement targeting of minority communities.

At the same time, cannabis has been used to create subcultural identities, from 1960s countercultural movements to current global cannabis lifestyle brands. Such identities tend to defy societal norms and espouse individual freedom, natural living, and spiritual consciousness. Yet, these expressions are not stigma-free. The historical connection of cannabis with criminality, deviance, and minority populations has led to social exclusion, legal persecution, and public misconceptions. Even while legalization expands, cultural stigmas still affect users—especially from historically marginalized communities, pointing to the enduring battle for social acceptance and cultural legitimacy.

7. Cannabis and Public Health

As cannabis becomes increasingly legally accepted across the globe, its public health implications have become a top priority for policymakers, healthcare professionals, and researchers. The cannabis debate has moved from one focused solely on prohibition or legalization to one that increasingly examines how cannabis can be incorporated into public health systems in a manner that maximizes benefits while minimizing harms. This more subtle method requires a sophisticated consideration of the plant's healing potential, risks, especially for vulnerable groups, and the general cultural effects of its use (Wilkinson et al. 2015).

7.1 Benefits vs. Risks: A Balanced Perspective

Cannabis possesses widely known therapeutic effects, especially in chronic pain patients, chemotherapy-induced vomiting, epilepsy, spasticity of multiple sclerosis, and other anxiety disorders. Its active elements—primarily tetrahydrocannabinol (THC) and cannabidiol (CBD)—interact with the body's endocannabinoid system to moderate mood, hunger, sleep, and pain. These therapeutic outcomes have prompted pharmaceutical cannabis derivatives, such as Epidiolex (CBD for seizure control) and Dronabinol (THC for the stimulation of appetite) (Matheson and Le Foll 2020).

But cannabis use comes with health dangers, especially if used irresponsibly or in the absence of medical supervision. Perhaps the best-researched danger is cannabis dependence. The World Health Organization estimates that about 1 in 10 adult users and 1 in 6 youths will develop cannabis use disorder (CUD). It is characterized by psychological dependence, withdrawal symptoms, and an inability to cut down despite negative effects (Leinen et al. 2023).

Teenagers are at special risk. Many studies that have employed neuroimaging technologies have concluded that early exposure to cannabis interferes with development, particularly in parts of the brain involved with executive function, memory, and emotions. Exposure to THC through critical developmental phases can have longstanding cognitive consequences, heightened psychotic potential, and inferior educational and labor market results. As a result, nearly all public health bodies strongly oppose usage before 25.

Another concern is drug-impaired driving by cannabis. While cannabis does not impair motor function as alcohol does, it impairs reaction time, coordination, and attention, which puts people at a higher risk of causing traffic accidents. In contrast to alcohol, THC may still be detected in the blood after impairment has passed, making roadside measurement and threshold determination in law a challenging task (Jacobus and Tapert 2014). Legalized cannabis jurisdictions have experienced varied outcomes: while some have observed spikes in cannabis-involved traffic crashes, others have noted no real change, implying that wider contextual elements, including education and enforcement, influence (Pearlson et al. 2021).

7.2 Strategies for Harm Reduction

Instead of supporting abstinence by itself, contemporary public health frameworks prioritize harm reduction, a realist strategy geared towards reducing the harms of drug consumption without necessarily ending it. The model proves useful for cannabis due to its prevalent use and rising legality (Farrelly et al. 2023).

A key approach is regulating the product. Legalized cannabis markets generally have caps on THC levels, child-resistant packaging requirements, and strict labeling with potency, origin, and health warnings. Some jurisdictions have implemented "seed-to-sale" tracking systems to track quality and avoid contamination with pesticides, mold, or heavy metals (Payne-James 2015).

Public consumption legislation also has harm reduction purposes. Governments seek to decrease secondhand exposure and deter youth normalization by limiting cannabis use in public or near minors. "Start low, go slow" policies are another example where governments teach consumers, particularly new or older users, how to prevent overuse and bad psychological reactions such as panic attacks or acute psychosis (Caulkins and Kilborn 2019).

Cannabis education programs, usually based on tobacco and alcohol campaigns, are designed to educate, not to scare. Stress is laid on learning about personal tolerance, staying away from poly-substance use (e.g., with alcohol), and knowing high-potency products such as edibles and concentrates, which pose a higher risk of overuse due to delayed effects.

Clinical practice guidelines have also appeared for clinicians, guiding how to advise patients on cannabis use, screen for cannabis use disorder, and recommend cannabis as part of an integrated treatment plan, especially in palliative care or chronic disease situations (Bell et al. 2024).

7.3 CBD Wellness Trends and Commercialization

Together with the recreational and medical markets, exists the lucrative world trade in CBD-infused health products. The non-intoxicating cannabinoid cannabidiol (CBD) has emerged as a new favorite for perceived anti-anxiety, anti-inflammatory, and insomnia-relieving activities. In 2025, CBD is featured in a vast array of products, including oils, capsules, cosmetics, beverages, pet products, and even clothes with CBD microcapsules inserted (Kicman and Toczek 2020).

CBD's business appeal is its wide marketability: it is not a "high," is typically well-tolerated, and can be sold as a natural health supplement. This is appealing to elderly individuals, athletes, and those with no cannabis experience. But regulatory surveillance of CBD products is erratic. In most places, over-the-counter CBD products are weakly regulated, so there is concern about incorrect labeling, inadequate dosing, and adulteration (Simei et al. 2024).

Clinical evidence for CBD is growing, but its applications are still in their infancy for most suggested uses. Whereas there is robust evidence for its therapeutic value in the management of some types of epilepsy, evidence of efficacy for anxiety, sleep disorders, and chronic pain continues to emerge. Health authorities have sounded an alarm that rash marketing often precedes scientific evidence, thereby confusing consumers and diverting them from evidence-based therapies (Singh et al. 2023).

In response, some nations have set quality standards for CBD products, mandating third-party testing and prohibiting unsubstantiated health claims. Others have begun to incorporate CBD into existing pharmaceutical models, mandating prescriptions for the higher-dose formulations but permitting low-dose formulations to be marketed openly (Baratta et al. 2025).

7.4 Educational Campaigns and Regulatory Warnings

With expanding legalization, education and public messaging have been essential elements in cannabis policy. Governments and public health agencies have the responsibility of educating the public about the possible benefits as well as the potential risks of cannabis in a simple, science-oriented, and stigma-free way (E. and M. H. and M. D. B. on P. H. and P. H. P. C. on the P. H. C. of C. in the C. P. L. National Academies of Sciences et al. 2024).

Contemporary public education campaigns are shifting away from the scare tactics of the "Reefer Madness" days, instead focusing on evidence-based strategies that balance respect for personal autonomy with a promotion of safe use. Campaigns generally address a number of target populations.

- Adolescents and young adults: Messaging focuses on delaying use, understanding risks to brain development, and resisting peer pressure.
- Pregnant and breastfeeding individuals: Warnings about the potential effects of THC on fetal development are emphasized, with campaigns advising complete abstinence.
- Older adults: Many seniors exploring cannabis for the first time are educated on dosing, interactions with medications, and risks such as falls or cardiovascular issues.
- Drivers: Public service announcements emphasize the dangers of cannabis-impaired driving and promote designated driver alternatives.

Cannabis packaging in regulated markets also includes health warnings, much like tobacco and alcohol. Labels often highlight potential side effects (e.g., dizziness, dry mouth, and anxiety), contraindications (e.g., use during pregnancy), and contact information for poison control centers or addiction support services (Narouze et al. 2024).

To ensure inclusivity and accessibility, some jurisdictions have launched multilingual campaigns or targeted outreach to communities historically criminalized for cannabis use. In doing so, public health efforts can contribute not only to safer use but also to restorative justice by addressing misinformation and historical inequities (Tyskiewicz et al. 2022).

8. Industrial Hemp and the Green Economy

Industrial hemp (*Cannabis sativa* L.) has emerged as a cornerstone of the green economy in the 21st century, driven by growing environmental concerns, the need for sustainable raw materials, and changing regulatory policies. In contrast to THC-laden cannabis, hemp has trace levels of tetrahydrocannabinol (usually less than 0.3% dry weight) and does not yield psychoactive effects. Its unique legal status and incredible versatility have made hemp an exciting solution for various industries, including construction, clothing, food production, and environmental rehabilitation.

Hemp is one of the oldest crops known to humanity. Its fibrous, strong stalks have been cultivated since ancient times. In ancient times, hemp was utilized to manufacture ropes, sailing vessels, paper, and garments throughout ancient world civilizations. Current hemp fibers are experiencing a modern-day renaissance in green lines of products (Ingrao et al. 2015). Bast fibers found on the outer stalk are as strong as those of flax and jute, and find applications in biodegradable textiles, composites, and insulation panels. Hurd (inner core) fibers of shorter lengths can be used to produce hempcrete, a lightweight, ventilated, and energy-efficient building material that serves as a carbon-sequestering substitute for concrete. Hempcrete has found applications in an increasing number of green building projects in Europe and North America (Neijat et al. 2016).

In addition to its fiber, hemp seeds contain a rich content of protein, omega-3 and omega-6 fatty acids, and essential nutrients, and are, therefore, an upmarket plant food in oil, protein powder, or shelled seed forms. The seeds lack cannabinoids and can be eaten without harm, making them an excellent crop for use in both food security and health. Furthermore, hemp seed oil has gained widespread use in the cosmetic, skincare, and nutraceutical industries, contributing significantly to its commercial applications (Manniche 1989).

From an environmental perspective, hemp has great sustainability benefits. Hemp is a low-input crop, as it grows quickly and has dense leaves that shade out weeds, requiring few pesticides and herbicides. Hemp has a brief cultivation cycle (around 90–120 days), and its extensive root system enhances the structure of the soil and stops erosion. Hemp is also a phytoremediator, which can absorb heavy metals and toxins from contaminated soils—a quality that has been utilized in land reclamation efforts, such as around the Chernobyl nuclear accident site. Additionally, hemp farming

Industrial Applications of Hemp and Their Environmental Benefits

APPLICATION AREA	HEMP-DERIVED PRODUCT	ENVIRONMENTAL BENEFITS
Construction	Hempcrete, insulation panels	Carbon-negative material Energy-efficient Blodegradable-a don-toxic
Textiles & Fabrics	Hemp fiber clothing, geotextiles	Requires less water than cotton Naturally pest-resistant
Paper & Packaging	Hemp pulp paper, biodegradable wraps	Faster-growing than trees Recyclable Reduces deforestation
Bioplastics	Hemp-based polymers	Renewable alternative to petroleum plastics Biodegradable
Food & Nutrition	Hemp seeds, oil protéin powder	High-yleld food crop Plant-based protein source Sustainable to cultivate
Cosmetics & Personal Care	Hemp seed oil in lotions, shampoos	Rich in omega fatty acids Eco-friendly formulations Supports organic farming practices
Biofuels	Hemp biodiesel and ethanol	Lower carbon emissions than fossil fuels Renewable and efficient in land use
Animal Bedding & Feed	Hemp hurds processed seed cake	Absorbent, compostable bedding Nutrient-rich animal feed byproduct

Figure 2: Industrial Applications of Hemp and their Environmental Benefits.

is beneficial for carbon sequestration, with estimates suggesting that it can absorb more CO_2 per hectare than most forests, and thus a valuable tool in climate mitigation efforts (Placido and Lee 2022). Figure 2 sumarizes industrial applications of hemp and their enviroemental benifits.

One of the key elements of hemp's industrial comeback has been the unambiguous legal separation of industrial hemp and psychoactive cannabis. Throughout most jurisdictions, this separation is enacted through the maximum THC content allowed—usually 0.2% in the European Union, 0.3% in the United States and Canada, and up to 1% in some nations such as Switzerland and Thailand. The capacity to control and screen hemp crops for THC content has made hemp legal to grow even in nations that still prohibit cannabis for medicinal or recreational purposes. This distinction is crucial not only for public image and compliance but also for international commerce, where the classification influences import/export authorization, tariffs, and certification (Fordjour et al. 2023).

International policy-making organizations have increasingly recognized the value of industrial hemp. Low-THC industrial hemp is not categorized by the United Nations in the same control group as high-THC cannabis, particularly since the 2020 vote of the UN Commission on Narcotic Drugs, which deleted cannabis from Schedule IV of the 1961 Single Convention. While cannabis is still a controlled substance under Schedule I, hemp or industrial hemp is considered an exception in international regulations, particularly when there is corresponding national-level legal support.

In the European Union, hemp production is promoted under the Common Agricultural Policy (CAP), and farmers are eligible for subsidies to grow certified hemp crops. The EU has also established standards for THC levels, seed certification, and industrial classification of permitted uses. Hemp is prominently featured in the EU's Green Deal and Circular Economy Action Plan, where it is seen as having the potential to replace fossil-fuel-based plastics, reduce agricultural emissions, and contribute to meeting bioeconomy objectives (Kaminski et al. 2024).

Hemp's reindustrialization is an increasing recognition of the plant's eco-industrial value. Startups and global giants are all investing in hemp-derived bioplastics, insulation, biofuels, animal bedding, and even car components, where hemp composites replace metal to lower vehicle weight and increase fuel efficiency. France, the Netherlands, and Canada are among the leading nations in hemp innovation, with ecosystems of growers, processors, researchers, and product developers emerging (Ahmed et al. 2022).

Despite this potential, several obstacles persist. Scale is prevented by the absence of processing infrastructure in most areas, and variable policies regarding THC testing, harvest, and end-use classification leave farmers and investors uncertain. Moreover, decades of prohibition for cannabis have given rise to a regulatory and social baggage that continues to criminalize hemp growth in some areas. Education, economic incentives, and more transparent policy settings are necessary to unlock hemp's full potential.

9. Future Directions and Perspectives

As the world of cannabis continues to shift, the future of the plant is not just in policy change and commodification but also in furthering scientific research, cultivation technology, social justice, and environmental responsibility. New frontiers are emerging quickly that will further our knowledge of cannabis' potential and transform how it is brought into society.

One of the brightest potential avenues for exploration is research on minor cannabinoids and terpene science. While THC and CBD have been the main focus of study and product development, the cannabis plant has more than 100 other cannabinoids like CBG, CBN, and THCV with distinct pharmacological profiles. Minor cannabinoids are being examined for uses in the treatment of conditions that range from neurodegenerative disease to metabolic disease (Walsh et al. 2021). Also, terpenes, the organic molecules responsible for the smell of cannabis, are becoming increasingly scientifically noted for their potential entourage effect, where they act synergistically with cannabinoids to maximize therapeutic effects. Unlocking these intricate phytochemical interactions could lead to the development of tailored formulations for specific medical conditions or user profiles (Laaboudi et al. 2024).

Alongside this, advances in artificial cultivation methods are transforming the way cannabis is cultivated. Vertical and controlled environment agriculture (CEA) enables year-round production on a minimal amount of land and water, maintaining consistent quality and phytochemical profiles. Still more sophisticated methods, including bioreactors and cell culture, are emerging for producing cannabinoids without the need to grow the plant at all (Heuvelink et al. 2025). These technologies utilize biosynthesis using yeast, algae, or genetically modified cells to produce cannabinoids such as THC and CBD on an industrial scale. This would decrease the environmental impact of cultivation and provide pharmaceutical-grade uniformity for medical use (Hussain et al. 2021).

Aside from laboratory technology, there is increasing acknowledgment of the significance of bioprospecting and native knowledge in cannabis science. Local cannabis varieties have been utilized by indigenous and traditional communities in Asia, Africa, and the Americas for centuries, usu ally with distinctive healing practices and strain selection (Große et al. 2021). These communities serve as a reservoir of ethnobotanical knowledge that can complement scientific studies. Yet, ethical frameworks are necessary to ensure that knowledge is not used without agreement or benefit-sharing. Principles such as Access and Benefit-Sharing (ABS) in the Nagoya Protocol promote responsible bioprospecting by demanding fair collaboration and compensation to traditional knowledge owners (Heinrich et al. 2020).

With cannabis emerging as an international commodity, questions of ethics, equity, and social justice are entering the limelight. Legal cannabis economies have disproportionately enriched investors and corporations at the expense of marginalized groups, with those most impacted by prohibition too often locked out of economic inclusion. Racial and economic inequalities continue in cannabis licensing, employment, and business ownership in most nations (Hendy et al. 2023). Equity-focused legalization platforms, as in states like Illinois and New York, seek to remedy gaps through the establishment of social equity programs, erasing prior convictions, and assisting minority cannabis businesses. However, implementation challenges remain, and broader international frameworks are needed to embed justice into the cannabis economy (Garriott and Garcia-Fuerte 2023).

In addition, international commercialization of cannabis poses corporate ethics, patent monopolies, and biodiversity conservation issues. Large agricultural and pharmaceutical corporations are increasingly patenting cannabis genetic material and cannabinoid formulations, raising issues of biopiracy and intellectual property disputes. There is an urgent need for open-access research, public domain strain databases, and legal safeguards that acknowledge communal knowledge and environmental stewardship.

Here, the future of cannabis is not just a scientific or commercial issue, but a multifaceted task including technology, ecology, culture, and justice. A future for cannabis that is inclusive and sustainable will demand collaborative governance, ethical innovation, and global solidarity, integrating old wisdom and new science, and balancing profit with planetary and social health.

10. Conclusion

Cannabis has followed an extraordinary historical trajectory—having been used for its earliest known purposes as an ancient medicinal plant and sacred plant, to being demonized in the 20th century, and now toward its resurgence as a scientifically established and commercially viable plant. Throughout civilizations in Asia, Africa, the Middle East, and Europe, cannabis was venerated for its medicinal value, spiritual properties, and industrial uses. But the arrival of colonialism and the emergence of prohibitionist thinking in the 20th century reconfigured cannabis as a marker of deviance, precipitating mass criminalization, stigmatization, and suppression of research.

The last three decades have seen a paradigm shift. Motivated by patient activism, scientific discovery, and socio-political change, cannabis has come back into the global limelight—not just as a medicine but as an economic driver, a driver of legal reform, and a symbol of cultural legitimacy. Contemporary science has debunked many of the myths surrounding the plant's pharmacology, isolating cannabinoid chemicals and their interaction with the human endocannabinoid system, thus authenticating traditional knowledge with scientific facts.

However, as cannabis is incorporated into legal and medical systems, there must be a balanced strategy—one that respects cultural heritage, encourages ethical commercialization, is guaranteed equitable access, and is responsive to the public health challenges entailed in its consumption. Policies should be based on science, but they should also be inclusive, redemptive, and future-oriented, especially in correcting the past injustices of prohibition.

The future of cannabis lies in interdisciplinary stewardship, one that spans ethnobotany and biotechnology, indigenous wisdom and regulatory acumen, as well as commercial potential and human rights. This way, society can transform cannabis from a divisive topic to a rallying point for health, sustainability, and social advancement.

References

Abdel-Salam, O. M. E., Galal, A. F., ElShebiney, S. A., and Gaafar, A. E. D. M. (2017). International Aspects of Cannabis Use and Misuse: Egypt. *Handbook of Cannabis and Related Pathologies: Biology, Pharmacology, Diagnosis, and Treatment*, 110–121. https://doi.org/10.1016/B978-0-12-800756-3.00013-2

Adebisi, Y. A., and Olaoye, D. Q. (2022). Medical Use of Cannabis in Africa: The Pharmacists' Perspective. *Innovations in Pharmacy*, 13(1): 10.24926/iip.v13i1.4430. https://doi.org/10.24926/IIP.V13I1.4430

Ahmed, A. T. M. F., Islam, M. Z., Mahmud, M. S., Sarker, M. E., and Islam, M. R. (2022). Hemp as a potential raw material toward a sustainable world: A review. *Heliyon*, 8(1): e08753. https://doi.org/10.1016/J.HELIYON.2022.E08753.

Ahmed, W., and Katz, S. (2016). Therapeutic Use of Cannabis in Inflammatory Bowel Disease. *Gastroenterology and Hepatology*, 12(11): 668. https://pmc.ncbi.nlm.nih.gov/articles/PMC5193087/

Baldwin, G. T., Vivolo-Kantor, A., Hoots, B., Roehler, D. R., and Ko, J. Y. (2024). Current Cannabis Use in the United States: Implications for Public Health Research. *American Journal of Public Health*, 114(Suppl 8), S624. https://doi.org/10.2105/AJPH.2024.307823

Balthazar, C., Joly, D. L., and Filion, M. (2022). Exploiting Beneficial Pseudomonas spp. for Cannabis Production. *Frontiers in Microbiology*, 12. https://doi.org/10.3389/FMICB.2021.833172/FULL

Bapat, S. N. (2016). Cannabis: The Forgotten Sacred Plant of India. *Journal of Ayurveda and Holistic Medicine*, 3(5): 92–96.

Baratta, F., Brusa, P., Firenzuoli, F., Jardim, C., and Begoña Delgado-Charro, M. (2025). The regulatory environment surrounding cannabis medicines in the EU, the USA, and Australia. *Pharmaceutics* 2025, Vol. 17, Page 635, 17(5), 635. https://doi.org/10.3390/PHARMACEUTICS17050635

Bell, A. D., MacCallum, C., Margolese, S., Walsh, Z., Wright, P., Daeninck, P. J. et al. (2024). Clinical practice guidelines for cannabis and cannabinoid-based medicines in the management of chronic pain and co-occurring conditions. *Cannabis and Cannabinoid Research*, 9(2): 669–687. https://doi.org/10.1089/CAN.2021.0156

Bonn-Miller, M. O., ElSohly, M. A., Loflin, M. J. E., Chandra, S., and Vandrey, R. (2018). Cannabis and Cannabinoid Drug Development: Evaluating Botanical Versus Single Molecule Approaches. *International Review of Psychiatry (Abingdon, England)*, *30*(3), 277. https://doi.org/10.1080/09540261.2018.1474730

Brand, E. J., and Zhao, Z. (2017). Cannabis in Chinese medicine: are some traditional indications referenced in ancient literature related to cannabinoids? *Frontiers in Pharmacology*, 8(MAR): 108. https://doi.org/10.3389/FPHAR.2017.00108

Caulkins, J. P., and Kilborn, M. L. (2019). Cannabis legalization, regulation, and control: a review of key challenges for local, state, and provincial officials. *American Journal of Drug and Alcohol Abuse*, 45(6): 689–697. https://doi.org/10.1080/00952990.2019.1611840

Charitos, I. A., Gagliano-Candela, R., Santacroce, L., and Bottalico, L. (2020). The cannabis spread throughout the continents and its therapeutic use in history. *Endocrine, Metabolic and Immune Disorders - Drug Targets*, 21(3): 407–417. https://doi.org/10.2174/1871530320666200520095900

Clark, P. A., Capuzzi, K., and Fick, C. (2011). Medical marijuana: Medical necessity versus political agenda. *Medical Science Monitor : International Medical Journal of Experimental and Clinical Research*, 17(12): RA249. https://doi.org/10.12659/MSM.882116

Crippa, J. A. S., Guimarães, F. S., Zuardi, A. W., and Hallak, J. E. C. (2023). Dr. Raphael Mechoulam, cannabis and cannabinoids research pioneer (November 5, 1930–March 9, 2023) and his legacy for Brazilian pharmacology. *Brazilian Journal of Psychiatry*, 45(3): 201. https://doi.org/10.47626/1516-4446-2023-0047

Crocq, M. A. (2020). History of cannabis and the endocannabinoid system. *Dialogues in Clinical Neuroscience*, 22(3): 223. https://doi.org/10.31887/DCNS.2020.22.3/MCROCQ

Del-Bel, E., Barros-Pereira, N., Moraes, R. P. de, Mattos, B. A. de, Alves-Fernandes, T. A., Abreu, L. B. de et al. (2024). A journey through cannabidiol in Parkinson's disease. *International Review of Neurobiology*, 177: 65–93. https://doi.org/10.1016/BS.IRN.2024.04.015

Farrelly, K. N., Wardell, J. D., Marsden, E., Scarfe, M. L., Najdzionek, P., Turna, J. et al. (2023). The impact of recreational cannabis legalization on cannabis use and associated outcomes: A systematic review. *Substance Abuse: Research and Treatment*, 17: 11782218231172054. https://doi.org/10.1177/11782218231172054

Fordjour, E., Manful, C. F., Sey, A. A., Javed, R., Pham, T. H., Thomas, R. et al. (2023). Cannabis: a multifaceted plant with endless potentials. *Frontiers in Pharmacology*, 14: 1200269. https://doi.org/10.3389/FPHAR.2023.1200269

Garriott, W., and Garcia-Fuerte, J. (2023). *The Social Equity Paradigm: The Quest for Justice in Cannabis Legalization.*

Große, M., Ruetalo, N., Layer, M., Hu, D., Businger, R., Rheber, S. et al. (2021). Quinine inhibits infection of human cell lines with sars-cov-2. *Viruses*, 13(4). https://doi.org/10.3390/V13040647

Heinrich, M., Scotti, F., Andrade-Cetto, A., Berger-Gonzalez, M., Echeverría, J., Friso, F. et al. (2020). Access and benefit sharing under the nagoya protocol—Quo Vadis? Six Latin american case studies assessing opportunities and risk. *Frontiers in Pharmacology*, 11: 765. https://doi.org/10.3389/FPHAR.2020.00765

Hendy, K., Mauri, A. I., and Creary, M. (2023). Bounded equity: The limits of economic models of social justice in cannabis legislation. *Contemporary Drug Problems*, 50(1): 121. https://doi.org/10.1177/00914509221147133

Heuvelink, E., Hemming, S., and Marcelis, L. F. M. (2025). Some recent developments in controlled-environment agriculture: on plant physiology, sustainability, and autonomous control. *Journal of Horticultural Science and Biotechnology*. https://doi.org/10.1080/14620316.2024.2440592; JOURNAL:JOURNAL:THSB18;WGROUP:STRING:PUBLICATION

Hossain, M. K., and Chae, H. J. (2024). Medical cannabis: From research breakthroughs to shifting public perceptions and ensuring safe use. *Integrative Medicine Research*, 13(4): 101094. https://doi.org/10.1016/J.IMR.2024.101094

Hussain, T., Jeena, G., Pitakbut, T., Vasilev, N., and Kayser, O. (2021). Cannabis sativa research trends, challenges, and new-age perspectives. *IScience*, 24(12): 103391. https://doi.org/10.1016/J.ISCI.2021.103391

Hyam, R. (1993). Britain's Imperial Century, 1815–1914. *Britain's Imperial Century,* 1815–1914. https://doi.org/10.1007/978-1-349-22784-6

Ingrao, C., Lo Giudice, A., Bacenetti, J., Tricase, C., Dotelli, G., Fiala, M. et al. (2015). Energy and environmental assessment of industrial hemp for building applications: A review. *Renewable and Sustainable Energy Reviews*, 51: 29–42. https://doi.org/10.1016/j.rser.2015.06.002

Jackson, F. (2024). *TURNING OVER NEW LEAVES: ACHIEVING EQUITY THROUGH CANNABIS LICENSURE REFORM IN NEW YORK.* https://doi.org/10.2139/SSRN.5172645

Jacobus, J., and Tapert, S. F. (2014). Effects of Cannabis on the Adolescent Brain. *Current Pharmaceutical Design*, 20(13): 2186. https://doi.org/10.2174/13816128113199990426

Jaiswal, Y. S., and Williams, L. L. (2016). A glimpse of Ayurveda – The forgotten history and principles of Indian traditional medicine. *Journal of Traditional and Complementary Medicine*, 7(1): 50. https://doi.org/10.1016/J.JTCME.2016.02.002

Kaminski, K. P., Hoeng, J., Goffman, F., Schlage, W. K., and Latino, D. (2024). Opportunities, Challenges, and Scientific Progress in Hemp Crops. *Molecules*, 29(10): 2397. https://doi.org/10.3390/MOLECULES29102397/S1

Kaul, M., Zee, P. C., and Sahni, A. S. (2021). Effects of Cannabinoids on Sleep and their Therapeutic Potential for Sleep Disorders. *Neurotherapeutics*, 18(1): 217. https://doi.org/10.1007/S13311-021-01013-W

Kicman, A., and Toczek, M. (2020). The Effects of Cannabidiol, a non-intoxicating compound of cannabis, on the cardiovascular system in health and disease. *International Journal of Molecular Sciences*, 21(18): 6740. https://doi.org/10.3390/IJMS21186740

Kühne, F., Becker, L. L., Bast, T., Bertsche, A., Borggraefe, I., Boßelmann, C. M., Fahrbach, J. et al. (2023). Real-world data on cannabidiol treatment of various epilepsy subtypes: A retrospective, multicenter study. *Epilepsia Open*, 8(2): 360. https://doi.org/10.1002/EPI4.12699

Laaboudi, F. Z., Rejdali, M., Amhamdi, H., Salhi, A., Elyoussfi, A., and Ahari, M. 'hamed. (2024). In the weeds: A comprehensive review of cannabis; its chemical complexity, biosynthesis, and healing abilities. *Toxicology Reports*, 13: 101685. https://doi.org/10.1016/J.TOXREP.2024.101685

Leinen, Z. J., Mohan, R., Premadasa, L. S., Acharya, A., Mohan, M., and Byrareddy, S. N. (2023). Therapeutic Potential of Cannabis: A Comprehensive Review of Current and Future Applications. *Biomedicines*, 11(10): 2630. https://doi.org/10.3390/BIOMEDICINES11102630

Lester, P. A., Shuster, K. A., Allen, P. S., Hish, G. A., and Myers, D. D. (2015). Controlled Substances: Maintaining Institutional Compliance. *Research Regulatory Compliance*, 159–186. https://doi.org/10.1016/B978-0-12-420058-6.00006-X

Lines, R., Elliott, R., Hannah, J., Schleifer, R., Avafia, T., and Barrett, D. (2017). The Case for International Guidelines on Human Rights and Drug Control. *Health and Human Rights*, 19(1): 231. https://pmc.ncbi.nlm.nih.gov/articles/PMC5473052/

Manniche, L. (1989). *An ancient Egyptian herbal*. 176.

Manthey, J., Rehm, J., and Verthein, U. (2024). Germany's cannabis act: a catalyst for European drug policy reform? *The Lancet Regional Health - Europe*, 42: 100929. https://doi.org/10.1016/J.LANEPE.2024.100929

Matheson, J., and Le Foll, B. (2020). Cannabis legalization and acute harm from high potency cannabis products: A narrative review and recommendations for public health. *Frontiers in Psychiatry*, 11: 591979. https://doi.org/10.3389/FPSYT.2020.591979/BIBTEX

McDonald, A. J., Cooper, A., Doggett, A., Halladay, J., Belisario, K., and MacKillop, J. (2025). Association of recreational cannabis legalization with changes in medical, illegal, and total cannabis expenditures in Canada. *International Journal of Drug Policy*, 139: 104793. https://doi.org/10.1016/J.DRUGPO.2025.104793

Metwaly, A. M., Ghoneim, M. M., Eissa, I. H., Elsehemy, I. A., Mostafa, A. E., Hegazy, M. M. et al. (2021). Traditional ancient Egyptian medicine: A review. *Saudi Journal of Biological Sciences*, 28(10): 5823. https://doi.org/10.1016/J.SJBS.2021.06.044

Mills, J. H. (2016). The IHO as Actor: The case of cannabis and the Single Convention on Narcotic Drugs 1961. *Hygiea Internationalis*, 13(1): 95. https://doi.org/10.3384/HYGIEA.1403-8668.1613195

Mücke, M., Phillips, T., Radbruch, L., Petzke, F., and Häuser, W. (2018). Cannabis-based medicines for chronic neuropathic pain in adults. *The Cochrane Database of Systematic Reviews*, 2018(3): CD012182. https://doi.org/10.1002/14651858.CD012182.PUB2

Nahas, G. G., and Greenwood, A. (1974). The first report of the National Commission on marihuana (1972): signal of misunderstanding or exercise in ambiguity. *Bulletin of the New York Academy of Medicine*, 50(1): 55. https://pmc.ncbi.nlm.nih.gov/articles/PMC1749335/

Narouze, S. N., Maccallum, C. A., and de Freitas, L. (2024). Cannabis Use Disorder. *Cannabinoids and Pain*, 313–316. https://doi.org/10.1007/978-3-030-69186-8_38

National Academies of Sciences, E. and M., Division, H. and M., Practice, B. on P. H. and P. H., and Agenda, C. on the H. E. of M. A. E. R. and R. (2017). *Challenges and Barriers in Conducting Cannabis Research.*

National Academies of Sciences, E. and M. H. and M. D. B. on P. H. and P. H. P. C. on the P. H. C. of C. in the C. P. L., Boyle, E. B., Hurd, Y. L., and Teutsch, S. M. (2024). Summary. *Cannabis Policy Impacts Public Health and Health Equity*, 1–341. https://doi.org/10.17226/27766

Nayak, P., Pantvaidya, G., Ranganathan, P., Jiwnani, S., Joshi, S., and Gogtay, N. (2023). Clinical studies with Cannabis in India – A need for guidelines for the investigators and ethics committees. *Perspectives in Clinical Research*, 14(3): 146. https://doi.org/10.4103/PICR.PICR_159_22

Neijat, M., Suh, M., Neufeld, J., and House, J. D. (2016). Hempseed products fed to hens effectively increased n-3 Polyunsaturated fatty acids in total lipids, Triacylglycerol and Phospholipid of Egg Yolk. *Lipids*, 51(5): 601–614. https://doi.org/10.1007/S11745-015-4088-7

Orenstein, D. G., and Glantz, S. A. (2020). Cannabis Legalization in State Legislatures: Public Health Opportunity And Risk. *Marquette Law Review*, 103(4): 1313. https://pmc.ncbi.nlm.nih.gov/articles/PMC8351589/

Pacula, R. L., and Smart, R. (2017). Medical Marijuana and Marijuana Legalization. *Annual Review of Clinical Psychology*, 13: 397. https://doi.org/10.1146/ANNUREV-CLINPSY-032816-045128

Payne-James, J. (2015). Substance Misuse: Substance Misuse and Crime. *Encyclopedia of Forensic and Legal Medicine: Second Edition*, 428–435. https://doi.org/10.1016/B978-0-12-800034-2.00364-5

Pearlson, G. D., Stevens, M. C., and D'Souza, D. C. (2021). Cannabis and Driving. *Frontiers in Psychiatry*, 12: 689444. https://doi.org/10.3389/FPSYT.2021.689444

Placido, D. F., and Lee, C. C. (2022). Potential of Industrial Hemp for Phytoremediation of Heavy Metals. *Plants*, 11(5): 595. https://doi.org/10.3390/PLANTS11050595

Pretorius, S. (2006). The significance of the use of ganja as a religious ritual in the Rastafari movement. *Verbum et Ecclesia*, 27(3): 1012–1030. https://doi.org/10.4102/VE.V27I3.199

Queirolo, R., Rossel, C., Álvarez, E., and Repetto, L. (2019). Why Uruguay legalized marijuana? The open window of public insecurity. *Addiction*, 114(7): 1313–1321. https://doi.org/10.1111/ADD.14523,

Ransing, R., de la Rosa, P. A., Pereira-Sanchez, V., Handuleh, J. I. M., Jerotic, S., Gupta, A. K. et al. (2022). Current state of cannabis use, policies, and research across sixteen countries: cross-country comparisons and international perspectives. *Trends in Psychiatry and Psychotherapy*, 44(Suppl 1): e20210263. https://doi.org/10.47626/2237-6089-2021-0263

Riboulet-Zemouli, K., and Clarke, M. (2025). A constitutional right to cannabis? Grassroots litigation and dagga policy reform in South Africa. *Authorea Preprints*. https://doi.org/10.22541/AU.173862410.09452161/V2

Riboulet-Zemouli, K. (2025). 1925–2025: a century of international pharmaceutical law. *Journal of Pharmaceutical Policy and Practice*, 18(1): 2470840. https://doi.org/10.1080/20523211.2025.2470840

Russo, E. (2005). Cannabinoids as Therapeutics. *Cannabinoids as Therapeutics, March* 2006. https://doi.org/10.1007/3-7643-7358-x

Russo, M., Calabrò, R. S., Naro, A., Sessa, E., Rifici, C., D'Aleo, G. et al. (2015). Sativex in the Management of Multiple Sclerosis-Related Spasticity: Role of the Corticospinal Modulation. *Neural Plasticity*, 2015: 656582. https://doi.org/10.1155/2015/656582

Satterlund, T. D., Lee, J. P., and Moore, R. S. (2015). Stigma among california's medical marijuana patients. *Journal of Psychoactive Drugs*, 47(1): 10. https://doi.org/10.1080/02791072.2014.991858

Schlag, A. K., Hindocha, C., Zafar, R., Nutt, D. J., and Curran, H. V. (2021). Cannabis based medicines and cannabis dependence: A critical review of issues and evidence. *Journal of Psychopharmacology (Oxford, England)*, 35(7): 773. https://doi.org/10.1177/0269881120986393

Schluttenhofer, C., and Yuan, L. (2017). Challenges towards Revitalizing Hemp: A multifaceted crop. *Trends in Plant Science*, 22(11): 917–929. https://doi.org/10.1016/j.tplants.2017.08.004

Schroeder, W. (2009). Cosmeceutical (Antiaging) products: Advertising rules and claims substantiation. *Global Regulatory Issues for the Cosmetics Industry*, 121–153. https://doi.org/10.1016/B978-0-8155-1569-2.50013-0

Shakya, D. R., Upadhaya, S. R., and Thapa, M. (2021). Cannabis Use and Abuse in Nepal: A Review of Studies. *JNMA: Journal of the Nepal Medical Association*, 59(241): 954. https://doi.org/10.31729/JNMA.6931

Simei, J. L. Q., Souza, J. D. R., Pedrazzi, J. F., Guimarães, F. S., Campos, A. C., Zuardi, A., Hallak, J. E. C., and Crippa, J. A. S. (2024). Research and Clinical Practice Involving the use of Cannabis Products, with Emphasis on Cannabidiol: A Narrative Review. *Pharmaceuticals*, (12): 1644. https://doi.org/10.3390/PH17121644

Simon, L., Baldwin, C., Kalea, A. Z., and Slee, A. (2021). Cannabinoid interventions for improving cachexia outcomes in cancer: A systematic review and meta-analysis. *Journal of Cachexia, Sarcopenia and Muscle*, 13(1): 23. https://doi.org/10.1002/JCSM.12861

Smith, R. T., Dahlgren, M. K., Sagar, K. A., Kosereisoglu, D., and Gruber, S. A. (2025). Clinical and cognitive improvement following treatment with a hemp-derived, full-spectrum, high-cannabidiol product in patients with anxiety: An open-label pilot study. *Biomedicines*, 13(8): 1874. https://doi.org/10.3390/BIOMEDICINES13081874/S1

Singh, K., Bhushan, B., Chanchal, D. K., Sharma, S. K., Rani, K., Yadav, M. K. et al. (2023). Emerging therapeutic potential of Cannabidiol (CBD) in Neurological Disorders: A comprehensive review. *Behavioural Neurology*, 2023: 8825358. https://doi.org/10.1155/2023/8825358

Smart, R., and Pacula, R. L. (2019). Early evidence of the impact of cannabis legalization on cannabis use, cannabis use disorder, and the use of other substances: Findings from state policy evaluations. *The American Journal of Drug and Alcohol Abuse*, 45(6): 644. https://doi.org/10.1080/00952990.2019.1669626

Sznitman, S. R., Meiri, D., Amit, B. H., Rosenberg, D., and Greene, T. (2022). Posttraumatic stress disorder, sleep and medical cannabis treatment: A daily diary study. *Journal of Anxiety Disorders*, 92: 102632. https://doi.org/10.1016/J.JANXDIS.2022.102632

Totelin, L. (2015). When foods become remedies in ancient Greece: The curious case of garlic and other substances. *Journal of Ethnopharmacology*, 167: 30. https://doi.org/10.1016/J.JEP.2014.08.018

Tyskiewicz, A. J., Arkfeld, P. A., Smith, E. E., Eilerman, J. K., and Conner, B. T. (2022). Does accessibility of cannabis mediate the relation between method of acquisition and cannabis use frequency among adolescents? *Cannabis*, 5(3): 61. https://doi.org/10.26828/CANNABIS/2022.03.006

Vasantha Rupasinghe, H. P., Davis, A., Kumar, S. K., Murray, B., and Zheljazkov, V. D. (2020a). Industrial Hemp (*Cannabis sativa* subsp. sativa) as an emerging source for value-added functional food ingredients and nutraceuticals. *Molecules*, 25(18): 4078. https://doi.org/10.3390/MOLECULES25184078

Vasantha Rupasinghe, H. P., Davis, A., Kumar, S. K., Murray, B., and Zheljazkov, V. D. (2020b). Industrial Hemp (*Cannabis sativa* subsp. sativa) as an emerging source for value-added functional food ingredients and nutraceuticals. *Molecules*, 25(18): 4078. https://doi.org/10.3390/MOLECULES25184078

Visković, J., Zheljazkov, V. D., Sikora, V., Noller, J., Latković, D., Ocamb, C. M. et al. (2023). Industrial Hemp (*Cannabis sativa* L.) agronomy and utilization: A review. *Agronomy*, 13(3): 931. https://doi.org/10.3390/AGRONOMY13030931

Ware, M. A., Daeninck, P., and Maida, V. (2008). A review of nabilone in the treatment of chemotherapy-induced nausea and vomiting. *Therapeutics and Clinical Risk Management*, 4(1): 99. https://doi.org/10.2147/TCRM.S1132

Walsh, K. B., McKinney, A. E., and Holmes, A. E. (2021). Minor Cannabinoids: Biosynthesis, molecular pharmacology and potential therapeutic uses. *Frontiers in Pharmacology*, 12: 777804. https://doi.org/10.3389/FPHAR.2021.777804

Wilkinson, S. T., Yarnell, S., Radhakrishnan, R., Ball, S. A., and D'souza, D. C. (2015). Marijuana Legalization: Impact on physicians and public health. *Annual Review of Medicine*, 67: 453. https://doi.org/10.1146/ANNUREV-MED-050214-013454

Zuardi, A. W. (2006). History of cannabis as a medicine: A review. *Revista Brasileira de Psiquiatria*, 28(2): 153–157. https://doi.org/10.1590/S1516-44462006000200015

CHAPTER 2

The Current State of Cannabis in the Asia-Pacific Region

*Rishabh Agade, Ujban Hussain, Aditya Wadalkar, Shweta Jaiswal, Veena S. Belgamwar** and *Prashant Puranik*

1. Introduction

The Asia-Pacific region, stretching from South Asia to East Asia and Oceania, has one of the most complex and contradictory cannabis landscapes. It encompasses both the world's most liberal and most prohibitive cannabis policies, reflecting deep cultural ties to the plant alongside strict modern regulations (Rafei et al. 2023). This contrast of ancient use and contemporary prohibition highlights the Asia-Pacific's unique position, as traditional reverence clashes with imported regulatory frameworks and colonial-era laws. Countries like India, China, and Thailand have millennia-long histories of cannabis use embedded in religion and medicine. For instance, the Atharva Veda (circa 1500 BCE) mentions cannabis as one of India's sacred plants, and cannabis (in the form of bhang) remains part of Hindu rituals today (Karki and Rangaswamy 2022). In Nepal, cannabis is traditionally used by Hindu ascetics during the Shivaratri festival, and in China, hemp has been cultivated and applied for food, fiber, and medicine since Neolithic times. Conversely, in countries like Singapore, Japan, Indonesia, and the Philippines, cannabis laws are among the world's strictest, with penalties from lengthy prison terms to death. Modern reforms further complicate this picture. Australia, New Zealand, and Thailand have trended toward liberal cannabis models, legalizing medical cannabis and, in some cases, decriminalizing adult use (S. F. Cheng et al. 2023). Australia legalized medical cannabis in 2016, and in 2020, the Australian Capital Territory decriminalized possession. Thailand, once known for very harsh drug laws, became the first Asian country to decriminalize cannabis in 2022 and has since been developing a regulated medical and commercial cannabis industry. Nonetheless, the region remains highly fragmented in cannabis policy. Many countries still rely on colonial-era drug laws and strict interpretations of the UN Single Convention on Narcotic Drugs (1961), frameworks that have historically discouraged reform and stigmatized users. In South Korea and Japan, even minor cannabis offenses can lead to arrest, public shaming, and severe social or professional penalties (Lines et al. 2017). This fragmentation reflects the political diversity of the Asia-Pacific region. Advanced democracies such as Australia and New Zealand have liberalized laws through public health advocacy, evidence-based policy, and civic activism. In contrast, conservative and authoritarian governments in parts of East and Southeast Asia treat drug

Department of Pharmaceutical Sciences, Rashtrasant Tukadoji Maharaj Nagpur University, Nagpur–440033.
* Corresponding author: vbelgamwar@gmail.com

DOI: 10.1201/9781003668190-3

use as a criminal or moral failing. Singapore and Malaysia classify cannabis in the most severe drug category, with trafficking punishable by a mandatory death sentence. Asia-Pacific nations are also among the original homelands of the cannabis plant. Traditional cannabis use has been widespread and sacred. In India, cannabis is integral to Ayurvedic medicine and temple ceremonies (Hourfane et al. 2023). Many communities with centuries-old cannabis traditions now find their practices ignored or criminalized by modern laws (Shakya et al. 2021). Much of the region is well-suited to cannabis cultivation, especially hemp. Nations like India, China, and Thailand are beginning to develop hemp cultivation and cannabis export industries targeting markets in Europe and North America (Caio Fernando de C Lambert et al. 2024). Australia's medicinal cannabis industry is growing rapidly for domestic and international markets. Thailand's policy even includes community-based growing and permits families to register a limited number of plants for medical or commercial use. With over half the world's population, Asia-Pacific represents a major market for cannabis-based medicines and wellness products (CBD oils, topicals, edibles, and nutraceuticals). As the middle classes rise and health awareness grows, demand for natural, plant-based therapies is increasing. For example, Japan and South Korea have vibrant CBD wellness markets despite restrictive regulations, indicating consumer interest. Indeed, these markets show acceptance of cannabis products despite restrictive laws. However, Asia-Pacific's cannabis future faces many hurdles. Inconsistent laws, international treaty constraints, cultural stigma, and poor public education continue to obstruct reform. Many countries lack the institutional capacity to implement legalization safely, and widespread confusion persists between hemp (industrial or medicinal) and higher-potency cannabis. Misinformation, stigma, and political inertia continue to be major challenges. Social equity is another pressing issue. Indigenous and rural communities with historic cannabis knowledge (e.g., tribal groups in India's northeast or Thailand's hill tribes) risk being marginalized by corporate interests and poorly designed licensing regimes. Social justice and benefit-sharing for these communities will be crucial in building ethical and sustainable cannabis economies. Diplomatic pressures shape Asia-Pacific cannabis policy. Countries are signatories to UN drug treaties, ASEAN agreements, and trade deals that can limit domestic liberalization or enable cross-border investment. Balancing these international commitments with national priorities is a delicate task. Some countries, such as Thailand and Australia, have implemented reforms in ways that respect global obligations, while others remain under strict punitive frameworks. Policy success will require political will.

2. Historical and Cultural Roots of Cannabis in Asia-Pacific

Cannabis has been deeply embedded in the cultural, spiritual, and medicinal traditions of numerous communities in the Asia-Pacific region for millennia. Before scientific investigation or global drug policy, cannabis was sacred as a healing, ritual, and economically significant plant. This region, with its varied civilizations and belief systems, made major contributions to the ethnobotanical history of cannabis, influencing how the plant was utilized and interpreted across continents (Zuardi 2006). The ascendance of colonial powers and global prohibitionist norms during the 19th and 20th centuries, though, upset these customary relationships, transforming cannabis from a sacred herb to a criminal substance. Comprehension of the historical and cultural origins of cannabis in the Asia-Pacific is essential to framing contemporary reforms and recovering indigenous knowledge systems.

2.1 India: Bhang, Ayurveda, and Shiva Traditions

India is likely one of the richest cultural sources of historical cannabis consumption globally. Cannabis is mentioned in the Atharva Veda (1500 BCE), where it is described as one of the five holy plants and "a source of happiness, a joy-giver." The plant was thought to have been gifted to humans by the gods, most notably Lord Shiva, who is regularly depicted smoking cannabis in the form of bhang, a ground paste of cannabis leaves mixed with milk, spices, and sugar. Bhang continues to be legally sold in numerous Indian states, particularly around the time of the Holi festival, and is found in government-sanctioned outlets.

Cannabis also holds a central position in Ayurvedic medicine, where it has been used for centuries to cure digestive problems, sleep disorders, pain, and neurological disorders. Ancient Ayurvedic texts placed cannabis (vijaya) in the category of strong herbs when used in the right way and cautioned against excess use, showing a sophisticated understanding of both its therapeutic and intoxicating properties. Physicians formulated mixtures that blended cannabis with other herbs to achieve synergistic effects, showing an early form of polyherbal pharmacology (Crocq 2020).

Notwithstanding this venerable history, cannabis was slowly criminalized under British colonialism, especially following the Indian Hemp Drugs Commission Report of 1894, which determined that moderate consumption was substantially innocuous but suggested regulation. In post-independence India, cannabis came to be outlawed by the Narcotic Drugs and Psychotropic Substances (NDPS) Act of 1985, driven by global pressure rather than by domestic policy. Nonetheless, the Act provided a legal exception for bhang, preserving its cultural value while prohibiting other types such as charas (resin) and ganja (flower) (Shamir and Hacker 2001).

2.2 Nepal: Cannabis in Religious Rituals and Himalayan Culture

Nepal also shares India's cultural heritage of cannabis use, specifically among Hindu sadhus and during Maha Shivaratri, the festival celebrating Lord Shiva. Cannabis is widespread in the Himalayan foothills and has long been included in shamanic and Tantric ceremonies, employed to induce altered states of consciousness and intensify meditative practice (Acharya et al. 2015).

Cannabis was grown legally in Nepal until the early 1970s, and Kathmandu was a destination for global cannabis tourism. Hashish shops were legal businesses under government license, selling their wares to locals and foreign visitors alike. But in 1976, under pressure from the United States at the peak of the worldwide "War on Drugs," Nepal passed strict anti-cannabis legislation and shut down these shops.

Today, though cannabis is technically illegal in Nepal, enforcement is hit-or-miss and culturally accepted, particularly at festival times and among specific rural and religious communities. That contradiction represents the dilemma between ancient tolerance and contemporary criminalization, a theme found repeatedly throughout much of the region.

2.3 China: Early Medicinal Use and Hemp Heritage

China is credited with being one of the earliest people to have used cannabis. The ancient Chinese medical pharmacopeia Shennong Ben Cao Jing, which is credited to the legendary Emperor Shennong (~2700 BCE), includes cannabis (ma) as a drug. The book describes the seeds as being nourishing and the resinous flowers as having mind-altering properties when ingested in large quantities. Cannabis was employed to cure numerous diseases, such as pain, menstrual ailments, rheumatism, and malaria (Brand and Zhao 2017).

Aside from therapeutic applications, hemp was a basis of early Chinese farming. Hemp was used to create clothing, ropes, nets, and paper, and hemp fabric dates back to the Neolithic era (5000 BCE). The manufacture of hemp paper dates back as early as the Han Dynasty (~200 BCE), marking a significant milestone in information storage technology.

Notwithstanding this rich tradition, psychoactive use of cannabis decreased over time, particularly during the Confucian period, which advocated moderation and was suspicious of intoxication. In the contemporary period, cannabis was made illegal by Chinese law, and possession or trafficking is a serious criminal act. Cultivation of industrial hemp is still allowed in some provinces (e.g., Yunnan, Heilongjiang) for the production of textiles, food, and cosmetics.

2.4 Southeast Asia: Indigenous Use and Tribal Traditions

Cannabis has been used for years by indigenous peoples in Southeast Asia, specifically in the highland regions of Thailand, Vietnam, Laos, and Cambodia. Within those communities, cannabis was consumed as a folk medicine, as a food spice, and as a post-labor relaxant. In Thailand, it was traditionally brewed in teas and soups to relieve muscle pain, promote sleep, and heal women's ailments (Sommano et al. 2022).

Among the ethnic minorities of Laos and Northern Thailand, cannabis was also ritually employed, particularly by shamans in healing rituals. These were transmitted through oral cultures and are part of the very fabric of ethnomedicinal knowledge in these areas. Cannabis was previously ubiquitous in Vietnamese and Cambodian cuisine, particularly in rural areas (Evrard et al. 2013).

Colonial incursions and later international drug treaties significantly dislocated these practices. Since the 1960s, U.S. military presence in Southeast Asia and the advent of the international narcotics trade have seen nations in the region implementing strict punishments for the cultivation and use of cannabis, typically at the expense of traditional customs and way of life.

2.5 Colonial Legacy and Criminalization

The criminalization of cannabis within the Asia-Pacific region was not locally initiated but was imported as a result of colonial and global pressures. Western legal systems brought by British, French, Dutch, and American colonial governments treated cannabis as a social evil and not as a culturally rooted or medicinal plant. In India, British colonialism initially accepted the use of cannabis but progressed towards regulation for political and moral purposes. In French Indochina (Vietnam, Laos, and Cambodia), cannabis was criminalized as part of wider attempts to suppress native traditions. In Australia and New Zealand, cannabis prohibition was in line with British and American patterns, ending in blanket prohibitions in the early 20th century.

This history of imposed prohibition was subsequently further entrenched by post-colonial states keen to prove modernity and conformity to global norms, most notably the UN Single Convention on Narcotic Drugs (1961). States signed these agreements without scrutiny in relation to their cultural context, leading to the erasure or marginalization of customary cannabis knowledge systems.

3. Legal and Regulatory Frameworks

The cannabis legal environment in the Asia-Pacific region is characterized by extreme contrasts—ranging from some of the globe's most restrictive drug laws to new models of medical access and decriminalization. This patchwork regulatory environment mirrors the heterogeneity of political systems, cultural attitudes, and international pressures throughout the region. Although a few nations have tentatively edged toward reform, many persist in maintaining rigorous prohibitionist approaches, frequently with severe sanctions for even minor cannabis-related crimes (Areesantichai et al. 2020).

Several Asia-Pacific countries are still strongly adhering to zero-tolerance drug enforcement, especially in Southeast and East Asia. Singapore, Indonesia, Malaysia, and the Philippines have some of the toughest cannabis laws globally. Possession, cultivation, or trafficking of cannabis in these nations is punished with harsh legal penalties, such as life imprisonment and, in most instances, the death penalty. For instance, Singapore has a mandatory death penalty for dealing with over 500 grams of cannabis, whereas Malaysia—albeit currently mulling some changes—continues to issue capital punishment for possession in large quantities. Long-term prison sentences are standard in Indonesia and the Philippines, and enforcement campaigns frequently feature active policing. These policies are embedded in both colonial legal histories and post-independence political ideologies that position drugs as threats to social order and national development.

Japan and South Korea, while less severe in sentencing, also have extremely punitive strategies. In both nations, people can be charged with a crime for personal possession, and no differentiation is made between medical and recreational use at the national level. Most striking, even CBD products that are embraced as non-intoxicating and medicinal elsewhere are prohibited or stringently regulated. In South Korea, nationals have been prosecuted for the legal use of cannabis outside the country, and in Japan, public figures arrested with cannabis usually face career-ending social ostracism. These nations' rigid positions are underpinned by conservative social norms and past anti-drug campaigns that focus on moral purity and national duty.

Conversely, an increasing number of Asia-Pacific nations are looking into more lax regulatory paradigms for cannabis, seeing the therapeutic potential of the plant as well as the international momentum toward legalization. Thailand is the most progressive country in the region in this context. In 2022, Thailand was the first Asian nation to decriminalize cannabis when it delisted it from its narcotics list and permitted large-scale medical, household, and community-based cultivation (Yimsaard et al. 2023). The government in Thailand has supported cannabis as an agricultural and economic resource, with scores of clinics authorized to write prescriptions for medical cannabis and a nationwide effort to make the nation a cannabis export and tourism hub in the region. Although the use of cannabis for recreation continues as a legal gray area, the Thai model represents a radical departure from the nation's previous war-on-drugs stance and has fuelled policy discussions throughout Southeast Asia (Assanangkornchai et al. 2022).

India, though a custodian of cannabis culture, is still trapped in a legal contradiction. The Narcotic Drugs and Psychotropic Substances (NDPS) Act of 1985 makes the cultivation and sale of cannabis resin (charas) and flowers (ganja) illegal, but leaves bhang, a classical preparation from cannabis leaves, legal in many Indian states. Although this exception has maintained cultural traditions, it has also generated regulatory uncertainty, particularly as popular interest in medical cannabis and CBD increases. No overall medical cannabis system exists in India, but scattered research projects and startups have started operating within state-level legal loopholes to provide Ayurvedic cannabis medicines. Inadequate policy still hinders both medical access and scientific progress, however.

Australia provides a more formalized example of contemporary cannabis control. In 2016, the nation legalized medicinal cannabis on a federal level and instituted a framework for cultivation, importation, prescription, and product approval. Medicinal cannabis is dispensed to patients by licensed doctors under the Therapeutic Goods Administration (TGA) Special Access Scheme. Further, the Australian Capital Territory (ACT) led the way in 2020 with the legalisation of private possession and cultivation of cannabis for adults, the first jurisdiction to legalise recreational use in a restricted form. Nevertheless, cannabis remains illicit under federal criminal law, leaving a legal anomaly that replicates the situation in the United States. Broader national reform has been held up, but public opinion and policy experimentation keep the debate alive (K. Cheng et al. 2023).

New Zealand has also progressed, albeit with more incremental cannabis reform. Medical cannabis was legalized in 2018, and the nation introduced a regulatory regime for cultivation, prescription, and product distribution in later years. Still, a 2020 national referendum seeking recreational legalization was narrowly defeated at the polls, with 50.7% opposing the measure. The administration has since proceeded gingerly, moving to broaden medical access but not to full legalization. The narrow outcome, however, indicated an expanding social receptivity to change, and reformers continue to advocate for wider change (Fischer and Hall 2021).

4. Medical Cannabis Programs

The Asia-Pacific region is experiencing a slow but considerable growth in the rollout of medical cannabis programs, but the speed and character of reform are highly variable across countries. While Australia and Thailand have established formal systems for medical access and product control, others, such as Japan, South Korea, and New Zealand, have taken more restrictive or conservative paths. Even with increasing international recognition and an expanding body of clinical data, most countries in the region remain plagued by regulatory, scientific, and societal hurdles that impede the universal integration of medical cannabis into public health systems.

In Australia, medical cannabis became legal at the federal level in 2016 with the Narcotic Drugs Amendment Act. The nation has built one of the most extensive and controlled medical cannabis markets on the continent. Patients can obtain cannabis-based products using the Therapeutic Goods

Administration (TGA)'s Special Access Scheme or Authorised Prescriber Scheme, as long as they have a prescription from an authorized medical practitioner (Castle et al. 2019). The schemes permit personalized patient treatment, especially for conditions like chronic pain, epilepsy, multiple sclerosis, and chemotherapy-induced nausea. The Australian market has also supported a booming pharmaceutical cannabis industry, with regulated domestic cultivation, production, and research facilities that comply with international Good Manufacturing Practice (GMP) standards (Baratta et al. 2022).

Thailand has been on a significantly different course, combining traditional medicine, public health, and economic development into its medical cannabis policy. Since the decriminalization of cannabis in 2022, Thailand has implemented an inclusive model of medicine in which government health clinics and hospitals have been licensed to prescribe cannabis. Thousands of families and community cooperatives are registered to grow cannabis legally, particularly in rural districts (Yimsaard et al. 2023). The government provides cannabis seedlings and promotes its use for economic development as well as domestic healthcare. Cannabis is part of the official Thai traditional medicine formulary, and education programs have been initiated for health professionals. This mass, public health-driven system contrasts with highly commercialized systems, such as those in the West, and represents a distinctly Southeast Asian model of legalization (Assanangkornchai et al. 2022).

Japan and South Korea, on the other hand, have very restrictive systems. Legalization of domestic medical cannabis cultivation has not occurred in either country. But both have granted limited exceptions for the importation of certain cannabis-based medicines like Epidiolex (CBD) and Sativex (THC: CBD), prescribed under medical supervision by a physician. In South Korea, the Ministry of Food and Drug Safety approved the importation in 2018, making it the first East Asian nation to do so. Yet access is scarce and tightly controlled, and general public consumption of even non-euphoric cannabinoids such as CBD can lead to criminal charges. Japan has indicated potential regulatory changes through 2023, but the political environment remains guarded, and drug use stigma within society is well ingrained.

New Zealand made medical cannabis legal in 2018, establishing a legal framework to allow patients to access products through the Medicinal Cannabis Scheme, which was implemented in 2020. The implementation has been criticized as complex, expensive, and with limited product availability. Physicians have to go through specific licensing processes, and most products are not available or not approved, so patients are being forced to self-medicate or seek unapproved imports. These hurdles notwithstanding, however, support among the general population for medical cannabis continues high, and the nation is likely to further adapt in the next few years (Fischer and Hall 2021).

Around the Asia-Pacific region, numerous shared hurdles keep medical cannabis initiatives from thriving. Research gaps—few clinical trials involving local populations—create doubts among clinicians. Physicians are unaware of cannabinoid pharmacology in many instances and are not enthusiastic about recommending medication without substantial national evidence. Additionally, bureaucratic hurdles like delays in licensing, import bans, and unclear wording in the law further hinder patient access. For most, costs are exorbitant, particularly in nations that do not provide public healthcare subsidies for cannabis medicines (National Academies of Sciences et al. 2017).

Ultimately, public opinion and cultural norms are important factors. In traditionally conservative cultures like South Korea, Japan, and some countries in Southeast Asia, entrenched stigma surrounding the use of cannabis persists, fuelled by years of prohibitionist rhetoric. Education and awareness campaigns are essential to changing these perceptions and developing a better-informed view of medical cannabis as a medicine rather than as a criminal menace (Faguet 2010).

5. Societal Attitudes and Public Health Perspectives

Social understanding of cannabis throughout the Asia-Pacific is slowly, yet significantly, shifting. More and more nations over the last decade have seen rising public demand for the legalization of cannabis, especially its use for medicine. Yet a significant number remain mired in entrenched stigma, myths, and cultural conservatism both among the people and in government policies. This divergence presents a multifaceted challenge to public health leaders, educators, and policymakers, who must reconcile social values, scientific realities, and regulation (Resko et al. 2019).

In Australia, New Zealand, and Thailand, public attitudes have dramatically changed in support of reform, promoted by increased education about the potential medical benefits of cannabis, publicity, and bottom-up activism. In Australia, regular polling shows that a majority of the population now favors legal adult use of cannabis, with even stronger support for medical cannabis. State-level reforms and prominent media reports of patients using cannabis to alleviate chronic conditions have served to destigmatize the plant (Lewis and Flood 2021).

New Zealand follows suit, with a majority of citizens favoring access to medical cannabis. Although a 2020 referendum to legalize recreational cannabis narrowly failed, the close result—49.3% in favor—signaled a growing openness to reform, especially among younger and urban populations. In Thailand, attitudes have changed rapidly since the nation made history in Asia by decriminalizing cannabis in 2022. Easy availability of cannabis products at stores and pharmacies and official cultivation programs sponsored by the government have made its use common in urban and rural areas.

Conversely, conservative cultures like Japan, South Korea, Singapore, and Indonesia have strong anti-cannabis stances where the use of cannabis is considered a moral failure or a social illness. These nations have cultural values of discipline, obedience, and national cleanliness that support an atmosphere in which cannabis users are highly stigmatized. Even for minor violations, social exclusion, public embarrassment, and prosecution are possible, which deters public discussion and patient inquiry. Public persons apprehended for use of cannabis—legal or otherwise—tend to invite career-destroying reaction.

Adding to the problem is the widespread dissemination of misinformation, as well as the lack of science-based public education. In nations with extensive histories of prohibition, most citizens lack knowledge regarding the distinction between hemp, CBD, and THC-containing cannabis. Educational programs are scarce, creating a void filled with government fear campaigns and media coverage that tends to exaggerate the harms of cannabis while minimizing its therapeutic uses.

From a public health point of view, adolescent use, mental health, and road safety remain at the core of current controversy. Although research indicates that legalization does not in itself result in increased youth consumption, high-cannabis-using adolescents have been associated with enhanced risk of psychosis, cognitive loss, and chronic dependency, particularly when high-THC cannabis is used. In transforming countries such as Australia and New Zealand, these issues have been addressed by incorporating cannabis education into school curricula, with a focus on age limits and awareness of the dangers (Donnelly et al. 2022).

Cannabis Driving Impairment is another issue of concern. THC impairs motor function, reaction time, and judgment; however, available roadside screening technologies often fail to differentiate between acute and chronic use. Consequently, some jurisdictions have implemented zero-tolerance policies, while others use behavioral tests or establish legal THC thresholds. Public education campaigns, such as those in Australia, aim to educate users about the dangers of driving under the influence and encourage safe use practices (Schiemer et al. 2025).

6. Economic and Industrial Developments

The Asia-Pacific region is set to become a major player in the new global cannabis economy, with many nations actively enacting economic and industrial approaches to capture value from the medical cannabis and industrial hemp industries. The region's enormous agricultural potential, low production costs, and increasing scientific capabilities make it well placed to meet growing global demand. However, these advances are uneven, influenced by competing regulatory models, cultural acceptance, and availability of capital and infrastructure. While nations such as Thailand,

Australia, China, and India are establishing legal cannabis and hemp industries, they face significant challenges related to regulatory environments, access to finance, international trade restrictions, and market sophistication (Sommano et al. 2022).

6.1 Export-Oriented Strategies: Thailand and the Lesotho Partnership

One of the most ambitious regional examples of export-oriented cannabis policy is Thailand, which in 2022 became the first Asian country to decriminalize cannabis production and use. Thailand has established itself as a hub for medical cannabis and wellness tourism in Southeast Asia, with a focus on rural production, public health applications, and low-cost manufacturing. The Thai government has released more than one million cannabis seedlings to homes and invited local farmers to apply for cultivation permits. Small- and medium-sized businesses have welcomed the opportunity to create cannabis-infused cosmetics, foods, and traditional medicines, backed by the nation's established herbal medicine sector.

Aside from meeting domestic demand, Thailand aims to become the export leader in the Asia-Pacific cannabis market. But because of global prohibitions on importing cannabis, particularly in nations that still regard cannabis as a narcotic, the immediate scope of such aspirations has been curtailed. Thai companies have had to rely on accessing countries with lawful export-import routes, like Lesotho in southern Africa, one of the earliest African countries to legalize the export of cannabis. Thai-African joint ventures are seeking to co-develop products and exchange cultivation and processing expertise, establishing South-South cooperation models in the cannabis industry that avoid traditional Western-controlled markets.

6.2 Australia's Cannabis Pharmaceutical Industry

Australia has pursued a more clinical, pharmaceutical-oriented approach to building its cannabis economy. Since the legalization of medical cannabis in 2016, the nation has established a strong, highly regulated medicinal cannabis industry. Licensed growers and manufacturers are licensed under Good Manufacturing Practice (GMP) conditions, regulated by the Therapeutic Goods Administration (TGA) and the Office of Drug Control (ODC). Australian companies are manufacturing cannabis oils, capsules, and extracts for domestic and export markets, focusing on countries such as Germany, the UK, and certain areas of Latin America.

The Australian approach emphasizes scientific research, product quality, and medical validity. The nation also hosts cutting-edge cannabis research centers and clinical trials into the use of cannabinoids to treat pain, epilepsy, and psychiatric conditions. Incorporation of cannabis into Australia's healthcare and pharmaceutical frameworks has created a multi-billion-dollar industry, one still restricted by patient access issues and a conservative medical establishment. Still, Australia is primed to emerge as a world supplier of pharmaceutical-grade cannabis, particularly as global regulations continue to ease.

6.3 Hemp Industry in India and China

Industrial hemp, being a non-psychoactive variety of Cannabis sativa, is a leading character in the economic drama of the region, especially in India and China. China is the global leader in hemp production, primarily cultivating it for fiber and textile purposes in provinces such as Heilongjiang and Yunnan. Chinese firms have been at the forefront of producing hemp-based textiles, ropes, bioplastics, and paper, exporting raw materials to other parts of the world. The government of China has promoted the growth of hemp under strict THC regulations, enabling it to thrive as a state-approved agricultural crop while maintaining high-THC cannabis (Graham et al. 2023).

India, with its long history of cannabis and growing textile industry, has only now started to consider hemp's economic value. States like Uttarakhand, Himachal Pradesh, and Uttar Pradesh have seen pilot projects and startup companies drawing on traditional knowledge as well as indigenous biodiversity to develop hemp-based products such as clothing, building materials, paper, and wellness items. Agritech companies and NGOs have also led efforts to revive hemp cultivation among tribal and hilly communities, promoting environmental benefits such as soil rejuvenation, reduced water usage, and carbon trapping. Nonetheless, the absence of a national hemp policy and uneven state-level regulations have hindered India's progress in becoming a significant participant in the industrial hemp supply chain (Castle et al. 2019).

6.4 Barriers to Scaling: Regulation, Banking, and Trade Policies

Despite these promising developments, the Asia-Pacific cannabis and hemp industries are confronted with several structural barriers that limit scalability and international competitiveness.

One significant issue is regulatory fragmentation. Policies regarding cannabis differ not just between nations but also domestically (like in Australia and India), confusing investors, business people, and consumers alike. Licensing holdups, uneven enforcement, and poorly defined distinctions among medical, wellness, and industrial cannabis complicate market entry and operations (Kiran P. Kolkar et al. 2025).

Financing and banking pose another major barrier. Banks across most Asia-Pacific countries are slow to provide services to cannabis companies due to concerns over the legality of their operations or potential damage to their reputations. This leaves entrepreneurs with limited options for private investment or venture capital financing, further reducing their access to financial instruments for growth. Lack of access to insurance, trade credit, and capital markets tightens the reins on growth, particularly for smallholder farmers and cooperatives based at a community level.

In international trade, exports of cannabis are tightly controlled by UN drug control conventions, import prohibitions in destination nations, and rigorous shipping rules. Although several nations have arranged legal medical export channels, these are limited in number and stringently regulated. Moreover, tariff classifications, phytosanitary regulations, and customs procedures frequently differentiate cannabis from other farm products, making logistics and compliance difficult as seen in Figure 1 Cannabis law reforms in the Asia–Pacific region have evolved gradually over the past two decades.

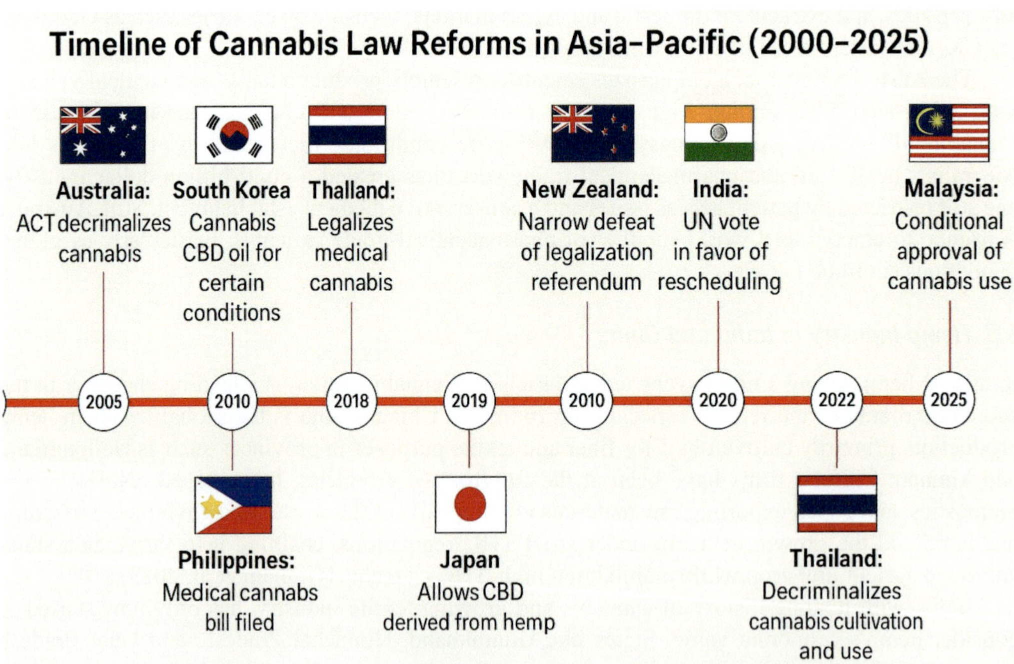

Figure 1: Timeline of Cannabis Law Reforms in the Asia-Pacific Regions.

Lastly, the lack of knowledge among regulators, medical practitioners, and consumers hinders sectoral growth. Insufficient domestic clinical studies, general mistrust, and technical talent shortages discourage it from establishing sustainable cannabis value chains in accordance with international standards (Kruk et al. 2018).

7. International Law and Regional Influence

An intricate network of regional alliances, international treaties, and geopolitical interests strongly shapes the political and legal path of cannabis legalization in the Asia-Pacific. Although many nations have started to seek domestic cannabis legalization, especially for industrial or medicinal purposes, these initiatives tend to be in tension with established regional political patterns and traditional international drug control conventions. It is necessary to understand the effect of UN conventions, ASEAN policy coherence, and international pressure on trade to appreciate the region-wide cautious and contradictory cannabis policies.

7.1 UN Conventions and Their Influence on Drug Policy

The strongest global framework influencing cannabis legislation across the globe is the United Nations Single Convention on Narcotic Drugs (1961), and its amendment through the 1971 Convention on Psychotropic Substances and the 1988 Convention Against Illicit Traffic in Narcotic Drugs and Psychotropic Substances. These treaties all categorize cannabis as a Schedule I drug, which puts it in the same legal class as heroin and cocaine—considered to have high abuse potential and no accepted medical use (at the time of classification).

Though the 2020 UN Commission on Narcotic Drugs de-scheduled cannabis from Schedule IV (which is reserved for the most dangerous drugs), it is still stringently controlled in Schedule I. Signatory countries are bound to limit its cultivation, trade, and use only to scientific and medical applications. For Asia-Pacific nations, several of which are signatories to the treaties, these conventions have been the de facto legal pillar of cannabis prohibition for decades and are frequently quoted to support domestic prohibitions.

However, as nations such as Thailand and Australia liberalize, they progressively operate in the gray zones of international law. The exception for medical and scientific purposes is permitted in the treaties; however, the definition and the application of the exception are open to the discretion of national authorities. This flexibility has made reform possible without violating the treaties, but it also subjects reformist governments to attacks in international arenas.

7.2 Role of ASEAN in Upholding Strong Regional Consensus

Aside from international agreements, the Association of Southeast Asian Nations (ASEAN) is important in enforcing the prohibition of cannabis throughout large parts of the region. ASEAN joint statements and regional drug control policy are strongly rooted in a zero-tolerance framework concerning narcotics. ASEAN Work Plan on Securing Communities Against Illicit Drugs (2016–2025) officially pledges member states to a "drug-free" region, and cannabis is always listed as one of the more hazardous drugs.

This regional unanimity has long dissuaded member states from seeking reform, even when public sentiment or economic incentives favor change. Nations such as Indonesia, Singapore, and Malaysia continue to adhere to ASEAN's hardline approach, often speaking out against any weakening of drug policy. These forces can cause diplomatic tension for nations such as Thailand, whose decriminalization attempts run counter to ASEAN's collective stance. Nonetheless, Thailand has justified its reforms as legal by international law and presented them as public health-driven rather than recreational legalization, indicating a possible shift in regional norms.

7.3 Conflicts Between Domestic Reform and International Obligations

As cannabis laws start diverging across the region, tensions have arisen between regional legalization drives and global commitments. Reforming nations are specifically confronted with legal and reputational challenges in balancing compliance under the treaty with national sovereignty. Australia's medical cannabis market exists within the uses allowed by the treaty, but ACT recreational legalization presents a legal grey area, as federal legislation and global obligations do not change.

In a similar vein, partial decriminalization of bhang and localized hemp initiatives in India challenge the limits of the NDPS Act and its conformity with international control paradigms. Legal contradictions can arise in certain instances with reform-oriented policies, particularly when federal and state governments adopt divergent policies or when enforcement practices diverge considerably.

These tensions could have diplomatic and economic implications. Nations wishing to increase cannabis exports might see their products prohibited by importing countries held to more austere treaty interpretations. Furthermore, uneven enforcement of policies will discourage foreign investment, hinder international research cooperation across borders, and pose compliance issues for international players in the cannabis industry (Wheeldon and Heidt 2023).

7.4 Foreign Investment and Geopolitics of Cannabis Trade

As cannabis becomes an ever-more valuable global commodity, geopolitical factors and foreign investment are increasingly influencing national cannabis strategies. Asian-Pacific countries with favorable climates and farming potential—such as Thailand, India, and Laos—are being targeted by multinational cannabis companies seeking to establish low-cost production hubs and gain access to Asian and Western markets.

Bilateral free trade agreements, intellectual property regulations, and regulatory openness frequently determine these investment streams. Nations that develop stable and investor-friendly legal frameworks—such as Australia—are better positioned to secure pharmaceutical partnerships and clinical trial investments. Nations with legal insecurity or lax enforcement, on the other hand, will struggle to expand their industries beyond domestic limits (Cooper et al. 2021).

There is also increasing awareness of neo-colonial dynamics in the cannabis industry. It is argued that liberalization disproportionately advantages Western corporations, while indigenous and local people, having grown and used cannabis for centuries, are excluded or marginalized from economic gains. This concerns ethical issues with regard to equity, biopiracy, and cultural appropriation, especially in post-colonial nations with a rich history of cannabis (Lee et al. 2021).

8. Future Outlook and Recommendations

As the world conversation on cannabis keeps evolving towards pragmatism from prohibition, the Asia-Pacific region is at a tipping point. With its rich cultural heritage, growing markets, and multicultural political landscape, the region is poised to drive global cannabis policy in significant directions. In the future, a prosperous and viable cannabis industry for the Asia-Pacific region will require an interdimensional response that accepts research, regulation, education, equity, and sustainability (Svrakic et al. 2012).

8.1 Opportunities for Medical Research and Public Health Innovation

One of the strongest frontiers is cannabis-related medicine. With the growing need for plant-based treatments and increasing amounts of international data, the Asia-Pacific nations can become the leaders in clinical trials, drug development research, and cannabinoid-based medicine research. Australian, South Korean, Indian, and Thai institutions are already researching cannabinoids to treat chronic pain, epilepsy, cancer therapy, and mental health conditions (Varin et al. 2023).

Yet, important gaps exist in regional evidence. Much of the existing cannabis research has been Western-oriented, with an underrepresentation of Asian populations. Scaling up locally initiated clinical trials and cross-border research partnerships could produce regionally applicable evidence to inform policy and healthcare practice. Public health systems must also invest in comprehensive cannabis care models, particularly in pain clinics, oncology wards, and mental health services, backed by adequate physician training and real-world data collection (Simei et al. 2024).

8.2 The Requirement for Even-Handed, Science-Informed Regulation

As cannabis is increasingly legalized or decriminalized for medicinal, industrial, or even recreational use, regulation needs to be evidence-informed, responsive, and proportionate. Blanket criminalization has been ineffectual and damaging, but unregulated markets pose their own dangers—especially to youth, vulnerable groups, and road safety (Kaur and Kander 2023).

Regulators must implement a tiered system of regulation that differentiates between medical, adult-use, and industrial cannabis, with context-specific standards applying to each. Safety regulations for products, labeling, testing, and potency caps must be enacted, while cooperative models and smallholder participation must be shielded from monopolies. Greatest care needs to be taken to harmonize national law with flexibility of international treaties, thereby reducing legal tensions while advancing health-driven reform (Bodwitch et al. 2021).

8.3 Focus on Public Education and Harm Reduction

No cannabis policy can be effective without public literacy and awareness. In nations where stigma and misinformation are prevalent, education campaigns are crucial for promoting educated attitudes and safe behaviors. Governments must invest in multi-language, culturally sensitive education presenting the risks and benefits of cannabis use, THC vs. CBD, and best practices for responsible consumption.

Harm reduction also needs to be emphasized. Approaches like age limits, smokeless alternatives, potency labels, secure storage, and prevention of driving while impaired need to be integrated into every cannabis program. Crucially, these approaches should not be enforced solely by the criminal system, but rather through public health outreach, education in schools, and peer support networks.

8.4 Respect for Traditional and Indigenous Cannabis Knowledge

Asia-Pacific's cannabis future must not only be high-tech it should also be culturally sensitive and historically conscious. The indigenous and traditional communities of India, Nepal, Thailand, and Southeast Asia have long cultivated and used cannabis for spiritual, medicinal, and agricultural reasons. Their knowledge systems provide an understanding of the long-term safety of cannabis, use as an ingredient in polyherbal remedies, and ecologically friendly cultivation methods.

Cannabis policy and research must acknowledge, defend, and engage traditional knowledge keepers. Benefit-sharing arrangements, local license assistance, and heritage seed bank conservation programs can guarantee that these communities remain part of the legitimate cannabis economy. Compliance with the Nagoya Protocol and ethical bioprospecting best practices should be integrated into national cannabis plans.

8.5 Recommendations for Sustainable Industrial Hemp Development

In addition to cannabinoids, industrial hemp offers a window into environmentally friendly growth. Hemp's diversity—utilized in textiles, food, bio-construction, and bioplastics—makes it a perfect crop for low-carbon economies. China, India, and Australia already have the agronomic capability to dominate this industry. To facilitate sustainable hemp development, nations ought to:

- Establish clear legal definitions and distinct regulations of low-THC hemp.
- Offer incentives for research, mechanization, and value-added processing.

- Encourage farmer cooperatives and rural integration, particularly in mountainous and tribal areas.
- Connect hemp with climate resilience and carbon credit programs under green economy initiatives.
- Investing in hemp R&D, certification regimes, and international trade standards will help Asia-Pacific countries to leverage global markets while supporting regenerative agriculture and sustainable industry.

9. Conclusion

The Asia-Pacific region's cannabis ecosystem is a study in contrasts—fragmented yet evolving, culturally rich yet politically cautious. From ancient traditions in India, China, and Nepal to contemporary regulatory experiments in Australia and Thailand, the region showcases a broad spectrum of cannabis engagements shaped by history, religion, science, and geopolitics.

On one end of the spectrum, countries like Singapore, Japan, and South Korea maintain strict prohibition rooted in conservative values and international treaty obligations. On the other hand, Thailand's decriminalization, Australia's regulated medical market, and New Zealand's public debates represent a growing shift toward science-based and socially responsive policy reform. Meanwhile, countries such as India and Nepal straddle the line—honoring traditional use in limited forms while grappling with modern legal and institutional challenges.

Despite this diversity, a clear trend is emerging: the inflexible prohibitionist model is slowly giving way to more nuanced, evidence-informed frameworks. These frameworks seek to balance the therapeutic potential and economic opportunities offered by cannabis with the need to manage public health risks, prevent misuse, and honor cultural norms.

For cannabis to be effectively and ethically integrated into Asia-Pacific societies, future policy must embrace pragmatism over ideology. This means recognizing cannabis as more than a commodity or controlled substance—it is a botanical medicine, cultural artifact, and economic resource. Policymakers must prioritize research, education, and equity, ensuring that cannabis reform is led by public health imperatives, not commercial interests alone.

Furthermore, any successful cannabis model in this region must respect indigenous knowledge, promote sustainable development, and be adaptable to local realities. The future of cannabis in Asia-Pacific lies in collaborative governance, science-driven regulation, and inclusive socio-cultural dialogue. Only through this balanced approach can the region move forward—transforming cannabis from a symbol of criminality into one of healing, heritage, and innovation.

References

Acharya, S. L., Howard, J., Panta, S. B., Mahatma, S. S., and Copeland, J. (2015). Cannabis, Lord Shiva and Holy Men: Cannabis Use Among Sadhus in Nepal. *Journal of Psychiatrists' Association of Nepal*, 3(2): 9–14. https://doi.org/10.3126/JPAN.V3I2.12379

Areesantichai, C., Perngparn, U., and Pilley, C. (2020). Current cannabis-related situation in the Asia-Pacific region. *Current Opinion in Psychiatry*, 33(4): 352–359. https://doi.org/10.1097/YCO.0000000000000616,

Assanangkornchai, S., Thaikla, K., Talek, M., and Saingam, D. (2022). Medical cannabis use in Thailand after its legalization: A respondent-driven sample survey. *PeerJ*, *10*, e12809. https://doi.org/10.7717/PEERJ.12809/SUPP-3

Baratta, F., Pignata, I., Ravetto Enri, L., and Brusa, P. (2022). Cannabis for medical use: Analysis of recent clinical trials in view of current legislation. *Frontiers in Pharmacology*, 13: 888903. https://doi.org/10.3389/FPHAR.2022.888903

Bodwitch, H., Polson, M., Biber, E., Hickey, G. M., and Butsic, V. (2021). Why comply? Farmer motivations and barriers in cannabis agriculture. *Journal of Rural Studies*, 86: 155–170. https://doi.org/10.1016/J.JRURSTUD.2021.05.006

Brand, E. J., and Zhao, Z. (2017). Cannabis in Chinese medicine: Are some traditional indications referenced in ancient literature related to Cannabinoids? *Frontiers in Pharmacology*, 8(MAR): 108. https://doi.org/10.3389/FPHAR.2017.00108

Caio Fernando de C Lambert, Evandro Alves Barbosa Filho, Karen Viviana Castaño Coronado, and Ravindra B. Malabadi. (2024). Exploring the potentialities of industrial hemp for sustainable rural development. *World Journal of Biology Pharmacy and Health Sciences*, 18(1): 305–320. https://doi.org/10.30574/WJBPHS.2024.18.1.0205

Castle, D. J., Strauss, N., Norman, A., and Bonomo, Y. (2019). Medical Marijuana: The Australian Experience. *Missouri Medicine*, 116(4): 270.

Cheng, K., Harnett, J., Davis, S., and Smith, L. (2023). Conversations about cannabis: The supply process in Australia. *Advances in Integrative Medicine*, 10(4): 190–197. https://doi.org/10.1016/J.AIMED.2024.01.001

Cheng, S. F., De Franco, G., and Lin, P. (2023). Marijuana liberalization and public finance: A capital market perspective on the passage of medical use laws. *Journal of Accounting and Economics*, 75(1). https://doi.org/10.1016/j.jacceco.2022.101516

Cooper, Z. D., Abrams, D. I., Gust, S., Salicrup, A., and Throckmorton, D. C. (2021). Challenges for clinical cannabis and cannabinoid research in the United States. *Journal of the National Cancer Institute. Monographs*, 2021(58): 114. https://doi.org/10.1093/JNCIMONOGRAPHS/LGAB009

Crocq, M. A. (2020). History of cannabis and the endocannabinoid system. *Dialogues in Clinical Neuroscience*, 22(3): 223. https://doi.org/10.31887/DCNS.2020.22.3/MCROCQ

Donnelly, J., Young, M., Marshall, B., Hecht, M. L., and Saldutti, E. (2022). Public health implications of cannabis legalization: An exploration of adolescent use and evidence based interventions. *International Journal of Environmental Research and Public Health*, 19(6): 3336. https://doi.org/10.3390/IJERPH19063336

Evrard, Olivier, ed, Guillaud, Dominique, and Vaddhanaphuti. (2013). *Mobility and heritage in Northern Thailand and Laos : past and present.*

Faguet, G. B. (2010). Pain Control and Drug Policy. *Pain Control and Drug Policy*. https://doi.org/10.5040/9798400694844

Fischer, B., and Hall, W. (2021). New Zealand's failed cannabis legalization referendum – implications for cannabis policy reform. *The Lancet Regional Health: Western Pacific*, 7: 100080. https://doi.org/10.1016/J.LANWPC.2020.100080

Graham, M., Chiu, V., Stjepanović, D., and Hall, W. (2023). A provisional evaluation of Australia's medical cannabis program. *International Journal of Drug Policy*, 122: 104210. https://doi.org/10.1016/J.DRUGPO.2023.104210

Hourfane, S., Mechqoq, H., Bekkali, A. Y., Rocha, J. M., and El Aouad, N. (2023). A Comprehensive Review on Cannabis sativa Ethnobotany, Phytochemistry, Molecular Docking and Biological Activities. *Plants*, 12(6): 1245. https://doi.org/10.3390/PLANTS12061245

Karki, P., and Rangaswamy, M. (2022). A review of historical context and current research on cannabis use in India. *Indian Journal of Psychological Medicine*, 45(2): 105. https://doi.org/10.1177/02537176221109272

Kaur, G., and Kander, R. (2023). The Sustainability of Industrial Hemp: A literature review of its economic, environmental, and social sustainability. *Sustainability*, 15(8), 6457. https://doi.org/10.3390/SU15086457

Kiran, P. Kolkar, Ravindra B. Malabadi, Raju K. Chalannavar, Divakar M. S., Swathi, Avinash A. Kamble, Kishore S. Karamchand et al. (2025). Industrial Cannabis sativa (Fiber or Hemp): Hemp Cottonization-Advantages and Current Challenges. *International Journal of Science and Research Archive*, 14(3): 1233–1267. https://doi.org/10.30574/IJSRA.2025.14.3.0755

Kruk, M. E., Gage, A. D., Arsenault, C., Jordan, K., Leslie, H. H., Roder-DeWan, S. et al. (2018). High-quality health systems in the Sustainable Development Goals era: time for a revolution. *The Lancet. Global Health*, 6(11): e1196. https://doi.org/10.1016/S2214-109X(18)30386-3

Lee, C., Round, J. M., Klarenbach, S., Hanlon, J. G., Hyshka, E., Dyck, J. R. B. et al. (2021). Gaps in evidence for the use of medically authorized cannabis: Ontario and Alberta, Canada. *Harm Reduction Journal*, 18(1): 1–9. https://doi.org/10.1186/S12954-021-00509-0/TABLES/2

Lewis, M., and Flood, J. (2021). The transition of cannabis into the mainstream of Australian healthcare: framings in professional medical publications. *Journal of Cannabis Research*, 3(1): 48. https://doi.org/10.1186/S42238-021-00105-W

Lines, R., Elliott, R., Hannah, J., Schleifer, R., Avafia, T., and Barrett, D. (2017). The Case for International Guidelines on Human Rights and Drug Control. *Health and Human Rights*, 19(1): 231.

National Academies of Sciences, E. and M., Division, H. and M., Practice, B. on P. H. and P. H., and Agenda, C. on the H. E. of M. A. E. R. and R. (2017). *Challenges and Barriers in Conducting Cannabis Research.*

Rafei, P., Englund, A., Lorenzetti, V., Elkholy, H., Potenza, M. N., and Baldacchino, A. M. (2023). Transcultural Aspects of Cannabis Use: a Descriptive Overview of Cannabis Use across Cultures. *Current Addiction Reports*, 10(3): 458–471. https://doi.org/10.1007/S40429-023-00500-8

Resko, S., Ellis, J., Early, T. J., Szechy, K. A., Rodriguez, B., and Agius, E. (2019). Understanding public attitudes toward cannabis legalization: Qualitative findings from a statewide survey. *Substance Use and Misuse*, 54(8): 1247–1259. https://doi.org/10.1080/10826084.2018.1543327

Schiemer, C., Horswill, M. S., Hill, A., Summers, M. J., and Stefanidis, K. B. (2025). The acute effects of vaporized cannabis on drivers' hazard perception and risk-taking behaviors in medicinal patients: A within-subjects experiment. *Journal of Safety Research*, 92: 385–392. https://doi.org/10.1016/J.JSR.2024.12.004

Shakya, D. R., Upadhaya, S. R., and Thapa, M. (2021). Cannabis Use and Abuse in Nepal: A Review of Studies. *JNMA: Journal of the Nepal Medical Association*, 59(241): 954. https://doi.org/10.31729/JNMA.6931

Shamir, R., and Hacker, D. (2001). Colonialism's Civilizing Mission: The Case of the Indian Hemp Drug Commission. *Law and Social Inquiry*, 26(2): 435–461. https://doi.org/10.1111/j.1747-4469.2001.tb00184.x

Simei, J. L. Q., Souza, J. D. R., Pedrazzi, J. F., Guimarães, F. S., Campos, A. C., Zuardi, A. et al. (2024). Research and clinical practice involving the use of cannabis products, with emphasis on Cannabidiol: A narrative review. *Pharmaceuticals*, 17(12): 1644. https://doi.org/10.3390/PH17121644

Sommano, S. R., Tangpao, T., Pankasemsuk, T., Ponpanumas, V., Phimolsiripol, Y., Rachtanapun, P. et al. (2022). Growing ganja permission: a real gate-way for Thailand's promising industrial crop? *Journal of Cannabis Research*, 4(1). https://doi.org/10.1186/S42238-022-00121-4

Svrakic, D. M., Lustman, P. J., Mallya, A., Lynn, T. A., Finney, R., and Svrakic, N. M. (2012). Legalization, Decriminalization and Medicinal Use of Cannabis: A Scientific and Public Health Perspective. *Missouri Medicine*, 109(2): 90.

Varin, M., Champagne, A., Venugopal, J., Li, L., McFaull, S. R., Thompson, W. et al. (2023). Trends in cannabis-related emergency department visits and hospitalizations among children aged 0–11 years in Canada from 2015 to 2021: spotlight on cannabis edibles. *BMC Public Health*, 23(1). https://doi.org/10.1186/S12889-023-16987-9

Wheeldon, J., and Heidt, J. (2023). Cannabis, research ethics, and a duty of care. *Research Ethics*, 19(3): 250–287. https://doi.org/10.1177/17470161231164530

Yimsaard, P., Lancaster, K. E., and Sohn, A. H. (2023). Potential impact of Thailand's cannabis policy on the health of young adults: current status and future landscape. *The Lancet Regional Health - Southeast Asia*, 10: 100145. https://doi.org/10.1016/J.LANSEA.2023.100145

Zuardi, A. W. (2006). History of cannabis as a medicine: A review. *Revista Brasileira de Psiquiatria*, 28(2): 153–157. https://doi.org/10.1590/S1516-44462006000200015

CHAPTER 3

Cannabis Cultivation for the Production of Secondary Metabolites

Agronomic Practices, Phytochemical Profiling, and Post-Harvest Processing

Francisco Mayron de Sousa e Silva,[1,*] *Sara da Silva Lima,*[2]
Paulo Jordão de Oliveira Cerqueira Fortes,[3] *Jamila Ferreira Rocha,*[4]
Maurício Pires de Moura do Amaral,[1,2] *Salomon Tinman*[5] and
Livio Cesar Cunha Nunes[1,2]

1. Introduction

Research on the genetic and agronomic factors influencing the biosynthesis of cannabinoids and terpenes in *Cannabis sativa* L. has emerged as a critical area of investigation due to the plant's significant medicinal, industrial, and economic value (Henry et al. 2020; Naim-Feil et al. 2023). Over the past few decades, advances in genomics and metabolomics have elucidated the complex biosynthetic pathways of cannabinoids and terpenes, emphasizing their synthesis in glandular trichomes and the key roles of enzymes such as THCAS, CBDAS, and CBCAS (Apicella et al. 2021; Yeo et al. 2022). The evolving legal landscape and growing market demand have intensified research efforts to optimize phytochemical profiles for both therapeutic efficacy and regulatory compliance (Siracusa et al. 2023; Trancoso et al. 2022). Notably, the wide chemotypic diversity, ranging from THC-dominant to CBD-dominant and balanced types, underscores the importance of understanding the relationships between genotype and phenotype relationships, as well as environmental modulation.

[1] Graduate Program in Pharmaceutical Sciences (PPGCF), Federal University of Piauí (UFPI), Teresina – PI
[2] Pharmacy Program, Federal University of Piauí (UFPI), Teresina – PI
[3] CCA/UFPI (Administration), Federal University of Piauí (UFPI), Teresina – PI
[4] BCY Association, INEAGRO/UFPI – Sala 01 Rua Dirce Oliveira, 3597 – Ininga, Teresina – PI, CEP 64048-550
[5] Piauí Hemp (CANNAPI) – Quadra 330 casa, 09 Dirceu 2 Teresina – PI, CEP 64.078-444
* Corresponding author: mayrondcf@gmail.com, mailto:mayrondcf@gmail.com

DOI: 10.1201/9781003668190-4

Despite considerable progress, the precise genetic determinants and environmental interactions governing cannabinoid and terpene profiles remain incompletely understood (Singh et al. 2021; Wenger et al. 2020). While gene copy number variation and single-nucleotide polymorphisms in cannabinoid synthase genes have been linked to chemotypic variability, the regulatory mechanisms and the impact of agronomic practices, such as light spectrum, nutrient management, and cultivation techniques, are still subjects of ongoing debate (Morello et al. 2022; Simonutti et al. 2024; Vergara et al. 2019).

Conflicting reports exist regarding the extent to which environmental stressors, including temperature and photoperiod, influence the accumulation of secondary metabolites and gene expression (Brousseau et al. 2021; Hahm et al. 2025; Peterswald et al. 2023). Additionally, the interaction between physiological traits, plant architecture, and phytochemical production constitutes a complex system that challenges breeding and cultivation strategies (Naim-Feil et al. 2023; Stack et al. 2022). The lack of consensus on these factors hinders the development of standardized cultivation protocols and consistent product quality (Tanney et al. 2021; Trancoso et al. 2022; Zandkarimi et al. 2023).

The conceptual framework of this review integrates the genetic regulation of cannabinoid biosynthesis, agronomic influences on phytochemical profiles, and physiological interactions that affect secondary metabolite production (Brousseau et al. 2021; Yeo et al. 2022). Key concepts include the enzymatic pathways responsible for cannabinoid and terpene synthesis, the genetic basis of chemotype determination, and the modulation of metabolite accumulation by environmental and cultivation-related factors. Understanding these relationships is essential for targeted breeding and optimized cultivation to enhance yield and consistency of therapeutic compounds (Naim-Feil et al. 2023; Yoosefzadeh Najafabadi and Torkamaneh 2025).

In this context, the present chapter provides the conceptual basis for applied research aimed at developing cannabis-based pharmaceutical formulations, particularly those involving alternative routes of administration such as transdermal systems. These systems have emerged as promising strategies for the targeted delivery of cannabinoids for analgesic and anti-inflammatory purposes, as they allow controlled release, bypass first-pass metabolism, and enhance bioavailability. However, the effectiveness of such formulations depends directly on the quality and consistency of the secondary metabolites extracted from the plant. Therefore, understanding the genetic, environmental, and agronomic determinants that modulate cannabinoid production is essential for ensuring suitable plant-derived raw materials for pharmaceutical compounding and achieving therapeutic efficacy in clinical applications such as the treatment of chronic pain and inflammation.

This systematic review aims to critically evaluate the current understanding of the genetic factors that control the biosynthesis of cannabinoids and terpenes in *Cannabis sativa* L., assess the impact of genotype selection and agronomic practices on phytochemical profiles, and elucidate the physiological and environmental interactions influencing secondary metabolite production. This review aims to bridge existing knowledge gaps by synthesizing multidisciplinary findings, thereby informing breeding programs and cultivation strategies that aim to enhance the quality and efficacy of medicinal cannabis (Henry et al. 2020; Simonutti et al. 2024; Trancoso et al. 2022).

The review employs a comprehensive survey of the literature, covering genomic, transcriptomic, metabolomic, and agronomic studies. Inclusion criteria focus on recent advances in genetic regulation, chemotype variability, cultivation techniques, and the effects of environmental stress on cannabinoid and terpene biosynthesis. Analytical frameworks integrate molecular genetics with physiological and agronomic data, organizing findings to delineate the multifactorial determinants of phytochemical profiles in *Cannabis sativa* L. (Brousseau et al. 2021; Trancoso et al. 2022; Yeo et al. 2022).

2. Methodology

To develop this chapter, which addresses the factors influencing the phytochemical profile of *Cannabis sativa* L., a narrative review of scientific and technical literature was conducted. Searches were performed in the PubMed, Web of Science, SciELO, Scopus, and Google Scholar databases using the following keywords: "environmental factors *Cannabis*," "cannabinoids and cultivation," "photoperiod *Cannabis*," "genetic influence on *Cannabis*," "post-harvest *Cannabis*," "phytochemical profile *Cannabis*," and "cannabinoid storage."

No publication date restrictions were applied to include both classical studies and the most recent research. Articles were selected in Portuguese, English, and Spanish. The selection process considered the relevance of titles and abstracts to the topics covered in the chapter and included experimental studies, systematic and narrative reviews, technical reports, regulatory guidelines, and operational manuals from medicinal cannabis producer associations.

In addition to scientific publications, supplementary references were included from the bibliographies of the reviewed articles, as well as from regulatory documents such as ANVISA legislation and guidelines, technical bulletins, institutional websites, and materials published by medicinal cannabis associations (ACMs). Pharmacopeias and official documents were also consulted to support the technical understanding of the cultivation, harvesting, drying, extraction, and quality control processes of cannabis-derived products.

This methodological approach enabled a comprehensive contextualization of the main genetic, environmental, agronomic, and technological factors that directly impact the expression and preservation of the plant's secondary metabolites, such as cannabinoids and terpenes, in alignment with the chapter's objectives.

3. Brief Historical Overview and Medicinal Relevance of Cannabis

Cannabis sativa has a millennia-old history of human use, with archaeological evidence indicating its cultivation and application as early as 4000 BCE in China, where it was utilized for various purposes, including fiber production, food, religious rituals, and, most notably, traditional medicine. Ancient records, both in the form of cannabis remnants and written texts, document its use in treating rheumatic pain, constipation, malaria, and even as an anesthetic during surgical procedures, as found in foundational Ayurvedic texts (circa 800 BCE) and in the earliest known pharmacopoeia, the Chinese *Shen Nung Pen Ts'ao Ching* (1st century BCE) (Crocq 2020; Nascimento and Dalcin 2019; Pisanti and Bifulco 2019).

Paleobotanical studies confirm that cannabis was present over 11,700 years ago in Central Asia, near the Altai Mountains (Pisanti and Bifulco 2019). In ancient Greece and Rome, the physician Pedanius Dioscorides, considered the father of pharmacology, described the medicinal use of this substance around 50 CE for relieving joint pain and inflammation. In the 19th century, Irish physician William Brooke O'Shaughnessy introduced cannabis to Western medicine after observing its therapeutic effects in India, publishing studies on its potential in treating seizures, muscle spasms, and chronic pain (Crocq 2020; Russo 2016).

However, the 20th century saw a drastic shift in the perception of cannabis. Beginning in the 1930s, a campaign in the United States, driven by racial, economic, and political prejudice, led to the enactment of the Marihuana Tax Act in 1937, effectively criminalizing its use (Hewitt 2020; King 2018). Subsequently, the 1961 United Nations Single Convention on Narcotic Drugs classified cannabis as a substance with high abuse potential and no recognized therapeutic value, prompting its removal from the U.S. Pharmacopeia in 1942 (Grinspoon and Bakalar 1995; Hewitt 2020).

The scientific rehabilitation of cannabis began in the 1990s with the discovery of the endocannabinoid system, a network of receptors (CB1 and CB2), enzymes, and endogenous ligands that regulate physiological functions such as pain, sleep, appetite, and mood (Kulkarni et al. 2025; Sampson 2021). This discovery reignited scientific interest in cannabis, laying the foundation for therapies based on its active compounds (Hill 2024).

The medicinal relevance of cannabis lies in its complex phytochemical composition, which includes hundreds of secondary metabolites, primarily cannabinoids, terpenes, and flavonoids. The most extensively studied cannabinoids are cannabidiol (CBD), which is non-psychoactive and known for its anxiolytic, anticonvulsant, and anti-inflammatory properties, and delta-9-tetrahydrocannabinol (Δ9-THC), which is psychoactive but also effective in reducing nausea, stimulating appetite, and alleviating pain (Blebea et al. 2024; O'Brien and Blair 2021). The synergistic interaction among these compounds, known as the entourage effect, enhances therapeutic outcomes and modulates clinical responses (Al-Khazaleh et al. 2024; O'Brien and Blair 2021).

Currently, medicinal cannabis is used in the management of several clinical conditions, including chronic pain, refractory epilepsy, multiple sclerosis, Parkinson's disease, autism spectrum disorder, generalized anxiety disorder, and sleep disorders. Countries such as Canada, the United Kingdom (2018), the Netherlands (2003), Italy (2006), Israel, Germany (2017), and Uruguay have regulated the cultivation, production, and medicinal use of cannabis, fostering research, pharmaceutical product development, and advancements in agricultural biotechnology (Pereira 2023; Silva and Figueiredo 2023).

In Brazil, although the National Health Surveillance Agency (ANVISA) has authorized the importation and commercialization of cannabis-based products under medical prescription (RDC No. 327/2019 and RDC N°. 660/2022), significant barriers remain, including the high cost of imported products, legal bureaucracy, and the prohibition of home cultivation. In response, the number of legal actions and preventive habeas corpus petitions has grown, as patients and families seek the right to self-cultivate or obtain products through collective cultivation associations.

This scenario highlights the urgent need for inclusive public policies, scientific research incentives, and specific regulations for the cultivation of medicinal cannabis in Brazil. Such measures would enable the development of a secure, traceable, and economically viable production chain.

Within this historical and scientific context, advances in the therapeutic use of *Cannabis sativa* are intrinsically linked to the quality of the plant's bioactive compounds, especially cannabinoids with analgesic and anti-inflammatory properties. Mastery over cultivation techniques, phytochemical characterization, and standardization of botanical raw materials becomes a fundamental requirement for the development of effective pharmaceutical formulations, such as transdermal systems designed to optimize the release and bioavailability of cannabinoids in the treatment of chronic pain and inflammation.

4. Types of Cannabis and the Phytochemical Profile

4.1 Subspecies and Chemotypes of Cannabis (sativa, indica, and ruderalis)

Cannabis sativa L. is an annual plant widely cultivated for its medicinal, industrial, and recreational properties. Although different subspecies, varieties, and cultivars have traditionally been recognized based on morphological and geographical traits, recent genomic studies indicate that such botanical classifications do not always align with the chemical diversity observed among different types of *Cannabis* (Raman et al. 2017; Rock and Parker 2021; Thomas and ElSohly 2016). Historically, the plant has been classified into three main subspecies, as illustrated in Figure 1.

Despite this traditional classification, most cannabis plants available on the market today are hybrids, resulting from extensive crossbreeding between these lineages. Such widespread hybridization has blurred botanical criteria, rendering the distinction between sativa and indica less scientifically and practically meaningful. A classification based on phytochemical composition (chemotypes) is now considered more informative (Benredjem and Pineyro 2023; Borroto

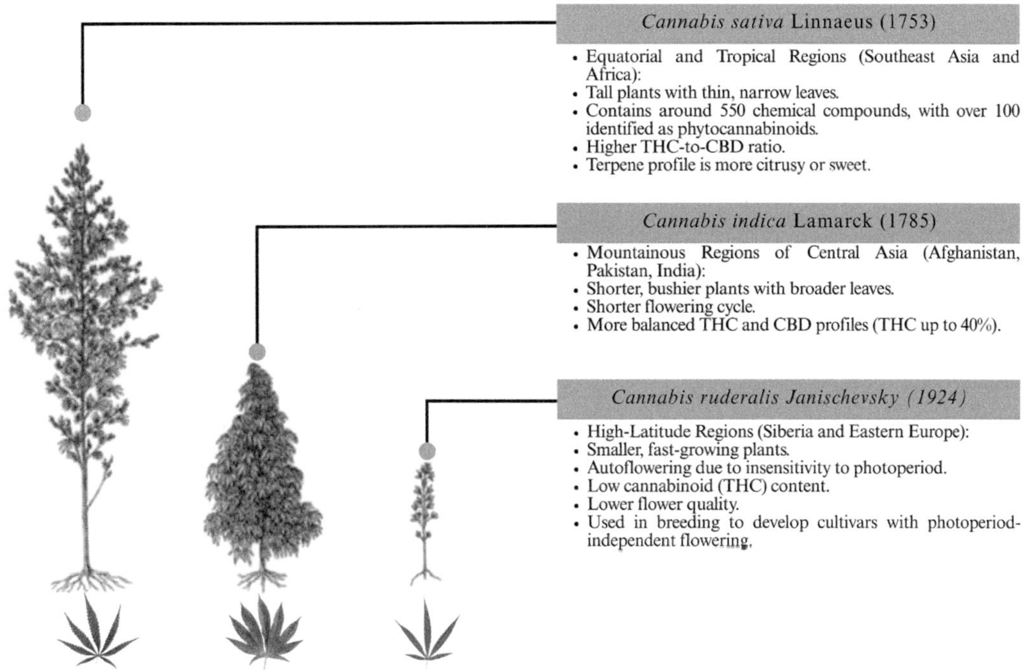

Figure 1: Main subspecies of *Cannabis sativa L.*

Source: Prepared by the authors based on the following references: *Cannabis sativa* Linnaeus (1753) (Raman et al. 2017; Rock and Parker 2021; Thomas and ElSohly 2016); *Cannabis indica* Lamarck (1785) (Chauhan et al. 2024; McPartland and Small 2020); *Cannabis ruderalis Janischevsky* (1924) (Kurtz et al. 2023; Leckie et al. 2023, 2024).

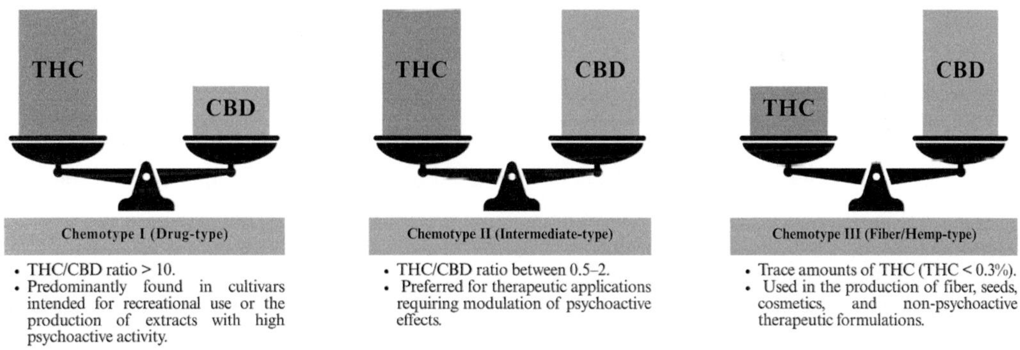

Figure 2: Classification of *Cannabis sativa* chemotypes based on the THC to CBD ratio.

Source: Prepared by the authors based on the references: Chemotype I (Benredjem and Pineyro 2023); Chemotype II (Benredjem and Pineyro 2023; Jin et al. 2021); Chemotype III (Borroto Fernandez et al. 2020).

Fernandez et al. 2020; Jin et al. 2021). For therapeutic, regulatory, and pharmacognostic purposes, the most relevant classification is that which considers phytocannabinoid content, particularly the ratio between THC and CBD. Three primary chemotypes are recognized, as shown in Figure 2.

Some authors also propose the existence of chemotypes IV and V. Chemotype IV (CBG-rich) is characterized by high levels of cannabigerol (CBG) and minimal THC content, presenting unique phytochemical properties and potential therapeutic benefits (Fournier et al. 1987; Gargiulo et al. 2024). Chemotype V (terpene-rich), on the other hand, exhibits low levels of cannabinoids but high terpene production, suggesting an emphasis on aromatic and flavor profiles rather than psychoactive effects (Jin et al. 2021). While interest in specific chemotypes, such as CBG- and terpene-rich strains, is increasing, it is essential to consider the broader implications of cannabis cultivation, including its potential for diverse applications in both medicine and industry. The interaction between genetics,

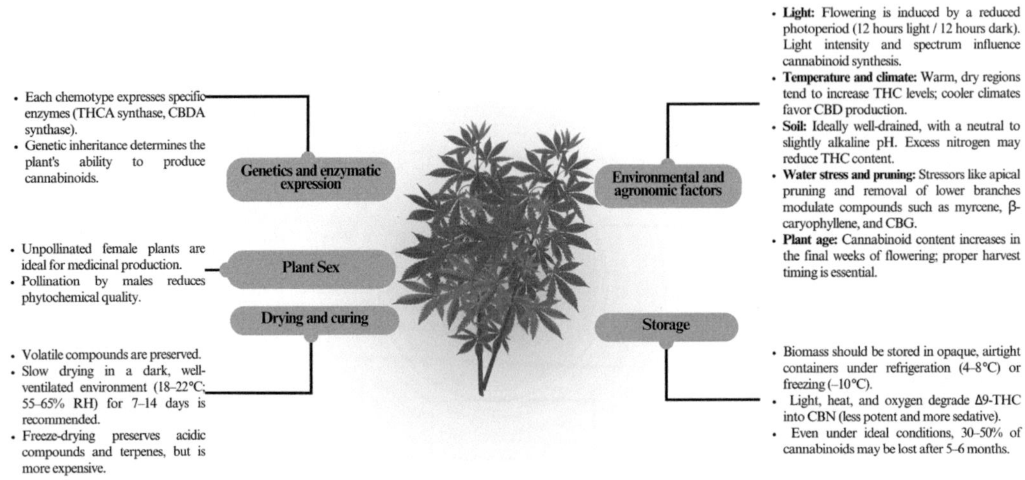

Figure 3: Critical variables for the production and stability of cannabinoids and terpenes in *Cannabis sativa*.
Source: Prepared by the authors (2025).

environment, and management practices continues to shape the future of cannabis research and product development (Figure 3) (Fournier et al. 1987; Gargiulo et al. 2024; Jin et al. 2021).

The high genetic plasticity of *Cannabis*, combined with rampant commercial hybridization and the lack of standardized botanical nomenclature, makes the traditional classification into "sativa" and "indica" insufficient for therapeutic purposes. Hybrid varieties often exhibit phytochemical profiles that diverge from their popular labels. For scientific, clinical, and industrial purposes, chemotype and standardized phytochemical profiling using chromatography (HPLC or GC-MS) are the most reliable approaches for categorizing cultivars and ensuring therapeutic consistency.

The plant *Cannabis sativa* L. is notable for its complex phytochemical composition, which includes hundreds of compounds, among them more than 60 types of cannabinoids. These molecules are characteristic of cannabis and act on the human endocannabinoid system, exerting various pharmacological and therapeutic effects. The two most well-known and studied cannabinoids, due to their scientifically proven therapeutic effects, are Δ9-THC and CBD. In addition to these, cannabis contains other cannabinoids, some of which are acidic precursors that convert into their neutral forms through decarboxylation, usually when exposed to heat.

Besides the cannabinoids described in Figure 4, their precursor acidic forms, such as Δ9-THCA, CBDA, CBGA, and CBCA, are also present. In the fresh plant, most cannabinoids are found in these acidic forms, which are converted into their neutral counterparts (such as Δ9-THC and CBD) through the decarboxylation process. This conversion occurs naturally over time or can be accelerated by heat or in alkaline environments. Elevated temperatures, such as 145°C for 30 minutes, are sufficient to promote the complete decarboxylation of compounds like Δ9-THCA, CBGA, and CBCA (L.-Y. Wang et al. 2016).

4.2 *Terpenes and Flavonoids and Their Therapeutic Influence*

Among the various secondary metabolites present in *Cannabis sativa* L., terpenes and flavonoids stand out for their significant contribution to the plant's phytochemical profile and therapeutic properties, especially when considered in combination with cannabinoids. These classes of compounds not only confer sensory characteristics to the plant, such as aroma and flavor, but also exert their own pharmacological effects and interact synergistically with cannabinoids, directly influencing the therapeutic potential of cannabis-derived products (Hourfane et al. 2023).

Terpenes are volatile organic compounds widely found in the resin of cannabis and are primarily responsible for its characteristic aroma. The first terpene isolated from cannabis was β-caryophyllene, historically associated with effects such as dizziness and euphoria in agricultural

Δ-9 THC

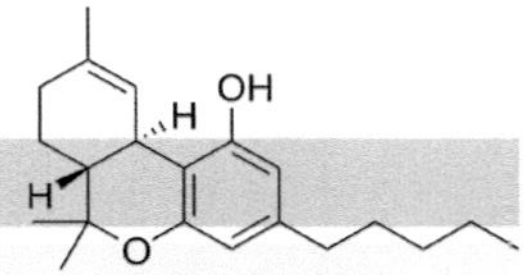

- Main psychoactive cannabinoid of the plant.
- Primarily acts on CB1 receptors.
- Highly lipophilic.
- Unstable in the presence of heat, light, acids, and oxygen.
- Exhibits antinociceptive, anti-inflammatory, and muscle-relaxant effects.
- Stimulates appetite, with antiemetic and neuroprotective actions.
- Enhances the analgesic effects of opioids.
- Approved by ANVISA at concentrations above 0.2% for palliative care.
- Produces hallucinogenic effects.
- May cause cognitive dysfunction and memory impairment.
- Inhibits NMDA receptors and reduces acetylcholine in the hippocampus.
- Activates CB1 receptors in parasympathetic neurons.
- Low doses can reverse cognitive decline in the elderly.
- Increases synaptic expression and dendritic spine density in the hippocampus.

CBN

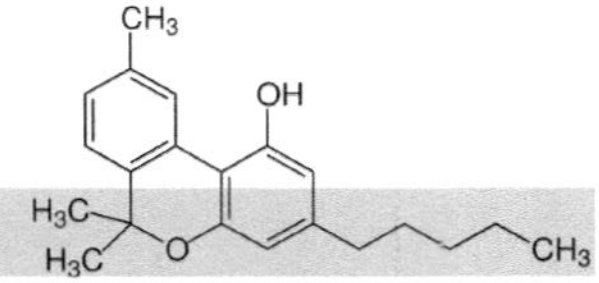

- Derived from the oxidative degradation of Δ9-THC.
- First non-psychoactive compound isolated from Cannabis.
- Used as an indicator of product aging and quality.
- Has mild psychoactive activity.
- Inactive on its own but enhances THC's sedative effects.
- Exhibits anti-inflammatory and anticonvulsant properties.
- Primarily acts on CB2 receptors.

CBG

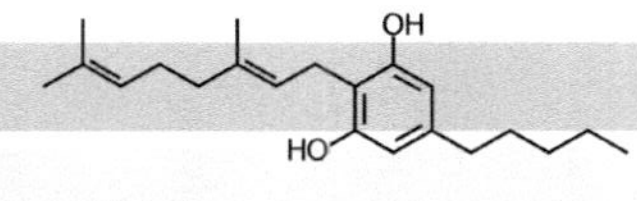

- Natural cannabinoid precursor to other phytocannabinoids.
- forms Δ9-THCA, CBDA, and CBCA via CBGA.
- Found in rare strains with low THC and CBD content.
- Exhibits antiproliferative activity.
- Reduces pain, erythema, and inflammation.
- Acts by inhibiting lipoxygenase and activating α2-adrenergic receptors.
- Inhibits anandamide reuptake.
- Functions as a moderate antagonist of 5-HT1a receptors.

CBD

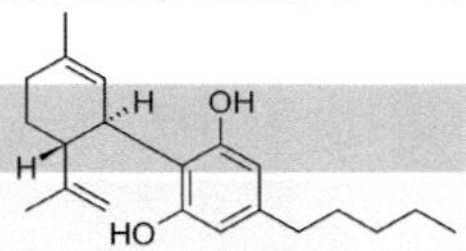

- Second most abundant cannabinoid.
- Non-psychoactive cannabinoid.
- Reclassified by ANVISA to Schedule C1 in 2015.
- Exhibits sedative, anti-inflammatory, anticonvulsant, and antipsychotic effects.
- Acts on neurological and psychiatric disorders.
- Reduces seizures as an adjuvant therapy.
- Anticonvulsant effect is independent of cannabinoid receptors.
- Acts on GABA-A and adenosine A1 receptors.
- Inhibits THC-induced tachycardia via adenosine A1 receptor.
- Has antipsychotic and neuroprotective effects.
- Protects against cardiotoxicity, fibrosis, and oxidative stress.
- Induces apoptosis in breast cancer cells.
- Enhances doxorubicin uptake via TRPV2 receptor.

THCV

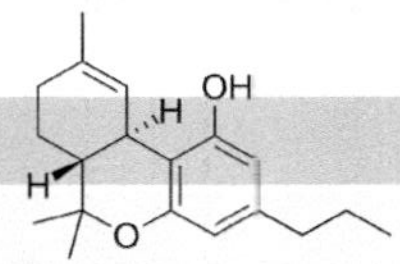

- Minor cannabinoid with a propyl side chain.
- Mild and short-lasting psychoactive effects.
- Acts as a CB1 antagonist at low doses and a partial agonist at high doses.
- Suppresses appetite.
- Exhibits anticonvulsant, anxiolytic, and antipsychotic effects.
- Shows potential for obesity, type 2 diabetes, and metabolic syndrome.
- Modulates glucose levels and insulin sensitivity.
- Promising for therapeutic use with fewer side effects.

CBC

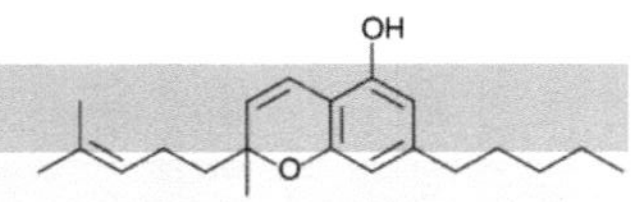

- Natural cannabinoid derived from CBGA.
- No affinity for CB1 or CB2 receptors.
- Exhibits anti-inflammatory and analgesic effects.
- Inhibits cyclooxygenase and prostaglandins.
- Does not have anticonvulsant action nor inhibits CYP enzymes.

Figure 4: Main cannabinoids of *Cannabis sativa*: chemical structures, target receptors, and pharmacological effects.

Source: Prepared by the authors based on (Maayah et al. 2020).

workers who handled the plant. Today, terpenes have received growing scientific attention due to their relevance in the so-called "entourage effect," a synergistic interaction between terpenes and phytocannabinoids that enhances the pharmacological activity of the plant. Terpenes are classified into monoterpenes and sesquiterpenes, the former being more volatile and thus more susceptible to loss during drying and storage processes. Factors such as exposure to oxygen and ultraviolet radiation can degrade or transform them into allergenic compounds, reducing their stability and therapeutic efficacy (Dalli et al. 2023; Hourfane et al. 2023).

Terpene concentrations in cannabis plants can vary significantly among different plant parts, such as flowers, leaves, stems, roots, and bark, and are strongly influenced by agronomic and environmental factors. Management practices, such as pruning of lower branches, can alter the chemical profile of terpenes like myrcene and β-caryophyllene, as can environmental conditions like light, temperature, and humidity during cultivation (Brousseau et al. 2021; Jurga et al. 2024). Changes in growth cycle duration, planting density, and moderate water stress also directly impact the production and stability of these volatile compounds. The choice of extraction method is another crucial factor: techniques such as supercritical fluid extraction (SFE) allow for terpene fractionation at lower pressures than those required for cannabinoid extraction, thus favoring their preservation (Baldino et al. 2020). Conversely, dry extraction methods may lead to the evaporation of lighter monoterpenes, reducing the total terpene content and aromatic complexity of extracts.

Several terpenes are present in varying proportions in cannabis strains, with the most common being myrcene, α-pinene, limonene, linalool, β-caryophyllene, α-humulene, bisabolol, and (E)-β-farnesene (Baldino et al. 2020). Among these, myrcene stands out as one of the most abundant monoterpenes, exhibiting therapeutic actions that include antipsychotic, antioxidant, analgesic, anti-inflammatory, sedative, muscle-relaxant, and potentially anticancer properties (Surendran et al. 2021). β-Caryophyllene, on the other hand, is considered the most relevant sesquiterpene, as it is the only one currently recognized as a dietary cannabinoid capable of selectively binding to the CB2 receptor of the endocannabinoid system (Hashiesh et al. 2020). This binding confers a wide range of pharmacological effects, including gastroprotective, analgesic, antifungal, antibacterial, anti-inflammatory, antioxidant, neuroprotective, and anxiolytic actions. *In vitro* studies have also shown its selectivity against the herpes simplex virus type 1 (Yasaghi et al. 2025).

The interaction between terpenes and cannabinoids, known as the entourage effect, is one of the most relevant concepts in the medicinal use of cannabis. Terpenes such as myrcene, linalool, and limonene can cross the blood-brain barrier and influence neurotransmitter activity, as well as modulate Δ9-THC binding affinity to CB1 receptors, thereby directly impacting the psychoactive and analgesic effects of the compound (Al-Ghezi et al. 2019; Andre et al. 2016). This complex chemical interaction not only enhances the therapeutic efficacy of phytocannabinoids but may also mitigate their adverse effects, contributing to a more balanced clinical response. A practical example of the entourage effect is the drug Sativex®, a full-spectrum *Cannabis sativa* L. extract containing Δ9-THC, CBD, minor cannabinoids, and terpenoids, indicated for the treatment of chronic pain and spasticity associated with multiple sclerosis (Javid et al. 2024).

In addition to terpenes, flavonoids also represent an important class of secondary metabolites in cannabis. These polyphenolic compounds play a role in plant defense mechanisms against environmental stress, contributing to coloration and protection against ultraviolet radiation (Laaboudi et al. 2024). In ecological interactions, flavonoids act antagonistically toward insects, influencing their feeding behavior, growth, and reproduction. These effects are partly due to the inhibition of enzymes such as acetylcholinesterase (AChE) and glutathione S-transferase (GST), as well as the modulation of hormone receptors like the ecdysone receptor (Pereira et al. 2024). *Cannabis sativa* L. essential oil, for instance, has demonstrated a stronger inhibitory effect on AChE than essential oils from other medicinal plants.

Flavonoids found in cannabis, such as apigenin, luteolin, kaempferol, and cannaflavins (A, B, and C), have been studied for their anti-inflammatory, antioxidant, neuroprotective, and even antineoplastic properties (Kratz and García de Palau 2018). Furthermore, evidence suggests that they may act as inhibitors of P-glycoprotein (P-gp), a transporter associated with multidrug resistance, indicating a potential role in overcoming pharmacokinetic barriers in combination therapies (Tinoush et al. 2020). Like terpenes, flavonoids do not act in isolation but contribute to cannabis's therapeutic spectrum by interacting with phytocannabinoids, reinforcing the notion that the plant's chemical complexity is essential for achieving more effective and safer therapeutic outcomes (André et al. 2024; Blebea et al. 2024).

Therefore, both terpenes and flavonoids are fundamental elements in understanding the pharmacology of *Cannabis sativa* L., not only due to their direct effects but also because of their synergistic roles with cannabinoids. Advancing knowledge of the chemical and physiological interactions between these compounds paves the way for more rational and precise formulations, capable of maximizing the plant's therapeutic potential while minimizing risks.

5. Agronomic Practices and Their Influence on the Phytochemical Profile

The expression of secondary metabolites in *Cannabis sativa* L., particularly cannabinoids and terpenes, results from a multifactorial interaction between genetic, physiological, and agronomic factors. These factors directly impact the plant's phytochemical profile, with significant repercussions for its potency, safety, and therapeutic efficacy (Nascimento and Dalcin 2019).

Genetics is the starting point for modulating the chemical composition of Cannabis. The appropriate choice of genotype, whether through selected seeds or clones from stabilized mother plants, determines the plant's biosynthetic potential. The genetic diversity of this species is reflected in its wide chemical variability, with over 80 identified phytocannabinoids and a diverse array of terpenes and flavonoids (Lynch et al. 2015, 2016). Three main genetic groups have been identified: narrow-leaf drug-type (NLDTs), broad-leaf drug-type (BLDTs), and hemp varieties, each with specific cannabinoid and terpenoid contents (Lynch et al. 2016). Chemotype classification helps guide production toward specific medicinal purposes (Tzimas et al. 2022).

The enzymatic expression related to the biosynthetic pathways of phytocannabinoids is also genetically determined, but influenced by environmental factors and plant management. Enzymes such as THCA synthase and CBDA synthase act directly in the conversion of precursors, and their activity can be modulated by environmental conditions, including temperature, light, and relative humidity (Bogdan et al. 2016; Fiorentino et al. 2024; Nabila et al. 2025).

The cultivation type—whether outdoor, greenhouse, or indoor—determines the level of control over environmental variables. Indoor systems, although more expensive, allow for precise control of photoperiod, light spectrum, and intensity, as well as humidity and temperature, enabling phytochemical standardization and up to four annual cycles. Meanwhile, outdoor or greenhouse cultivation is more susceptible to climatic fluctuations and seasonality, which affects the consistency of chemical profiles (Andre et al. 2016; Trancoso et al. 2022).

Among environmental factors, light (especially UVB radiation), temperature, humidity, and even wind have a significant influence on cannabinoid and terpene synthesis. Sunnier, warmer regions favor Δ^9-THC production, while colder and cloudier environments tend to increase CBD levels. Low relative humidity and mild water stress may induce the accumulation of secondary metabolites as an adaptive response (Bogdan et al. 2016).

Photoperiod modulation is critical since cannabis is a short-day plant whose flowering is induced by decreasing daylight hours. In indoor cultivation, a 12h light/12h dark cycle is used to trigger and maintain flowering, and light spectrum (especially blue and UVB) plays a key role in stimulating trichome production and, consequently, phytocannabinoids (Brousseau et al. 2021; Flores-Sanchez and Verpoorte 2008; Namdar et al. 2019).

Plant sex also significantly affects chemical composition: unpollinated female plants (*sinsemilla*) have inflorescences rich in glandular trichomes, which are specialized structures for cannabinoid biosynthesis. The presence of male plants should be avoided, as pollination reduces trichome density and may compromise the chemical quality of the final product (Bogdan et al. 2016; Flores-Sanchez and Verpoorte 2008; Lynch et al. 2015).

Agronomic management includes strategies such as apical pruning, lower branch pruning, and low-stress training, which direct energy and metabolic resources to the most productive plant parts. Pruning has a particularly significant impact on light distribution and ventilation, affecting both vegetative growth and the accumulation of bioactive metabolites (Bevan et al. 2021; Yazici 2023).

Management also involves precisely determining the harvest time, which can be based on trichome coloration analysis. Studies show that between days 84 and 94 of the vegetative phase, there is a significant increase in cannabinoid content, even without a substantial increase in biomass (Bevan et al. 2021; Yazici, 2023).

Mineral nutrition is another critical component. The balanced supply of macronutrients (N, P, and K) and micronutrients (Fe, Zn, Mn, B, Cu, and Mo) at different plant stages influences the expression of genes involved in the biosynthesis of bioactive compounds. Excessive nitrogen fertilization, for instance, may reduce Δ^9-THC concentrations in the leaves, while disrupting the balance between vegetative growth and trichome production (Campiglia et al. 2017; Malík et al. 2025; Yazici 2023).

Phytosanitary control is crucial for maintaining the phytochemical integrity of plant biomass. Cannabis is susceptible to pests such as mites, thrips, whiteflies, aphids, and pathogens like *Fusarium* spp. and *Botrytis cinerea*. The use of biopesticides and natural plant compounds, such as certain insecticidal terpenes, is a promising approach that reduces the risk of toxic residues and maintains the safety of cannabis for medical use (Bogdan et al. 2016; McPartland 2018; Nolan et al. 2025).

In addition, the selection of superior genotypes, the maintenance of vigorous mother plants, and the production of genetically stable clones are practices that ensure the repeatability of the production process. Using clones enables chemical and phenotypic uniformity, thereby reducing batch variability and facilitating pharmaceutical standardization (Mipeshwaree Devi et al. 2023; Zheng 2022).

Organic and sustainable cultivation practices, with proper soil management, crop rotation, composting, and the use of biological controls, promote regenerative agriculture, increase biodiversity, and contribute to the stability of phytochemical profiles (Figure 5). Standardizing cultivation conditions, alongside traceability and quality control, is essential to ensure the safety, efficacy, and reproducibility of cannabis-derived products intended for therapeutic use.

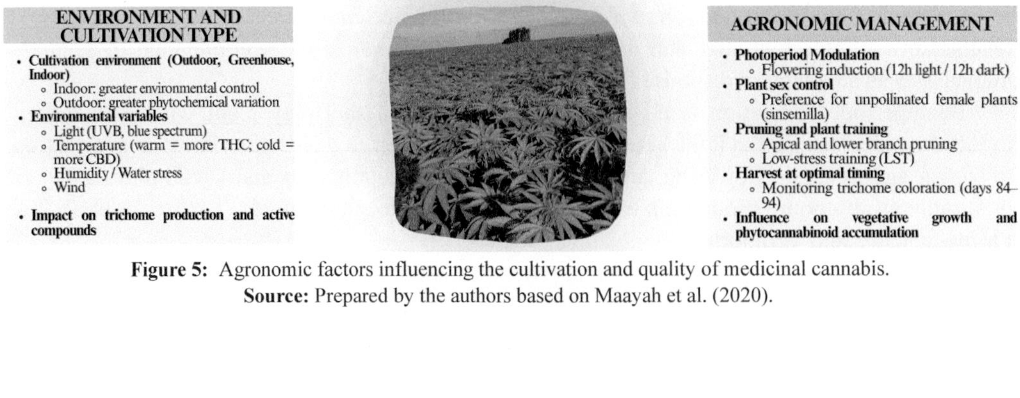
GENETICS AND GENOTYPE SELECTION
Genotype selection
Selected seeds / stabilized clones
Chemotypes (NLDTs, BLDTs, hemp)
Defined biosynthetic potential
Diversity of cannabinoids and terpenes
NUTRITION AND FERTILIZATION
Macronutrients (N, P, K)
Micronutrients (Fe, Zn, Mn, B, Cu, Mo)
Influence on Gene Expression and
Compound Synthesis
Excess Nitrogen: reduced THC content
Imbalance: lower trichome production
PEST MANAGEMENT AND SUSTAINABLE CULTIVATION
Pest and pathogen control
Biopesticides, terpenes with insecticidal activity
Reduction of toxic residues / medicinal safety
Sustainable and organic cultivation
Crop rotation, composting, biodiversity
Traceability and standardized quality
ENVIRONMENT AND CULTIVATION TYPE
Cultivation environment (Outdoor, Greenhouse, Indoor)
Indoor: greater environmental control
Outdoor: greater phytochemical variation
Environmental variables
Light (UVB, blue spectrum)
Temperature (warm = more THC; cold = more CBD)
Humidity / Water stress
Wind
Impact on trichome production and active compounds
AGRONOMIC MANAGEMENT
Photoperiod Modulation
Flowering induction (12h light / 12h dark)
Plant sex control
Preference for unpollinated female plants (sinsemilla)
Pruning and plant training
Apical and lower branch pruning
Low-stress training (LST)
Harvest at optimal timing
Monitoring trichome coloration (days 84–94)
Influence on vegetative growth and phytocannabinoid accumulation

Figure 5: Agronomic factors influencing the cultivation and quality of medicinal cannabis.
Source: Prepared by the authors based on Maayah et al. (2020).

6. Post-Harvest Processes

After the cultivation and development of *Cannabis sativa* L., post-harvest processes play a central role in maintaining the plant's therapeutic quality. It is during this phase that the phytochemical profile is either consolidated or compromised, especially concerning the preservation of cannabinoids and terpenes. Improper handling of these compounds can lead to their degradation through physicochemical processes, such as oxidation, volatilization, and uncontrolled decarboxylation, which negatively impact the effectiveness of cannabis-derived products (Andre et al. 2016; Bogdan et al. 2016). Therefore, the harvest point, drying methods, storage conditions, and exposure to degradation factors are key determinants for ensuring the stability of secondary metabolites (Potter 2014; Trancoso et al. 2022).

The determination of the ideal harvest time is based on the biosynthetic dynamics of phytocannabinoids throughout the plant's life cycle (Tanney et al. 2021). In the early vegetative stages, cannabinoid concentrations are still low. However, in the final weeks of this phase, particularly between days 84 and 94, there is a significant increase in the acidic precursors Δ9-THCA and CBDA, even without notable biomass growth. The maturation of trichomes, glandular structures responsible for synthesizing and storing these compounds, enhances this accumulation. Understanding and respecting this cycle is essential for maximizing phytochemical yield and ensuring the therapeutic potency of the plant material (Melzer et al. 2022; Nascimento et al. 2022).

Once the harvest is complete, cannabis drying must be conducted with care to avoid microbial growth, allow for long-term storage, and preserve the plant's sensory and pharmacological characteristics. Among the most commonly used methods, air drying is the most traditional, involving the exposure of plants in dark environments with controlled temperatures between 18°C and 25°C and relative humidity between 45% and 55% (Kanabus et al. 2024). This process, often referred to as curing, allows for the gradual oxidation of compounds like Δ9-THC into CBN and the conversion of terpenes such as myrcene into secondary products like hashishene, while also reducing microbial activity. On the other hand, oven drying, although faster, may compromise the phytochemical profile. Studies indicate that high temperatures (e.g., 105°C) promote decarboxylation and subsequent degradation of Δ9-THC into CBN, a less potent cannabinoid, thus decreasing the therapeutic efficacy of the product. Freeze-drying (lyophilization), considered the gold standard for chemical preservation, removes moisture by sublimation under vacuum at low temperatures, preserving volatile compounds and the acidic forms of cannabinoids intact (Baek et al. 2025). However, its high energy and operational costs limit its large-scale application.

In addition to drying, proper storage is essential to prevent the gradual loss of cannabinoids and terpenes over time. Ground biomass should be stored in opaque, hermetically sealed drums with internal polyethylene liners, at temperatures between 18°C and 20°C for short-term storage, and at –10°C for long-term preservation. Exposure to light, oxygen, and humidity, as well as storage duration, are critical factors in the chemical degradation of extracts (Lumu et al. 2024). Studies show that even under ideal conditions, cannabinoid levels can decline by up to 50% after five months, making therapeutic dose adjustments over time indispensable. Trials have demonstrated that resins stored at –20°C in the dark retain their levels of Δ9-THC, CBD, and CBN for up to a year, whereas samples exposed to artificial light experience degradation of over 10% (Milay et al. 2020).

Among the most relevant degradation mechanisms is decarboxylation, a process in which acidic cannabinoids, such as THCA and CBDA, lose a carboxyl group and convert into their neutral forms, THC and CBD. This can occur spontaneously over time or be triggered by exposure to heat, light, or alkaline pH (Filer 2022). Experiments have shown that temperatures around 145°C for 30 minutes are sufficient to decarboxylate Δ9-THCA, CBGA, and CBCA. Moreover, equipment such as gas chromatographs may induce partial inadvertent decarboxylation when operated at high temperatures (e.g., 300°C), reducing the initial CBD concentration by up to 20% and promoting the conversion of Δ9-THC into Δ8-THC or CBN (Wang et al. 2016). Oxidation, in turn, transforms terpenes into allergenic products and cannabinoids into less active compounds, such as CBN, particularly in environments with excessive UV light and oxygen. The volatility of terpenes, especially monoterpenes, poses another challenge, as these compounds are easily lost during drying or evaporation and may degrade to nearly undetectable levels through methods such as rotary evaporation or speed vac (André et al. 2024; Baek et al. 2025; Jin et al. 2021).

To properly preserve the plant's chemical profile after harvest, good practices must integrate technical knowledge and operational measures. Harvesting should occur at the peak of cannabinoid concentration. Drying should be conducted under conditions that minimize thermal and oxidative losses, and storage must protect against light, heat, and humidity. Whenever possible, drying methods such as freeze-drying should be preferred to preserve volatile compounds (Djilali et al. 2022). Additionally, analytical standardization is essential: techniques like high-performance liquid chromatography (HPLC) are recommended for quantifying phytocannabinoids and terpenes, as they do not induce decarboxylation as thermal chromatographic methods (Giovannoni et al. 2023).

Adopting Good Manufacturing Practices (GMP), as established by regulatory agencies such as ANVISA, is also essential to ensure the safety, quality, and traceability of cannabis-derived products. These practices include process validation, strain identity and purity control, and stability studies. In summary, maintaining the phytochemical profile of cannabis post-harvest is a multifactorial process that requires planning, technical rigor, and continuous quality control. Only through this integrated approach can the final product retain its therapeutic value, with reproducible efficacy and pharmacological safety.

7. Brazilian Cultivation Model Through Associations

The Brazilian model of cannabis cultivation through associations emerged as an alternative in the context of the lack of clear regulation for cultivating the plant for medicinal purposes in Brazil, combined with the high cost of imported medications. Although Brazilian legislation permits the federal government to authorize the planting, cultivation, and harvesting of plants for medicinal or scientific purposes under supervision, such regulation has never been specifically established (Pereira 2025; Philbin et al. 2019).

The movement of Medicinal Cannabis Associations (ACMs) in Brazil began in 2014 with the founding of *Abrace Esperança* in the state of Paraíba. This organization became a national reference after obtaining a judicial authorization to cultivate and produce cannabis derivatives three years after its creation. Since then, other ACMs have emerged in various states, following a similar model: they initially organize their operations with community support and later resort to the judiciary to legalize their activities. This process reflects the absence of specific regulations that recognize and standardize the cultivation and production of medicinal cannabis in the country, resulting in legal uncertainty, operational challenges, and limitations on the sector's growth (Decorte 2015).

Inspired by European Cannabis Social Clubs (CSCs), Brazilian ACMs operate under a community-driven, non-commercial, and collaborative framework, providing cultivation, distribution, therapeutic guidance, and research exclusively to their members (Belackova et al. 2023; Decorte 2015). A survey conducted in 2025 identified 118 active associations in the country, with the majority concentrated in the Northeast and Southeast regions (38 ACMs each), followed by the South (20), Central-West (12), and North (10). Figure 6 illustrates this geographical distribution.

Brazilian Cannabis Medicinal Associations (ACMs) have been classified into three productive profiles: small (serving up to 100 patients/month), medium (around 300 patients), and large (over 800 patients). *Abrace Esperança* and *Santa Cannabis* are examples of large ACMs, with 45,000 and 8,000 patients, respectively. Based on the cost structure, the average price of a 30 mL bottle was estimated at R$300, with MCT oil being one of the main raw materials used, costing approximately R$9.00 per bottle. Although this input accounts for only about 3% of annual revenue, it highlights the relevance of indirect costs in the production chain of cannabis derivatives.

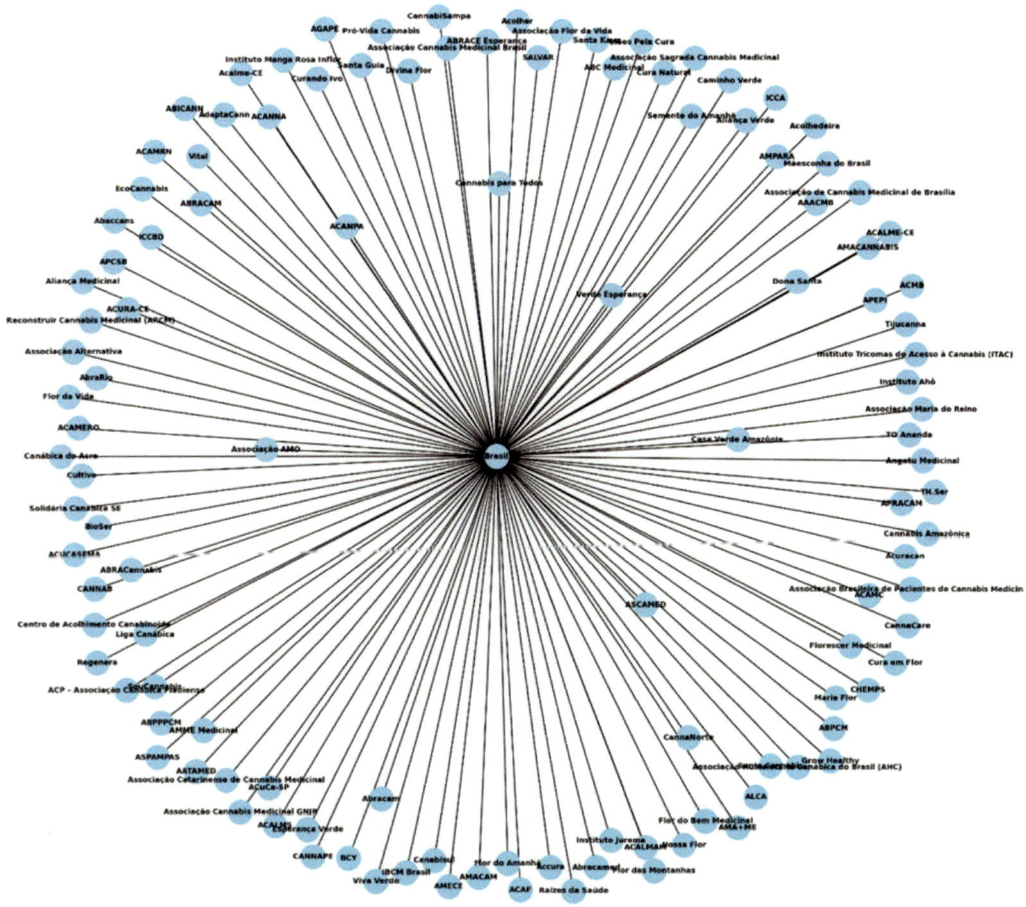

Figure 6: Network of Medicinal *Cannabis* Associations in Brazil.
Source: Prepared by the authors (2025).

To assess equity in ACM distribution, the Associative Density Indicator (ACMs per 100,000 inhabitants) was developed. As shown in Table 1, the Central-West region has the highest density (0.70), followed by the Northeast (0.66) and South (0.64), all of which are classified as high to very high. The North has a medium density (0.54), whereas the Southeast (despite being the most populous region) has only 0.43, which is also considered medium density. This may be due to greater reliance on formal healthcare services or underreporting of ACMs in the database used.

Despite recent progress, the main challenge faced by ACMs remains the lack of a specific regulatory framework. Currently, ANVISA regulations (RDC No. 327/2019 and 660/2022) permit the importation of cannabis products, but do not cover national cultivation by companies, patients, or associations (Brazil 2019; Brazil 2022). This regulatory gap compels associations to operate based on individual court rulings, in contrast to countries like Uruguay and Germany, which recognize collective cultivation (Pardal 2018; Pardo 2014; Tarkowski et al. 2025).

The international literature is unanimous in asserting that self-regulation, while important, is insufficient to ensure adequate sanitary standards, traceability, and therapeutic safety. The absence of structured public policies exacerbates operational asymmetries and undermines the sustainability of ACMs (Belackova et al. 2023; Decorte 2015; Obradors-Pineda et al. 2021). Therefore, regulating cultivation is an urgent and strategic demand to guarantee legal security, align Brazil with international standards, and strengthen the right to health through legitimate and controlled organizational practices.

Table 1: Critical synthesis of scientific advances and challenges in the cultivation and genetic improvement of *Cannabis sativa* L.

Aspect	Strengths	Weaknesses
Genetic determinants of cannabinoid and terpene biosynthesis	• The use of high-density SNP genotyping and genome-wide association studies has elucidated key genetic loci and gene copy number variations that regulate cannabinoid synthase genes such as THCAS and CBDAS, providing a robust framework for breeding programs targeting specific chemotypes (Grassa et al. 2021; Henry et al. 2020; Singh et al. 2021; Vergara et al. 2019). • Transcriptomic analyses have identified differential gene expression patterns and novel transcription factors that influence cannabinoid biosynthesis, thereby deepening our understanding of the regulatory mechanisms (Alberto et al. 2014; Apicella et al. 2021; Innes and Vergara 2023; Liu et al. 2021).	• Despite advances, genetic regulation remains incompletely understood, with some studies suggesting post-transcriptional regulation and unclear roles of additional metabolic pathway genes. • The complexity of gene-environment interactions and the presence of large repetitive genomic regions complicate mapping efforts (Laverty et al. 2019). • Furthermore, molecular markers for chemotype prediction show variable discriminative power across populations, thereby limiting their universal applicability (Murovec et al. 2022).
Agronomic practices and cultivation techniques	• Controlled-environment studies have shown that light quality, intensity, and photoperiod significantly influence cannabinoid and terpene concentrations, with specific spectra modulating metabolite profiles and plant morphology (Ahsan et al. 2024; Morello et al. 2022; Reichel et al. 2021). • Fertilization and nutrient management have been linked to phytochemical composition and biological activity, emphasizing the importance of tailored agronomic inputs (Simonutti et al. 2024). • Innovative treatments, such as plasma-activated water, melatonin, and nano-zinc, show promise in enhancing secondary metabolite production via physiological modulation (Oloumi et al. 2024).	• Many agronomic studies are limited by short-term or single-factor experimental designs, which may not capture the complex interactions among environmental variables (Konvalina et al. 2024; Trancoso and de Souza et al. 2022). • The variability in cultivar responses and the lack of standardized protocols hinder reproducibility and generalizability (Reichel et al. 2021, 2022). • Additionally, the mechanistic basis of some agronomic effects on metabolite biosynthesis remains speculative or underexplored (Ahsan et al. 2024; Desaulniers Brousseau et al. 2021).
Physiological and environmental stress interactions	• Research has highlighted the role of physiological factors such as uptake force, nutrient allocation, and diurnal rhythms in modulating cannabinoid and terpene biosynthesis, linking metabolic fluxes to developmental stages and environmental stimuli (Dimopoulos et al. 2025; Jost et al. 2025; Naim-Feil et al. 2023). • Thermal stress studies show that heat can upregulate key biosynthetic genes and alter cannabinoid profiles, offering insights into stress-induced metabolic plasticity (Hahm et al. 2025).	• The complexity of physiological responses and their integration with environmental stressors remains unresolved, as many studies focus on isolated factors rather than multifactorial stress scenarios (Jost et al. 2025). • The temporal dynamics of metabolite accumulation and gene expression require further elucidation to understand regulatory hierarchies (Dimopoulos et al. 2024). • Moreover, the influence of biotic stress and microbiome interactions remains largely unexplored (Bitežnik et al. 2023).

Chemotypic variability and therapeutic implications	• Comprehensive metabolomic profiling of diverse chemotypes has identified distinct cannabinoid and terpene signatures that correlate with genetic backgrounds and potential therapeutic effects, facilitating chemotaxonomic discrimination and quality standardization (Eržen et al. 2021; Ghosh et al. 2025; Jin et al. 2021; Mudge et al. 2019). • Studies comparing THC- and CBD-dominant chemotypes reveal differential accumulation of minor cannabinoids and terpenes, informing clinical and breeding applications (Jin et al. 2021; Mishchenko et al. 2021).	• Despite detailed profiling, the functional implications of chemotypic variability for therapeutic efficacy are often inferred rather than directly tested, which limits their translational impact (Jin et al. 2021; Mudge et al. 2019). • Heterogeneity within chemotypes and intra-plant variation complicate consistent characterization (Stack et al. 2022). • Additionally, the biosynthetic regulation of minor cannabinoids remains less understood, posing challenges for targeted breeding (Mishchenko et al. 2021).
Molecular and biochemical pathways underlying genotype impact	• Integrated genomic and transcriptomic analyses have outlined key enzymes and pathways, such as the MEP and MVA pathways for terpene biosynthesis and the polyketide pathway for cannabinoids, with evidence of coordinated regulation in glandular trichomes (Fulvio et al. 2025; Innes and Vergara 2023; Marks et al. 2009; Yeo et al. 2022). • The identification of gene duplications, copy number variations, and enzyme localization enhances mechanistic understanding (Fulvio et al. 2025; Innes and Vergara 2023; Marks et al. 2009; Yeo et al. 2022).	• The precise molecular mechanisms governing enzymatic activity, substrate channeling, and pathway flux are only partially characterized, with some regulatory factors and transcriptional networks still unidentified (Innes and Vergara 2023; Liu et al. 2021). • Spatial and temporal regulation of biosynthetic genes during flower development and under environmental modulation requires further investigation (Apicella et al. 2022). • The functional validation of candidate genes and transcription factors is limited, restricting definitive conclusions.
Methodological approaches and data quality	• The application of multi-omics approaches, including genomics, transcriptomics, metabolomics, and machine learning-enhanced genomic prediction, represents a methodological strength, allowing for comprehensive data integration and predictive breeding (Welling et al. 2020; Yeo et al. 2022; Yoosefzadeh Najafabadi and Torkamaneh 2025). • Controlled-environment experiments enable precise manipulation of variables such as light and nutrients (Morello et al. 2022; Reichel et al. 2021).	• Variability in experimental designs, sample sizes, and analytical techniques across studies limits comparability. Some studies rely heavily on correlative data without functional validation, weakening causal inference. • The predominance of greenhouse or indoor studies may limit ecological validity for outdoor cultivation scenarios (Zandkarimi et al. 2023). • Additionally, the rapid evolution of cannabis genomics demands continual updates to reference genomes and annotations.
Integration of multidisciplinary findings for breeding and cultivation optimization	• The synthesis of genetic, physiological, and environmental data provides a foundation for informed breeding strategies and cultivation practices aimed at enhancing targeted secondary metabolite production (Ahsan et al. 2024; Henry et al. 2020; Naim-Feil et al. 2023; Yoosefzadeh Najafabadi and Torkamaneh 2025). • The identification of key genetic markers and environmental modulators supports precision agriculture and product standardization (Trancoso and de Souza et al. 2022).	• Despite integrative efforts, the translation of these findings into practical breeding and cultivation protocols is still emerging, with gaps in understanding genotype-by-environment interactions and long-term trait stability (Naim-Feil et al. 2023; Trancoso and De Souza et al. 2022). • The complexity of secondary metabolism and its regulation presents challenges for predictable manipulation, requiring further research and multidisciplinary validation in diverse contexts.

Source: Prepared by the authors (2025).

8. Case Study: BCY Association

The initiative began with the implementation of a macroprocess for quality control based on thin-layer chromatography (TLC), using Alpha-CAT kits. This quality control approach became transversal to all organizational processes. Chromatographic analysis, conducted under strict standardization of samples and reagents, enabled the identification and quantification of cannabinoids, including THC, CBD, CBG, and their acidic precursors at various stages of production. Traceability was enhanced through the use of photographic documentation of the chromatographic plates and systematic recording of results, allowing for analytical validation of seeds, clones, flowers, extracts, and final products.

The genetic selection and cultivation stage involved the development of a planting macroprocess focused on traceability and standardization. Seeds with higher phytogenetic potential were tested for their phytochemical profiles, and selected individuals formed part of the mother plant bank, ensuring controlled clonal propagation. Identification of female plants, preferred due to their higher cannabinoid concentration in inflorescences, and removal of male plants prevented cross-pollination, thereby promoting consistency in results (Bogdan et al. 2016; Flores-Sanchez and Verpoorte 2008; Lynch et al. 2015, 2016). Clones were also managed under controlled environmental conditions until released for production cycles.

After cultivation, harvesting was preferably carried out early in the morning, followed by sanitary sorting and controlled drying. Each batch was weighed and sampled for chromatographic analysis, then transferred to refrigerated chambers (4ºC) under standardized storage conditions. This system allowed for monitoring post-harvest variations in cannabinoid profiles, especially the expected increase in THC, CBD, and CBG levels during dehydration. Precisely determining the harvest time was crucial to avoid loss of active compounds and errors in subsequent stages, such as extraction and fractioning.

In the extraction stage, BCY employed two main methods: mechanical extraction using Rosin presses and chemical extraction with ethanol, assisted by ultrasonic technology. Quality control determined the destination of the extracts based on their cannabinoid composition, ensuring the production of four main profiles: high-CBD, high-THC, balanced 1:1 THC to CBD, and high-CBG. This segmentation enabled precise direction into therapeutic formulations and reduced losses due to a mismatch with desired standards.

The macroprocess of fractioning was the final critical stage in the production cycle, responsible for dosage calculation, homogenization of the extract in MCT oil, and bottling into 30 mL flasks. Batch acceptance was subject to a maximum tolerance deviation of 3% from the reference value. Any deviation beyond this threshold requires batch correction or disposal, according to Good Manufacturing Practices (GMP). This strict control resulted in a 100% product compliance rate following the implementation of the new procedures.

Among the key outcomes achieved were a reduction in the batch rejection rate from 12% to 5%, the elimination of losses from laboratory testing of unsuitable extracts, and a decrease in average production time from 30 to 21 days. Improved accuracy in harvest timing, along with the preservation of genetic and chemical plant characteristics, contributed to these results. Formalizing the processes also strengthened the association's legal security by providing robust technical documentation for presentation in court cases.

Furthermore, the use of BPMN flowcharts and VAC models in training the operational team, composed mostly of workers with limited formal education, enabled an accessible understanding of the procedures. This improved handling and sanitization efficiency, reduced pest incidence, and promoted genetic and phytochemical consistency of the plants. The experience of the BCY Association demonstrates that, even in a limited regulatory context, adopting rigorous agronomic practices, analytical controls, and process-based management is a viable strategy to ensure quality, standardization, and safety in the cultivation and processing of medicinal cannabis.

9. Critical Analysis and Synthesis

The reviewed literature explores the genetic, agronomic, physiological, and environmental factors that influence the biosynthesis of cannabinoids and terpenes in *Cannabis sativa* L. Strengths of the current body of research include the integration of advanced genomic tools, transcriptomic analyses, and metabolomic profiling, which collectively enhance our understanding of the molecular and biochemical pathways underlying phytochemical variability. Furthermore, studies employing controlled environmental manipulations provide valuable insights into the impact of cultivation practices and abiotic stressors on the production of secondary metabolites.

However, limitations arise from the variability in experimental designs, the incomplete elucidation of regulatory networks, and challenges in consistently correlating genotype with chemotype across different cultivars. Additionally, the complexity of physiological interactions and environmental influences often complicates the interpretation of results, underscoring the need for standardized methodologies and multifactorial approaches. Overall, while significant progress has been made, critical gaps remain in fully deciphering the intricate controls of cannabinoid and terpene biosynthesis and their implications for therapeutic efficacy.

10. Final Considerations

The present discussion highlights that the production of *Cannabis sativa* L. derivatives with therapeutic quality depends on the careful integration of genotype selection, cultivation practices, and post-harvest processes, all of which directly influence the concentration and stability of phytocannabinoids and terpenes. Scientific literature emphasizes that the plant's metabolic expression is deeply associated with agronomic and environmental conditions, making the standardization of these elements essential to ensure product efficacy.

In the Brazilian context, the progress made by Medicinal Cannabis Associations (ACMs) demonstrates the potential of community organization and innovation in the absence of comprehensive legislation. However, regulatory challenges still pose significant barriers to technical and scientific advancement, especially when aiming to ensure quality, safety, and traceability in a sensitive and high-impact therapeutic production chain. The lack of specific technical standards weakens product reproducibility and undermines confidence in clinical and scientific findings.

In this regard, the development of national guidelines becomes urgent. These guidelines should cover everything from genetic selection and agronomic criteria to protocols for drying, curing, storage, and quality control. The traceability of raw materials, combined with detailed and standardized phytochemical analysis, is a key step not only for meeting regulatory requirements but also for ensuring that final formulations consistently contain the desired concentrations of bioactive compounds.

These considerations become even more critical in the scope of research involving alternative delivery systems, such as transdermal administration, which require matrices with a high degree of purity and stability. The cutaneous bioavailability and therapeutic efficacy of transdermally applied phytocannabinoids depend directly on the rigorous control of all preceding stages. Therefore, the continuation of this research will benefit greatly from a more standardized and technically regulated production system, reinforcing the importance of coordinated efforts among science, cultivation, and regulation.

References

Ahsan, S., Hoque, M., Kumar, A., Shaffique, S., Rahman, M., and Choi, H. (2024). Plant improvement and metabolite production in *Cannabis sativa*: Recent biotechnological advances. *Plant Trends*, 2(3): 74. https://doi.org/10.5455/pt.2024.07

Ahsan, S., Injamum-Ul-Hoque, Md., Shaffique, S., Ayoobi, A., Rahman, M. A., Rahman, Md. M. et al. (2024). Illuminating *Cannabis sativa* L.: The Power of Light in Enhancing *C. sativa* growth and secondary metabolite production. *Plants*, 13(19): 2774. https://doi.org/10.3390/plants13192774

Alberto, G. N., Marcos, E. G.-C., and Julia Rosl, W. (2014). Control genético del quimiotipo en *Cannabis sativa*: Más allá de las sintasas de cannabinoides. 13 o Workshop en Investigación Agroalimentaria para jóvenes investigadores. 13 o Workshop en Investigación Agroalimentaria para jóvenes investigadores. https://doi.org/10.31428/10317/17365

Al-Ghezi, Z. Z., Miranda, K., Nagarkatti, M., and Nagarkatti, P. S. (2019). Combination of Cannabinoids, Δ9-Tetrahydrocannabinol and Cannabidiol, Ameliorates Experimental Multiple Sclerosis by Suppressing Neuroinflammation Through Regulation of miRNA-Mediated Signaling Pathways. *Frontiers in Immunology*, 10, 1921. https://doi.org/10.3389/fimmu.2019.01921

Al-Khazaleh, A. K., Zhou, X., Bhuyan, D. J., Münch, G. W., Al-Dalabeeh, E. A., Jaye, K. et al. (2024). The Neurotherapeutic Arsenal in *Cannabis sativa*: Insights into Anti-Neuroinflammatory and Neuroprotective Activity and Potential Entourage Effects. *Molecules*, 29(2): 410. https://doi.org/10.3390/molecules29020410

Andre, C. M., Hausman, J.-F., and Guerriero, G. (2016). *Cannabis sativa*: The plant of the thousand and one molecules. *Frontiers in Plant Science*, 7. https://doi.org/10.3389/fpls.2016.00019

André, R., Gomes, A. P., Pereira-Leite, C., Marques-da-Costa, A., Monteiro Rodrigues, L., Sassano, M. et al. (2024). The entourage effect in cannabis medicinal products: A comprehensive review. *Pharmaceuticals*, 17(11): 1543. https://doi.org/10.3390/ph17111543

Apicella, P. V., Sands, L. B., Ma, Y., and Berkowitz, G. A. (2021). Delineating the genetic regulation of cannabinoid biosynthesis during female flower development in *Cannabis sativa*. *Cold Spring Harbor Laboratory*. https://doi.org/10.1101/2021.11.05.464876

Apicella, P. V., Sands, L. B., Ma, Y., and Berkowitz, G. A. (2022). Delineating genetic regulation of cannabinoid biosynthesis during female flower development in *CANNABIS SATIVA*. *Plant Direct*, 6(6). https://doi.org/10.1002/pld3.412

Baek, Y., Grab, H., and Chen, C. (2025). Postharvest drying and curing affect cannabinoid contents and microbial levels in industrial Hemp (*Cannabis sativa* L.). *Plants*, 14(3): 414. https://doi.org/10.3390/plants14030414

Baldino, L., Scognamiglio, M., and Reverchon, E. (2020). Supercritical fluid technologies applied to the extraction of compounds of industrial interest from *Cannabis sativa* L. and to their pharmaceutical formulations: A review. *The Journal of Supercritical Fluids*, 165: 104960. https://doi.org/10.1016/j.supflu.2020.104960

Belackova, V., Rychert, M., Wilkins, C., and Pardal, M. (2023). Cannabis social clubs in contemporary legalization reforms: talking consumption sites and social justice. *Clinical Therapeutics*, 45(6): 551–559. https://doi.org/10.1016/j.clinthera.2023.03.017

Benredjem, B., and Pineyro, G. (2023). A type II cannabis extract and a 1:1 blend of Δ(9)-tetrahydrocannabinol and cannabidiol display distinct antinociceptive profiles and engage different endocannabinoid targets when administered into the subarachnoid space. *Frontiers in Pharmacology*, 14. https://doi.org/10.3389/fphar.2023.1235255

Bevan, L., Jones, M., and Zheng, Y. (2021). Optimization of N, P, K for Soilless Production of <em>*Cannabis sativa*</em> in the Flowering Stage Using Response Surface Analysis. *MDPI AG*. https://doi.org/10.20944/preprints202108.0460.v1

Biteżnik, L., Dermastia, M., and Trdan, S. (2023). Sekundarni metaboliti v navadni konoplji (*Cannabis sativa* L.) in njihova vloga pri obrambi rastline pred škodljivci in patogeni. *Acta Biologica Slovenica*, 66(1). https://doi.org/10.14720/abs.66.1.12521

Biteżnik, L., Štukelj, R., and Flajšman, M. (2024). The efficiency of CBD production using grafted *Cannabis sativa* L. plants is highly dependent on the type of rootstock: A study. *Plants*, 13(8): 1117. https://doi.org/10.3390/plants13081117

Blebea, N. M., Pricopie, A. I., Vlad, R.-A., and Hancu, G. (2024). Phytocannabinoids: Exploring pharmacological profiles and their impact on therapeutical use. *International Journal of Molecular Sciences*, 25(8): 4204. https://doi.org/10.3390/ijms25084204

Bogdan, R., Winstone, J. M., and Agrawal, A. (2016). Genetic and environmental factors associated with cannabis involvement. *Current addiction reports*, 3(2): 199–213. https://doi.org/10.1007/s40429-016-0103-1

Borroto Fernandez, E., Peterseil, V., Hackl, G., Menges, S., De Meijer, E., and Staginnus, C. (2020). Distribution of Chemical phenotypes (Chemotypes) in European Agricultural Hemp (*Cannabis sativa* L.) Cultivars. *Journal of Forensic Sciences*, 65(3): 715–721. https://doi.org/10.1111/1556-4029.14242

Brousseau, V., Wu, B.-S., MacPherson, S., Morello, V., and Lefsrud, M. (2021). Cannabinoids and Terpenes: How production of photo-protectants can be manipulated to enhance *Cannabis sativa* L. phytochemistry. *Frontiers in Plant Science*, 12. https://doi.org/10.3389/fpls.2021.620021

Campiglia, E., Radicetti, E., and Mancinelli, R. (2017). Plant density and nitrogen fertilization affect agronomic performance of industrial hemp (*Cannabis sativa* L.) in Mediterranean environment. *Industrial Crops and Products*, 100: 246–254. https://doi.org/10.1016/j.indcrop.2017.02.022

Chauhan, J., Bastia, B. K., Kohli, K., Chaudhary, B., Chikara, G., Gupta, A. et al. (2024). Phytocannabinoid profile and potency of cannabis resin (hashish) of northwest Himalayas of India. *Journal of Forensic Sciences*, 69(5): 1918–1925. https://doi.org/10.1111/1556-4029.15583

Crocq, M.-A. (2020). History of cannabis and the endocannabinoid system. *Dialogues in Clinical Neuroscience*, 22(3): 223–228.https://doi.org/10.31887/DCNS.2020.22.3/mcrocq

Dalli, M., Azizi, S., Azghar, A., Saddari, A., Benaissa, E., Lahlou, Y. B. et al. (2023). *Cannabis sativa* L.: A Comprehensive review on legislation, decriminalization, phytochemistry, antimicrobial activity, and safety. *Journal of Food and Drug Analysis*, 31(3): 408–435. https://doi.org/10.38212/2224-6614.3471

Decorte, T. (2015). Cannabis social clubs in Belgium: Organizational strengths and weaknesses, and threats to the model. *International Journal of Drug Policy*, 26(2): 122–130. https://doi.org/10.1016/j.drugpo.2014.07.016

Dimopoulos, N., Guo, Q., Purdy, S. J., Nolan, M., Halimi, R. A., Mieog, J. C. et al. (2025). From dawn 'til dusk: Daytime progression regulates primary and secondary metabolism in Cannabis glandular trichomes. *Journal of Experimental Botany*, 76(1): 134–151. https://doi.org/10.1093/jxb/erae148

Djilali, E., Pappalardo, L., Posadino, A. M., Giordo, R., and Pintus, G. (2022). Effects of the storage conditions on the stability of natural and synthetic cannabis in biological matrices for forensic toxicology analysis: An update from the literature. Metabolites, 12(9): 801. https://doi.org/10.3390/metabo12090801

Eržen, M., Košir, I. J., Ocvirk, M., Kreft, S., and Čerenak, A. (2021). Metabolomic analysis of cannabinoid and essential oil profiles in different Hemp (*Cannabis sativa* L.) phenotypes. *Plants*, 10(5): 966. https://doi.org/10.3390/plants10050966

Filer, C. N. (2022). Acidic Cannabinoid Decarboxylation. *Cannabis and Cannabinoid Research*, 7(3): 262 273. https://doi.org/10.1089/can.2021.0072

Fiorentino, N., Formisano, C., Delfine, S., and Chianese, G. (2024). Editorial: Environmental and agronomic factors affecting the chemical composition and biological activity of cannabis extracts. *Frontiers in Plant Science*, 15. https://doi.org/10.3389/fpls.2024.1407262

Flores-Sanchez, I. J., and Verpoorte, R. (2008). Secondary metabolism in cannabis. *Phytochemistry Reviews*, 7(3): 615–639. https://doi.org/10.1007/s11101-008-9094-4

Fournier, G., Richez-Dumanois, C., Duvezin, J., Mathieu, J.-P., and Paris, M. (1987). Identification of a new chemotype in *Cannabis sativa*: Cannabigerol - Dominant Plants, Biogenetic and agronomic prospects. *Planta Medica*, 53(03): 277–280. https://doi.org/10.1055/s-2006-962705

Fulvio, F., Pieracci, Y., Ascrizzi, R., Bassolino, L., Flamini, G., and Paris, R. (2025). Insights into terpenes profiling and transcriptional analyses during flowering of different *Cannabis sativa* L. chemotypes. *Phytochemistry*, 229: 114294. https://doi.org/10.1016/j.phytochem.2024.114294

Gargiulo, E., Moriello, A. S., Benetti, E., Pagni, L., Arnoldi, L., De Petrocellis, L. et al. (2024). Phytochemical Characterization and TRPA1/TRPM8 Modulation Profile of the Cannabigerol-Rich *Cannabis sativa* L. Chemotype IV. *Journal of Natural Products*, 87(4): 722–732. https://doi.org/10.1021/acs.jnatprod.3c00831

Ghosh, D., Kundu, A., Chaudhary, N., Gupta, D., Dwivedi, M., Verma, R. S. et al. (2025). Unveiling Cannabinoids and Terpenes diversity in *Cannabis sativa* L. from northern India for future breeding strategies. *Chemistry & Biodiversity*, 22(6). https://doi.org/10.1002/cbdv.202402278

Giovannoni, S., Lancioni, C., Vaccarini, C., Sedan, D., Andrinolo, D., and Castells, C. (2023). Determination of variability of terpenes and terpenoids in *Cannabis sativa* by gas chromatography-flame ionization detection and gas chromatography-mass spectrometry. *Journal of Chromatography A*, 1687: 463669. https://doi.org/10.1016/j.chroma.2022.463669

Grassa, C. J., Weiblen, G. D., Wenger, J. P., Dabney, C., Poplawski, S. G., Timothy Motley, S. et al. (2021). A new Cannabis genome assembly associates elevated cannabidiol (CBD) with hemp introgressed into marijuana. *New Phytologist*, 230(4): 1665–1679. https://doi.org/10.1111/nph.17243

Grinspoon, L., and Bakalar, J. B. (1995). Marihuana as Medicine: A plea for reconsideration. *JAMA*, 273(23), 1875–1876. https://doi.org/10.1001/jama.1995.03520470083037

Hahm, S., Lee, J. Y., Im, H. M., Lee, H. J., and Park, J. (2025). Influence of temperature stress on the major cannabinoid contents and biosynthesis gene expression levels in industrial Hemp (*Cannabis sativa* L.). *Horticultural Science and Technology*, 43(2): 221–233. https://doi.org/10.7235/hort.20250024

Hashiesh, H. M., Meeran, M. F. N., Sharma, C., Sadek, B., Kaabi, J. A., and Ojha, S. K. (2020). Therapeutic potential of β-Caryophyllene: A dietary cannabinoid in diabetes and associated complications. *Nutrients*, 12(10): 2963. https://doi.org/10.3390/nu12102963

Henry, P., Khatodia, S., Kapoor, K., Gonzales, B., Middleton, A., Hong, K. et al. (2020). A single nucleotide polymorphism assay sheds light on the extent and distribution of genetic diversity, population structure and functional basis of key traits in cultivated north American cannabis. *Journal of Cannabis Research*, 2(1). https://doi.org/10.1186/s42238-020-00036-y

Hewitt, K. (2020). History and Cultural Context of Marijuana in the United States. Em Understanding Medical Cannabis. *Routledge*. https://www.taylorfrancis.com/chapters/edit/10.4324/9780429343803-4/history-cultural-context-marijuana-united-states-kim-hewitt

Hill, A. (2024). Health, Wellness, and a Balanced Endocannabinoid System. *Caring for the Ages*, 25(1): 15. https://doi.org/10.1016/j.carage.2023.12.011

Hourfane, S., Mechqoq, H., Bekkali, A. Y., Rocha, J. M., and El Aouad, N. (2023). A comprehensive review on *Cannabis sativa* ethnobotany, phytochemistry, molecular docking and biological activities. *Plants*, 12(6): 1245. https://doi.org/10.3390/plants12061245

Innes, P. A., and Vergara, D. (2023). Genomic description of critical cannabinoid biosynthesis genes. *Botany*, 101(7): 270–283. https://doi.org/10.1139/cjb-2022-0140

Javid, F. A., Alam, A., Williams, E., Malik, S. S., Mohayuddin, U., and Hasan, S. S. (2024). Trends in prescription and cost of Sativex, a cannabinoid-based medicine, in treating patients with multiple sclerosis in England. *Journal of Pharmaceutical Policy and Practice*, 17(1): 2342318. https://doi.org/10.1080/20523211.2024.2342318

Jin, D., Henry, P., Shan, J., and Chen, J. (2021). Identification of chemotypic markers in three chemotype categories of cannabis using secondary metabolites profiled in inflorescences, leaves, stem bark, and roots. *Frontiers in Plant Science*, 12. https://doi.org/10.3389/fpls.2021.699530

Jost, R., Berkowitz, O., Pegg, A., Hurgobin, B., Tamiru-Oli, M., Welling, M. T. et al. (2025). Sink strength, nutrient allocation, cannabinoid yield, and associated transcript profiles vary in two drug-type Cannabis chemovars. *Journal of Experimental Botany*, 76(1): 152–174. https://doi.org/10.1093/jxb/erae367

Jurga, M., Jurga, A., Jurga, K., Kaźmierczak, B., Kuśmierczyk, K., and Chabowski, M. (2024). Cannabis-Based Phytocannabinoids: Overview, mechanism of action, therapeutic application, production, and affecting environmental factors. *International Journal of Molecular Sciences*, 25(20): 11258. https://doi.org/10.3390/ijms252011258

Kanabus, J., Bryła, M., and Roszko, M. (2024). Effect of selected drying methods on the cannabinoid profile of *Cannabis sativa* L. var. Sativa inflorescences and leaves. *Polish Journal of Food and Nutrition Sciences*, 408–418. https://doi.org/10.31883/pjfns/195594

King, R. (2018). The Resurgence of American Nativism In The Early-Twentieth Century And Its Effects On Industrial Hemp Production In The United States [Fort Hays State University]. https://doi.org/10.58809/rbis5013

Konvalina, P., Neumann, J., Hoang, T. N., Bernas, J., Trojan, V., Kuchař, M. et al. (2024). Effect of light intensity and two different nutrient solutions on the yield of flowers and Cannabinoids in *Cannabis sativa* L. grown in controlled environment. *Agronomy*, 14(12): 2960. https://doi.org/10.3390/agronomy14122960

Kratz, J. W., and García de Palau, M. (2018). Manual sobre cannabis medicinal: Formación en el uso profesional y responsable de cannabinoides y terpenos. Kalapa Clinic - 1a ed. https://kalapa.academy/wp-content/uploads/2021/09/Manual-Kalapa-Clinic-primera-edicion.pdf

Kulkarni, V. A., Nimje, H. P., Varhade, P. P., Chopade, R. K., Jatale, S. V., Mhaske, S. D. et al. (2025). Cannabinoid pharmacology: Research on medicinal cannabins and its therapeutic application. *Journal of Pharmaceutical and Biological Sciences*, 12(2): 135–143. https://doi.org/10.18231/j.jpbs.2024.020

Kurtz, L. E., Brand, M. H., and Lubell-Brand, J. D. (2023). Gene dosage at the autoflowering locus effects flowering timing and plant height in Triploid cannabis. *Journal of the American Society for Horticultural Science*, 148(2): 83–88. https://doi.org/10.21273/jashs05293-23

Laaboudi, F.-Z., Rejdali, M., Amhamdi, H., Salhi, A., Elyoussfi, A., and Ahari, M. 'hamed. (2024). In the weeds: A comprehensive review of cannabis; its chemical complexity, biosynthesis, and healing abilities. *Toxicology Reports*, 13: 101685. https://doi.org/10.1016/j.toxrep.2024.101685

Laverty, K. U., Stout, J. M., Sullivan, M. J., Shah, H., Gill, N., Holbrook, L. et al. (2019). A physical and genetic map of *Cannabis sativa* identifies extensive rearrangements at the THC/CBD acid synthase loci. *Genome Research*, 29(1): 146–156. https://doi.org/10.1101/gr.242594.118

Leckie, K. M., Sawler, J., Kapos, P., MacKenzie, J. O., Giles, I., Baynes, K. et al. (2024). Loss of daylength sensitivity by splice site mutation in Cannabis pseudo-response regulator. *The Plant Journal*, 118(6): 2020–2036. https://doi.org/10.1111/tpj.16726

Leckie, K. M., Sawler, J., Kapos, P., Mackenzie, J. O., Giles, I., Baynes, K. et al. (2023). Loss of daylength sensitivity by splice site mutation in Cannabis. *Cold Spring Harbor Laboratory*. https://doi.org/10.1101/2023.03.10.532103

Liu, Y., Zhu, P., Cai, S., Haughn, G., and Page, J. E. (2021). Three novel transcription factors involved in cannabinoid biosynthesis in *Cannabis sativa* L. *Plant Molecular Biology*, 106(1-2): 49–65. https://doi.org/10.1007/s11103-021-01129-9

Lumu, S., Hatterman-Valenti, H., Hammed, A., and Monono, E. (2024). Effect of short-term storage on cannabinoid content of dried floral hemp (*Cannabis sativa* L) inflorescence. *Journal of Applied Research on Medicinal and Aromatic Plants*, 42: 100567. https://doi.org/10.1016/j.jarmap.2024.100567

Lynch, R. C., Vergara, D., Tittes, S., White, K., Schwartz, C. J., Gibbs, M. J. et al. (2015). Genomic and chemical diversity in cannabis. *Cold Spring Harbor Laboratory*. https://doi.org/10.1101/034314

Lynch, R. C., Vergara, D., Tittes, S., White, K., Schwartz, C. J., Gibbs, M. J. et al. (2016). Genomic and chemical diversity in cannabis. *Critical Reviews in Plant Sciences*, 35(5-6): 349–363. https://doi.org/10.1080/07352689.2016.1265363

Maayah, Z. H., Takahara, S., Ferdaoussi, M., and Dyck, J. R. B. (2020). The molecular mechanisms that underpin the biological benefits of full-spectrum cannabis extract in the treatment of neuropathic pain and inflammation. Biochimica et Biophysica Acta (BBA) - *Molecular Basis of Disease*, 1866(7): 165771. https://doi.org/10.1016/j.bbadis.2020.165771

Malík, M., Praus, L., Kuklina, A., Velechovský, J., Janatová, A. K., Klouček, P. et al. (2025). Cannabis yield and cannabinoid profile affected by plant nutrition and planting density. *Industrial Crops and Products*, 223: 120293. https://doi.org/10.1016/j.indcrop.2024.120293

Marks, M. D., Tian, L., Wenger, J. P., Omburo, S. N., Soto-Fuentes, W., He, J. et al. (2009). Identification of candidate genes affecting Δ9-tetrahydrocannabinol biosynthesis in *Cannabis sativa*. *Journal of Experimental Botany*, 60(13): 3715–3726. https://doi.org/10.1093/jxb/erp210

McPartland, J. M. (2018). Cannabis systematics at the levels of family, genus, and species. *Cannabis and Cannabinoid Research*, 3(1): 203–212. https://doi.org/10.1089/can.2018.0039

McPartland, J. M., and Small, E. (2020). A classification of endangered high-THC cannabis (*Cannabis sativa* subsp. Indica) domesticates and their wild relatives. *PhytoKeys*, 144: 81–112. https://doi.org/10.3897/phytokeys.144.46700

Melzer, R., McCabe, P. F., and Schilling, S. (2022). Evolution, genetics and biochemistry of plant cannabinoid synthesis: A challenge for biotechnology in the years ahead. *Current Opinion in Biotechnology*, 75: 102684. https://doi.org/10.1016/j.copbio.2022.102684

Milay, L., Berman, P., Shapira, A., Guberman, O., and Meiri, D. (2020). Metabolic profiling of cannabis secondary metabolites for evaluation of optimal postharvest storage conditions. *Frontiers in Plant Science*, 11: 583605. https://doi.org/10.3389/fpls.2020.583605

Mipeshwaree Devi, A., Khedashwori Devi, K., Premi Devi, P., Lakshmipriyari Devi, M., and Das, S. (2023). Metabolic engineering of plant secondary metabolites: Prospects and its technological challenges. *Frontiers in Plant Science*, 14. https://doi.org/10.3389/fpls.2023.1171154

Mishchenko, S. V., Kyrychenko, H. I., and Laiko, I. M. (2021). Genotype screening of *Cannabis sativa* L. based on the specifics of minor cannabinoids manifestation. *Plant varieties studying and protection*, 17(3): 218–225. https://doi.org/10.21498/2518-1017.17.3.2021.242949

Morello, V., Brousseau, V. D., Wu, N., Wu, B.-S., MacPherson, S., and Lefsrud, M. (2022). Light quality impacts vertical growth rate, phytochemical yield and cannabinoid production efficiency in *Cannabis sativa*. *Plants*, 11(21): 2982. https://doi.org/10.3390/plants11212982

Mudge, E. M., Brown, P. N., and Murch, S. J. (2019). The terroir of cannabis: terpene metabolomics as a tool to understand *Cannabis sativa* selections. *Planta Medica*, 85(09/10): 781–796. https://doi.org/10.1055/a-0915-2550

Murovec, J., Eržen, J. J., Flajšman, M., and Vodnik, D. (2022). Analysis of morphological traits, cannabinoid profiles, THCAS gene sequences, and photosynthesis in wide and narrow leaflet high-cannabidiol breeding populations of medical cannabis. *Frontiers in Plant Science*, 13. https://doi.org/10.3389/fpls.2022.786161

Nabila, C. I. B., Ramona, Y., Wirasuta, I. M. A. G., and Karsono, J. (2025). Factors affecting cannabidiol and tetrahydrocannabinol production in Cannabis: Internal mechanisms and environmental factors – A systematic review. *Journal of Pharmacy & Pharmacognosy Research*, 13(4): 1178–1190. https://doi.org/10.56499/jppres24.2184_13.4.1178

Naim-Feil, E., Elkins, A. C., Malmberg, M. M., Ram, D., Tran, J., Spangenberg, G. C. et al. (2023). The cannabis plant as a complex system: interrelationships between cannabinoid compositions, morphological, physiological and phenological traits. *Plants*, 12(3): 493. https://doi.org/10.3390/plants12030493

Namdar, D., Voet, H., Ajjampura, V., Nadarajan, S., Mayzlish-Gati, E., Mazuz, M. et al. (2019). Terpenoids and Phytocannabinoids Co-Produced in *Cannabis sativa* strains show specific interaction for cell cytotoxic activity. *Molecules*, 24(17): 3031. https://doi.org/10.3390/molecules24173031

Nascimento, A. G. T. P. D., and Dalcin, M. F. D. (2019). Uso terapêutico da *Cannabis sativa*: Uma breve revisão. *Brazilian Journal of Surgery and Clinical Research - BJSCR*, 2: 164–169. https://www.mastereditora.com.br/periodico/20190704_103122.pdf

Nascimento, Leme, and Teixeira. (2022). Morphological diversity of glandular trichomes in Urticalean Rosids. *Acta Botanica Brasilica*, 36. https://doi.org/10.1590/0102-33062022abb0061

Nolan, M., Guo, Q., Liu, L., Dimopoulos, N., Garcia-de Heer, L., Barkla, B. J. et al. (2025). Characterisation of Cannabis glandular trichome development reveals distinct features of cannabinoid biosynthesis. *Plant Cell Reports*, 44(2): 30. https://doi.org/10.1007/s00299-024-03410-9

Obradors-Pineda, A., Bouso, J.-C., Parés-Franquero, Ò., and Romaní, J.-O. (2021). Harm reduction and cannabis social clubs: Exploring their true potential. *International Journal of Drug Policy*, 97: 103358. https://doi.org/10.1016/j.drugpo.2021.103358

O'Brien, K., and Blair, P. (2021). Overview of medicinal cannabis. pp. 89–129. Em K. O'Brien and P. Blair (Orgs.). Medicinal Cannabis and CBD in Mental Healthcare. Springer International Publishing. https://doi.org/10.1007/978-3-030-78559-8_4

Oloumi, H., Nasibi, F., Poorsheikhali, Z., and Malekpourzadeh, L. (2024). Changes on growth and secondary metabolite production in *Cannabis sativa* L. by simultaneous treatment of plasma activated water, melatonin and nano-zinc. *Springer Science and Business Media LLC*. https://doi.org/10.21203/rs.3.rs-4898263/v1

Pardal, M. (2018). An analysis of Belgian Cannabis Social Clubs' supply practices: A shapeshifting model? *International Journal of Drug Policy*, 57: 32–41. https://doi.org/10.1016/j.drugpo.2018.03.027

Pardo, B. (2014). Cannabis policy reforms in the Americas: A comparative analysis of Colorado, Washington, and Uruguay. *International Journal of Drug Policy*, 25(4): 727–735. https://doi.org/10.1016/j.drugpo.2014.05.010

Pereira. (2023). O avanço internacional da regulação da cannabis e o injustificável atraso brasileiro. *Boletim IBCCRIM*, 31(369), Artigo 369. https://publicacoes.ibccrim.org.br/index.php/boletim_1993/article/view/608

Pereira. (2025). Civil disobedience and bottom-up governance of cannabis for medicinal use in Brazil: The role of patient associations. *Contemporary Drug Problems*, 52(2): 234–254. https://doi.org/10.1177/00914509241309233

Pereira, V., Figueira, O., and Castilho, P. C. (2024). Flavonoids as insecticides in crop protection—A review of current research and future prospects. *Plants*, 13(6): 776. https://doi.org/10.3390/plants13060776

Peterswald, T. J., Mieog, J. C., Azman Halimi, R., Magner, N. J., Trebilco, A., Kretzschmar, T. et al. (2023). Moving away from 12:12; the effect of different photoperiods on biomass yield and cannabinoids in medicinal cannabis. *Plants*, 12(5): 1061. https://doi.org/10.3390/plants12051061

Philbin, M. M., Mauro, P. M., Santaella-Tenorio, J., Mauro, C. M., Kinnard, E. N., Cerdá, M. et al. (2019). Associations between state-level policy liberalism, cannabis use, and cannabis use disorder from 2004 to 2012: Looking beyond medical cannabis law status. *International Journal of Drug Policy*, 65: 97–103. https://doi.org/10.1016/j.drugpo.2018.10.010

Pisanti, S., and Bifulco, M. (2019). Medical Cannabis: A plurimillennial history of an evergreen. *Journal of Cellular Physiology*, 234(6): 8342–8351. https://doi.org/10.1002/jcp.27725

Potter, D. J. (2014). A review of the cultivation and processing of cannabis (*Cannabis sativa* L.) for production of prescription medicines in the UK. *Drug Testing and Analysis*, 6(1-2): 31–38. https://doi.org/10.1002/dta.1531

Raman, V., Lata, H., Chandra, S., Khan, I. A., and ElSohly, M. A. (2017). Morpho-anatomy of marijuana (*Cannabis sativa* L.). Em S. Chandra, H. Lata, and M. A. ElSohly (Orgs.). *Cannabis sativa* L. - Botany and Biotechnology (p. 123–136). Springer International Publishing. https://doi.org/10.1007/978-3-319-54564-6_5

Reichel, P., Munz, S., Hartung, J., Kotiranta, S., and Graeff-Hönninger, S. (2022). Impacts of different light spectra on CBD, CBDA and Terpene Concentrations in Relation to the Flower Positions of Different *Cannabis sativa* L. Strains. *Plants*, 11(20): 2695. https://doi.org/10.3390/plants11202695

Reichel, P., Munz, S., Hartung, J., Präger, A., Kotiranta, S., Burgel, L. et al. (2021). Impact of three different light spectra on the yield, morphology and growth trajectory of three different *Cannabis Sativa* L. Strains. Plants, 10(9): 1866. https://doi.org/10.3390/plants10091866

Rock, E. M., and Parker, L. A. (2021). Constituents of *Cannabis sativa*. Em E. Murillo-Rodriguez, S. R. Pandi-Perumal, and J. M. Monti (Orgs.). Cannabinoids and Neuropsychiatric Disorders (p. 1–13). Springer International Publishing. https://doi.org/10.1007/978-3-030-57369-0_1

Russo, E. B. (2016). Current therapeutic cannabis controversies and clinical trial design issues. *Frontiers in Pharmacology*, 7. https://doi.org/10.3389/fphar.2016.00309

Sampson, P. B. (2021). Phytocannabinoid pharmacology: Medicinal properties of *Cannabis sativa* constituents aside from the "Big Two". *Journal of Natural Products*, 84(1): 142–160. https://doi.org/10.1021/acs.jnatprod.0c00965

Silva, R. F. D. O. E., and Figueiredo, E. N. (2023). Legislação atual sobre cannabis medicinal na União Europeia: Históricos, movimentos, tendências e contratendências. Lições para o Brasil. Brazilian Journal Of Pain. https://doi.org/10.5935/2595-0118.20230052-pt

Simonutti, M., Seimandi, G., Richard, G., Zabala, J. M., and Derita, M. (2024). Correlation between chemical fertilization practices, phytochemical response, and biological activities of *Cannabis sativa* L. *Combinatorial Chemistry & High Throughput Screening*, 27. https://doi.org/10.2174/0113862073319590240801112332

Singh, A., Bilichak, A., and Kovalchuk, I. (2021). The genetics of Cannabis—Genomic variations of key synthases and their effect on cannabinoid content. *Genome*, 64(4), 490–501. https://doi.org/10.1139/gen-2020-0087

Siracusa, L., Ruberto, G., and Cristino, L. (2023). Recent research on *Cannabis sativa* L.: Phytochemistry, New matrices, cultivation techniques, and recent updates on its brain-related effects (2018–2023). *Molecules*, 28(8): 3387. https://doi.org/10.3390/molecules28083387

Stack, G. M., Carlson, C. H., Toth, J. A., Philippe, G., Crawford, J. L., Hansen, J. L. et al. (2022). Plant architecture is correlated with variation in cannabinoid concentration and biomass production in *Cannabis sativa*. *Cold Spring Harbor Laboratory*. https://doi.org/10.1101/2022.12.02.518916

Surendran, S., Qassadi, F., Surendran, G., Lilley, D., and Heinrich, M. (2021). Myrcene—what are the potential health benefits of this flavouring and aroma agent? *Frontiers in Nutrition*, 8: 699666. https://doi.org/10.3389/fnut.2021.699666

Tanney, C. A. S., Backer, R., Geitmann, A., and Smith, D. L. (2021). Cannabis glandular trichomes: A cellular metabolite factory. *Frontiers in Plant Science*, 12. https://doi.org/10.3389/fpls.2021.721986

Tarkowski, P., Kopecký, P., Riboulet-Zemouli, K., and Frébort, I. (2025). Where are you heading to, Cannabis research? *Phytochemistry Reviews*. https://doi.org/10.1007/s11101-024-10052-y

Thomas, B. F., and ElSohly, M. A. (2016). The Botany of *Cannabis sativa* L. Em B. F. Thomas and M. A. ElSohly (Orgs.), The Analytical Chemistry of Cannabis (p. 1–26). *Elsevier*. https://doi.org/10.1016/B978-0-12-804646-3.00001-1

Tinoush, B., Shirdel, I., and Wink, M. (2020). Phytochemicals: Potential Lead Molecules for MDR Reversal. *Frontiers in Pharmacology*, 11: 832. https://doi.org/10.3389/fphar.2020.00832

Trancoso, I., De Souza, G. A. R., Dos Santos, P. R., Dos Santos, K. D., De Miranda, R. M. D. S. N., Da Silva, A. L. P. M. et al. (2022). *Cannabis sativa* L.: Crop management and abiotic factors that affect phytocannabinoid production. *Agronomy*, 12(7): 1492. https://doi.org/10.3390/agronomy12071492

Tzimas, P., Petrakis, E. A., Beteinakis, S., Martini, A. N., Papafotiou, M., Bilalis, D. et al. (2022). Exploring the dynamics of developmental stages of micropropagated medical cannabis (*Cannabis sativa* L.) through chemical characterization and optimal plant regeneration. *Planta Medica*, 88. https://doi.org/10.1055/s-0042-1759238

Vergara, D., Huscher, E. L., Keepers, K. G., Givens, R. M., Cizek, C. G., Torres, A. et al. (2019). Gene copy number is associated with phytochemistry in*Cannabis sativa*. Cold Spring Harbor Laboratory. https://doi.org/10.1101/736181

Wang, L.-Y., OuYang, L., Tong, F., Zhang, X.-J., Li, X.-D., Wang, C.-C. et al. (2016). The effect of contraceptive methods on reproductive tract infections risk: A cross-sectional study having a sample of 52,481 women. *Archives of Gynecology and Obstetrics*, 294(6): 1249–1256. https://doi.org/10.1007/s00404-016-4172-0

Wang, M., Wang, Y.-H., Avula, B., Radwan, M. M., Wanas, A. S., Van Antwerp, J. et al. (2016). Decarboxylation study of acidic cannabinoids: A novel approach using ultra-high-performance supercritical fluid chromatography/photodiode array-mass spectrometry. *Cannabis and Cannabinoid Research*, 1(1): 262–271. https://doi.org/10.1089/can.2016.0020

Welling, M. T., Liu, L., Kretzschmar, T., Mauleon, R., Ansari, O., and King, G. J. (2020). An extreme-phenotype genome-wide association study identifies candidate cannabinoid pathway genes in Cannabis. *Scientific Reports*, 10(1). https://doi.org/10.1038/s41598-020-75271-7

Wenger, J. P., Dabney, C. J., ElSohly, M. A., Chandra, S., Radwan, M. M., Majumdar, C. G. et al. (2020). Validating a predictive model of cannabinoid inheritance with feral, clinical, and industrial *Cannabis sativa*. *American Journal of Botany*, 107(10): 1423–1432. https://doi.org/10.1002/ajb2.1550

Yasaghi, M., Dolatabadi, S. B., Yamchi, A., Tabarraei, A., Moradi, A., and Hosseini, S. D. (2025). Insights into the antiviral mechanisms of β-caryophyllene: Inhibiting viral spread and its synergy with acyclovir. *BMC Complementary Medicine and Therapies*, 25(1): 245. https://doi.org/10.1186/s12906-025-04964-1

Yazici, L. (2023). Optimizing plant density for fiber and seed production in industrial hemp (*Cannabis sativa* L.). *Journal of King Saud University - Science*, 35(1): 102419. https://doi.org/10.1016/j.jksus.2022.102419

Yeo, H. C., Reddy, V. A., Mun, B.-G., Leong, S. H., Dhandapani, S., Rajani, S. et al. (2022). Comparative transcriptome analysis reveals coordinated transcriptional regulation of central and secondary metabolism in the trichomes of cannabis cultivars. *International Journal of Molecular Sciences*, 23(15): 8310. https://doi.org/10.3390/ijms23158310

Yoosefzadeh Najafabadi, M., and Torkamaneh, D. (2025). Machine learning-enhanced multi-trait genomic prediction for optimizing cannabinoid profiles in cannabis. *The Plant Journal*, 121(1). https://doi.org/10.1111/tpj.17164

Zandkarimi, F., Decatur, J., Casali, J., Gordon, T., Skibola, C., and Nuckolls, C. (2023). Comparison of the cannabinoid and terpene profiles in commercial cannabis from natural and artificial cultivation. *Molecules*, 28(2), 833. https://doi.org/10.3390/molecules28020833

Zheng, Y. (Org.). (2022). Handbook of Cannabis Production in Controlled Environments. CRC Press. https://doi.org/10.1201/9781003150442

Chapter 4

Cannabis From Farm to Pharmacy

Juliane M. S. Silva, Silvânia N. A. Lima, Enaianny R. S. Frankenberger, Carla F. C. Rodrigues, Tarcísio C. L. Araújo, Cristiane dos S. C. Alves, João V. M. Silva, Pedro G. S. Sá, Pedro J. Rolim-Neto and *Larissa A. Rolim**

1. Introduction

Cannabis sativa L. is a herbaceous species native to Central Asia, also known as hemp or marijuana (Andre et al. 2016; Kovalchuk et al. 2020), recognized for its chemical diversity and therapeutic potential. It can be cultivated for various purposes (Figure 1), either for the production of industrial fibers (such as hemp) or for medicinal use (Hurgobin et al. 2021; Balant et al. 2021). The literature highlights its chemical complexity, presenting more than 560 chemical compounds in its composition, including cannabinoids, alkaloids, terpenes, phenols, amino acids, carbohydrates, and other secondary metabolites (Bonini et al. 2018; Duczmal et al. 2024).

There is no consensus on the classification of species within the genus Cannabis, and many scientists consider their differentiation primarily based on the content of cannabinoids produced or their intended use for industrial or medicinal purposes (McPartland 2018). However, the most recent evidence, combined with the application of genomic studies, corroborates the idea that there is a single species, *Cannabis sativa*, which is chemically very diverse (Lapierre et al. 2023).

Although most studies focus on leaves and inflorescences, which are a significant source of cannabinoids, other parts of the plant, such as seeds, stems, resin glands, and roots, also contain relevant bioactive compounds (Ryz et al. 2017).

The chemotype of the species must also be considered, as genetic variations can lead to the production of specific metabolites. Currently, Cannabis species are still primarily classified by the content and type of cannabinoids they produce (Singh et al. 2021; Herwig et al. 2025). For the proper identification of varieties, studies of the chemical composition of plants of this genus must be complemented by genetic analyses of each cultivar, which broadens the parameters of comparison and ensures greater rigor in the characterization of the raw material—a fundamental step in ensuring the quality and consistency of the final product (Monti et al. 2022).

Research and Extension Group on Medicinal Cannabis, Federal University of Pernambuco, Post Office Box 50670-901, Recife-PE, Brazil.

* Corresponding author: larissa.rolim@univasf.edu.br

DOI: 10.1201/9781003668190-5

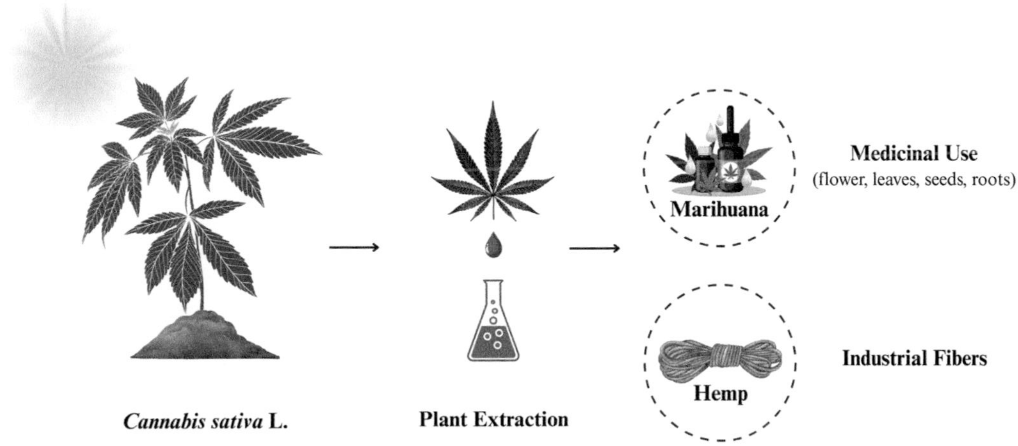

Figure 1: From plant to product: cultivation, extraction, and applications of *Cannabis sativa* L.
Source: Prepared by the authors (2025).

2. From Cultivation to Herbal Drug Production

The search for medicines derived from medicinal plants involves several fundamental steps, including the collection of plant materials, proper preservation, and taxonomic identification by a botanist in a herbarium, which ensures the authenticity of the species (Bitwell et al. 2023).

Plants used to obtain herbal medicines contain natural compounds with therapeutic potential that must be preserved during the processing stages to obtain the herbal medicine. *Cannabis sativa* has a rich and diverse chemical composition, and its main secondary metabolites—cannabinoids, terpenes, and polyphenols—are widely found in its leaves and inflorescences. Other parts of the plant, such as the stem and roots, are also being investigated for their potential therapeutic applications (Hourfane et al. 2023; Siracusa et al. 2023).

After the identification process, plant structures used as active pharmaceutical ingredients (APIs) must undergo controlled drying, fragmentation, and stabilization processes. All these steps must follow a rigorous methodology to ensure the chemical stability of bioactive metabolites, as well as their reproducibility (Simões et al. 2017).

During the cultivation stage, environmental factors such as seasonality, temperature, water availability, exposure to ultraviolet radiation, access to nutrients, altitude, harvest season, plant development stage, air pollution, and the presence of pathogens can affect the quantity and quality of secondary metabolites produced by the plant (Bezerra et al. 2017; Qaderi et al. 2023; Laaboudi et al. 2024). Studies show the direct influence of these factors on the biological activity presented by the plant extract. For example, climate, altitude, and soil characteristics influence the antioxidant efficiency of plant extracts, with significant variations observed in the production of phenolic compounds (Zargoosh et al. 2019; Fiorentino et al. 2024).

As for *Cannabis sativa*, a study by Ferrini et al. (2021) evaluated the influence of different cultivation methods on the content and presence of certain metabolites contained in the roots. Root extracts from specimens grown in soil and in aeroponic cultivation were analyzed. Aeroponic cultivation showed advantages over soil cultivation, resulting in a considerable increase in plant growth and a 20-fold increase in the quantification of metabolites of interest.

In the study by Linder et al. (2022), it was observed that the concentration of THC peaked at the junction of the leaves and inflorescences, before the plant's maturation process. In contrast, CBD levels increased progressively, reaching their maximum concentration during maturation and remaining stable after the peak. Given this, the high variability of conditions that can affect the metabolic composition of *C. sativa* highlights the need to standardize cultivation practices to ensure the quality, reproducibility, and safety of the plant's medicinal use.

The application of modern cultivation techniques in a controlled environment can be an alternative for more efficient management of environmental factors, thereby optimizing the production of secondary metabolites of interest (Fleming et al. 2023; Pérez-Bermúdez and Rognoni Martínez 2023; Selwal et al. 2023). To mitigate these issues and improve the yield of compounds of biological interest, studies are already underway using modern cultivation techniques in controlled environments, such as soilless cultivation systems, plant tissue cultures, light-emitting diode (LED) lighting techniques, and the association of symbiotic microorganisms with cannabis (Salachas et al. 2015; Espinosa-Leal et al. 2018; Dastogeer et al. 2020; Marchev et al. 2020; Fazili et al. 2022; Siracusa et al. 2023; Kaminsky et al. 2024). Thus, the application of technology in cultivation favors the production of higher-quality plant drugs for the development of active pharmaceutical ingredients (APIs).

3. From Extract to Active Plant Pharmaceutical Ingredient

When the plant material is obtained and processed, selected parts of the plant undergo extraction methods to isolate the active constituents, aiming to obtain the phytocannabinoids of interest for pharmaceutical applications (Bowen et al. 2021).

Different extraction methods can impact the chemical composition and biological activity of plant extracts (Oliveira et al. 2016; Torres et al. 2018; Rožanc et al. 2021; Oliveira et al. 2023). A study of the aerial parts of the species corroborates this idea, as extracts obtained using different extraction protocols, varied not only in the concentration of the main phytocannabinoids such as CBD and THC, but also in the abundance of less-researched phytocannabinoids (Bowen et al. 2021).

In addition to conventional methods, such as cold and hot extraction, with or without agitation, the technique of extraction with supercritical CO_2 fluid applied to *Cannabis sativa* L. stands out due to its efficiency in recovering bioactive compounds, especially cannabinoids and phytochemicals of interest (Aguiar et al. 2023; Bowen et al. 2021). Most studies that utilize the supercritical fluid extraction process mainly involve inflorescences or mixtures of aerial parts of the plant, such as stems, leaves, and flowers (Aguiar et al. 2023).

Conventional extraction techniques are often limited by long extraction times or low yields (Azwanida 2015). As such, they can be highly damaging to the environment, mainly due to the types of solvents used. A growing search for faster and more efficient techniques to replace the use of toxic organic solvents, such as hexane and chloroform, has been the increasing focus of research aimed at developing plant-based active pharmaceutical ingredients (AVPIs) (Bitwell et al. 2023), with priority given to methodologies that use green solvents (Ražić et al. 2023).

In addition to supercritical fluid extraction (Atwi-Ghaddar et al. 2023), solvent-accelerated extractions (Kryževičiūtė et al. 2016; Ahmed et al. 2024), microwave-assisted extractions (Ismail-Suhaimy et al. 2021), ultrasound-assisted (Yang et al. 2021), pressurized hot water (Cheng et al. 2021), and enzyme-assisted (Shi et al. 2022) extractions may be promising strategies for optimizing the extraction of cannabis extracts for conversion into standardized AVPIs. However, it is still essential to consider the criteria for industrial feasibility, yield, cost-effectiveness, and safety.

4. Quality Control and Development of Herbal Medicines

A prior study of critical variables is necessary for standardizing plant production, including knowledge of the soil, seed authentication, pesticide use, harvest season, and other important factors to ensure sample homogeneity (Singh et al. 2022). In the cultivation of *Cannabis sativa* L., the timing of harvest has a direct impact on phytocannabinoid concentrations (Linder et al. 2022).

Quality control and stability studies of natural products contribute significantly to ensuring the safety of herbal medicines. These processes are essential in the initial stages, such as the extraction and standardization of plant inputs, through to the final formulation. The active pharmaceutical ingredient (API) is subjected to analyses that verify its identity, purity, potency, and stability. Using advanced chromatographic methods, such as high-performance liquid chromatography (HPLC) coupled with data array detectors (DAD) or mass spectrometers (LC-MS), in addition to the gas chromatography (GC) platform, is beneficial for characterizing phytocannabinoids (Stefkov et al. 2022).

The development of herbal medicines involves formulating appropriate pharmaceutical forms, such as tablets, solutions, suspensions, and capsules, with the establishment of the bioavailability, stability, and efficacy of the formulation. Quality control is maintained throughout the production process, from cultivation to dispensing at the pharmacy, ensuring the safety, efficacy, and therapeutic reliability of herbal medicines (Baratta et al. 2021).

The phytochemical richness of *Cannabis sativa* translates into a wide diversity of metabolites identified in various parts of the plant (Figure 2), among which cannabinoids, terpenes, alkaloids, and flavonoids stand out—many of them associated with potential pharmacological activities (Bonini et al. 2018; Duczmal et al. 2024; Laaboudi et al. 2024). Interest in the molecules that comprise the plant has increased significantly since the discovery of the endocannabinoid system

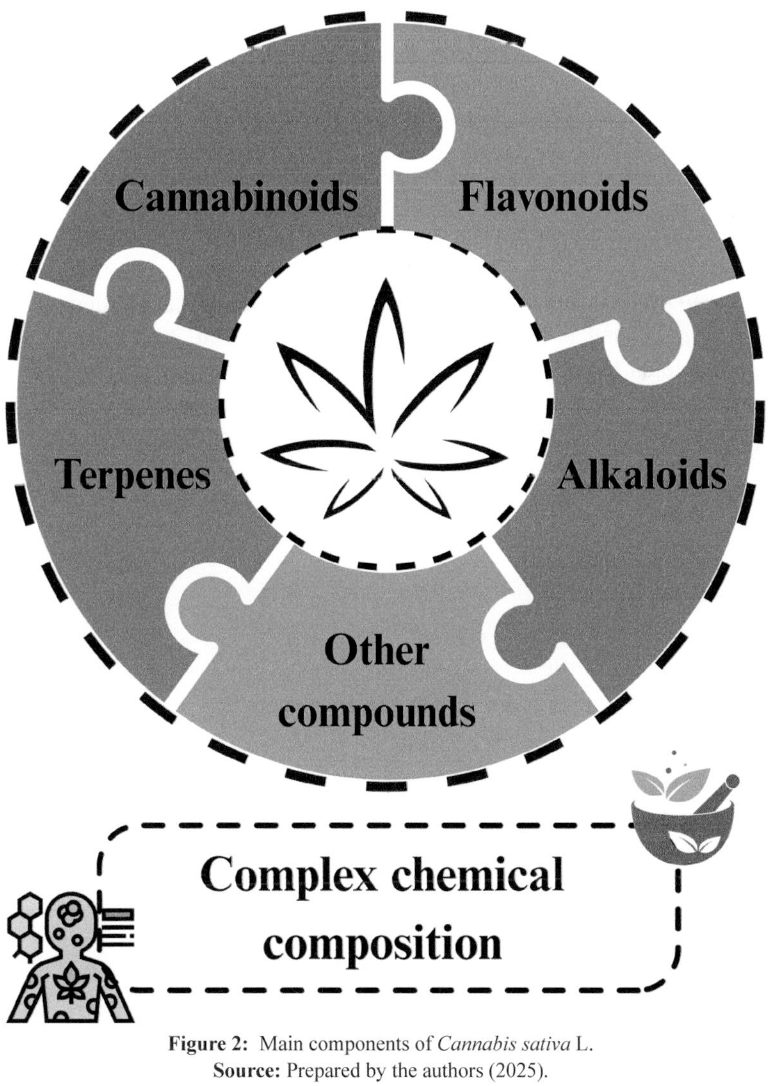

Figure 2: Main components of *Cannabis sativa* L.
Source: Prepared by the authors (2025).

and cannabinoid receptors in the human body (Siracusa et al. 2023), paving the way for research into a widely prohibited species.

The classification of cannabinoids, secondary metabolites representative of the species, is based on their chemical structure (Figure 3) and the effects they produce in the body (Radwan et al. 2021), and is currently the most widely investigated group. Among these compounds, cannabidiol (CBD) and tetrahydrocannabinol (THC) stand out due to their biological actions and abundance.

Studies indicate that CBD has comprehensive biological properties ranging from analgesic and anti-inflammatory actions (Wang et al. 2023; Safi et al. 2024), to potential effects for the treatment of various conditions, such as nausea and vomiting (Rock et al. 2021), sleep regulation (Kisiolek et al. 2023), anxiety (O'Sullivan et al. 2023), epilepsy, Rett syndrome (Desnous et al. 2023), diabetes, cardiovascular diseases, cancer, Alzheimer's, and skin diseases (Duczmal et al. 2024), among other clinical conditions.

THC is a psychoactive cannabinoid that exhibits analgesic and anti-inflammatory properties, as well as controlling nausea and vomiting and stimulating appetite (Duczmal et al. 2024). In addition to these, tetrahydrocannabivarin (THCV), cannabinol (CBN), cannabigerol (CBG), and cannabichromene (CBC) are other phytocannabinoids identified in *C. sativa* that have therapeutic potential of interest (Radwan et al. 2021).

Terpenes are the main compounds identified in the roots of the species and have been widely studied due to their diverse biological properties (Wróblewska-Łuczka et al. 2023), including antimicrobial (Barros et al. 2023), anti-inflammatory, and antitumor actions (Rivera Rodríguez and Johnson 2023). Friedelin and β-caryophyllene are the main representatives in the species (Huang et al. 2019; Kornpointner et al. 2021; Ferrini et al. 2021). Friedelin exhibits antioxidant, hepatoprotective, antiulcerogenic, antidiabetic, antiproliferative, proapoptotic, neuroprotective, antimicrobial, and antiparasitic properties (Joshi et al. 2023; Singh et al. 2023; Sandhu et al. 2023). β-caryophyllene, in turn, has antitumor (Wróblewska-Łuczka et al. 2023), anti-inflammatory (Scandiffio et al. 2020), and immunomodulatory activities, with potential therapeutic applications in the treatment of emotional and cognitive disorders (Ricardi et al. 2024).

Some alkaloids have also been described in the species, including those found in the rhizomes and resin, such as cannabinine, tetanocannabin, and cannabisativine (Lowe et al. 2021; Radwan et al. 2021). The pharmacological effects of alkaloids such as cannabisativine and anhydrocannabisativine derivatives have not yet been investigated in isolation; however, extracts containing these metabolites have demonstrated antidismenorrheic, antiasthmatic, analgesic, and

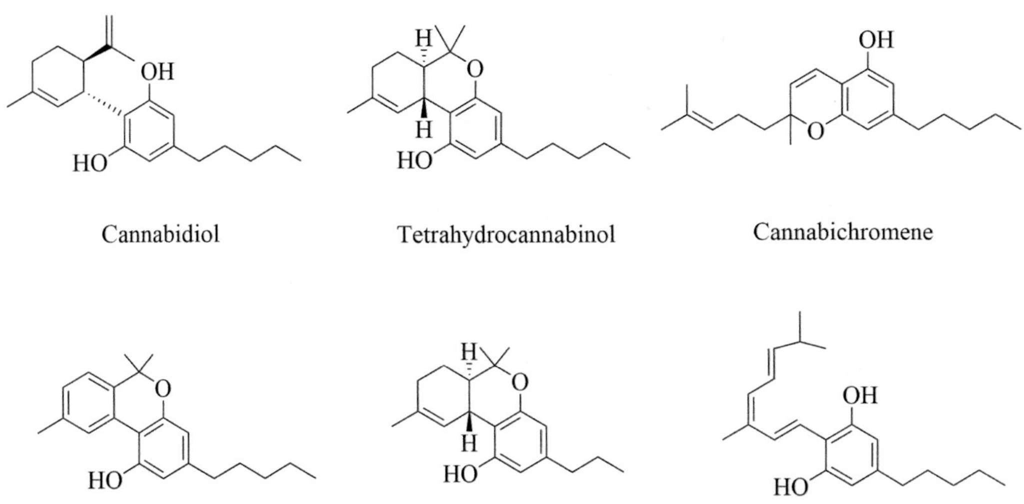

Figure 3: Structure of the main cannabinoids representative of the species *Cannabis sativa* L.
Source: Prepared by the authors (2025).

anti-inflammatory properties in animal models (Lima et al. 2021; Menezes et al. 2021; Araújo et al. 2024).

Flavonoids represent about 10% of the molecules that make up the Cannabis genus and are found in the leaves, stems, inflorescences, seeds, and pollen. These secondary metabolites serve to enhance the medicinal effects of the plant, and their concentrations are directly linked to variations between subspecies and other components of the plant, as well as being influenced by environmental factors. Kaempferol, quercetin, and caniflavin are representatives of this group (Siracusa et al. 2023; Laaboudi et al. 2024).

Cannabis sativa stands out for its complex phytochemical composition, comprising hundreds of already identified compounds that include several classes of bioactive metabolites. This diversity contributes to a wide range of therapeutic effects, and the synergistic interaction between these compounds strengthens the plant's pharmacological potential. In this scenario, ongoing scientific research is crucial for deepening knowledge about these interactions and broadening understanding of their therapeutic applications, contributing to the development of safe and effective medicines, as well as ensuring the quality of products derived from the plant.

5. Pharmaceutical Forms and Routes of Administration

Traditionally, the most common form of cannabis consumption was the dried inflorescence, usually consumed by inhalation, either through smoking or vaporization (Tarlovski et al. 2025). However, with increasing legalization and market expansion, there has been a growing demand for more standardized, potent, and diverse formulations (Blake and Nahtigal 2019).

Cannabinoids are currently available in multiple dosage forms, including oral (tablets, capsules, oily solutions), buccal (lozenges), sublingual (oromatous sprays), rectal (suppositories), topical (ointments, oils, soaps), ophthalmic (eye drops), and systemic (intramuscular or intravenous injections) (Figure 4) (Bidwell et al. 2022; Jaipakdee et al. 2022; O'Brien and Blair 2021; Tarlovski et al. 2025). The choice of administration route should consider not only pharmacokinetic aspects, but also patient preferences and needs, as these are essential factors for promoting greater treatment adherence and a better quality of life (Capano et al. 2020).

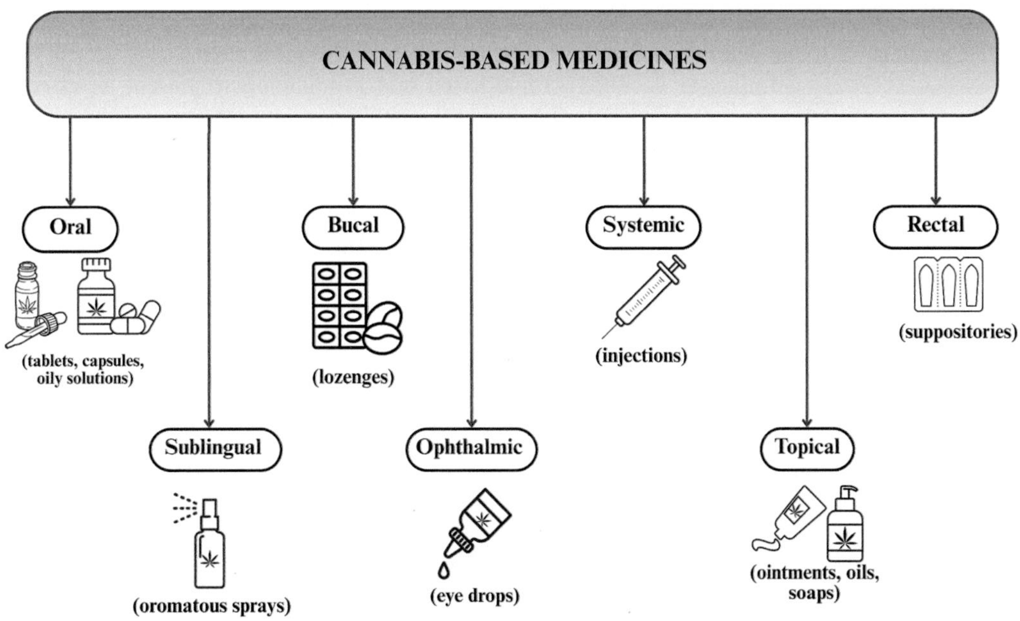

Figure 4: Presentations of products based on *Cannabis sativa* L.
Source: Prepared by the authors (2025).

The inhalation route may offer some advantages in drug administration, such as rapid onset of action (Hartman et al. 2015; Bruni et al. 2018). However, in the case of cannabis, this route shows high interindividual variability, difficulty in precisely controlling the dose administered, and low adherence by patients (Lucas et al. 2018). In contrast, the oral route remains the most widely used in cannabinoid therapy due to its practicality, ease of administration, possibility of standardizing the dose, and greater acceptance by patients (Stella et al. 2021).

Oral formulations of cannabis are especially advantageous for pediatric and elderly populations, as well as for patients with eating difficulties, such as in cases of anorexia, palliative care, post-surgery, and dental conditions (Tagsold et al. 2024; Doucette et al. 2024). Additionally, the preparation of oils from the plant is generally straightforward and does not require sophisticated equipment, which enhances its viability (Romano and Hazekamp 2013). On the other hand, the development of inhalable formulations presents more complex technological challenges, particularly concerning the need for particles of small size (between 0.5 and 5 μm) to ensure adequate deposition of the active ingredient in the target regions of the lungs (Gutowski 2021).

One of the main limitations of oral cannabis formulations is related to the high lipophilicity of cannabinoids, resulting in low water solubility and, consequently, reduced bioavailability (MacCallum and Russo 2018). These compounds are sensitive to degradation by factors such as light, oxidation, and heat, which compromise their stability over time (Fraguas-Sánchez et al. 2020).

Oral cannabinoids are primarily formulated in oil solutions (Herrera et al. 2024), but they are also found in other pharmaceutical forms, such as soft capsules, oral solutions, or mouth sprays. According to the labels of imported products, the most commonly used vehicle is medium-chain triglyceride (MCT). In artisanal preparations, cannabis resin is typically dissolved in oils such as olive oil, coconut oil, or sunflower oil (Carvalho et al. 2020; Herrera et al. 2024). In Brazil, olive and sunflower oils are the most commonly used in the development of these preparations (Carvalho et al. 2020).

Studies show that the bioavailability of oily cannabis formulations can be significantly increased by incorporating lipids, with this effect depending on the type of lipid used. For example, sesame oil can increase bioavailability by up to three times compared to lipid-free formulations (Banerjee et al. 2024; Feng et al. 2021). In addition, Romano and Hazekamp (2013) highlighted the effectiveness of olive oil in extracting compounds from cannabis, particularly terpenes, due to the ability of lipids to solubilize and protect these compounds against degradation and evaporation.

Cannabis oil is the pharmaceutical form that has received the most attention in recent years (Costa et al. 2025; Grimling et al. 2025). Lipid-based oral formulations represent an effective strategy for optimizing the systemic bioavailability of lipophilic drugs by increasing solubility and permeability. In cases where intestinal lymphatic transport is involved, it is possible to avoid first-pass metabolism in the liver (Feeney et al. 2016).

Depending on the fatty acid composition, including chain length and degree of saturation, certain lipids, such as those found in canola, sesame, and coconut oils, can affect the permeability of the blood-brain barrier (Brookes et al. 2022). Therefore, when administered in the correct concentrations, they can reach different regions of the brain (Brookes et al. 2022; Brookes et al. 2023).

Zgair et al. (2016) observed that the oral administration of THC and CBD in lipophilic formulations resulted in a 2.5 and 3-fold increase in absolute bioavailability and plasma concentration profiles over time, respectively, when compared to lipid-free vehicle formulations. In a subsequent study, the same authors demonstrated that co-administration of cannabinoids with lipids significantly increased intestinal lymphatic transport in rats. CBD concentrations in lymph were 250 times higher than in plasma, while THC concentrations were 100 times higher (Zgair et al. 2017).

Chesney et al. (2024) conducted a double-blind, crossover study with healthy fasting volunteers, comparing the pharmacokinetics of a single 1000 mg dose of CBD in both lipid and powder formulation. Animal models received CBD in lipid formulation or dissolved in water via oral gavage. As a result, they observed that plasma exposure to CBD was nine times higher for the lipid formulation than for the powder formulation. After administration of the lipid formulation, measurable concentrations of CBD were detected in all organs evaluated. In contrast, the aqueous formulation showed tissue levels of CBD below the limit of quantification.

Triglycerides are fatty constituents that represent between 95% and 98% of the composition of vegetable oils. They are widely used in the development of lipid formulations due to their simple structure and widespread presence in the human diet (Chernova et al. 2018; Guidoni et al. 2019; Vergallo 2020).

Medium-chain triglycerides (MCTs), such as those found in coconut oil, consist of a mixture of saturated fatty acids with 6–12 carbon atoms. MCTs are mainly composed of caprylic acid (80%), capric acid (20–50%), caproic acid, and lauric acid (1–2%). In contrast, long-chain triglycerides (LCTs), such as those found in sesame and canola oil, are composed of fatty acids ranging from 12 to 18 carbons in length. Consequently, MCTs have smaller molecular sizes, lower melting points, and lower viscosity, but are more soluble in water than LCTs. The oil obtained from coconuts contains about 46–54% lauric acid, 5–10% caprylic acid, and 5–8% capric acid (Jadhav and Annapure 2023).

MCTs, composed of medium-chain fatty acids (MCFAs) that are bound to a glycerol molecule, have distinct metabolic characteristics compared to LCTs (Figure 5). The digestion of MCTs begins in the mouth and stomach, where they undergo partial hydrolysis by the action of lingual and gastric lipase. Subsequently, in the small intestine, they are hydrolyzed more efficiently by pancreatic lipase (a), a process that is faster than that observed with LCTs (Lee et al. 2022; Jadhav and Annapure 2023). After hydrolysis, ACMs are released from the glycerol structure. Due to their shorter carbon chain and greater water solubility, these fatty acids are rapidly absorbed and transported to the liver (b), without the need for packaging in chylomicrons, as occurs with TCLs. MCTs (e.g., C8:0, C10:0) are rapidly hydrolyzed, and their fatty acids (MCFAs) quickly go to the liver for metabolism (Jadhav and Annapure 2023).

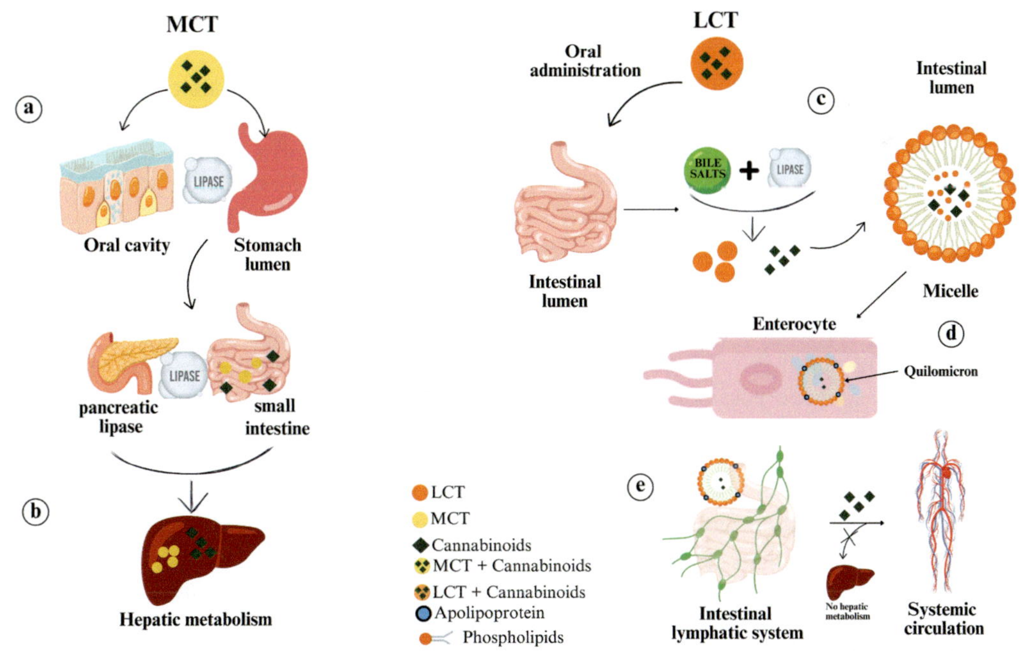

Figure 5: Proposed mechanism for intestinal lymphatic transport of THC and CBD after oral administration with MCT and LCT. MCT, after degradation by lipases (a), proceeds to metabolism in the liver (b). For LCT, solubilization of THC and CBD (c) in mixed micelles after lipid digestion in the small intestine. (d) Uptake of chylomicrons into enterocytes. (e) Chylomicrons transport THC and CBD to the systemic circulation via the intestinal lymphatic system, bypassing first-pass hepatic metabolism.

Source: Prepared by authors based on (Jadhav and Annapure 2023).

Whereas in the absorption of LCTs, such as those found in sesame oil, there is no significant influence of first-pass metabolism even when administered orally. It is believed that after ingestion, LCTs are broken down by pancreatic enzymes and lipases in the intestinal lumen, after which triglycerides undergo reacylation and are incorporated, together with cannabinoids, into micelles (c), which, after being absorbed by enterocytes, are incorporated into chylomicrons (d). Finally, chylomicrons act as transporters for THC and CBD through the epithelial layer to the intestinal lymphatic system, carrying them into the systemic circulation via the thoracic duct (e) (Zgair et al. 2016).

Differences in digestion and absorption pathways can result in distinct effects on the blood-brain barrier, including the time after administration until an effect on the barrier is observed. However, substantial gaps in understanding the impact of lipids on blood-brain barrier permeability after oral administration (Brookes et al. 2022).

A wide range of products containing cannabinoids is currently available on the market, with CBD oil being one of the most common. These oils can be classified into three main categories: CBD isolates (without other cannabinoids or terpenes), broad-spectrum products, which contain all cannabinoids and terpenes except Δ^9-tetrahydrocannabinol (THC), and full-spectrum products, which include all compounds present in the plant, with up to 0.3% THC by dry weight. Sativex ® (USAN: nabiximols), an ethanol-based oral preparation containing 2.7 mg of THC and 2.5 mg of cannabidiol (CBD) per spray, was the first cannabis product to obtain regulatory approval as a pharmaceutical product in 29 countries, having met the required standards of safety, efficacy, and consistency (MacCallum and Russo 2018).

Dronabinol (Marinol® and Syndros®), a synthetic form of THC dissolved in sesame oil, has been approved as an appetite stimulant, mainly in AIDS patients, and as an antiemetic in cases of chemotherapy. More recently, Epidiolex®, a strawberry-flavored syrup containing CBD, also dissolved in sesame oil, has been approved for seizures associated with Lennox-Gastaut syndrome and Dravet syndrome. Commercial formulations typically utilize LCT or MCT as lipophilic vehicles (Chen and Rogers 2019).

Thus, the development of oral formulations represents a promising strategy to overcome challenges such as those faced by patients with swallowing difficulties and children. Due to the physicochemical properties of cannabinoids, significant challenges arise in developing effective pharmaceutical forms for oral administration. However, the use of lipid-based systems, such as oil solutions, has proven effective in overcoming these obstacles, promoting greater solubility, absorption, and bioavailability.

6. Conclusions

Cannabis sativa spp. has received considerable attention due to its numerous constituents that offer broad therapeutic possibilities for various clinical conditions, making it a source for the development of medicines. The variability in the concentration of secondary metabolites stems from the existence of different chemotypes of the plant. For this reason, the cultivation of this genus needs to be standardized, and the establishment of a rigorous standard for the isolation and identification of biologically interesting molecules is an essential procedure for a better understanding of the chemical composition of the species.

The literature has highlighted a plurality of therapeutic properties derived from this genus, with research demonstrating promising characteristics of the compounds and various parts of the plant, highlighting its versatility.

Given the growing scientific interest, it is essential to adopt plant production practices that are associated with appropriate extraction processes and robust quality control methods in order to ensure the standardization and safety of final products with therapeutic potential.

From cultivation to formulation, which ultimately reaches the patient, systematic monitoring of the stages is a determining factor in ensuring the reproducibility of therapeutic effects and the rational use of the plant in clinical practice. Investments in multidisciplinary research based on scientific evidence are crucial for harnessing the potential of *C. sativa* spp. into safe, effective, and accessible therapies, promoting advances in the treatment of various clinical conditions.

References

Ahmed, O. S., Tahanout, F., Marti-Mestres, G., Weber, J.-F., and Waffo-Téguo, P. (2024). An automated accelerated salting-out assisted solvent extraction (A-ASASE) of stilbenoids from *Vitis vinifera* L. branches: False proof or a proof of concept. *Talanta*, 266: 124935

Aguiar, A. C., Vardanega, R., Viganó, J., and Silva, E. K. (2023). Supercritical carbon dioxide technology for recovering valuable phytochemicals from *Cannabis sativa* L. and valorization of its biomass for food applications. *Molecules*, 28: 3849.

Andre, C. M., Hausman, J. F., and Guerriero, G. (2016). Cannabis sativa: The Plant of the Thousand and One Molecules. *Frontiers in Plant Science*, 4: 7–19.

Araújo, T. C. L., Menezes, P. M. N., Ribeiro, T. F., Macêdo, C. A. F., Souza, N. A. C., Lima, K. S. B. et al. (2024). *Cannabis sativa* L. roots from Northeast Brazil reduce abdominal contortions in a mouse model of primary dysmenorrhea. *Journal of Ethnopharmacology*, 318: 116891.

Atwi-Ghaddar, S., Destandau, E., and Lesellier, E. (2023). Integrated supercritical fluid extraction and pre-formulation process of *Punica granatum* L. Pericarp Polar Compounds. *Molecules*, 28: 8110.

Azwanida, N. N. (2015). A review on the extraction methods use in medicinal plants, principle, strength and limitation. *Med Aromat Plants* (Los Angel), 04: 196.

Balant, M., Gras, A., Ruz, M., Vallès, J., Vitales, D., and Garnatje, T. (2021). Traditional uses of Cannabis: An analysis of the CANNUSE database. *Journal of Ethnopharmacology*, 279: 114362.

Banerjee, S., Saharan, V. A., Banerjee, D., Ram, V., Kulhari, H., Pooja, D. et al. (2024). A comprehensive update on cannabidiol, its formulations and drug delivery systems. *Phytochemistry Reviews*, 24: 2723–2757.

Baratta, F., Simiele, M., Pignata, I., Enri, L. R., D'avolio, A., Torta, R. et al. (2021). Cannabis-based oral formulations for medical purposes: Preparation, quality and stability. *Pharmaceuticals*, 14: 171.

Barros, D. B., Nascimento, N. S., Sousa, A. P., Barros, A. V., Borges, Y. W. B. et al. (2023). Antifungal activity of terpenes isolated from the Brazilian Caatinga: a review. *Brazilian Journal of Biology*, 83: e270966.

Bezerra, R. C. F., Neto, F. B. O., Silva, F. F. M., Bertini, L. M., and Alves, L. A. (2017). Seasonal effect in essential oil composition and antioxidant activity of *Plectranthus amboinicus* leaves. *Bioscience Journal*, 33: 1608–1616.

Bidwell, L. C., Karoly, H. C., Torres, M. O., Master, A., Bryan, A. D., and Hutchison, K. E. (2022). A naturalistic study of orally administered vs. inhaled legal market cannabis: cannabinoids exposure, intoxication, and impairment. *Psychopharmacology*, 239: 385–397.

Bitwell, C., Indra, S. S., Luke, C., and Kakoma, M. K. (2023). A review of modern and conventional extraction techniques and their applications for extracting phytochemicals from plants. *Scientific African*, 19: e01585.

Blake, A., and Nahtigal, I. (2019). The evolving landscape of cannabis edibles. *Current Opinion in Food Science*, 28: 25–31.

Bonini, S. A., Premoli, M., Tambaro, S., Kumar, A., Maccarinelli, G., Memo, M. et al. (2018) *Cannabis sativa*: A comprehensive ethnopharmacological review of a medicinal plant with a long history. *Journal of Ethnopharmacology*, 227: 300–315.

Bowen, J. K., Chaparro, J. M., McCorkle, A. M., Palumbo, E., and Prenni, J. E. (2021). The impact of extraction protocol on the chemical profile of cannabis extracts from a single cultivar. *Scientific Reports*, 1: 21801.

Brookes, A., Jewell, A., Feng, W., Bradshaw, T. D., Butler, J., and Gershkovich, P. (2023). Oral lipid-based formulations alter delivery of cannabidiol to different anatomical regions in the brain. *International Journal of Pharmaceutics*, 635: 122651.

Brookes, A., Ji, L., Bradshaw, T. D., Stocks, M., Gray, D., Butler, J. et al. (2022). Is oral lipid-based delivery for drug targeting to the brain feasible? *European Journal of Pharmaceutics and Biopharmaceutics*, 172: 112–122.

Bruni, N., Della Pepa, C., Oliaro-Bosso, S., Pessione, E., Gastaldi, D., and Dosio, F. (2018). Cannabinoid Delivery Systems for Pain and Inflammation Treatment. *Molecules*, 23: 2478.

Capano, A., Weaver, R. and Burkman, E. (2020). Evaluation of the effects of CBD hemp extract on opioid use and quality of life indicators in chronic pain patients: a prospective cohort study. *Postgraduate Medicine*, 132: 56–61.

Carvalho, V. M., Aguiar, A. F. L., Baratto, L. C., Souza, F. L. C., and Rocha, E. D. (2020). Cannabinoids quantification in medicinal cannabis extracts by high performance liquid chromatography. *Química Nova*, 43: 90–97.

Cheng, Y., Xue, F., Yu, S., Du, S., and Yang, Y. (2021). Subcritical Water Extraction of Natural Products. *Molecules*, 26: 4004.

Chen, P. X., and Rogers, M. A. (2019). Opportunities and challenges in developing orally administered cannabis edibles. *Current Opinion in Food Science*, 28: 7–13.

Chernova, A., Gubaev, R., Mazin, P., Goryunova, S., Demurin, Y., Gorlova, L. et al. (2018). UPLC–MS triglyceride profiling in sunflower and rapeseed seeds. *Biomolecules*, 9: 9.

Chesney, E., Mazibuko, N., Oliver, D., Minichino, A., Lamper, A. D., Chester, L. et al. (2024). Novel lipid formulation increases absorption of oral Cannabidiol (CBD). *Pharmaceutics*, 16: 1537.

Costa, M. C., Gomes, A. P., Vinhas, I., Rosa, J., Pereira, F., Moniz, S. et al. (2025). Process development for GMP-grade full extract cannabis oil: Towards standardized medicinal use. *Pharmaceutics*, 17: 848.

Dastogeer, K. M. G., Tumpa, F. H., Sultana, A., Akter, M. A., and Chakraborty, A. (2020). Plant microbiome–an account of the factors that shape community composition and diversity. *Current Plant Biology*, 23: 100161.

Desnous, B., Beretti, T., Muller, N., Neveu, J., Villeneuve, N., Lépine, A. et al. (2023). Efficacy and tolerance of cannabidiol in the treatment of epilepsy in patients with Rett syndrome. *Epilepsia Open*, 9: 397–403.

Doucette, M. L., Hemraj, D., Casarett, D. J., Macfarlan, D. L., and Fisher, E. (2024). Use of cannabis-based medical products for pediatric health conditions: a systematic review of the recent literature. *Med Cannabis Cannabinoids*, 7: 257–267.

Duczmal, D., Bazan-Wozniak, A., Niedzielska, K., and Pietrzak, R. (2024). Cannabinoids-multifunctional compounds, applications and challenges-mini review. *Molecules*, 29: 4923.

Espinosa-Leal, C. A., Puente-Garza, C. A., and García-Lara, S. (2018). *In vitro* plant tissue culture: means for production of biological active compounds. *Planta*, 248: 1–18.

Fazili, M. A., Bashir, I., Ahmad, M., Yaqoob, U., and Geelani, S. N. (2022). *In vitro* strategies for the enhancement of secondary metabolite production in plants: a review. *Bulletin of the National Research Centre* (Online), 46: 35.

Feeney, O. M., Crum, M. F., McEvoy, C. L., Trevaskis, N. L., Williams, H. D., Pouton, C. W. et al. (2016). 50 years of oral lipid-based formulations: Provenance, progress and future perspectives. *Advanced Drug Delivery Reviews*, 101: 167–194.

Feng, W., Qin, C., Chu, Y. J., Berton, M., Lee, J. B., Zgair, A. et al. (2021). Natural sesame oil is superior to pre-digested lipid formulations and purified triglycerides in promoting the intestinal lymphatic transport and systemic bioavailability of cannabidiol. *European Journal of Pharmaceutics and Biopharmaceutics*, 162: 43–49.

Ferrini, F., Fraternale, D., Donati Zeppa, S., Verardo, G., Gorassini, A., Carrabs, V. et al. (2021). Yield, characterization, and possible exploitation of *Cannabis Sativa* L. roots Grown under Aeroponics Cultivation. *Molecules*, 26: 4889.

Fiorentino, N., Formisano, C., Delfine, S., and Chianese, G. (2024). Editorial: Environmental and agronomic factors affecting the chemical composition and biological activity of cannabis extracts. *Frontiers in Plant Science*, 15: 1407262.

Fleming, H., Chamberlain, Z., Zager, J. J., and Lange, B. M. (2023). Controlled environments for cannabis cultivation to support "omics" research studies and production. *Methods in Enzymology*, 680: 353–380.

Fraguas-Sánchez, A. I., Fernández-Carballido, A., Martin-Sabroso, C., and Torres-Suárez, A. I. (2020). Stability characteristics of cannabidiol for the design of pharmacological, biochemical and pharmaceutical studies. *Journal of Chromatography B*, 1150: 122188.

Guidoni, M., Scherer, C. M. M., Figueira, M. M., Schmitt, E. F. P., Almeida, L. C., Scherer, R. et al. (2019). Fatty acid composition of vegetable oil blend and in vitro effects of pharmacotherapeutical skin care applications. *Brazilian Journal of Medical and Biological Research*, 52: e8209.

Grimling, B., Fast, M., Okoniewska, M., Owczarek, A., and Karolewicz, B. (2025). Optimization and Evaluation of Cannabis-Based Magistral Formulations: A Path to Personalized Therapy. *Pharmaceuticals*, 18: 73.

Gutowski, T. (2021). Inhalable Cannabidiol: Formulation Considerations for Extremely Lipophilic, UV-Labile Substances. Christian-Albrechts-Universität zu Kiel, Kiel.

Hartman, R. L., Brown, T. L., Milavetz, G., Spurgin, A., Gorelick, D. A., Gaffney, G. et al. (2015). Controlled Cannabis Vaporizer Administration: Blood and Plasma Cannabinoids with and without Alcohol. *Clinical Chemistry*, 61: 850–869.

Herrera, J. G., Rolim, L. A., Honorato, R. S., and Pimentel, M. F. (2024). Analysis of cannabinoids in medicinal cannabis products: a comprehensive review. *Journal of the Brazilian Chemical Society*, 35: 20240129.

Herwig, N., Utgenannt, S., Nickl, F., Möbius, P., Nowak, L., Schulz, O. et al. (2025). Classification of cannabis strains based on their chemical fingerprint-a broad analysis of chemovars in the german market. *Cannabis and Cannabinoids Research*, 10: 409–419.

Hourfane, S., Mechqoq, H., Bekkali, A. Y., Rocha, J. M., and Aouad, N. A. (2023). Comprehensive review on *Cannabis sativa* ethnobotany, phytochemistry, molecular docking and biological activities. *Plants*, 12: 1245.

Huang, H. T., Lin, C. C., Kuo, T. C., Chen, S. J., and Huang, R. N. (2019). Phytochemical composition and larvicidal activity of essential oils from herbal plants. *Planta*, 250: 59–68.

Hurgobin, B., Tamiru-Oli, M., Welling, M. T., Doblin, M. S., Bacic, A., Whelan, J. et al. (2021). Recent advances in *Cannabis sativa* genomics research. *New Phytologist*, 230: 73–89.

Ismail-Suhaimy, N. W., Gani, S. S. A., Zaidan, U. H., Halmi, M. I. E., and Bawon, P. (2021). Optimizing conditions for microwave-assisted extraction of polyphenolic content and antioxidant activity of *Barleria lupulina* Lindl. *Plants*, 10: 682.

Jadhav, H. B., and Annapure, U. S. (2023). Triglycerides of medium-chain fatty acids: a concise review. *Journal of Food Science and Technology*, 60: 2143–2152.

Jaipakdee, N., Tabboon, P., and Limpongsa, E. (2022). Application of a liquisolid technique to *Cannabis sativa* extract compacts: Effect of liquid vehicles on the dissolution enhancement and stability of cannabinoids. *International Journal of Pharmaceutics*, 612: 121277.

Joshi, B. P., Bhandare, V. V., Vankawala, M., Patel, P., Patel, R., Vyas, B et al. (2023). Friedelin, a novel inhibitor of CYP17A1 in prostate cancer from *Cassia tora*. *Journal of Biomolecular Structure and Dynamics*, 41: 9695–9720.

Kaminsky, N., Hubert, J., Guerin, C., Mazlani, M., Kotland, A., Pozzobon, V. et al. (2024). Deciphering the phytochemical potential of hemp hairy roots: a promising source of cannabisins and triterpenes as bioactive compounds. *Molecules*, 29: 5792.

Kisiolek, J. N., Flores, V. A., Ramani, A., Butler, B., Haughian, J. M., and Stewart, L. K. (2023). Eight weeks of daily cannabidiol supplementation improves sleep quality and immune cell cytotoxicity. *Nutrients*, 15: 4173.

Kornpointner, C., Sainz Martinez, A., Marinovic, S., Haselmair-Gosch, C., Jamnik, P., Schröder, K. et al. (2021). Chemical composition and antioxidant potential of *Cannabis sativa* L. roots. *Industrial Crops and Products*, 165: 113422.

Kovalchuk, I., Pellino, M., Rigault, P., van Velzen, R., Ebersbach, J., Ashnest, J. R. et al. (2020). The genomics of cannabis and its close relatives. *Annual Review of Plant Biology*, 71: 713–739.

Kryževičiūtė, N., Kraujalis, P., and Venskutonis, P. R. (2016). Optimization of high pressure extraction processes for the separation of raspberry pomace into lipophilic and hydrophilic fractions. *The Journal of Supercritical Fluids*, 108: 61–68.

Laaboudi, F. Z., Rejdali, M., Amhamdi, H., Salhi, A., Elyoussfi, A., and Ahari, M. (2024). In the weeds: A comprehensive review of cannabis; its chemical complexity, biosynthesis, and healing abilities. *Toxicology Reports*, 13: 101685.

Lapierre, É., Monthony, A. S., and Torkamaneh, D. (2023). Genomics-based taxonomy to clarify cannabis classification. *Genome*, 66: 202–211.

Lee, Y. Y., Tang, T. K., Chan, E. S., Phuah, E. T., Lai, O. M., Tan, C. P. et al. (2022). Medium chain triglyceride and medium-and long chain triglyceride: metabolism, production, health impacts and its applications - a review. *Critical Reviews in Food Science and Nutrition*, 62: 4169–4185.

Lima, K. S. B., Silva, M. E. G. C., Araújo, T. C. L., Silva, C. P. da F., Santos, B. L., Ribeiro, L. A. A. et al. (2021). Cannabis roots: Pharmacological and toxicological studies in mice. *Journal of Ethnopharmacology*, 271: 113868.

Linder, E. R., Young, S., Li, X., Henriquez Inoa, S., and Suchoff, D. H. (2022). The effect of harvest date on temporal cannabinoid and biomass production in the floral Hemp (*Cannabis sativa* L.) cultivars BaOx and cherry wine. *Horticulturae*, 8: 959.

Lowe, H., Steele, B., Bryant, J., Toyang, N., and Ngwa, W. (2021). Non-cannabinoid metabolites of *Cannabis sativa* L. with therapeutic potential. *Plants* (Basel), 10: 400.

Lucas, C. J., Galettis, P., and Schneider, J. (2018). The pharmacokinetics and the pharmacodynamics of cannabinoids. *British Journal of Clinical Pharmacology*, 84: 2477–2482.

MacCallum, C. A., and Russo, E. B. (2018) Practical considerations in medical cannabis administration and dosing. *European Journal of Internal Medicine*, 49: 12–19.

Marchev, A. S., Yordanova, Z. P., and Georgiev, M. I. (2020). Green (cell) factories for advanced production of plant secondary metabolites. *Critical Reviews in Biotechnology*, 40: 443–458.

McPartland, J. M. (2018). *Cannabis* systematics at the levels of family, genus, and species. *Cannabis and Cannabinoid Research*, 3: 203–212.

Menezes, P. M. N., Araújo, T. C. L., Pereira, E. C. V., Neto, J. A., Silva, D. S., Brito, M. C. et al. (2021). Investigation of antinociceptive, antipyretic, antiasthmatic, and spasmolytic activities of Brazilian *Cannabis sativa* L. roots in rodents. *Journal of Ethnopharmacology*, 278: 114259.

Monti, M. C., Frei, P., Weber, S., Scheurer, E., and Mercer-Chalmers-Bender, K. (2022). Beyond Δ9-tetrahydrocannabinol and cannabidiol: chemical differentiation of cannabis varieties applying targeted and untargeted analysis. *Analytical and Bioanalytical Chemistry*, 414: 3847–3862.

O'Brien, K., and Blair, P. (2021). Routes of Administration, Pharmacokinetics and Safety of Medicinal Cannabis. *Medicinal Cannabis and CBD in Mental Healthcare*, 8: 11.

Oliveira, I., Chrysargyris, A., Heleno, S. A., Carocho, M., Calhelha, R. C., Dias, M. I. et al. (2023). Effects of the extraction techniques on the chemical composition and bioactive properties of lemon balm (*Melissa officinalis* L.) plants grown under different cropping and irrigation regimes. *Food Research International*, 170: 113044.

Oliveira, V. B., Zuchetto, M., Oliveira, C. F., Paula, C. S., Duarte, A. F. S., Miguel, M. D. et al. (2016). Effect of different extraction techniques on the yield, antioxidant activity, total dosages, and profile by hplc-dad of *Dicksonia sellowiana* (Presl.). Hook, dicksoniaceae. *Brazilian Journal of Medicinal Plants*, 18: 230–239.

O'Sullivan, S. E., Jensen, S. S., Nikolajsen, G. N., Bruun, H. Z., Bhuller, R., and Hoeng, J. (2023). The therapeutic potential of purified cannabidiol. *Journal of Cannabis Research*, 5: 21.

Pérez-Bermúdez, P., and Rognoni Martínez, A. (2023). Strategies to improve Cannabis cultivation: optimizing plant growth and phytocannabinoid biosynthesis. In: *Current Applications, Approaches, and Potential Perspectives for Hemp*. Elsevier: p. 77–108.

Qaderi, M. M., Martel, A. B., and Strugnell, C. A. (2023). Environmental factors regulate plant secondary metabolites. *Plants*, 12: 447.

Radwan, M. M., Chandra, S., Gul, S., and Elsohly, M. A. (2021). Cannabinoids, Phenolics, Terpenes and Alkaloids of Cannabis. *Molecules*, 26: 2774.

Ražić, S., Arsenijević, J., Đogo Mračević, S., Mušović, J., and Trtić-Petrović, T. (2023). Greener chemistry in analytical sciences: from green solvents to applications in complex matrices. Current challenges and future perspectives: a critical review. *Analyst*, 148: 3130–3152.

Ricardi, C., Barachini, S., Consoli, G., Marazziti, D., Polini, B., and Chiellini, G. (2024). Beta-caryophyllene, a cannabinoid receptor type 2 selective agonist, in emotional and cognitive disorders. *International Journal of Molecular Sciences*, 25: 3203.

Rivera, R. R., and Johnson, J. J. (2023). Terpenes: Modulating anti-inflammatory signaling in inflammatory bowel disease. *Pharmacology & Therapeutics*, 248: 108456.

Rock, E. M., Limebeer, C. L., Pertwee, R. G., Mechoulam, R., and Parker, L. A. (2021). Therapeutic potential of cannabidiol, cannabidiolic acid, and cannabidiolic acid methyl ester as treatments for nausea and vomiting. *Cannabis and Cannabinoid Researsh*, 6: 266–274.

Romano, L. L., and Hazekamp, A. (2013). Cannabis oil: Chemical evaluation of an upcoming cannabis- based medicine. *Cannabinoids*, 1: 1–11.

Rožanc, J., Kotnik, P., Milojević, M., Gradišnik, L., Knez Hrnčič, M., Knez, Ž. et al. (2021). Different *Cannabis sativa* extraction methods result in different biological activities against a colon cancer cell line and healthy colon cells. *Plants* (Basel), 10: 566.

Ryz, N. R., Remillard, D. J., and Russo, E. B. (2017). Cannabis roots: A traditional therapy with future potential for treating inflammation and pain. *Cannabis and Cannabinoid Researsh*, 2: 210–216.

Safi, K., Sobieraj, J., Błaszkiewicz, M., Żyła, J., Salata, B., and Dzierżanowski, T. (2024) Tetrahydrocannabinol and cannabidiol for pain treatment—an update on the evidence. *Biomedicines*, 12: 307.

Salachas, G., Savvas, D., Argyropoulou, K., Tarantillis, P., and Kapotis, G. (2015). Yield and nutritional quality of aeroponically cultivated basil as affected by the available root-zone volume. *Emirates Journal of Food and Agriculture*, 27: 911–8.

Sandhu, M., Irfan, H. M., Arshad, L., Ullah, A., Shah, S. A., and Ali, H. (2023). Friedelin and Glutinol induce neuroprotection against ethanol induced neurotoxicity in pup's brain through reduction of TNF-α, NF-kB, caspase-3 and PARP-1. *Neurotoxicology*, 99: 274–281.

Scandiffio, R., Geddo, F., Cottone, E., Querio, G., Antoniotti, S., Gallo, M. P. et al. (2020). Protective effects of (E)-β-Caryophyllene (BCP) in chronic inflammation. *Nutrients*, 12: 3273.

Selwal, N., Rahayu, F., Herwati, A., Latifah, E., Supriyono, Suhara, C., Kade Suastika, I. B. et al. (2023). Enhancing secondary metabolite production in plants: Exploring traditional and modern strategies. *Journal of Agriculture and Food Research*, 14: 100702.

Shi, X., Zhao, L., Niu, L., Wei, J., Li, X., and Jin, Y. (2022). Enzyme-assisted extraction of narirutin from citri reticulatae pericarpium and anti-allergic asthma activity. *Iranian Journal of Immunology*, 19: 385–394.

Simões, C. M. O., Schenkel, E. P., Mello, J. C. P., Mentz, L. A., and Petrovick, P. R. (2017). *Farmacognosia: do produto natural ao medicamento*. Porto Alegre: Artmed.

Singh, A., Bilichak, A., and Kovalchuk, I. (2021). The genetics of Cannabis-genomic variations of key synthases and their effect on cannabinoid content. *Genome*, 64: 490–501.

Singh, P. A., Bajwa, N., Chinnam, S., Chandan, A., and Baldi, A. (2022). An overview of some important deliberations to promote medicinal plants cultivation. *Journal of Applied Research on Medicinal and Aromatic Plants*, 31: 100400.

Singh, S. K., Shrivastava, S., Mishra, A. K., Kumar, D., Pandey, V. K., Srivastava, P. et al. (2023) Friedelin: Structure, Biosynthesis, Extraction, and Its Potential Health Impact. *Molecules*, 28: 7760.

Siracusa, L., Ruberto, G., and Cristino, L. (2023). Recent research on *Cannabis sativa* L.: Phytochemistry, new matrices, cultivation techniques, and recent updates on its brain-related effects (2018–2023). *Molecules*, 28: 3387.

Stefkov, G., Karanfilova, I. C., Gjorgievska, V. S., Trajkovska, A., Geskovski, N., Karapandzova, M. et al. (2022). Analytical Techniques for Phytocannabinoid Profiling of Cannabis and Cannabis-Based Products-A Comprehensive Review. *Molecules*, 27: 975.

Stella, B., Baratta, F., della Pepa, C., Arpicco, S., Gastaldi, D., and Dosio, F. (2021). Cannabinoid Formulations and Delivery Systems: Current and Future Options to Treat Pain. *Drugs*, 81: 1513–1557.

Tagsold, D., Toni, I., Trollmann, R., Woelfle, J., and Gravou-Apostolatou, C. (2024). The use of cannabinoids in pediatric palliative care-a retrospective single-center analysis. *Children* (Basel), 11: 234.

Tarlovski, S., Bar Kadmon, A., Goldberg, E., Segal, D., Gavish, D., and Stepensky, D. (2025). Comparative pharmacokinetic assessment of innovative sublingual, rectal and vaporizer cannabis products versus approved cannabis products in healthy volunteers. *Cannabis and Cannabinoid Research*, 10: E289–e298.

Torres, D., Pereira, E., Sampaio, P., Souza, N., Ferraz, C., Oliveira, A. et al. (2018). Influence of extraction process on flavonoid content from *Cnidoscolus quercifolius* pohl (Euphorbiaceae) and antioxidant activity. *Quimica Nova*, 41: 743–747.

Vergallo, C. (2020) Nutraceutical vegetable oil nanoformulations for prevention and management of diseases. *Nanomaterials* (Basel), 10: 1232.

Wang Xue, Lin, C., Jin, S., Wang, Y., Peng, Y., and Wang, X. (2023). Cannabidiol alleviates neuroinflammation and attenuates neuropathic pain via targeting FKBP5. *Brain, Behavior, and Immunity*, 111: 365–375.

Wróblewska-Łuczka, P., Cabaj, J., Bargieł, J., and Łuszczki, J. J. (2023). Anticancer effect of terpenes: focus on malignant melanoma. *Pharmacological Reports*, 75: 1115–1125.

Yang, J., Li, N., Wang, C., Chang, T., and Jiang, H. (2021). Ultrasound-homogenization-assisted extraction of polyphenols from coconut mesocarp: Optimization study. *Ultrasonics Sonochemistry*, 78: 105739.

Zargoosh, Z., Ghavam, M., Bacchetta, G., and Tavili, A. (2019). Effects of ecological factors on the antioxidant potential and total phenol content of *Scrophularia striata* Boiss. *Scientific Reports*, 9: 16021.

Zgair, A., Lee, J. B., Wong, J. C. M., Taha, D. A., Aram, J., di Virgilio, D. et al. (2017). Oral administration of cannabis with lipids leads to high levels of cannabinoids in the intestinal lymphatic system and prominent immunomodulation. *Scientific Reports*, 7: 14542.

Zgair, A., Wong, J. C. M., Lee, J. B., Mistry, J., Sivak, O., Wasan, K. M. et al. (2016). Dietary fats and pharmaceutical lipid excipients increase systemic exposure to orally administered cannabis and cannabis-based medicines. *American Journal of Translational Research*, 8: 3448.

Section 2
Secondary Metabolites and Therapeutic Potential

Chapter 5

Secondary Metabolites in *Cannabis sativa*

Illa Fernanda Mesquita Silva,[1,3] *Herbert Gonzaga Sousa,*[1,2] *Natasha Alves Rocha,*[1] *Penina Sousa Mourão,*[1] *Wellington Silva Aguiar,*[1] *Isaac Bruno Paz Santos,*[1,3] *Patrícia e Silva Alves,*[1,2] *Rosemarie Brandim Marques*[1,3] and *Valdiléia Teixeira Uchôa*[1,*]

1. Introduction

Cannabis is an endemic plant of the Indian subcontinent and Asia. It is believed to have originated in the East and Central Asia, spreading throughout Asia and reaching Europe. Considered one of the first plants cultivated by humans, *Cannabis sativa* has evidence of early use in China, where it served both as food and as a raw material for the production of paper and cooking oil. Additionally, its medicinal potential was explored in China, where it was prescribed for pain relief, malaria treatment, and as an anesthetic in surgical procedures, as documented in the world's first pharmacopeia (Berardo et al. 2024; Almeida et al. 2021).

Cannabis sativa L., popularly known as marijuana, is a dicotyledonous plant of the Cannabaceae family and belongs to the Rosales order. It is an annual, erect herb with palmate-shaped leaves and small, yellowish-green flowers, growing between 1 and 6 meters in height. It has separate male and female inflorescences (dioecious), requiring it to undergo cross-pollination. The female flowers are particularly rich in acidic cannabinoids. Considered one of the fastest-growing plants in the world, it has a complex leaf structure. *Cannabis sativa* has various applications in industries such as textiles, construction, paper, food, pharmaceuticals, and cosmetics. It is used for fiber production, oil, and edible seeds, and has medicinal properties, making it also employed as a drug. Traditionally, the plant has been used for pain relief, malaria treatment, and as an anesthetic in surgical procedures, as recorded in the world's first pharmacopeia (Malabadi et al. 2023; Hancock et al. 2024).

Cannabis contains hundreds of specialized metabolites with bioactive potential, including cannabinoids, terpenes, and flavonoids, which are produced and accumulated in glandular trichomes, especially in the female inflorescences. Among the cannabinoids, cannabidiol (CBD) and tetrahydrocannabinol (THC) are the most prominent. CBD, in particular, has attracted increasing attention due to its anxiolytic, anti-inflammatory, anticonvulsant, neuroprotective, analgesic, and

[1] PPGQ - Department of Chemistry, Piaui State University, Teresina, PI, CEP-64002-150, Brazil.
[2] PPGQ - Department of Chemistry, Federal University of Piaui, Teresina, PI CEP-64049-550, Brazil.
[3] NPBio - Piaui State University, Teresina, PI, CEP 64003-120, Brazil.
* Corresponding author: valdileiatexeira@ccn.uespi.br

DOI: 10.1201/9781003668190-7

antitumor properties, and is widely investigated for its therapeutic potential in treating psychiatric disorders. In addition to its therapeutic applications, cannabis has also been explored for innovative uses, such as bioplastics, biofuels, and biopesticides. Its compounds and derivatives have been used in the treatment of various pathological conditions, including cancer, Alzheimer's disease, multiple sclerosis, chronic pain, inflammation, glaucoma, and other diseases (Almeida et al. 2021; Raihan and Bijoy 2023).

For many years, negative or skeptical views regarding alternative therapies hindered the development of an effective therapeutic alliance and limited research on *Cannabis sativa*. The widespread prohibition of the plant prevented the development of agricultural policies and guidelines that could mitigate its negative environmental impacts. However, in the last two decades, the legalization and decriminalization of *Cannabis sativa* L. have significantly advanced in several regions around the world. Advocates for legalization highlight the environmental, industrial, and health benefits of the plant, as well as its wide range of uses, arguing that it should be considered a viable and profitable cash crop for farmers. This progress has enabled a more comprehensive and balanced analysis of the benefits and risks associated with the plant's use, which was previously limited by the scarcity of research and appropriate regulations (Malabadi et al. 2023).

2. Popular Use and Ethnobotanical Study

C. sativa is a species of notable pharmacological and industrial relevance; however, its use is not limited to these domains, also assuming historical, cultural, and symbolic significance among various peoples throughout history (Bonini et al. 2018). It is further estimated that *C. sativa* is one of the first plants domesticated by humanity, with cultivation records dating back approximately 12,000 years (Malabadi et al. 2023). Its multiple by-products are obtained from the flowers, stems, and seeds, and have been used for therapeutic, ritualistic, dietary, and textile purposes in different sociocultural contexts (Karche 2019).

The earliest records of the medicinal use of *C. sativa* date back to the Chinese Emperor Shen Neng, around 2,737 BC. In his manuscripts, compiled in the *Pen Tsao*, considered the first pharmacopoeia in the world, he recommended infusions of the plant's parts in tea form for the treatment of various ailments, such as intestinal and joint pain (Almeida et al. 2021). Later, around 1,500 BC, the *Ebers Papyrus*, a medical compendium developed by the Egyptians, described more than 700 substances and therapeutic formulations, among which was "Shemshemet," a preparation based on *C. sativa* recognized for its anti-inflammatory and antioxidant properties (Cvijic and Bauer 2024). In the 15th century, in the Middle East, the physician Al-Bradi documented in 1464 CE the use of *C. sativa* in the treatment of refractory epilepsy, marking a historical milestone in the therapeutic application of the plant in neurological disorders (Carvalho et al. 2017).

In addition to its medicinal use, *C. sativa* has a long trajectory of use in spiritual and religious contexts. Archaeological evidence and sacred texts indicate that the plant was revered as sacred in various ancient cultures (Berardo et al. 2024). In India, for example, records in the *Atharva Veda*, one of the four Vedas of Hinduism, dated approximately 1,400 BCE, mention *C. sativa* as one of five sacred plants used to invoke divine benevolence and achieve expanded states of consciousness (Malabadi et al. 2023).

In the Middle East, archaeological findings in Israeli sites, such as the Temple of Tel Arad (8th century BCE), revealed cannabinoid residues in incense altars, suggesting ritualistic use of the plant in the ancient Kingdom of Judah (Charitos et al. 2021). In the Rastafarian tradition, which emerged in Jamaica in the 20th century, *C. sativa* is regarded as a sacramental herb, used in meditation and spiritual communion rituals, serving as a means of connection with the divine (Malabadi et al. 2023).

In the Brazilian context, the earliest records of *C. sativa* use date back to the colonial period, when the plant was introduced into the country by Portuguese colonizers and, primarily, by enslaved African peoples, who already utilized the herb in their religious rituals and medicinal practices (Charitos et al. 2021).

During the 19th century, its use spread among the lower classes, especially in urban peripheries, where it was consumed for pain relief, sleep disturbances, and as a form of socialization (Cvijic and Bauer 2024). However, with the rise of hygienist, racist, and moralist discourses, its consumption became criminalized.

Throughout the 20th century, the repression of the cultivation, trade, and consumption of *C. sativa* intensified, with the criminalization of the plant becoming increasingly strict and widespread. The law criminalized the consumption and trade of *C. sativa*, as well as imposed severe penalties for trafficking and use, contributing to the marginalization of those who used the plant. The adoption of this legislation was part of a broader trend observed in several countries around the world, aiming to control the consumption of psychoactive substances and combat drug trafficking (Bonini et al. 2018).

This repression intensified over time, with *C. sativa* being associated with risky behaviors and a public safety issue, rather than being viewed from a public health or even individual freedom perspective (Shakil et al. 2021). This shift in approach, now more focused on criminalizing trafficking and treating users, reflected the global movement seeking a more intense response to the so-called "war on drugs" (Koram 2022).

In recent years, there has been progress in discussions about its regulation, particularly in the health field, with court decisions allowing domestic cultivation for medicinal purposes and the use of CBD-based medications (cannabidiol) under medical prescription, thus demonstrating the need for more studies that address the scientific, legal, and medical interests to fill gaps in the debates about the free consumption of the plant (Rezende et al. 2023).

3. Phytochemical study of *C. sativa* L.

The phytochemical characterization of *C. sativa* plays a crucial role in elucidating its biological properties, controlling the quality of derivatives, and expanding its therapeutic applications (Hourfane et al. 2023). Its pharmacological value lies mainly in the complexity of the chemical compounds it produces, especially secondary metabolites such as cannabinoids, terpenes, and flavonoids (Adams et al. 2021).

The plant contains more than 550 bioactive molecules, the most characteristic of which are cannabinoids, found mainly in the female flowers. However, it also exhibits a diversity of phytocannabinoids with biological potential (Welling et al. 2022; Tzimas et al. 2024).

C. sativa produces a variety of phytocannabinoids, the main ones being Δ9-tetrahydrocannabinol (Δ9-THC), CBD, cannabigerol (CBG), and cannabinol (CBN). These molecules have chemical structures derived from carboxylic acids, such as tetrahydrocannabinolic acid (THCA), cannabidiolic acid (CBDA), and cannabigerolic acid (CBGA), which are precursor forms biosynthesized in the plant's inflorescences (Birenboim et al. 2022; Tzimas et al. 2024). THC is known for its psychoactive effects, while CBD exhibits anxiolytic, anti-inflammatory, and anticonvulsant properties and has been widely studied due to its good clinical tolerability (Welling et al. 2022).

Recently, dimeric phytocannabinoids have been identified, further expanding the plant's chemical diversity. Cannabisol, a THC dimer, and cannabitwinol (CBDD), a CBD dimer, have structures linked by a methylene bridge. Initial studies indicate that CBDD exhibits affinity for TRP-type channels, which are involved in detecting stimuli such as temperature and pain. These channels have been widely investigated as promising targets in the development of new analgesic and anti-inflammatory drugs, although the *in vivo* effects of CBDD are not yet fully understood (Welling et al. 2022).

Terpenes are one of the main classes of secondary metabolites in *C. sativa* and are responsible for a large part of its characteristic aroma. Among the most abundant compounds are myrcene, (E)-caryophyllene, and α-pinene, as well as others such as limonene, terpinolene, and linalool (Mazzara et al. 2022; Birenboim et al. 2022). Myrcene is an earthy-smelling monoterpene included in CBD formulations that have shown improved sleep quality in patients with insomnia, while (E) β-caryophyllene is a spicy-scented sesquiterpene with anti-inflammatory action mediated by the CB2 receptor (Dickson et al. 2023; Wang et al. 2025).

Terpenes interact functionally with cannabinoids, potentiating or modulating their pharmacological effects in a phenomenon known as the entourage effect. This synergistic effect has been proposed as an explanation for the more pronounced analgesic, anxiolytic, and anti-inflammatory activities observed in whole-plant extracts, compared to the use of isolated compounds (Simei et al. 2024).

The essential oils extracted from the flowers and inflorescences of *C. sativa* are mainly composed of volatile terpenes. Studies show marked variations between varieties and cultivation methods: some oils have a predominance of trans-caryophyllene, while others have more α-pinene or nerolidol (Rezghiyan et al. 2025). These differences are associated with the genetics of the plant, the part of the plant analyzed, and the extraction and storage conditions.

In addition to cannabinoids and terpenes, *C. sativa* produces a wide range of secondary metabolites with pharmacological relevance, including flavonoids, alkaloids, and lignans. The flavonoids found in the plant belong mainly to the flavone and flavonol subclasses, such as apigenin, luteolin, kaempferol, and quercetin, as well as the unique prenylated flavones called canflavins (Tzimas et al. 2024). These compounds have antioxidant, anti-inflammatory and neuroprotective activities, thereby contributing to the plant's therapeutic effects.

The identified alkaloids include compounds such as cannabisativine, cannabimine C, and anhydrocannabisativine, which are primarily located in the leaves and are likely involved in defense against herbivory and regulation of plant growth (Hourfane et al. 2023). Lignans, like cannabisins, also possess antioxidant properties and are involved in protecting cells against oxidative stress (Tzimas et al. 2024).

The lipid composition of *C. sativa* is a notable feature, particularly in the seeds, which contain a high proportion of polyunsaturated fatty acids. Linoleic acid is the most abundant, followed by oleic acid and palmitic acid (Raoui et al. 2024). This composition gives the seeds high nutritional value and potential use in nutraceutical formulations. The seeds also contain various phenolic compounds, such as epicatechin and phenolic acids, as well as flavonoids and lignanamides, including cannabisin B, which enhance the plant's antioxidant activity and therapeutic potential (El-Mernissi et al. 2024).

The phytochemical composition of *C. sativa* is highly variable and depends on a combination of genetic, environmental, and cultivation factors. This variation directly affects the levels of cannabinoids, terpenes, and other secondary metabolites, influencing both the therapeutic properties and sensory aspects of the plant (Tzimas et al. 2024).

4. Cannabinoids

Among the various secondary metabolites produced by *Cannabis sativa* L. are cannabinoid (terpenophenolic) compounds, which are categorized into three types: phytocannabinoids, synthetic cannabinoids, and endogenous cannabinoids, also known as endocannabinoids (Carvalho et al. 2020). It is worth noting that this class of metabolites has only been identified in cannabis to date (Akhtar et al. 2016). These metabolites can be found in the resin glands, with the highest concentration of cannabinoids in the flowering tips, followed by the leaves, stem, and roots, but not in the seeds (Dinis-Oliveira 2016).

Phytocannabinoids are lipophilic terpenoid compounds derived from resorcinol, with structures that are distinct from, yet pharmacologically similar to, endogenous ligands and synthetic cannabinoids (Carvalho et al. 2017; Carvalho et al. 2020). Synthetic cannabinoids are analogues of phytocannabinoids, i.e., they have similar chemical structures to phytocannabinoids. Endocannabinoids, on the other hand, are described as endogenous ligands and cannabinoid receptors 1 (CB1) and 2 (CB2), which together with their respective metabolic enzymes and membrane transporters, make up the endocannabinoid system (ECS) (Carvalho et al. 2020, Fonseca et al. 2019), the best known endocannabinoids being 2-arachidonoylglycerol and anandamide (Figure 1).

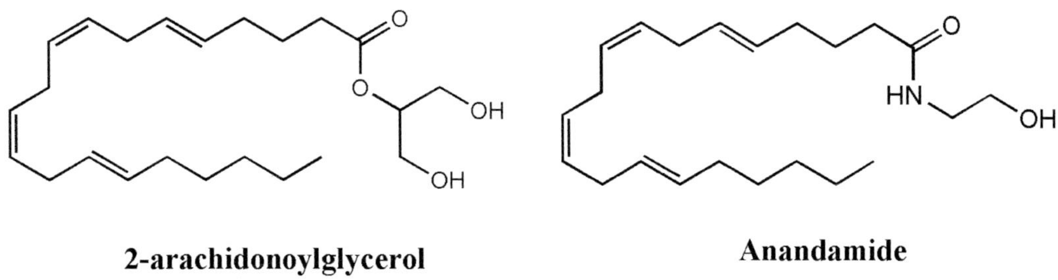

Figure 1: Structure of the most reported endocannabinoids. Source: Authors

CB1 cannabinoid receptors are located in the central nervous system, particularly in regions that mediate cognitive functions, pain, short-term memory, coordination, motor control, hypothermia, and hyperflagia. CB2 receptors, on the other hand, are found in the peripheral system and play a role in the immune system, including T cells, B cells, the spleen, tonsils, and activated microglial cells (Bonfá et al. 2008).

Around 60 substances make up the cannabinoid class, the most commonly found in extracts being: tetrahydrocannabinolic acid (THCA) and cannabidiolic acid (CBDA), which can be converted, by heating as a decarboxylation process, to their neutral forms: tetrahydrocannabinol (THC) and cannabidiol (CBD) (Carvalho et al. 2020; Garcia and Barbosa Neto 2023). THCA and CBDA are often detected in the flowering tops of rich pistillate (female) specimens. THC and CBD were the first phytocannabinoids to be isolated and identified (Castillo-Arellano et al. 2023). Another well-known compound is cannabinol (CBN), a degradation product of THC (Carvalho et al. 2020). However, other phytocannabinoids have been identified, including cannabigerol, cannabichromene, cannabivarin, tetrahydrocannabivarin, cannabichromenevarin, and cannabigerovarin (Figure 2; Carvalho et al. 2017).

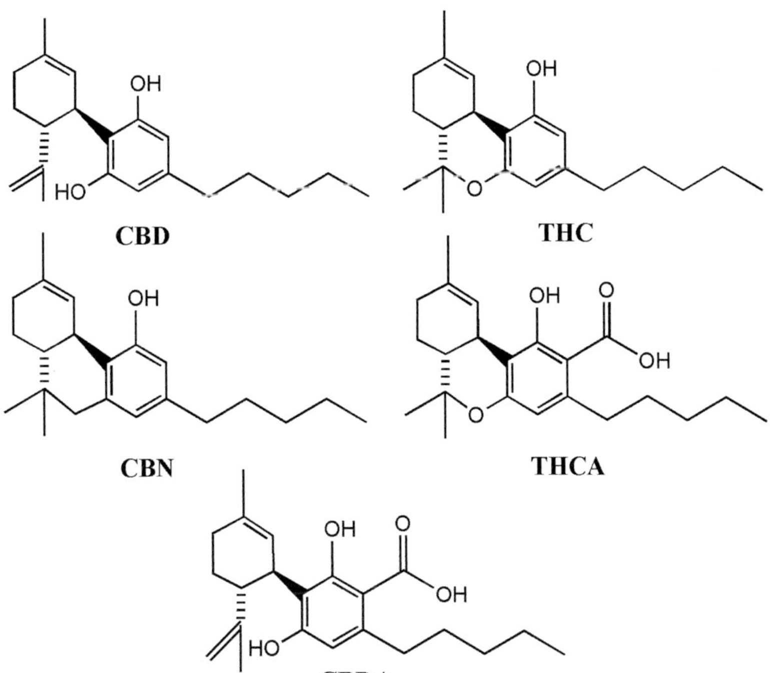

Figure 2: Main cannabinoids found in *Cannabis sativa* L. Source: Authors

Explaining a little about the chemical structure of cannabinoids, most of them have three rings in their structure (A, B, and C). Ring A is similar to resorcinol (mentioned above), ring B is similar to a terpenoid fraction, and ring C can be formed through intramolecular cyclisation (Figure 3). A widely used nomenclature system for cannabinoids is the benzopyran numbering system, in addition to the monoterpene system (Akhtar et al. 2016). As such, the cannabinoid THC can be labelled D^9-THC, following the benzopyran numbering system, and can also be known as D^1-THC, using the monoterpene numbering system (Akhtar et al. 2016).

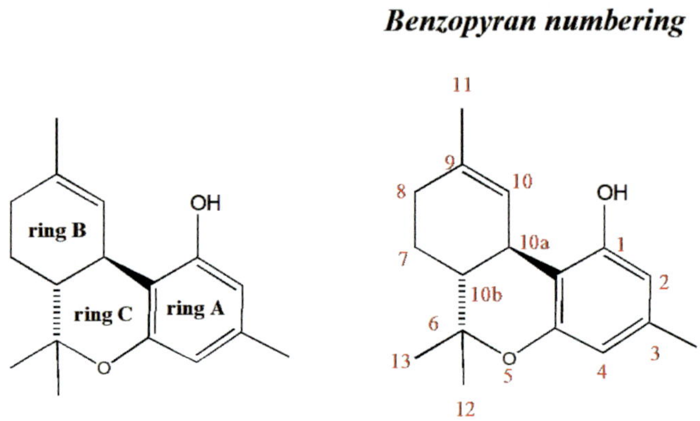

Figure 3: Structure and benzopyran numbering of cannabinoids. Source: Authors.

A biosynthetic route for cannabinoids, THC, and cannabidiol, being the most abundant in cannabis, is presented by Bloemendal et al. (2020) in a review paper that also presents various synthesis routes for THC analogues (i.e., synthetic cannabinoids). The biosynthesis of cannabinoids begins by obtaining geranyl pyrophosphate (GPP), one of the precursors of most terpenoids, which is derived from the coupling of dimethylallyl pyrophosphate (DMAPP) and isopentenyl pyrophosphate (IPP) via (non)-mavalonate and geranyl pyrophosphate synthase (Bloemendal et al. 2020). After obtaining GPP, it is coupled with olivetolic acid by geranyl transferase to produce cannabigerolic acid (CBGA), followed by stereoselective cyclisation induced by CBDA or THCA synthase, leading to the formation of cannabidiolic acid (CBDA) and Δ^9-tetrahydrocannabinolic acid (Δ^9-THCA) (Bloemendal et al., 2020; Figure 4).

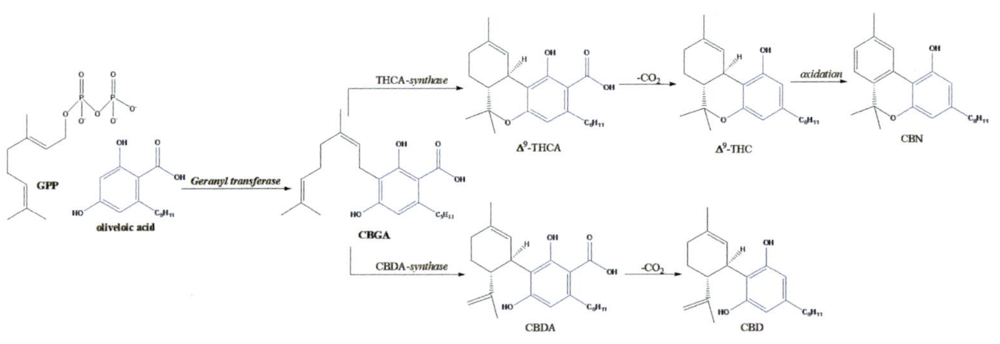

Figure 4: Biosynthetic route for obtaining cannabinoids. Source: Authors

Synthetic cannabinoids can not only have similar structures to phytocannabinoids, but are designed to target the endocannabinoid system and exert a higher affinity for cannabinoid receptors than Δ^9-THC, but with more intense effects and shorter duration (Roque-Bravo et al. 2023). They can be categorised into groups, some of which are shown in Figure 5.

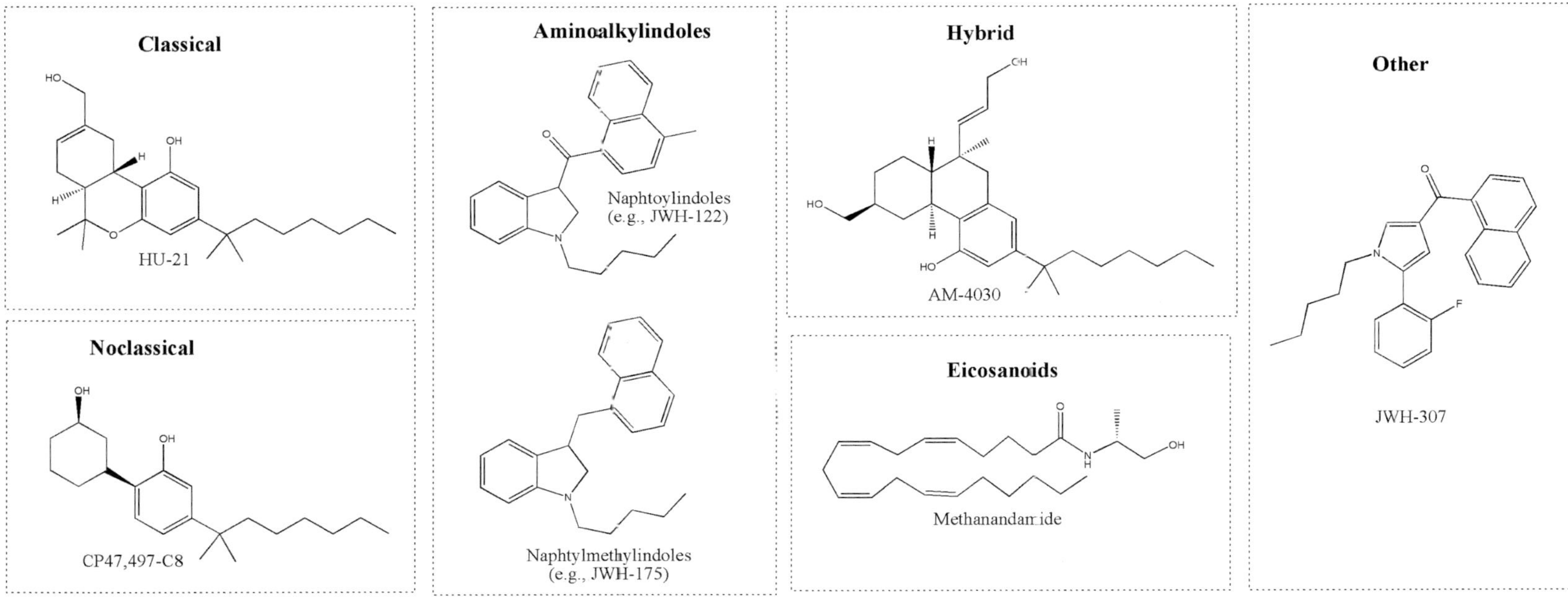

Figure 5. Some of the groups that use synthetic cannabinoids. Source: Authors.

Cannabinoids are widely used in medicine to treat various diseases, such as glaucoma (to reduce intraocular pressure), multiple sclerosis, and to help increase appetite, increase body fat, reduce nausea, and improve functional status. Antioxidant, anti-inflammatory, anticonvulsant, and analgesic properties have been observed (Fonseca et al. 2019). D^9-THC is the most psychoactive component of the cannabis plant, with its (-)-*trans* form more potent than the (+)-*trans* isomer, while the other constituents are not very psychoactive, such as CBD, CBN, cannabigerol, and cannabichromene (Akhtar et al. 2016; Dinis-Oliveira 2016). Acid cannabinoids are also not psychotropic (Akhtar et al. 2016). The mechanism of action of cannabinoids is based on the activation of the endocannabinoid system, via the cannabinoid receptors mentioned above, which results in the release of neurotransmitters, particularly glutamate (Camargo Filho et al. 2019).

Mechoulam et al. (2002) presented a review of the chemistry of CBD and discussed its anticonvulsant, anxiolytic, antipsychotic, antinausea, and anti-arthritic properties. We also suggest reading the work by Araujo et al. (2023), which discusses the mechanism of action of cannabinoids. They emphasise that the recreational use of cannabis due to the high THC content in humans can lead to addiction, mental, gastrointestinal, and cardiovascular problems for a limited period of time, as well as car accidents, among others.

Finally, we will comment a little on the methods used to identify cannabinoids. Chromatographic techniques, such as GC-MS and HPLC, are the most widely used in chemistry for identifying compounds. Antunes et al. (2023) compiled a review on the identification of cannabinoids in various biological specimens, including blood (and its derivatives), urine, and others. Highlighting the use of LC-MS as an effective technique for this type of analysis, given that the identification and quantification of acidic cannabinoids, such as THC-COOH, CBGA, and CBDA, can be difficult since they are decarboxylated into their neutral forms during GC analysis.

Rantaša and colleagues (2024) discuss the use of supercritical fluid extraction of cannabinoids and their analysis by liquid chromatography and supercritical fluid chromatography in their literature review. They point out that processes using supercritical fluids offer the possibility of ecologically correct, simple, and economical operation (using CO_2 as a solvent, for example), leading to exceptional solvent-free extracts of greater purity.

5. Flavonoids

One of the main secondary metabolites present in plants is flavonoids, also known as polyphenolic compounds, whose primary functions include biological activities such as protection and nutrition, as well as therapeutic actions found in plants, including anti-inflammatory, antioxidant, and antifungal activity, among others (Moreau et al. 2019). They are produced in large quantities by some plants and exhibit an exponential diversity within the flavonoid class, with thousands of flavonoids having specific characteristics for each plant (Martin et al. 2022).

The biosynthesis of flavonoids begins via the shikimate pathway, starting with the presence of phenylalanine. When phenylalanine comes into contact with the enzyme phenylalanine ammonia lyase (PAL), it removes the amine group from the compound, forming cinnamic acid. It then undergoes a hydroxylation process, and the presence of three molecules of malonyl-CoA, which promotes the formation of a chalcone (initial flavonoid for the formation of the other classes), and from these new reactions results in new polyphenolic compounds, as shown in Figure 6.

With a fundamental architecture of 15 carbon atoms, called phenylbenzopyran, flavonoids have three interconnected rings (A, B, and C) in their composition. These rings correspond to an aromatic system, a phenyl group, and a central heterocyclic ring (C6 – C3 – C6) (Martin et al. 2022). The numbering of the carbons in this structure makes it possible to identify the positions where different substituents can bind. The aromatic ring A and the heterocyclic ring C are fused, while the phenyl group B connects to carbon 2 of the heterocyclic ring. In addition to this structure, there is a carbonyl group, which can be present in several flavonoid compounds, on carbon 4 of the heterocyclic ring, and there is also the potential for several branches on carbons 3 to 8 of ring A and carbons 3' to 5'

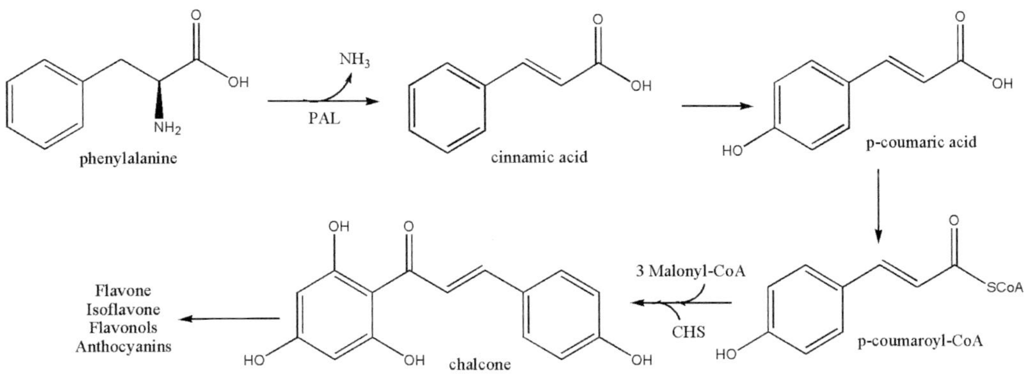

Figure 6: Flavonoid biosynthesis. Source: Authors

of ring B, where these specifications lead to the formation of classes of these phenolic compounds (Pereira et al. 2016).

According to Martin et al. (2022), there are more than twenty flavonoids that have been found in *Cannabis sativa* through HPLC analysis, where the most abundant are flavones, which include apigenin and luteolin, flavonoids such as kaempferol and quercetin, as well as aglycones and glycosides. In addition, prenylated and geranylated flavones, canflavin A, B, and C, which were isolated from *C. sativa* and are exclusive to this species.

Studies carried out on the extract of this plant have shown some of the main phenolic compounds, such as gallic acid, rosmarinic acid, caffeic acid, p-OH-benzoic acid, p-coumaric acid, as well as some flavonoids such as caniprene, canflavin, catechin, naringenin, resveratrol, and apigenin (Table 1) in extracts of *C. Sativa* (Allegrone et al. 2017).

Flavonoids are widely recognized for their antioxidant properties and have attracted considerable interest due to their potential in preventing and treating various pathologies. In addition, studies suggest that flavonoids may exhibit antiviral properties against a variety of viruses, including HIV, poliomyelitis, and respiratory viruses, among others. Due to their antioxidant properties and potential anticarcinogenic effects, flavonoids have been the subject of increasing attention in scientific research (Rea et al. 2019).

C. sativa has a rich phytochemical composition, highlighted in the literature, with canflavin being one of the main flavonoids identified. Canflavins A and B have been characterized as having a low cannabinoid content (Werz et al. 2014). A distinctive feature is that canflavins represent a class of flavonoids unique to the *Cannabis* plant and belong to the group of flavonoids called flavones. Flavones perform multiple crucial functions in plants, including modulating physiological processes, displacing compounds, and interacting with pathogenic organisms (Rea et al. 2019).

In structural terms, canflavins feature the addition of hydrophobic molecules, and these compounds are derived from luteolin, a flavonoid common in several plant species, including legumes and fruits consumed in human food (Rea et al. 2019). They can be identified in cannabis, demonstrating antioxidant, anti-inflammatory, and apparently also anticancer activities (Moreau et al. 2019). The mechanism of action of these two canflavins involves inhibiting the production of two crucial inflammatory mediators: prostaglandin E2 and leukotrienes (Werz et al. 2014). Furthermore, it is important to note that the occurrence and quantity of flavonoids can vary significantly between different strains of cannabis and depend on the cultivation practices adopted.

6. Terpenes

They are aromatic and lipophilic molecules, responsible for the characteristic aroma of *Cannabis sativa*, representing the second largest class of secondary metabolites found in the plant, behind phytocannabinoids. Terpenoids (terpenes with oxygen in their structure) play important roles in the

Table 1: Flavonoids are found in *C. sativa* extracts. Source: Adapted from Allegrone et al. (2017).

Compound	**Structure**	**Compound**	**Structure**
gallic acid	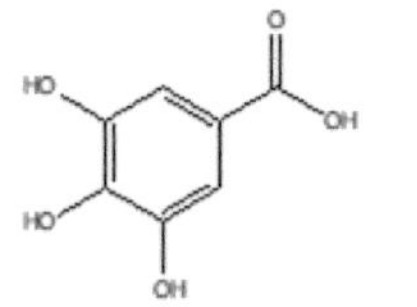	cannflavin A	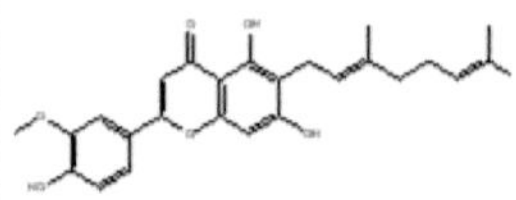
rosmarinic acid	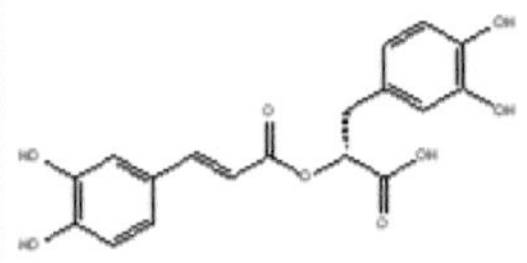	cannflavin B	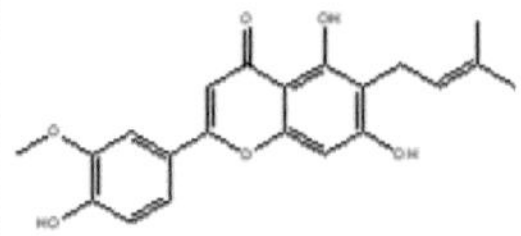
caffeic acid	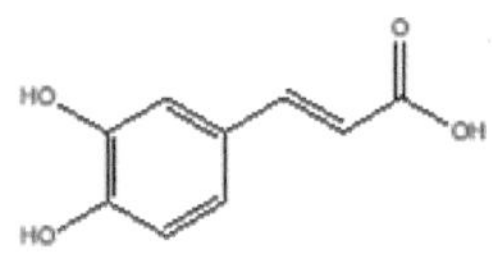	catechin	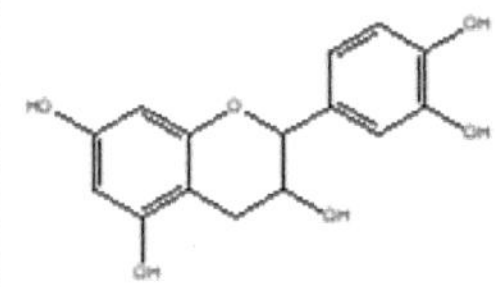
p-OH-benzoic acid	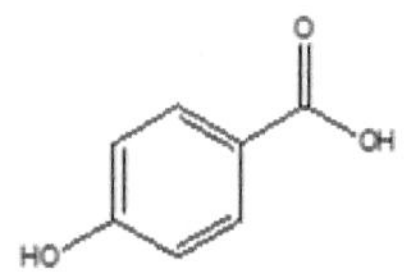	narigenin	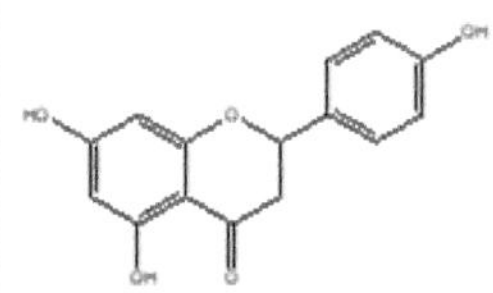
p-coumaric acid	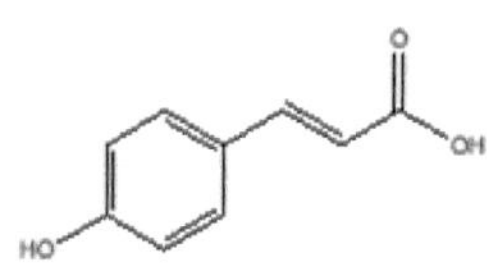	resveratrol	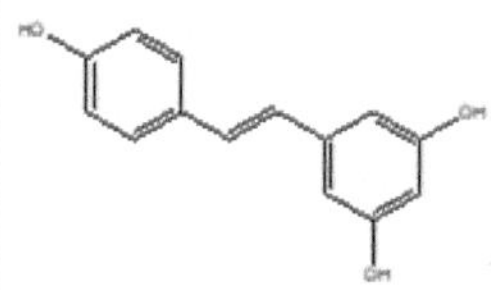
canniprene	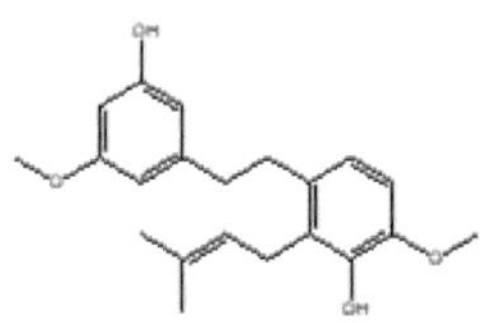	apigenin	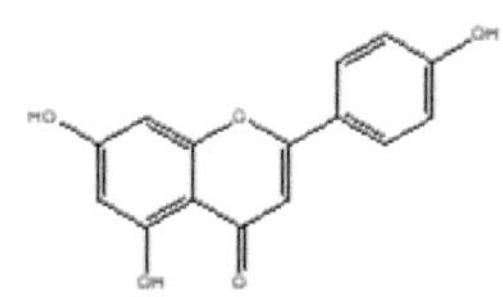

plant, including acting as phytohormones, membrane stabilizers, and participating in respiration, photosynthesis, cell signaling, and protective mechanisms (Laaboud et al. 2024). Their composition varies according to the plant's genetics, environmental factors, and stage of maturity. This is particularly important in the current context, as the increase in the medicinal use of the plant on an industrial and domestic scale, especially in the production of oils, has been driven by the synergistic effects between terpenes and cannabinoids, which potentiate their actions on the nervous system (Caruso et al. 2024).

Since the composition is highly susceptible to variability, it is challenging to determine the main terpenes in *C. sativa*. However, one study analyzed 33 samples of psychoactive cannabis (chemotype I) and light cannabis (chemotype III), and in agreement with other data in the literature, defined the main terpenes/terpenoids of *C. sativa* as: β-caryophyllene, β-myrcene, terpinolene, α-humulene, D-limonene, α-pinene, β-pinene, and cis-β-ocimene, which are present in both chemotypes and account for more than 80% of the total terpene content (Dei Cas et al. 2021). These compounds were also found in abundance in the inflorescences of three *C. sativa* genotypes collected at three stages of maturity, and in five different commercial cultivars of medicinal cannabis produced by Bedrocan International (Bedica®, Bediol®, Bedrobinol®, Bedrocan®, and Bedrolite®) (Francisco et al. 2024; Fulvio et al. 2025). Except for cis-β-Ocimene (Figure 7), the other terpenes have been extensively investigated for their biological activities and therapeutic potential.

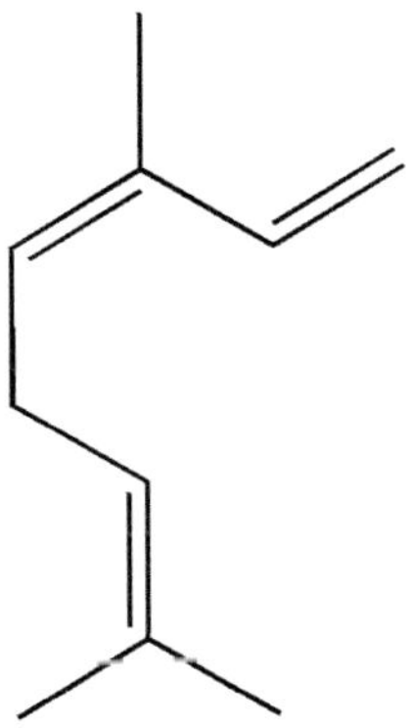

Figure 7: Structure of cis-β-Ocymene. Source: Authors.

β-Caryophyllene (Figure 8) is a sesquiterpene (15C) with important biological activities reported, both alone and in combination with other compounds (synergistic effects), including on the endocannabinoid system (CB2) (Klauke et al. 2014). Anti-inflammatory activity is among the most frequently reported, having been demonstrated in various models, including murine macrophages, rats, and mice (Weimer et al. 2023). It has also shown potential in treating depression, due to its antioxidant and anti-inflammatory effects (Al-Shudifat et al. 2024). In addition, neuroprotective properties are frequently reported, with promising therapeutic potential for Alzheimer's disease and perioperative neurocognitive disorders (PND) (Brand-Rubalcava et al. 2023).

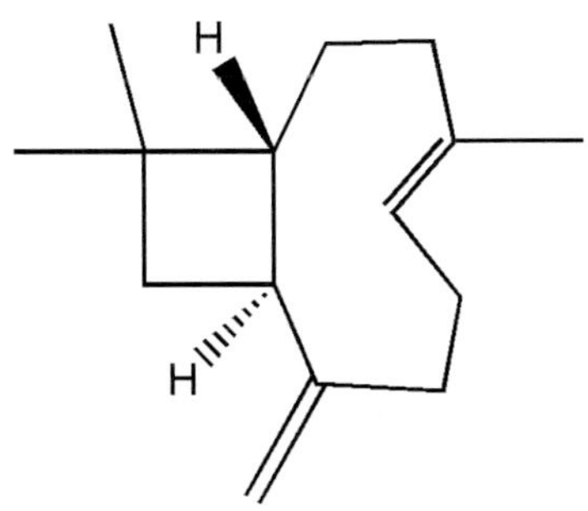

Figure 8: Structure of β-Caryophyllene. Source: Authors.

β-Myrcene (Figure 9) is a monoterpene (10C) widely used as a flavoring in foods in various regions of the world, and occurs naturally at high levels. It exhibits various biological activities, including anti-ulcer properties, and has been shown to protect against oxidative and histological damage in cardiac tissue following global ischemia-reperfusion (Bonamin et al. 2014). The most recent studies demonstrate its neuroprotective effects, with potential for treating Alzheimer's disease, as well as anti-inflammatory effects by inhibiting the activity of inflammatory cytokines and pro-inflammatory signals *in vivo* (Kumar et al. 2021).

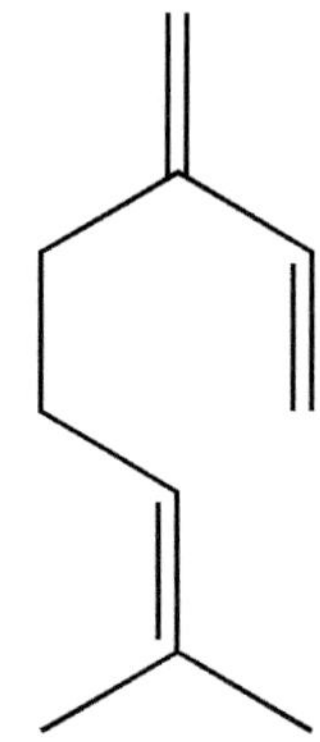

Figure 9: Structure of β-Myrcene. Source: Authors.

Terpinolene (Figure 10) is a monoterpene (10 C) widely used in the food industry as a flavoring agent. In an *in vitro* study, it attenuated inflammation and oxidative stress and may contribute to expanding wound treatment options. More recently, it has demonstrated significant anti-inflammatory activity in mouse models of paw edema induced by different phlogistic agents, by inhibiting acute inflammatory responses and reducing the development of granulomas (Menezes et al. 2021).

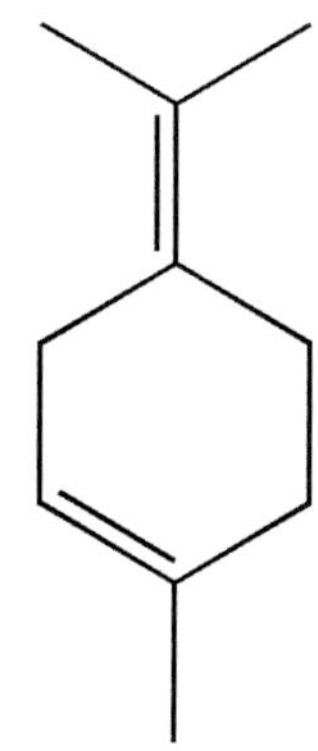

Figure 10: Structure of Terpinolene. Source: Authors.

α-Humulene (Figure 11), an isomer of β-Caryophyllene, is also a sesquiterpene with diverse biological potentials, such as antibacterial and antibiofilm effects against enterotoxigenic *Bacteroides fragilis*, which is associated with inflammatory bowel diseases (Jang et al. 2020). Its anticancer potential is widely reported; most recently, its antiproliferative effects have been demonstrated, alone, against hepatocellular carcinoma (HCC) cells, inducing apoptosis by inhibiting Akt signaling, both *in vitro* and *in vivo*, and coadministration with sclereol was effective in inhibiting the growth of pancreatic cancer (Kang et al. 2022).

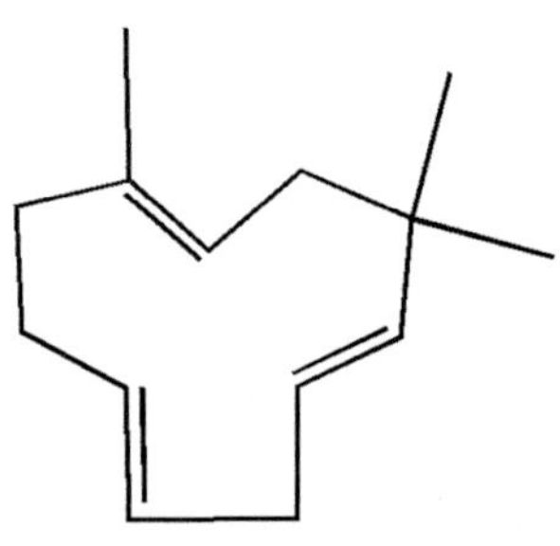

Figure 11: Structure of α-Humulene. Source: Authors.

D-Limonene (Figure 12), the primary component of citrus oils, is a monoterpene widely used in the food industry due to its aroma, antioxidant and antimicrobial properties. Its antibiofilm effect was effective in controlling the bacteria *Bacillus amyloliquefaciens* in soy-based products (Lü et al. 2024). More recently, it has demonstrated therapeutic potential in reducing ovarian damage caused by ischemia and reperfusion, as well as in the treatment of atopic dermatitis due to its anti-inflammatory properties (Chu et al. 2025). It has also potentiated the anti-cancer effects of Cisplatin in breast and bladder cancer cell lines (Laws III and Smid 2024).

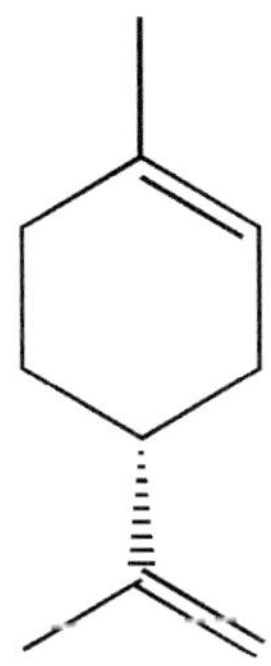

Figure 12: Structure of D-Limonene. Source: Authors.

α-Pinene and β-Pinene (Figure 13) are monoterpenes with important biological activities. These include neuroprotective effects against beta-amyloid-mediated neurotoxicity, as well as antimicrobial, anti-inflammatory, and antioxidant properties (Wei et al. 2025). In addition, α-pinene effectively attenuated oxidative damage, cognitive deficits, and depressive and anxious behaviors in the brains of mice treated with ketamine in a ketamine-induced mouse model of schizophrenia (Moghaddam et al. 2024). On the other hand, β-pinene inhibited adenovirus type 3 more effectively than the reference antiviral drug (ribavirin), but had no protective effects on cells (Qiu et al. 2022).

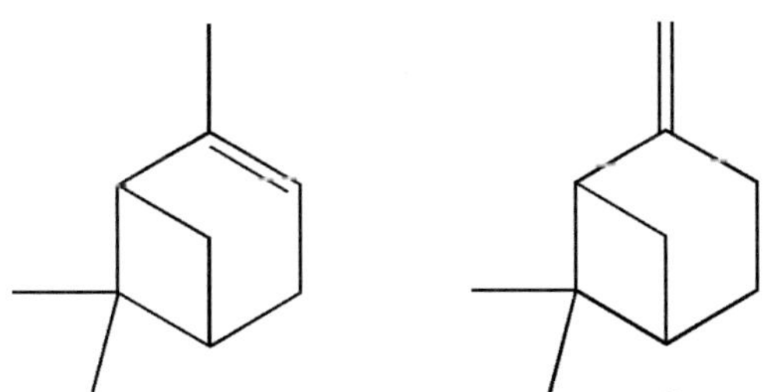

α β

Figure 13: Pinene structures. Source: Authors.

C. sativa terpenes show great therapeutic potential due to their wide range of biological activities, including anti-inflammatory, antioxidant, neuroprotective, and antimicrobial effects. A synergistic effect has also been demonstrated, reinforcing the concept of the "entourage effect" and underscoring the need for more targeted formulations for different clinical conditions. Furthermore, knowledge about many terpenes, such as cis-β-ocimene, remains limited, underscoring the need for further research to elucidate their mechanisms of action and their therapeutic potential. Continued research into the pharmacological profile of terpenes could therefore open up new horizons for *C. sativa* medicine and boost the development of new herbal medicines.

6.1 Structure-Activity Relationship of Cannabinoids

Cannabinoids, both natural and synthetic, have been shown to exhibit a wide range of biological effects due to their interactions with various molecular targets (Cortez-Resendiz et al. 2025).

Modifying their chemical structures can optimize important pharmacological aspects, such as selectivity and potency, while also improving their safety profile (Rao et al. 2025). In order to target these modifications and broaden therapeutic applications, structure-activity relationship (SAR) studies play a crucial role, enabling the development of more effective compounds with fewer side effects (Davis et al. 2025).

CBN is a promising cannabinoid for inhibiting ferroptosis, a type of iron-dependent cell death that is associated with neuronal degeneration in diseases such as Alzheimer's and Parkinson's (Liang et al. 2022). CBN's action as a ferroptosis inhibitor is related to its ability to prevent lipid peroxidation and preserve mitochondrial integrity, which contributes to its neuroprotective activity. The CP1 analogue, developed from CBN (Figure 14), exhibits optimized pharmacological properties and demonstrates superior efficacy *in vivo* models of brain damage in *Drosophila melanogaster*, highlighting its therapeutic potential in the treatment of neurological disorders (Liang et al. 2024).

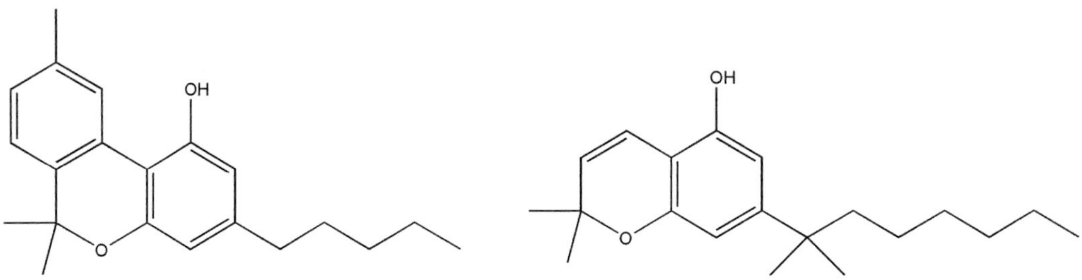

CBN **CP1**

Figure 14: CBN and CP1. Source: Authors.

Based on synthetic cannabinoids such as JWH-015, analogue compound 17 (Figure 15) was synthesized with potential anti-cancer activity and evaluated in different tumor cell lines. This analog has shown a preferential affinity for the CB2 receptor, and molecular modeling studies indicate that activation of the CB2 receptor is associated with the inhibition of cell proliferation, without the psychoactive effects characteristic of CB1 receptor activation (Hanlon et al. 2016; Doganc et al. 2024). JWH-015, derived from *Δ*9-THC, does not share obvious structural similarities with THC, but both have similar effects in modulating cannabinoid receptors (Henriquez et al. 2019). On the other hand, compound 17, an analogue of JWH-015, shares structural similarities with its precursor and has been designed to optimize selectivity for the CB2 receptor, thereby reducing the risks of psychoactive side effects, which are common with CB1 activation. These more optimized synthetic compounds offer greater specificity for CB2, making them promising for anti-tumour therapies (Doganc et al. 2024).

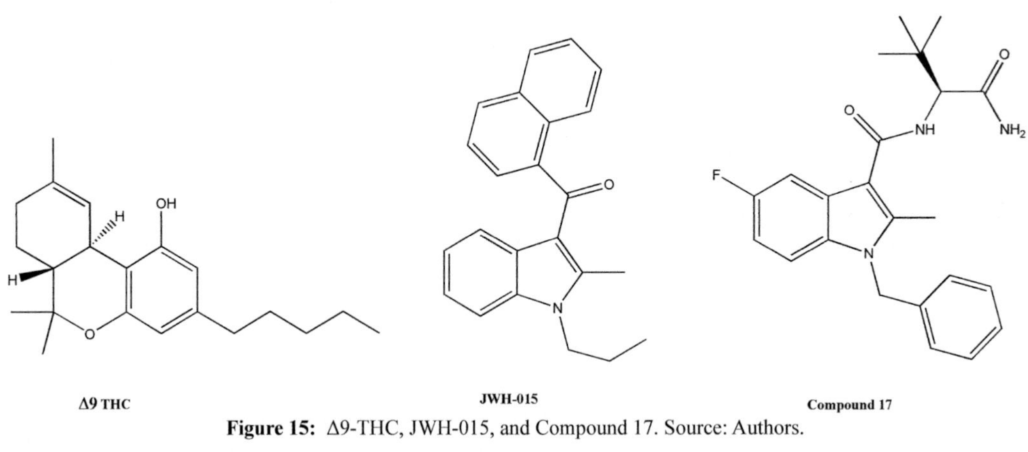

Δ9 THC **JWH-015** **Compound 17**

Figure 15: Δ9-THC, JWH-015, and Compound 17. Source: Authors.

In the case of CB1 receptor agonists, changes such as the introduction of halogens, subtle modifications to the carbon skeleton, or the substitution of functional groups result in significant variations in agonist potency (Mulvihill et al. 2024). Some compounds lose their activity completely when they undergo discrete modifications, highlighting the high conformational specificity required by the receptor for effective interaction with its ligands (Wouters et al. 2019).

The high lipophilicity of cannabinoids enables these ligands to cross the plasma membrane and interact with multiple intracellular targets, adding complexity to the SAR. The observed activity may result from the activation of different signaling pathways or additional targets, rather than just affinity for the CB1 receptor. In addition, SAR studies involving cannabinoids must consider not only the structural properties of the ligands but also the lipid microenvironment of the membrane, which can modulate receptor activity and influence the functional bias (Mulvihill et al. 2024; Tian et al. 2025).

Detailed SAR studies involving CBD stereoisomers have demonstrated that small changes in stereochemistry have a significant impact on biological activity. The synthetic (+)-CBD isomer showed greater affinity for CB1 receptors compared to the natural (-)-CBD isomer, and was up to ten times more effective at reducing neuron activation following electrical stimuli (Figure 16). This enantiomer also modulates alternative pathways; it not only acts on cannabinoid receptors, but also activates other receptors (Rao et al. 2025). This ability to act on multiple targets can be advantageous in complex therapeutic contexts, such as neurological and inflammatory diseases, where the simultaneous modulation of different pathways can amplify the beneficial effects.

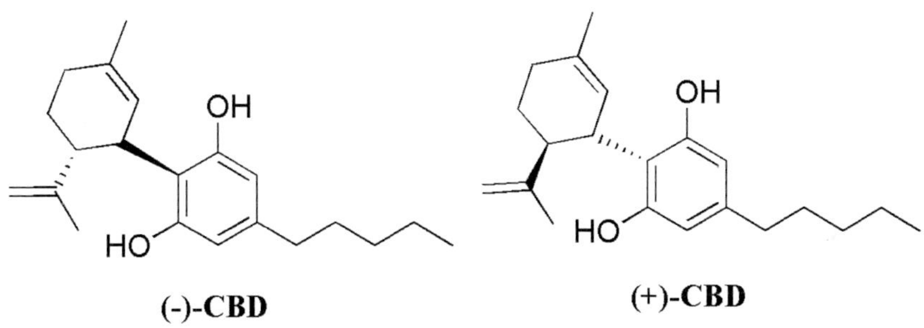

Figure 16: (-)-CBD and (+)-CBD. Source: Authors.

The synthesis of new tricyclic derivatives of indol-2-carboxamides, based on the structure of the synthetic cannabinoid WIN 55212-2, resulted in compounds with a significant loss of affinity for CB1 and CB2 receptors. Despite this, one of the analogues (compound 23) demonstrated potent antitumor activity in pediatric brain cancer cells (Figure 17) (Hamilton et al. 2024). Although structural modification of cannabinoids is a common strategy for improving selectivity and potency, its effects on pharmacological activity are not always predictable. An example of this was observed in the study of new dual-steric ligands, obtained by combining an orthosteric agonist and an allosteric modulator of the CB1 receptor. Although designed to act as agonists or positive modulators, these compounds behaved as antagonists or inverse agonists at the CB1 receptor and as positive modulators of CB2, demonstrating that the function of cannabinoid ligands cannot be predicted solely based on structural characteristics (Ferrisi et al. 2025).

SAR studies are essential for the synthesis of synthetic cannabinoids with improved selectivity, potency, and a safer profile. By identifying which structural modifications affect affinity for cannabinoid receptors and activity in different signaling pathways, these studies inform the development of more effective compounds with fewer side effects (Davis et al. 2025). In addition, the analysis of stereoisomers and derivatives enables the exploration of new biological activities and mechanisms of action, expanding the therapeutic potential of synthetic cannabinoids in conditions such as epilepsy, chronic pain, and inflammatory diseases (Rezende et al. 2023; Jiang et al. 2025).

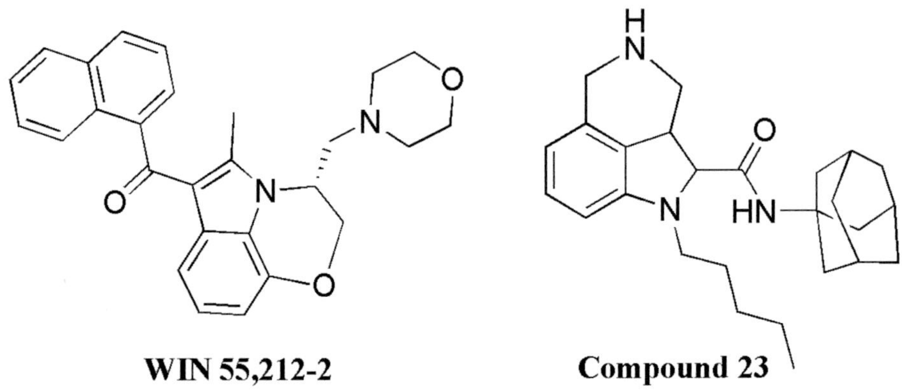

WIN 55,212-2 **Compound 23**

Figure 17: WIN 55212-2 and Compound 23. Source: Authors.

7. Conclusion

This study demonstrated that *Cannabis sativa* played an important role in ancient Chinese uses, including as a food source, an ingredient for papermaking, and edible oils mentioned in Egyptian records, as well as in medical prescriptions for treating epilepsy. Although limited by the prohibition policy, its therapeutic use has emerged in recent research, particularly in accordance with the varying laws of different countries.

From a chemical perspective, more than 550 bioactive substances have been identified. In addition, although other cannabinoids such as CBG, CBN, and various dimeric molecules (like CBDD) have the potential for analgesic and anti-inflammatory applications through their affinity for TRP channels, further preclinical and clinical research is needed to enhance our understanding.

Terpenes are responsible for most of the distinctive fragrances of various strains and affect the biological activity of cannabinoids (entourage effect). Compounds such as *β-caryophyllene*, *β-myrcene*, *terpinolene*, *α-humulene*, *D-limonene*, *α-pinene*, and *β-pinene* exhibit promising biological activities, including anti-inflammatory and neuroprotective activities.

Flavonoids are available in small quantities but possess antioxidant, anti-inflammatory, and sometimes anti-cancer properties. In particular, the canflavins A and B, unique to C. sativa, block inflammatory mediators such as prostaglandin E2 and leukotrienes. This highlights the need to use standardized and well-characterized extracts for medical purposes.

Therefore, *C. sativa* presents a complex panorama that combines ancestral use, diversified pharmacology, and regulatory challenges. The synergistic effects of cannabinoids, terpenes, and flavonoids have led to increased interest in health, agriculture, and industry. However, it is important to evaluate rigorous clinical research, establish standardized extraction processes, and develop public guidelines that complement safe medical use.

References

Adams, T. K., Masondo, N. A., Malatsi, P., and Makunga, N. P. (2021). *Cannabis sativa*: from therapeutic uses to micropropagation and beyond. *Plants*, 10: 2078.

Akhtar, M. T., Shaari, K., and Verpoorte, R. (2016) Biotransformation of tetrahydrocannabinol. *Phytochemistry Reviews*, 15: 921–934.

Al-Shudifat, A. E., Qnais, E., Bseiso, Y., Wedyan, M., Gammoh, O., Alqudah, M. et al. (2024). Antidepressant potential of β-caryophyllene in maternal separation-induced depression-like in mice: A focus on oxidative stress and nitrite levels, *Phytomedicine Plus*, 4: 100624.

Allegrone, G., Pollastro, F., Magagnini, G., Taglialatela-Scafati, O., Seegers, J., Koeberle, A. et al. (2017). Bibenzyl caniprene inhibits pro-inflammatory eicosanoid production and selectively accumulates in some *Cannabis sativa* strains. *Journal of Natural Products*, 80: 731–734.

Almeida, M. T. C., Costa, D. D., Ribeiro, E. de M., de Carvalho, M. A., de Oliveira, C. C., de Souza, A. P., et al. (2021). Tratamento dos sintomas e comorbidades associados ao Transtorno do Espectro Autista utilizando Cannabis sativa. *Revista Eletrônica Acervo Saúde*, 13(4): e6922.

Antunes, M., Barroso, M., and Gallardo, E. (2023). Analysis of cannabinoids in biological specimens: an update. *International Journal of Environmental Research and Public Health*, 20: 2312.

Araújo, M., Almeida, M. B., and Araújo, L. L. N. (2023). Mecanismo de ação dos canabinoides: visão geral. *Brazilian Journal of Pain*, 6: S109–13.

Berardo, M. E. V., Mendieta, J. R., Villamonte, M. D., Colman, S. L., and Nercessian, D. (2024) Antifungal and antibacterial activities of *Cannabis sativa* L. resins. *Journal of Ethnopharmacology*, 318: 116839.

Birenboim, M., Chalupowicz, D., Maurer, D., Barel, S., Chen, Y., Fallik, E. et al. (2022). Multivariate classification of cannabis chemovars based on their terpene and cannabinoid profiles. *Phytochemistry*, 200: 113215.

Bloemendal, V. R. L. J., Hest, J. C. M., and Rutjes, F. P. J. T. (2020). Synthetic pathways to tetrahydrocannabinol (THC): an overview. *Organic & Biomolecular Chemistry*, 18: 3203–3215.

Bonamin, F., Moraes, T. M., Dos Santos, R. C., Kushima, H., Faria, F. M., Silva, M. A. et al. (2014). The effect of a minor constituent of essential oil from *Citrus aurantium*: the role of β-myrcene in preventing peptic ulcer disease. *Chemico-Biological Interactions*, 212: 11–9.

Bonfá, L., Vinagre, R. C. O., and Figueiredo, N. V. (2008). Uso de canabinóide na dor crônica e em cuidados paliativos. *Revista Brasileira de Anestesiologia*, 58: 267–279.

Bonini, S. A., Premoli, M., Tambaro, S., Kumar, A., Maccarinelli, G., Memo, M. et al. (2018). *Cannabis sativa*: A comprehensive ethnopharmacological review of a medicinal plant with a long history. *Journal of Ethnopharmacology*, 227: 300–315.

Brand-Rubalcava, P. A., Tejeda-Martínez, A. R., González-Reynoso, O., Nápoles-Medina, A. Y., Chaparro-Huerta, V., and Flores-Soto, M. E. (2023). β-Caryophyllene decreases neuroinflammation and exerts neuroprotection of dopaminergic neurons in a model of hemiparkinsonism through inhibition of the NLRP3 inflammasome. *Parkinsonism & Related Disorders*, 117: 105906.

Calina, D. (2021). A pharmacological perspective on plant-derived bioactive molecules for epilepsy. *Neurochemical Research*, 46: 2205–2225.

Camargo Filho, M. F. A., Romanini, A. P., Pyrich, B. C., Pedri, E., Fontoura, G. C., Zorrer, L. A. et al. (2019) Canabinoides como uma nova opção terapêutica nas doenças de Parkinson e de Alzheimer: uma revisão de literatura. *Revista Brasileira de Neurologia*, 55: 17–32.

Caruso, S. J., Acquaviva, A., Müller, J. L., and Castells, C. B. (2024) Simultaneous analysis of cannabinoids and terpenes in *Cannabis sativa* inflorescence using full comprehensive two-dimensional liquid chromatography coupled to smart active modulation. *Journal of Chromatography A*, 1720: 464810.

Carvalho, C. R., Hoeller, A. A., Franco, P. L. C., Eidt, I., and Walz, R. (2017). Canabinoides e Epilepsia: potencial terapêutico do canabidiol. *Revista de Ciências da Saúde*, 29: 54–63.

Carvalho, V. M., Aguiar, A. F. L., Baratto, L. C., Souza, F. L. C., and Rocha, E. D. (2020) Quantificação de canabinoides em extratos medicinais de *cannabis* por cromatografia líquida de alta eficiência. *Quimica Nova*, 43: 90–97.

Castillo-Arellano, J., Canseco-Alba, A., Cutler, S. J., and León, F. (2023). The polypharmacological effects of cannabidiol. *Molecules*, 28: 3271.

Charitos, I. A., Gagliano-Candela, R., Santacroce, L., and Bottalico, L. (2021). The Cannabis spread throughout the continents and its therapeutic use in history. *Endocrine & Metabolic Disorders*, 21: 407–417.

Chu, T. W., Ho, C. C., Chiu, H. C., Hsu, Y. J., Hung, C. T., Sung, C. H. et al. (2025). d-Limonene inhibits cytokines and chemokines expression by regulating NF-kappaB and STAT in HaCat cells and DNCB-induced atopic dermatitis in BALB/c mice. *International Immunopharmacology*, 148: 114082.

Cortez-Resendiz, A., Leiter, T. J., Riela, S. M., Graziane, N. M., Raup-Konsavage, W. M., and Vrana, K. E. (2025). The pharmacology of cannabinoids in chronic pain. *Medical Cannabis and Cannabinoids*, 8: 31–46.

Cvijic, A., and Bauer, B. (2024). History and medicinal properties of cannabis. *Pharmacognosy Reviews*, 18: 159–164.

Davis, R. L., Grotjahn, S., Koenig, B., Buck, D. J., and Weaver, J. D. (2025) Novel fluorinated cannabinoid analogs modulate cytokine expression in human C20 microglial cells. *Pharmacological Reports*, 77: 295–301.

Dei Cas, M., Arnoldi, S., Monguzzi, L., Casagni, E., Morano, C., Vieira de Manincor, E., Bolchi, C. et al. (2021). Characterization of chemotype-dependent terpenoids profile in cannabis by headspace gas-chromatography coupled to time-of-flight mass spectrometry. *Journal of Pharmaceutical and Biomedical Analysis*, 203: 114180.

Dickson, K., Scott, C., White, H., Zhou, J., Kelly, M., and Lehmann, C. (2023). Antibacterial and analgesic properties of beta-caryophyllene in a murine urinary tract infection model. *Molecules*, 28: 4144.

Dinis-Oliveira, R. J. (2016). Metabolomics of Δ^9-tetrahydrocannabinol: implications in toxicity. *Drug Metabolism Reviews*, 48: 80–7.

Doganc, F., Ozkan, T., Farhangzad, N., Mavideniz, A., Celik, I., Sunguroglu, A. et al. (2024). Synthesis of novel indol-3-acetamido analogues as potent anticancer agents, biological evaluation and molecular modeling studies. *Bioorganic Chemistry*, 148: 107429.

El-Mernissi, R., El Menyiy, N., Metouekel, A., Zouhri, A., El-Mernissi, Y., Siddique, F. et al. (2024). Characterization of phenolic compounds and evaluation of anti-diabetic potential in *Cannabis sativa* L. seeds: *in vivo*, *in vitro*, and *in silico* studies. *Open Life Sciences*, 19: 20221024.

Ferrisi, R., Polini, B., Smolyakova, A. M., Migone, C., Giammattei, G., Banti, M. et al. (2025). Novel orthosteric/allosteric ligands of cannabinoid receptors: an unexpected pharmacological profile. *Journal of Medicinal Chemistry*, 68: 1280–1299.

Fulvio, F., Pieracci, Y., Ascrizzi, R., Bassolino, L., Flamini, G., and Paris, R. (2025). Insights into terpenes profiling and transcriptional analyses during flowering of different *Cannabis sativa* L. chemotypes. *Phytochemistry*, 229: 114294.

Fonseca, B. M., Soares, A., Teixeira, N., and Correia-da-Silva, G. (2019). Canábis e Canabinoides para Fins Medicinais. *Revista Portuguesa de Farmacoterapia*, 11: 21–31.

Francisco, V. P., Cerny, M., Valentin, R., Milone-Delacourt, F., Paillard, A. et al. (2024). Development of GC-MS coupled to GC-FID method for the quantification of *Cannabis* terpenes and terpenoids: Application to the analysis of five commercial varieties of medicinal *Cannabis*. *Journal of Chromatography B*, 1247: 124316.

Garcia, J. B. S., and Barbosa Neto, J. O. (2023). Efeitos adversos do uso dos canabinoides: qual o paradigma de segurança? *Brazilian Journal of Pain*, 6: S38–43.

Hamilton, A. J., Lane, S., Werry, E. L., Suri, A., Bailey, A. W., Mercé, C. et al. (2024). Synthesis and antitumour evaluation of tricyclic indole-2-carboxamides against paediatric brain cancer cells. *ChemMedChem*, 19(19): e202400098.

Hancock, J., Livingston, S. J., and Samuels, L. (2024) Building a biofactory: Constructing glandular trichomes in *Cannabis sativa*. *Current Opinion in Plant Biology*, 80: 102549.

Hanlon, K. E., Lozano-Ondoua, A. N., Umaretiya, P. J., Symons-Liguori, A. M., Chandramouli, A., Moy, J. K. et al. (2016). Modulation of breast cancer cell viability by a cannabinoid receptor 2 agonist, JWH-015, is calcium dependent. *Breast Cancer*, 8: 59–71.

Henriquez, J. E., Crawford, R. B., and Kaminski, N. E. (2019). Suppression of CpG-ODN-mediated IFNα and TNFα response in human plasmacytoid dendritic cells (pDC) by cannabinoid receptor 2 (CB2)-specific agonists. *Toxicology and Applied Pharmacology*, 369: 82–89.

Hourfane, S., Mechqoq, H., Bekkali, A. Y., Rocha, J. M., and El Aouad, N. (2023). A comprehensive review on *Cannabis sativa* ethnobotany, phytochemistry, molecular docking and biological activities. *Plants*, 12(6): 1245.

Jang, H. I., Rhee, K. J., and Eom, Y. B. (2020) Efeitos antibacterianos e antibiofilme do α-humuleno contra *Bacteroides fragilis* . *Revista Canadense de Microbiologia*, 66: 389–399.

Jiang, B. E., He, Y., Chen, J., Jiang, X. W., Qiu, Z. L., Liang, Q. W. et al. (2025). Design, synthesis, and biological evaluations of 5-aryl-pyrazole-3-carboxamide derivatives as selective CB2 receptor agonists for the treatment of colitis, *European Journal of Medicinal Chemistry*, 283: 117117.

Kang, Y., Wang, X., Wei, X., Li, D., Gan, L., Jin, J. et al. (2022). Synergistic inhibitory effect of α-humulene and sclareol on human pancreatic cancer cells. *Journal of Functional Foods*, 89: 104958.

Karche, T. (2019). The application of hemp (*Cannabis sativa* L.) for a green economy: A review. *Turkish Journal of Botany*, 43: 710–723.

Klauke, A. L., Racz, I., Pradier, B., Markert, A., Zimmer, A. M., Gertsch, J. et al. (2014). The cannabinoid CB_2 receptor-selective phytocannabinoid beta-caryophyllene exerts analgesic effects in mouse models of inflammatory and neuropathic pain. *Euripean Neuropsychopharmacology*, 24: 608–20.

Koram, K. (2022). The legalization of cannabis and the question of reparations. *Journal of International Economic Law*, 25: 294–311.

Kumar, R., Kumar, R., Sharma, N., and Khurana, N. (2021) Ameliorative effect of myrcene in mouse model of Alzheimer's disease. *European Journal of Pharmacology*, 911: 174529.

Laaboudi, F. Z., Rejdali, M., Amhamdi, H., Salhi, A., Elyoussfi, A., and Ahari, M. (2024). In the weeds: A comprehensive review of cannabis; its chemical complexity, biosynthesis, and healing abilities. *Toxicology Reports*, 13: 101685.

Laws III, J. S., and Smid, S. D. (2024) Characterizing cannabis-prevalent terpenes for neuroprotection reveal a role for α and β-pinenes in mitigating amyloid β-evoked neurotoxicity and aggregation *in vitro*. *Neurotoxicology*, 100: 16–24.

Liang, Z., Candib, A., Soriano-Castell, D., Fischer, W., Finley, K., and Maher, P. (2024). Fragment-based drug discovery and biological evaluation of novel cannabinol-based inhibitors of oxytosis/ferroptosis for neurological disorders. *Redox Biology*, 72: 103138.

Liang, Z., Soriano-Castell, D., Kepchia, D., Duggan, B. M., Currais, A., Schubert, D. et al. (2022). Cannabinol inhibits oxytosis/ferroptosis by directly targeting mitochondria independently of cannabinoid receptors. *Free Radical Biology and Medicine*, 180: 33–51.

Lü, X., Zhang, Y., Yang, L., Chen, A., Zhang, Z., and Shen, G. (2024). Antibiofilm activity of d-limonene against spoilage *Bacillus amyloliquefaciens*. *Food Bioscience*, 61: 104568.

Malabadi, R. B., Kolkar, K. P., and Chalannavar, R. K. (2023). *Cannabis sativa*: Ethnobotany and phytochemistry. *International Journal of Innovation Scientific Research and Review*. 5: 3990–3998.

Martin, E. M. S., Marrassini, C., Peralta, I. N., Cogoi, L. C., Alonso, M. D. R., and Anesini, C. A. (2022). El efecto de la decarboxilación de Cannabis sativa sobre su actividad antioxidante y el perfil de flavonoides: Un estudio preliminar. *Medicinal Plant Communications*, 5: 38–47.

Mazzara, E., Torresi, J., Fico, G., Papini, A., Kulbaka, N., Dall'Acqua, S. et al. (2022). A comprehensive phytochemical analysis of terpenes, polyphenols and cannabinoids, and micromorphological characterization of 9 commercial varieties of *Cannabis sativa* L. *Plants*, 11: 891.

Mechoulam, R., Parker, L. A., and Gallily, R. (2002). Cannabidiol: an overview of some pharmacological aspects. The *Journal of Clinical Pharmacology*, 42: 11S–19S.

Menezes, I. O., Scherf, J. R., Martins, A. O. B. P. B., Ramos, A. G. B., Quintans, J. S. S., Coutinho, H. D. M. et al. (2021). Biological properties of terpinolene evidenced by *in silico*, *in vitro* and *in vivo* studies: A systematic review. *Phytomedicine*, 93: 153768.

Moghaddam, H. Á., Hasan, T. A., Estalkhi, F. M., Farhadi-Pahnedari, S., Jelodar, S. K., and Karimian, M. (2024). Neuroprotective effects of alpha-pinene against behavioral deficits in ketamine-induced mice model of schizophrenia: Focusing on oxidative stress status. IBRO *Neuroscience Reports*, 16: 182–189.

Moreau, M., Ibeh, U., Decosmo, K., Bih, N., Yasmin-Karim, S., Toyang, N. et al. (2019). Cannabis flavonoid derivative demonstrates therapeutic potential in preclinical models of metastatic pancreatic cancer. *Frontiers in Oncology*, 9: 660.

Mulvihill, C. J., Lutgens, J. D., Gollihar, J. D., Bachanová, P., Tramont, C., Marcotte, E. M. et al. (2024). A humanized CB1R yeast biosensor enables facile screening of cannabinoid compounds. *International Journal of Molecular Sciences*, 25: 6060.

Pereira, I. S., Rodrigues, V. F., and Vega, M. R. G. (2016). Flavonoids from the genus *Solanum*. *Revista Virtual de Química*, 8: 4–26.

Qiu, B., Wei, F., Su, J., Hao, W., Zhou, J., Zhao, J. et al. (2022). The Effects of β-Pinene, a Pine Needle Oil Monoterpene, on Adenovirus Type 3. *Bulletin of Experimental Biology and Medicine*, 172: 345–351.

Raihan, A., and Bijoy, T. R. (2023). A review of the industrial use and global sustainability of *Cannabis sativa*. *Global Sustainability Research*, 2: 1–29.

Rantaša, M., Slaček, Gal, Knez, Ž., and Marevci, M. K. (2024). Supercritical fluid extraction of cannabinoids and their analysis by liquid chromatography and supercritical fluid chromatography: A short review. *Journal of CO_2 Utilization*, 86: 102907.

Rao, V. K., Lewis-Bakker, M. M., Wasilewski, E., Clarke, H. A., and Kotra, L. P. (2025). Stereoisomers of cannabidiols and their pharmacological activities—a potentially novel direction for cannabinoids. *Bioorganic & Medicinal Chemistry*, 117: 118019.

Raoui, K., Kabdy, H., Ettitaou, A., Aitbaba, A., Baslam, A., Benrazzouk, K. et al. (2024). Assessment of Moroccan *Cannabis sativa* seed oil: chemical analysis and evaluation of antioxidant, toxicological, and antinociceptive effects. *Chemistry & Biodiversity*, 21: e202400591.

Rea, K. A., Casaretto, J. A., Al-Abdul-Wahid, M. S., Sukumaran, A., Geddes-McAlister, J., Rothstein, S. J. et al. (2019). Biosynthesis of canflavins A and B from *Cannabis sativa* L. *Phytochemistry*, 164: 162–171.

Rezende, B., Alencar, A. K. N., Bem, G. F., Fontes-Dantas, F. L., and Montes, G. C. (2023) Endocannabinoid system: chemical characteristics and biological activity. *Pharmaceuticals*, 16: 148.

Rezghiyan, A., Esmaeili, H., and Farzaneh, M. (2025) Nanosilicon application changes the morphological attributes and essential oil compositions of hemp (*Cannabis sativa* L.) under water deficit stress. *Scientific Reports*, 15: 3400.

Roque-Bravo, R., Silva, R. S., Malheiro, R. F., Carmo, H., Carvalho, F., Silva, D. D. et al. (2023). Synthetic Cannabinoids: A Pharmacological and Toxicological Overview. *Annual Review of Pharmacology and Toxicology*, 63: 187–209.

Shakil, S. S., Gowan, M., Hughes, K., Azam, M. N. K., and Ahmed, M. N. (2021). A narrative review of the ethnomedicinal usage of *Cannabis sativa* Linnaeus as traditional phytomedicine by folk medicine practitioners of Bangladesh. *Journal of Cannabis Research*, 3: 1–12.

Simei, J. L. Q., Souza, J. D. R., Lisboa, J. R., Campos, A. C., Guimarães, F. S., Zuardi, A. et al. (2024). Does the "Entourage Effect" in cannabinoids exist? A narrative scoping review. *Cannabis and Cannabinoid Research*, 9: 1202–1216.

Tian, L., Qiang, T., Liu, S., Zhang, B., Zhang, Y., Zhang, B. et al. (2025). Cannabinoid receptor 1 ligands: Biased signaling mechanisms driving functionally selective drug discovery. *Pharmacology & Therapeutics*, 267: 108795.

Tzimas, P. S., Beteinakis, S., Petrakis, E. A., Papastylianou, P. T., Kakabouki, I., Small-Howard, A. L. et al. (2024). Uncovering the metabolite complexity and variability of cultivated hemp (*Cannabis sativa* L.): a first phytochemical diversity mapping in Greece. *Phytochemistry*, 222: 114076.

Wang, M., Faust, M., Abbott, S., Patel, V., Chang, E., Clark, J. I. et al. (2025). Effects of a cannabidiol/terpene formulation on sleep in individuals with insomnia: a double-blind, placebo-controlled, randomized, crossover study. *Journal of Clinical Sleep Medicine*, 21:69–80.

Wei, S. Y., Li, Y. L., Wang, L., Chu, Z. Y., Qin, Y. C., and Zeng, H. (2025) α-Pinene: Inhibitor of *Acinetobacter baumannii* biofilms and potential therapeutic agent for pneumonia. *International Immunopharmacology*, 151: 114287.

Weimer, P., Kirsten, C. N., de Araújo Lock, G., Nunes, K. A. A., Rossi, R. C., and Koester, L. S. (2023). Co-delivery of beta-caryophyllene and indomethacin in the oily core of nanoemulsions potentiates the anti-inflammatory effect in LPS-stimulated macrophage model *European Journal of Pharmaceutics and Biopharmaceutics*, 191: 114-123.

Welling, M. T., Deseo, M. A., Bacic, A., and Doblin, M. S. (2022). Biosynthetic origins of unusual cannabimimetic phytocannabinoids in *Cannabis sativa* L: a review. *Phytochemistry*, 201: 113282.

Werz, O., Seegers, J., Schaible, A. M., Weinigel, C., Barz, D., Koeberle, A. et al. (2014). Cannflavins from hemp sprouts, a novel cannabinoid-free hemp food product, target microsomal prostaglandin E2 synthase-1 and 5-lipoxygenase. *PharmaNutrition*, 2: 53–60.

Wouters, E., Walraed, J., Banister, S. D., and Stove, C. P. (2019). Insights into biased signaling at cannabinoid receptors: synthetic cannabinoid receptor agonists. *Biochemical Pharmacology*, 169: 113623.

CHAPTER 6

Non-Cannabinoid Metabolites of *Cannabis sativa* in Therapy

Sabrin R. M. Ibrahim,[1,2] *Mahmoud A. Elfaky,*[3,4,*] *Gamal A. Mohamed*[3] and *Hossam M. Abdallah*[3,5]

1. Introduction

Natural products, such as medicinal plants, also referred to as "green medicine," are becoming more and more well-liked globally because of their efficacy, safety, acceptance within cultures, and reduced risk of negative side effects as compared to synthetic medications (Fordjour et al. 2023). Interestingly, more than 80% of people worldwide rely on traditional plant remedies to cure their health issues (Howes et al. 2020).

Cannabis sativa (also known as weed or hemp; family Cannabaceae) is one of the ancient crops that people cultivated in central and eastern Asia many millennia ago. Its seeds have been used as food, and its stems have been frequently employed for textiles, fibers, and ropes (Crini et al., 2020). Its therapeutic potential was recognized by ancient civilizations, including the Greeks, Egyptians, and Chinese medicine practitioners, as a potential medication for treating a wide array of diseases and conditions that target the human body's various systems (Leinen et al. 2023).

Cannabis was used in ancient China as a remedy for gynecological disorders, rheumatic pain, gout, malaria, and constipation in the pharmacopoeia of Emperor Shen Nung (Pisanti and Bifulco 2019). In Egypt, cannabis products were first utilized to treat glaucoma. By the 1800s, cannabis tinctures and extracts were known in the West for their ability to prevent nausea and relieve migraine headaches (Walsh et al. 2021). Also, the traditional Ayurvedic medicine in India incorporated cannabis to treat pain, anxiety, and gastrointestinal disorders (Pathak et al. 2024). Its extract has been used in Arabic-Islamic medicine for its therapeutic benefits, including antiemetic, diuretic, antiepileptic, antiparasitic, anti-inflammatory, antipyretic, antitumor, antibacterial, vermifugal, dermatic, pain-killing, and carminative effects (Shakil et al. 2021). Despite the medicinal benefits of cannabis, many countries banned it in the early 1930s due to the recreational or narcotic use of its inflorescences that contain psychoactive cannabinoids (Riboulet-Zemouli 2020).

[1] Preparatory Year Program, Department of Chemistry, Batterjee Medical College, Jeddah 21442, Saudi Arabia.
[2] Department of Pharmacognosy, Faculty of Pharmacy, Assiut University, Assiut 71526, Egypt.
[3] Department of Natural Products and Alternative Medicine, Faculty of Pharmacy, King Abdulaziz University, Jeddah 21589, Saudi Arabia.
[4] Centre for Artificial Intelligence in Precision Medicines, King Abdulaziz University, Jeddah 21589, Saudi Arabia.
[5] Department of Pharmacognosy, Faculty of Pharmacy, Cairo University, Cairo, 11562, Egypt.
* Corresponding author: melfaky@kau.edu.sa

DOI: 10.1201/9781003668190-8

A significant breakthrough in the knowledge of cannabis pharmacology was observed after the separation and structural analysis of the phyto-cannabinoids, mainly Δ^9-THC (Δ9-tetrahydrocannabinol) and CBD (cannabidiol). These metabolites were first identified as the most bioactive constituents of cannabis that have been thoroughly investigated for their potential therapeutic benefits (Leinen et al. 2023; Riboulet-Zemouli 2020). Apart from Δ^9-THC and CBD, the plant synthesizes more than 120 additional phyto-cannabinoids in its glandular trichomes (Hanuš et al. 2016; Leinen et al. 2023).

Beyond cannabinoids, the plant produces a vast array of non-cannabinoid secondary metabolites, including terpenes, flavonoids, phenylpropanoids, glycoproteins, dihydrophenanthrenes, dibenzyls, phenols, fatty acids, stilbenes, lignans, and alkaloids with anticancer, analgesic, anti-inflammatory, neuroprotective, antimicrobial, and antioxidant capabilities, which collectively contribute to the overall therapeutic profile of the plant (Boucher et al. 2025; Liu et al. 2025; Wozniczka et al. 2025; Leinen et al. 2023; Lowe et al. 2021). It was reported that non-cannabinoid metabolites, most notably terpenes and flavonoids, can modulate the effects of cannabinoids, as well as the combinations of cannabinoids and non-cannabinoid substances, augmenting the overall effectiveness, which is called "the entourage effect" (Laaboudi et al. 2024). This work focuses on the major non-cannabinoid compounds and their potential therapeutic effects.

2. Classification of Non-Cannabinoid Metabolites and Their Therapeutic Effect

2.1 *Phenolics*

Lignans, flavonoids, and stilbenes are the three major categories of phenolics found in cannabis (Isidore et al. 2021). Lignans are mostly found in fruits, seeds, and roots, while flavonoids and stilbenes are primarily found in inflorescence, leaves, and stalks. As the plant grows, its levels decrease due to their condensation with terpenoids to generate cannabinoids (Isidore et al., 2021)

2.1.1 Lignans

C. sativa's lignans include two types: lignanamides (Figures 1 and 2) and phenolic amides (Figure 3). The phenylpropionamide moiety is a common part of these metabolites. Some lignanamides have been found to possess acetylcholinesterase inhibitory and antioxidant capacities; therefore, they could be promising potential medicines for multifaceted therapy for Alzheimer's disease. On the other hand, the capacity of cannabisin F (**6**) and grossamide (**12**) to control inflammation had been established.

Zhou et al. (2018) reported that lignanamides safeguarded mice against LPS-induced deleterious effects on learning and spatial memory by decreasing elevated TNF-α and IL-1β, and -6 brain levels and hippocampus neuron damage in the LPS-induced animals. Additionally, they reduced the harm that LPS caused to the mice's hippocampus neurons (Zhou et al. 2018). Additionally, Yan et al. stated that **1**, **3**, **4**, **8**, **13**, **19**, and **20** possessed marked antioxidant capacities, whereas **13**, **14**, and **19** *in vitro* prohibited acetylcholinesterase. These compounds, with their acetylcholinesterase-inhibiting and antioxidant properties, could be beneficial candidates as multitarget anti-Alzheimer's disease (Yan et al. 2015).

Additionally, **6** exhibited anti-oxidative and anti-neuroinflammatory properties by suppressing the NF-κB signaling pathway activation and modulating SIRT1 expression and Nrf2 signaling pathway activation, respectively, in BV2 microglia cells activated by LPS (Wang et al. 2019). Hence, it may be a promising therapeutic drug for neurodegenerative disorders (Wang et al. 2019).

A study by Bourjot et al. (2016) afforded a new lignanamide, cannabisin I (**7**), along with 1–3, 6, 8, 12, 13, 19, and 23 from the seed cakes (Figure 3). Among them, 19 displayed higher inhibition activity (IC_{50} 20.9 μM) on mammal arginase, compared to S-(2- 2-boronoethyl)-l-cysteine (IC_{50} 4.3 μM). Additionally, all cannabisins had marked antioxidant potential, comparable to or better than standard compounds in the ORACFL method.

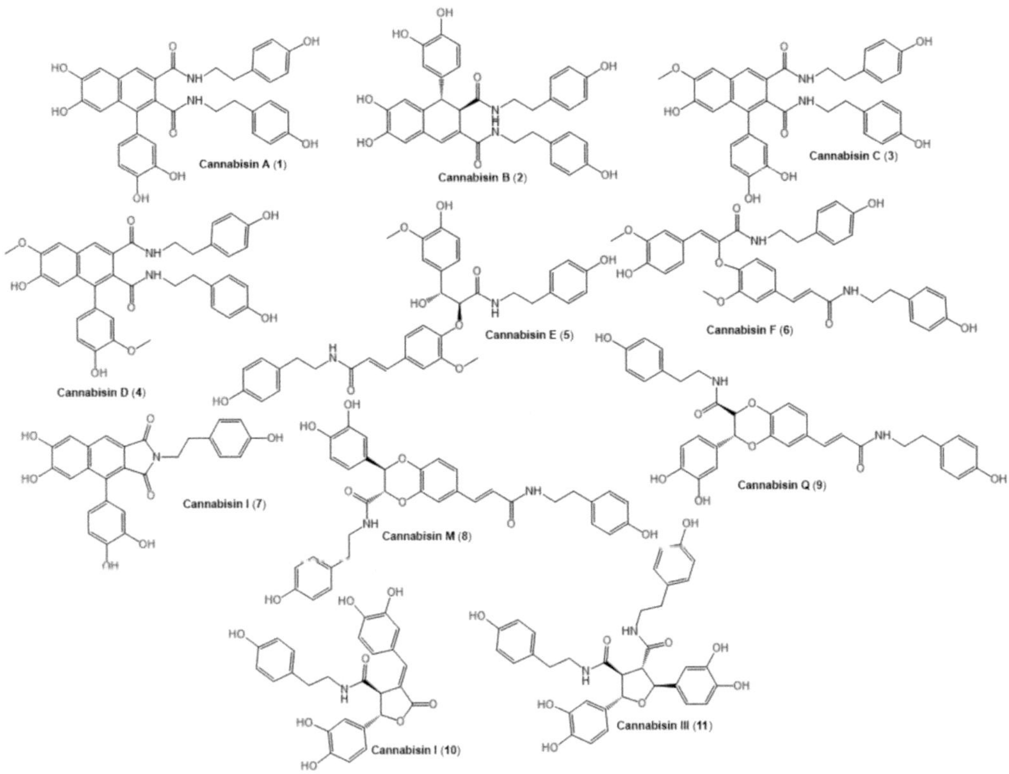

Figure 1: Examples of bioactive lignanamides reported from cannabis (Compounds 1–11).

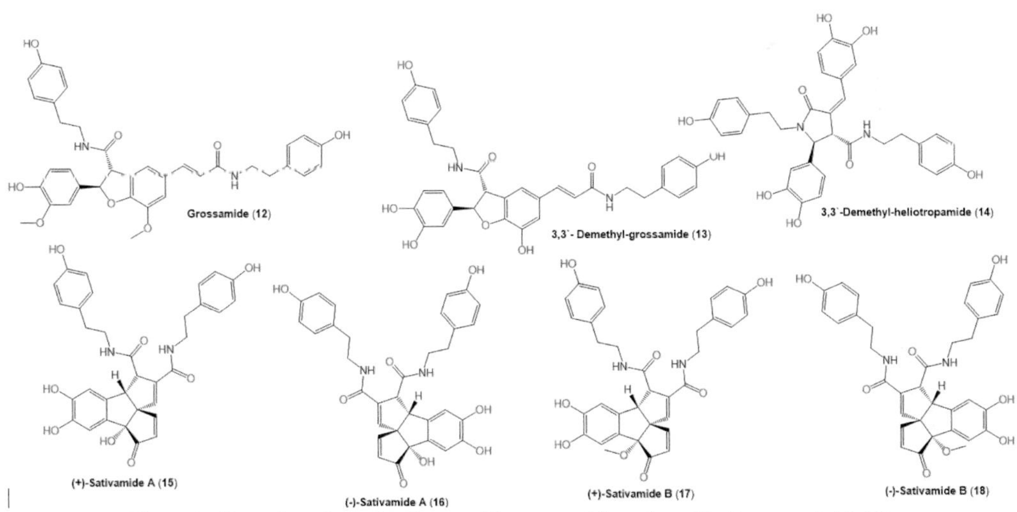

Figure 2: Examples of bioactive lignanamides reported from Cannabis (Compounds 12–18).

Furthermore, N-transcaffeoyltyramine's antioxidant and arginase inhibitory properties make it a potential lead for developing medications to address cardiovascular disorders associated with endothelial dysfunction (Bourjot et al. 2016).

Furthermore, **12** markedly reduced LPS-caused release of IL-6 and TNF-α, impeded the NF-κB p65 translocation into the nucleus, and lowered NF-κB subunit p65 phosphorylation levels (Luo et al. 2017). It significantly reduced the expression of MyD88 (myeloid differentiation factor 88) and TLR4 (Toll-like receptor 4), which were stimulated by LPS (Luo et al. 2017). Consequently,

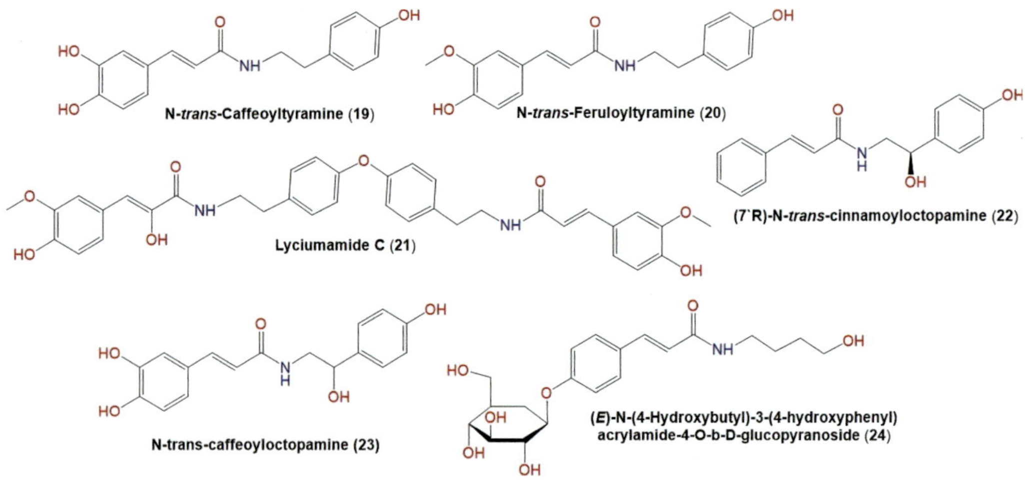

Figure 3: Examples of bioactive phenolic amides reported from cannabis.

it might be a potential treatment for reducing neuroinflammation in neurodegenerative illnesses (Luo et al. 2017). Also, **9** and **24** demonstrated anti-neuroinflammatory potential by inhibiting LPS-induced TNF-α release from BV2 microglia cells (Zhou et al. 2018).

Zhou et al. (2018) reported the isolation and identification of (±)-sativamides A (**15/16**) and B (**17/18**), two pairs of norlignanamide enantiomers characterized by a distinctive benzo-angular triquinane structure using chiral HPLC and NMR/ECD analyses, respectively (Zhou et al. 2018). It was found that the pretreatment of neuroblastoma cells (SH-SY5Y and PC12 cells) with compounds **15–18** protected them against tunicamycin and thapsigargin-caused endoplasmic reticulum (ER) stress, suggesting that these compounds could be neuroprotective and ER stress-inhibiting agents for treating neurodegenerative conditions (Zhou et al. 2018). Neurodegenerative disorders are greatly impacted by ER stress. Thus, targeting the ER stress signaling system has emerged as an effective therapy for several neurodegenerative illnesses, including Alzheimer's and Parkinson's (Zhou et al. 2018).

In vitro assessment against H_2O_2-mediated damage in PC12 cells revealed that seed extract (Conc. 6.125, 12.5, and 25 μg/mL) and **1**, **5**, **8**, **10**, **11**, **13**, **21**, and **22** possessed neuroprotective potential, whereas **13** was the most active compound. It effectively minimized ROS (reactive oxygen species) formation, elevated SOD and GSH-Px activity, reversed MDA (malondialdehyde) production, and boosted antioxidant levels, as well as prohibited PC12 cells' apoptosis rate (Zhang et al. 2024).

2.1.2 *Stilbenes*

Cannabis contains several stilbenes, all of which are structurally dihydrostilbenoids, about half of which possess a prenyl moiety (O'Croinin et al. 2023; Turner et al. 1980). These metabolites revealed a range of therapeutic benefits, including antioxidant, antiviral, anti-inflammatory, and anti-cancer properties. However, the possible health benefits of many of the identified stilbenes have only been partially studied (O'Croinin et al. 2023).

In 2018, Guo et al. identified the new stilbenoids: HM1–HM3 (**25–27**), using LC-MS/NMR/IR analyses of cannabis leaves obtained from Yunnan Province, China (Guo et al. 2018) (Figure 4).

Compound **25** exhibited selective inhibition for the A549 and MCF-7 cell lines, preventing the cancer cells from proliferating in the MTT method (Guo et al. 2018). Compound **26** demonstrated the strongest inhibition against MCF-7, whereas compound **27** revealed the same selectivity to MCF-7 and A549 (Guo et al. 2018). Thus, **25–27** might prove advantageous as antitumor therapy, particularly for lung and breast cancer (Guo et al. 2018).

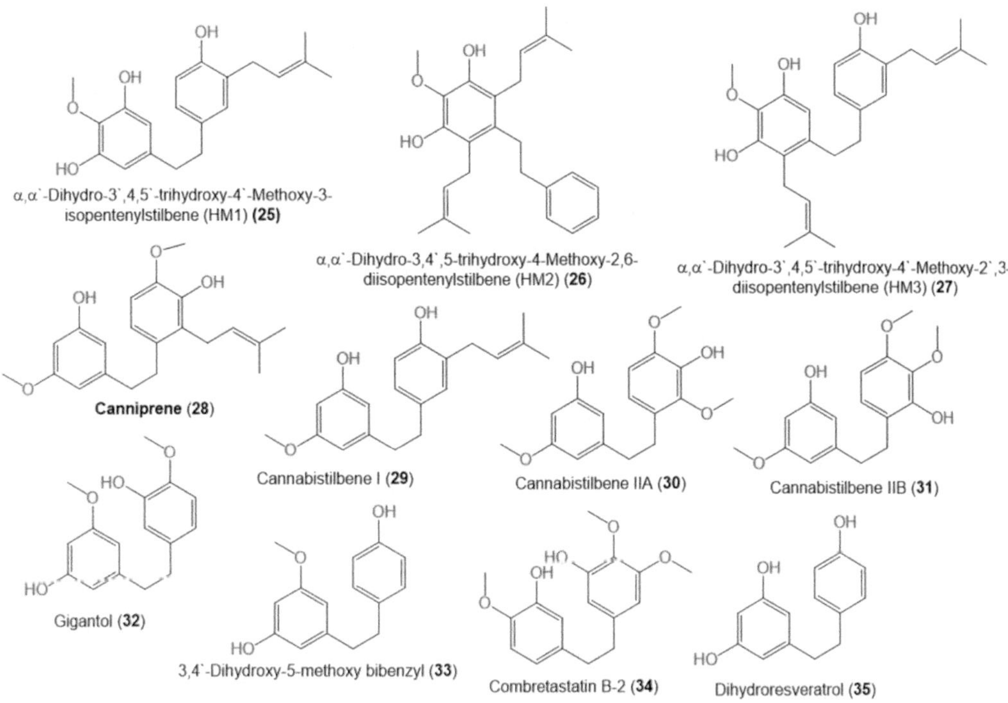

Figure 4: Examples of bioactive stilbenes reported from cannabis.

The cholesterol transporters SR-B1 and ABCG1 are crucial for removing cholesterol from cells and its conversion to high-density lipoprotein (HDL) cholesterol (Guo et al. 2018). All compounds demonstrated cardioprotective action by increasing the protein expression of these transporters, which enhanced RCT (reverse cholesterol transport). Compounds **25** and **27** stimulated cholesterol uptake by an indirect way of transport, and all these dihydrostilbenes elevated the SR-B1 protein expression in hepatocytes (Guo et al. 2018). Compound **25** was found to elevate the expression of CYP7A1, which is a crucial enzyme for the liver's conversion of cholesterol to bile acid. These findings highlighted their cardioprotective potential for minimizing atherosclerotic heart disease (Guo et al. 2018).

Canniprene (**28**) is the first prenylated dihydrostilbene identified from Thailand and Panamanian cannabis and elucidated using NMR analyses (Crombie et al. 1978; ElSohly and Turner 1982a). Canniprene possessed a powerful anti-inflammatory capacity through the inhibition of 5-LO that exceeded that of zileuton. 5-LO is crucial for arachidonic acid breakdown and the subsequent synthesis of inflammatory eicosanoids (Rubin and Mollison 2007). 5-LO inhibition has positive health effects in the management of idiopathic pulmonary fibrosis, asthma, COPD, and allergic rhinitis (Rubin and Mollison 2007). Additionally, canniprene inhibited mPEGS-1, which catalyzes the final stage of prostaglandin E2 production from arachidonic acid (Allegrone et al. 2017). The *in silico* investigation also demonstrated its potential for inhibiting COX2 and COX2 (inhibition constants of 0.21 and 14.53 μM, respectively) (Romero Salamanca and Castañeda Castellanos 2019). These outcomes indicated a strong rationale for canniprene's potential as a medication to reduce inflammation. Guo et al. stated that canniprene demonstrated cytotoxic effectiveness against A549 (human lung adenocarcinoma), MCF-7 (human breast cancer), HT-29 (human colorectal adenocarcinoma), and HepG2 (human liver carcinoma) cells, with inhibition rates above 80% agent (Guo et al. 2018). Khattab and Teleb (2022) examined 29 cannabis phytoligands, including canniprene, for potential interactions with the viral replication path or the SARS-CoV-2 binding site employing *in silico* modeling. Canniprene demonstrated highly effective antiviral efficacy among the tested compounds by preventing the virus from replicating, targeting the Mpro (major protease), which is crucial in the production of viral nonstructural (Khattab and Teleb 2022).

Cannabistilbene was reported by ElSohly et al. from cannabis grown in Panama. This compound was identified by spectral analysis and synthesis to exist in three forms: cannabistilbene I (**29**), IIa (**30**), and IIb (**31**), with **29** being prenylated (ElSohly et al. 1984).

Warner et al. studied the inhibitory effects of the three forms on COX1 and COX2 using an *in silico* study (Romero Salamanca and Castañeda Castellanos 2019). Compound **31** had the most powerful inhibitory potential on COX1, followed by **29** and **30** (inhibition constants 1.37, 2.27, and 14.53 μM, respectively) (Romero Salamanca and Castañeda Castellanos 2019). Whilst **29** and **30** were potent COX2 inhibitors (inhibition constant 0.21 μM), **31** (inhibition constant 2.69 μM) was less effective, with a value of 2.69 μM (Romero Salamanca and Castañeda Castellanos 2019). Compounds **29** and **30**'s higher COX2 inhibition than COX1 inhibition, which is advantageous because COX2 inhibition is anti-inflammatory, while COX1 inhibition has adverse gastric implications (Romero Salamanca and Castañeda Castellanos 2019).

Gigantol (**32**), a non-prenylated derivative, was separated from Mexican cannabis. Ahammed et al. revealed that gigantol demonstrated a marked inhibitory potential against hydroxyl and DPPH radicals (IC_{50}s of 4.16 and 6.61 μg/mL, respectively), as well as lipid peroxidation inhibition and total antioxidant activity, supporting gigantol as an antioxidant; however, further investigation is required (Ahammed et al. 2021). In an *in silico* study, it was demonstrated to possess anti-inflammatory properties marked by the inhibition of COX1 and COX2 (inhibition constants of 2.27 and 1.37 μM, respectively) (Romero Salamanca and Castañeda Castellanos 2019).

Additionally, it inhibited the growth of hepatocellular carcinoma cells as well as their metastases and migration (Li et al. 2022). Gigantol prevented cervical cancer from growing by inducing oxidative stress, which increased apoptosis and inhibited proliferation by generating reactive oxygen species in the mitochondria (Kang et al. 2022).

Gigantol suppressed the proliferation of breast cancer cells, including the cell lines MDA-MB-468 and MCF-7 (Huang et al. 2021). Co-administration of 60 μM gigantol with cisplatin significantly increased toxicity towards MCF-7 and MDA-MB-468, with changes in IC_{50s} from 22.66 μM to 8.36 μM and from 12.29 μM to 2.92 μM, respectively (Huang et al. 2021), as well as increased apoptosis caused by cisplatin (Huang et al. 2021).

Gigantol reduced the proliferation and survival of cancer stem cells, which are crucial for tumor regeneration and growth (Bhummaphan and Chanvorachote 2015; Losuwannarak et al. 2020). In a xenograft model, lung cancer tumor size and density, as well as tumor integrity, were significantly decreased by gigantol (Losuwannarak et al. 2020). Gigantol halted the growth of lung cancer cells by downregulating MYC, a proto-oncogene and transcription factor that stimulates the growth of cancer cells (Losuwannarak et al. 2020), and blocked mesenchymal-epithelial transition factor, a tyrosine kinase that facilitates cancer spread (Aksorn et al. 2021). These findings suggested that gigantol could be an effective anti-cancer for liver, cervical, lung, and breast cancers.

Rahman et al. assessed, using *in silico* molecular docking, the efficiency of gigantol's binding to sterol 24-C methyltransferase, an enzyme essential to *Leishmania donovani's* survival (Rahman et al. 2021). Gigantol was able to hinder it in a dose-dependent manner by generating reactive oxygen species (Rahman et al. 2021). It also showed binding (binding energy –6.9 Kcal/mol) to sterol 24-C methyltransferase (Rahman et al. 2021).

Basque et al. reported that gigantol impacted the generation of progesterone from cholesterol by Leydig cells of the male testes (Basque et al. 2021). Gigantol induced the overexpression of genes involved in cholesterol and steroid synthesis in Leydig cells *in vitro* (Basque et al. 2021), thereby significantly affecting progesterone synthesis. Thus, gigantol could prevent age-related hypogonadism (Basque et al. 2021).

Kettenes-van den Bosch and Salemink identified 3,4'-dihydroxy-5-methoxy bibenzyl (**33**) from Mexican cannabis, which is a non-prenylated analog assigned by spectral methods/synthesis (Kettenes-van den Bosch and Salemink 1978). Su et al. proved its anti-inflammatory capacity through inhibiting IL-1β, nitric oxide, and TNF-α induced by lipopolysaccharide in macrophages (Su et al. 2020). Further, it prohibited COX2 and COX1 (inhibition constants 1.62 and 10.37 μM, respectively) in an *in silico* study (Romero Salamanca and Castañeda Castellanos 2019).

A study by Wirth et al. was conducted to identify the chemicals responsible for the estrogenic effect of *Cannabis* (Wirth et al. 1981). It was found that **33** (doses 50 and 250 mg/kg) notably increased the uterine weight (Wirth et al. 1981), indicating the estrogenic potential of **33** (Wirth et al. 1981).

Guo et al. identified combretastatin B-2 (**34**), a non-prenylated stilbene in cannabis (Guo et al. 2018). The anti-cancer properties of combretastatin B-2 by Guo et al. revealed that the proliferation of MCF-7, A549, HepG2, and HT-29 cell lines was moderately inhibited by combretastatin B-2, as MCF-7 and HT-29 were more significantly inhibited than A549 and HepG2 (Guo et al. 2018). Combretastatin B-2 also showed an intense inhibitory action against murine P388 lymphocytic leukemia cells (Pettit and Singh 2011).

Dihydroresveratrol (**35**) is the most extensively studied stilbene found in cannabis. It is a non-prenylated dihydrostilbene and a phase I hydrogenated metabolite of resveratrol, which is similarly metabolized by human gut bacteria (Bode et al. 2013). Dihydroresveratrol has shown potential anti-inflammatory effects, similar to resveratrol, by reducing proinflammatory cytokines such as IL-6 and members of the IL-1 family (IL-1β and IL-18), which are involved in various inflammatory and autoimmune conditions (Kaneko et al. 2019; Roupe et al. 2008; Tanaka et al. 2014; Zhang et al. 2023). Notably, Zhang et al. (2023) demonstrated reduced IL-1β in a colitis mouse model, although TNF-α expression was increased during *in vitro* experiments, potentially offsetting the observed anti-inflammatory benefits. Studies also indicated that higher ratios of **35** relative to resveratrol amplified anti-inflammatory effects by upregulating the aryl hydrocarbon receptor, which aids intestinal integrity, and downregulating intestinal 5HT7 receptors, a potential biomarker for the effectiveness of colitis improvement (Fei et al. 2022).

Additionally, *in silico* models suggested **35** inhibited COX1 and COX2 (COX1 (inhibition constants 3.77 and 1.37 μM, respectively) (Romero Salamanca and Castañeda Castellanos 2019). Another study reported that nitric oxide is unaffected by **35** in an *in vitro* model unless it is combined with dihydrostilbene lunularin (Li et al. 2022).

Acute pancreatitis is an inflammatory disorder in which the pancreas self-digests due to digestive zymogens' early activation (Tsang et al. 2016). Oxidative stress is widely acknowledged as a contributing factor to acute pancreatitis (Tsang et al. 2016). The authors showed that **35** effectively decreased the severity of acute pancreatitis in rat models by reducing pancreatic leukocyte infiltration, plasma α-amylase levels, and edema (Tsang et al. 2016). They also examined the NADPH oxidase system, a primary source of ROS. It was noted that **35**-treated rats had reduced NADPH oxidase activity and decreased NF-κB expression (Tsang et al. 2016). Lin et al. also noted decreased lung injury and reduced NF-κB activation in rats with acute pancreatitis treated with **35** (Lin et al. 2016). These results underscore the anti-inflammatory effects of **35** by modulating the NADPH oxidase/NF-κB pathway, suggesting its potential as a target for the treatment of acute pancreatitis (Lin et al. 2016; Tsang et al. 2016).

Maintaining intestinal barrier integrity is crucial for gut health, particularly because disruptions in barrier integrity are linked to autoimmune reactions in Type I diabetes (Zhang et al. 2022). It was found that resveratrol restored tight junction proteins in the intestinal wall, whereas **35** did not have a similar effect (Sorini et al. 2019; Zhang et al. 2022).

Type II diabetes has been associated with elevated levels of the lipid chaperone fatty acid binding protein 4 (FABP4), which also plays a role in insulin resistance (Rodríguez-Calvo et al. 2019). Lowering FABP4 levels is similarly linked to enhanced ventricular function and increased cardiomyocyte pathology; diabetic-induced cardiomyopathy is caused by elevated FABP4 levels (Rodríguez-Calvo et al. 2019). Azorín-Ortuño et al. studied **35**'s impact on FABP4 levels in peripheral blood cells and observed a slight but statistically meaningful reduction in FABP4 levels at low **35** concentrations, suggesting a potential role in protecting against diabetic cardiomyopathy (Azorín-Ortuño et al. 2012).

2.1.3 Flavonoids

Flavonoids are an abundant class of natural constituents, particularly in higher plants, with significant structural diversity that are categorized into six subgroups: chalcones, flavonols, flavones, flavanols, anthocyanins, and proanthocyanidins. The variations in their ring structure arise from differences in the degree of oxidation and reduction of the aglycone, hydroxylation, and the positioning and diversity of hydroxyl groups and substitution patterns.

More than 30 flavonoids were isolated from *Cannabis sativa,* including glycosylated (O or C glycosides), prenylated, methylated, or geranylated structural types (Figure 5) (Chen et al. 2012; Cheng et al. 2008; Clark and Bohm 1979; Di Giacomo et al. 2021; Ingallina et al. 2020; Ross et al. 2005; Turner et al. 1980). These compounds were separated using various chromatographic methods, including silica gel, VLC, macroreticular resin, Sephadex-LH-20, RP-HPLC, and identified by TLC, hydrolysis, UV, NMR, MS, and HPLC-PDA, and HPLC-DAD-MS analyses. Some of the cannabis flavonoids have been shown to possess biological activities beneficial to humans.

Crombie and Barrett, along with their groups, isolated canniflavins A (**36**) and B (**37**), two prenylated and geranylated flavones, using advanced spectroscopic methods (Barrett et al. 1986; Crombie and Crombie 1982).

Tomko et al. (2022) reported that **36** reduced cell viability in bladder cancer cell lines in a concentration-dependent manner. Additionally, when combined with cisplatin or gemcitabine, it showed varying effects, ranging from antagonistic to additive, with occasional synergism depending on the drugs and concentrations. Compound **36** also reduced cell invasion by 50% and triggered apoptosis through caspase-3 cleavage. Notably, it demonstrated synergistic effects with other cannabinoids, including cannabidiol, Δ9-tetrahydrocannabinol, cannabivarin, and cannabichromene in bladder cancer cells. These findings suggested that compound **36** could be cytotoxic to bladder transitional carcinoma cells and could enhance the effects of other medications (Tomko et al. 2022).

Caroli et al. assessed the *in vitro* anti-proliferative potential of an enriched polyphenol fraction (PEF) and the isolated **36** and **37** against human colon adenocarcinoma cell lines: Caco-2 and SW480. PEF demonstrated promising inhibitory potential, with IC_{50} values comparable to those of the standard drug. It was noted that **36** exhibited the strongest antiproliferative effect on both cell

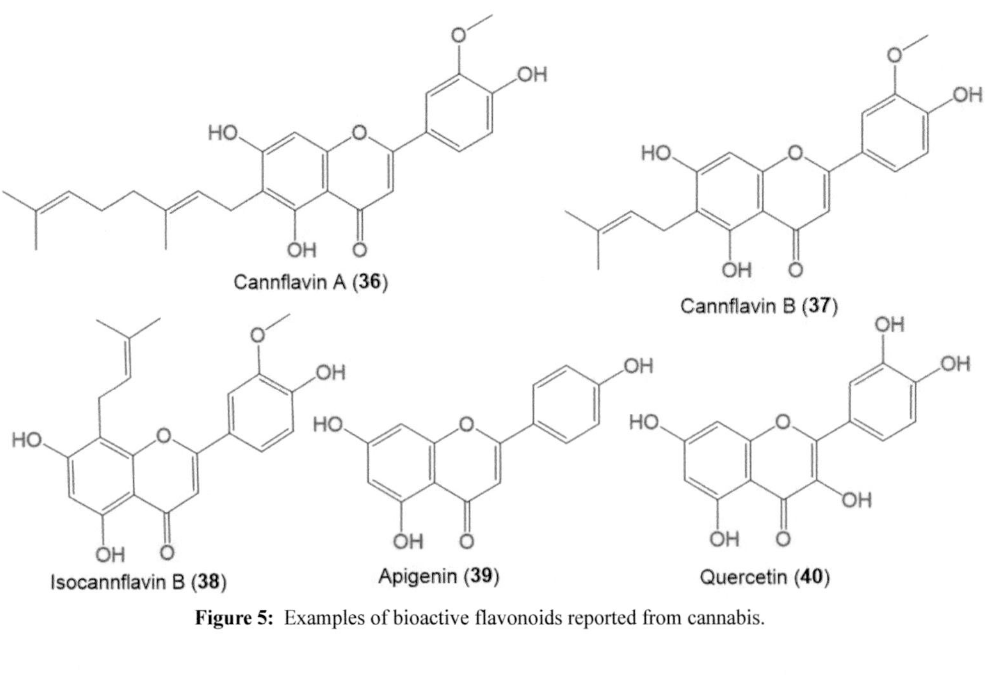

Figure 5: Examples of bioactive flavonoids reported from cannabis.

lines, even outperforming cisplatin, while **37** also demonstrated efficacy, though less than cannflavin A (Caroli et al. 2023). The key structural difference between **36** and **37** is the length of their attached groups, with cannflavin A's longer geranyl tail making it more hydrophobic; this higher lipophilicity may contribute to its stronger antiproliferative capacity. Additionally, the enhanced antiproliferative effects of PEF may be due to the synergistic interaction of its multiple components (Caroli et al. 2023).

Additionally, **36** has a neuroprotective effect, promoting PC12 cell viability against amyloid β-caused toxicity by minimizing Aβ1-42 aggregation at concentrations of 10 μM or less (Eggers et al. 2019). Enzyme assays by Werz et al. showed that **36** and **37** possessed anti-inflammatory capacities by inhibiting 5-lipoxygenase and microsomal PGE2 synthase-1, resulting in reducing leukotriene and PGE2 levels, respectively (Werz et al. 2014). Notably, **36** minimally inhibited COX-1 and COX-2, lacking the potential COX inhibitors' gastrointestinal side effects (Werz et al. 2014). Cannflavins A and B suppressed PGE2 production in human rheumatoid synovial cells triggered by the proinflammatory agent TPA (Barrett et al. 1985). They also demonstrated about 30 times the efficacy of aspirin in PGE2 release inhibition in human rheumatoid cells (Barrett et al. 1985).

Besides, **36** and **37** demonstrated moderate (IC_{50}s 4.5 and 5.0 μg/mL, respectively) anti-leishmanial potential against *Leishmania donovani* promastigotes (Radwan et al. 2008a). This was supported by a strong docking energy of -144.0 kJ/mol for cannflavin A binding to *Leishmania pteridine* reductase-1, a protein target in *L. donovani* (Ogungbe et al. 2014). In addition to its effect on *L. donovani*, **36** (IC_{50} 1.9 μg/mL) was moderately active against *Trypanosoma brucei brucei* (Salem et al. 2011).

Compound **36** also displayed efficient docking predictions to several Zika virus proteins: helicase (ATP site, –134.6 kJ/mol), helicase (RNA site, –131.7 kJ/mol), RNA-dependent RNA polymerase (–120.3 kJ/mol), and methyltransferase (–126.9 kJ/mol) (Byler et al. 2016). It exhibited a comparatively high reactivity (0.114 kcal/mol) and a high binding affinity (–9.7 kcal/mol) in the DFT (density functional theory) analysis against HIV-1 protease, an enzyme that makes HIV infectious (Akhtar et al. 2019). Further, it was identified as a potent docking ligand (docking energy –125.7 kJ/mol) for the Dengue virus envelope protein in a molecular docking analysis of several virus protein targets (Powers and Setzer 2016).

Isocannflavin B (**38**), a synthetic 8-prenylated isomer of **37,** induced a G0/G1 cell cycle arrest in estrogen-dependent T47-D human breast cancer cells, resulting in growth inhibition (Brunelli et al. 2009). An *in vitro* study by Moreau et al. (2019) revealed that **38** markedly increased apoptosis and reduced survival of Panc-02 and KPC pancreatic cancer cell lines. Furthermore, the *in vivo* experiment demonstrated a delayed progression of both local and metastatic tumors in pancreatic cancer animal models using FBL-03G delivered via smart radiotherapy biomaterials (Moreau et al. 2019).

Apigenin (**39**) exhibited little estrogenic activity and prevented the growth of breast cancer cells caused by estradiol, despite its strong affinity for the β-estrogen receptor (Wang and Kurzer 1997). Compound **39** and other flavonoids were found to interact with estrogen receptors, acting as primary estrogenic agents in cannabis smoke (Sauer et al. 1983). Smeriglio et al. (2016) demonstrated that Finola seed oil exhibited a notable antioxidant potential, likely due to its flavonoids, such as quercetin (**40**). A recent study by Curtasu et al. investigated the polyphenolic contents in different parts (buds, leaves, stems) of five cannabis cultivars (Finola, Ferimon, Fedora 17, Futura 75, and Santhica) using microflow LC-MS and spectrophotometry. The buds were found to contain the highest diversity and abundance of polyphenols, particularly catechin, epicatechin, and procyanidin B1 (Curtasu et al. 2025).

2.2 Terpenes

Terpenes are a diverse class of organic compounds composed primarily of carbon and hydrogen atoms. Their molecular structure is based on repeating isoprene units (C_5H_8), placing them within a larger family of hydrocarbons known as isoprenoids (Ashour et al. 2010). Terpenes are produced by a variety of plants and some animals, and play essential roles in both their biological processes and ecological interactions. Terpenes are classified based on the number of isoprene units into monoterpenes (two isoprene units; $C_{10}H_{16}$), sesquiterpenes (three isoprene units; $C_{15}H_{24}$), diterpenes (20 carbon atoms), and triterpenes (six isoprene units; $C_{30}H_{48}$).

Terpenes are synthesized via the mevalonate pathway (Zhu et al. 2014) or the methylerythritol phosphate (MEP) Pathway (Shi et al. 2020).

Cannabis sativa is recognized for its diverse range of chemical compounds, including terpenes and terpenoids (Figures 6 and 7), which contribute significantly to the plant's distinctive aroma, flavor, and potential therapeutic effects.

These compounds play important roles in the plant's interactions with its environment, such as attracting pollinators or deterring pests (Duggan 2021). They are primarily located within the glandular trichomes of the inflorescences and play a crucial role in defining their characteristic aroma (Laaboudi et al. 2024). Due to the varying composition of cannabis terpene profiles, distinct 'strains' can evoke diverse fragrance impressions, potentially influencing consumer preferences.

More than 200 unique terpenes have been recognized in cannabis, with the majority obtained by steam distillation (Fordjour et al. 2023). The terpenes found in cannabis include monoterpenes, as well as sesquiterpenes that have different levels based on genetic factors. In cannabis blooms, terpene concentrations ranged from 1% to 10% within trichomes. Nevertheless, through selective breeding, terpene concentrations have increased in recent years, with certain varieties showing concentrations of 3.5% or more (Lipson Feder et al. 2021).

Monoterpenes (10 C) contribute to the distinct, characteristic scent of cannabis (El-Feraly et al. 1977; Hendriks et al. 1975; Hood et al. 1973; Nigam et al. 2011; Radwan et al. 2021; Ross and ElSohly 1996; Simonsen and Todd 1942; Strömberg 1976). The key compounds include limonene (**46**), β-myrcene (**41**), α, β-pinene (**47** and **48**), linalool (**49**), α-terpinolene (**44**), borneol (**55**),

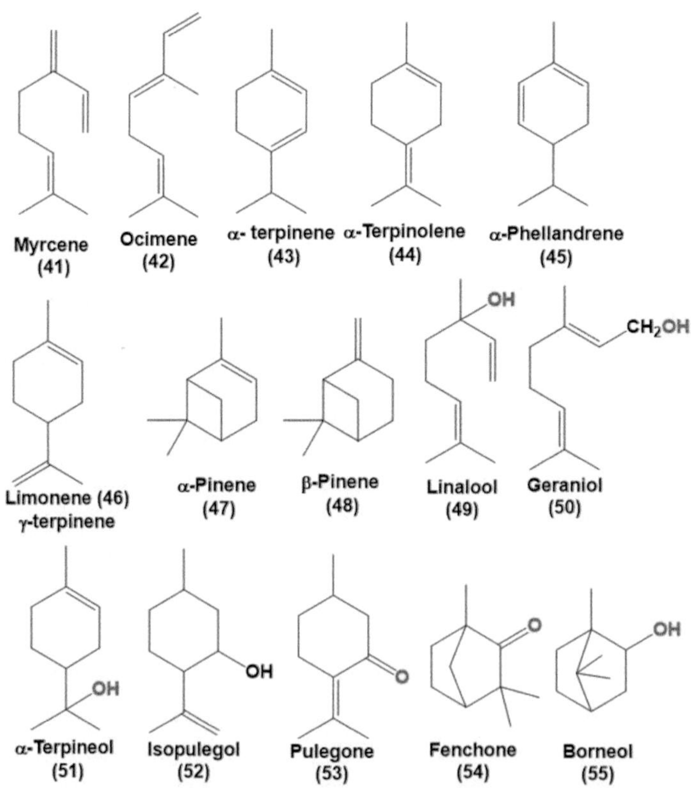

Figure 6: Examples of bioactive monoterpenes reported from cannabis.

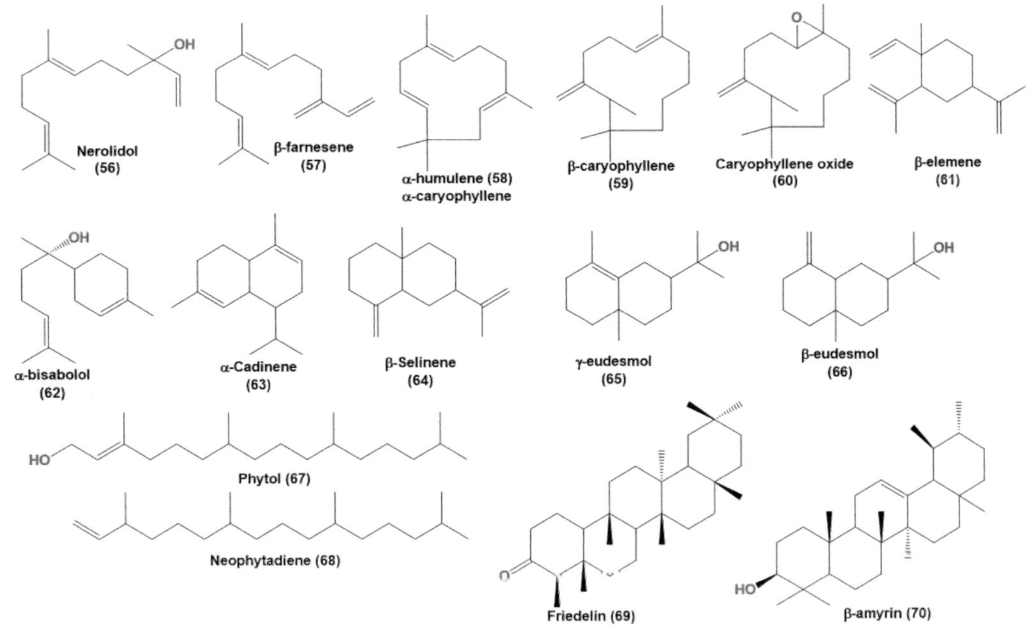

Figure 7: Examples of bioactive sesqui- and triterpenes reported from cannabis.

geraniol (**50**), and trans-ocimene (**42**) (Zheljazkov and Maggi 2021). Their presence in the plant intensifies during the late stages of the harvest (Isidore et al. 2021; Lowe et al. 2021).

Sesquiterpenes (15 C) play a role in the plant`s unique scent (Hendriks et al. 1975; Hood et al. 1973; Ingallina et al. 2020; Malingré et al. 1975; Menghini et al. 2021; Nigam et al. 2011; Radwan et al. 2021; Zheljazkov and Maggi 2021) They are exemplified by β-farnesene (**57**), caryophyllene oxide (**60**), α-humulene (α-caryophyllene) (**58**), bisabolol, β-selinene (**64**), α-cadinene (**63**), Ƴ-eudesmol (**65**), β-eudesmol (**66**), and β-caryophyllene (**59**), with their concentration peaking during the initial stages of the harvest (Isidore et al. 2021).

Diterpenes (20 C) are exemplified by only two compounds: phytol (**67**) and neophytadiene (**68**) (Ingallina et al. 2020; Radwan et al. 2021). Triterpenes are found in the stems, leaves, or roots of the plant. This group comprises friedelin (**69**) and smaller quantities of β-amyrin (**70**), which have been identified (Isidore et al. 2021; Radwan et al. 2021).

2.2.1 Interaction With Key Biological Targets (Receptors)

Cannabis terpenes have been found to interact non-selectively with a range of G-protein–coupled receptors (GPCRs), including opioid receptors, CB1/2 receptors, GPR55, dopamine receptors, muscarinic receptors, adrenergic receptors, adenosine receptors, and others. They also target ion channels, including transient receptor potential (TRP) channels, N-methyl-D-aspartate (NMDA) receptors, α-amino-3-hydroxy-5-methyl-4-isoxazolepropionic acid (AMPA) receptors, kainate receptors, nicotinic receptors, and potassium channels. These terpenes can activate both pro- and anti-inflammatory pathways, influencing the transmission of nociceptive signals at synapses, thereby either alleviating or contributing to pain perception (Liktor-Busa et al. 2021).

2.2.2 Analgesic and Anti-Inflammatory Activity of Monoterpenes

Limonene is known for its anxiolytic and anti-inflammatory effects. It is effective in providing pain relief at high doses, although results vary across pain types. It shows potential to reduce inflammation-related pain and anxiety by modulating serotonin and dopamine (Laaboudi et al. 2024; Liktor-Busa et al. 2021). α-Terpineol demonstrates significant pain relief in animal models, possibly interacting with opioid receptors and potassium channels (Liktor-Busa et al. 2021). α-Pinene also offers pain-relief, anti-inflammatory, and anti-swelling effects through essential oils rather than pure form studies (Liktor-Busa et al. 2021).

β-Pinene is known for its sedative, antihypertensive, and anti-nociceptive properties, potentially targeting the monoaminergic system, opioid receptors, and calcium channels (Duggan 2021; Nuutinen 2018).

Linalool exhibits marked efficacy in various pain models, acting through multiple receptor systems, including opioid and GABA receptors, suggesting a multifaceted mechanism of antinociception, involving both central and peripheral components (Liktor-Busa et al. 2021; Nuutinen 2018). β-Myrcene shows anti-nociceptive and anti-hyperalgesic effects in neuropathic pain models, involving opioid-related mechanisms (Liktor-Busa et al. 2021; Nuutinen 2018). Geraniol provides pain and inflammation relief without relying on opioid receptors. It has neuroprotective effects in spinal cord injury models (Liktor-Busa et al. 2021; Nuutinen 2018).

Terpinolene has anticancer potential and reduces neuron and neuroblastoma cell proliferation without causing genotoxicity. It also has antioxidant effects, protecting against LDL oxidation, which may benefit cardiovascular health. It possesses anti-inflammatory and pain-relieving properties, particularly when combined with NSAIDs, such as diclofenac (Liktor-Busa et al. 2021; Nuutinen 2018).

α-Terpinene is a fragrance compound and strong antioxidant that protects erythrocytes and lipids from oxidative damage. Although it shows no embryotoxicity and is not mutagenic, it may cause memory deficits with repeated use (Liktor-Busa et al. 2021; Nuutinen 2018).

Borneol has diverse therapeutic properties and is low-toxicity. It is traditionally used in Chinese medicine to enhance the drug effects and is known for its pain-relieving, anti-inflammatory, and neuroprotective properties (Liktor-Busa et al. 2021; Nuutinen 2018).

β-Caryophyllene is a bicyclic sesquiterpene abundant in cannabis and valued for its low toxicity and safety profile. It has anti-inflammatory, anticancer, and pain-relieving (antinociceptive) properties. It is a full agonist of the CB2 receptor, but shows minimal activity at the CB1 receptor, potentially targeting other molecular pathways (Liktor-Busa et al. 2021; Nuutinen 2018).

Caryophyllene oxide is a non-toxic terpene that is commonly used as a preservative in food, drugs, and cosmetics, and also serves as an insecticide. It lacks CB2 affinity but offers analgesic, anti-inflammatory, and anticancer properties (Liktor-Busa et al. 2021; Nuutinen 2018).

β-Elemene enhances chemotherapy and radiotherapy by inducing cancer cell apoptosis, cell cycle arrest, and autophagy, while being less toxic to normal cells. Beyond cancer, it shows protective effects against atherosclerosis by inhibiting inflammatory pathways (e.g., NF-κB and MAPK) and reducing oxidative stress (Liktor-Busa et al. 2021; Nuutinen 2018).

Fenchone demonstrates anticancer properties by inhibiting tumor growth through cell cycle arrest, and it enhances wound healing by promoting collagen synthesis and reducing inflammation. Additionally, it reveals antimicrobial and anti-diabetic properties (Liktor-Busa et al. 2021; Nuutinen 2018).

Pulegone exhibits a range of biological activities, including antimicrobial, anti-parasitic, anti-inflammatory, spasmolytic, antipyretic, anti-nociceptive, and antihistaminic effects (Chacon et al. 2022). While it displays promise as an anti-nociceptive agent, its adverse effects on heart, liver, and kidney function limit its suitability for long-term use or high doses (Liktor-Busa et al. 2021; Nuutinen 2018).

α-Phellandrene reveals prominent therapeutic potential, including immunomodulatory, anti-inflammatory, and antimicrobial effects. Additionally, it exhibits anti-nociceptive and anti-depressive effects, reducing pain sensitivity in neuropathic pain models through mechanisms involving multiple signaling systems (Liktor-Busa et al. 2021; Nuutinen 2018).

β-eudesmol exhibits various therapeutic effects, particularly as an anticancer, anti-inflammatory, and anticonvulsive agent. Additionally, it stimulates appetite and gastric emptying by increasing ghrelin levels and activating TRPA1 channels (transient receptor potential ankyrin 1), supporting its role in gastrointestinal and appetite regulation (Liktor-Busa et al. 2021; Nuutinen 2018).

Bisabolol demonstrates significant antinociceptive (pain-relieving) and anti-inflammatory effects, although its full dose-dependent mechanisms remain unclear, suggesting a nonspecific action. It also synergizes with diclofenac, enhancing pain relief while it reduces diclofenac-induced gastric damage (Liktor-Busa et al. 2021; Nuutinen 2018).

Nerolidol exhibits antinociceptive (pain-relieving) and anti-inflammatory effects, as demonstrated in animal studies using models like acetic acid-induced contractions, formalin, and carrageenan-induced paw edema (Liktor-Busa et al. 2021; Nuutinen 2018). Additionally, terpenes such as β-caryophyllene, limonene, and α-pinene displayed neuroprotective capacities due to their capability to boost antioxidant defenses, prohibit Aβ aggregation, and limit ROS-caused apoptosis (Doumar et al. 2025). A recent study by Singh et al. reported that Cannabis essential oil exhibited significant anti-inflammatory capacity by inhibiting NF-α, IL-6, and IL-1β in LPS-activated alveolar macrophages (MH-S), which was attributed to its high terpenes content (Singh et al. 2025).

2.2.3 Interaction of Terpenes With Cannabinoids

Terpenes can work synergistically with cannabinoids, such as THC and CBD, to influence the plant's overall effects. This interaction is known as the "entourage effect," where various cannabis compounds, aside from THC, work together to modulate the plant's psychoactive and therapeutic effects (Ferber et al. 2020). This synergy has been shown to enhance the effectiveness of cannabinoids in treating conditions such as inflammation, addiction, cancer, epilepsy, pain, and fungal or bacterial infections. Additionally, terpenes themselves possess analgesic and anxiolytic effects, enhancing stress relief, boosting energy, supporting concentration, improving mood through aromatherapy, and helping manage anxiety. Their therapeutic potential extends to various diseases and conditions affecting the nervous and gastrointestinal systems, owing to their antioxidative, anti-inflammatory, gastroprotective, antidepressant, antiproliferative, antipyretic, anticonvulsant, and neuroprotective properties (Laaboudi et al. 2024).

In laboratory settings, all terpenes have been shown to activate the CB1 receptor, with some also activating additional targets. These results imply that these terpenes from cannabis act as versatile cannabimimetic agents, lending conceptual backing to the entourage effect theory and potentially enhancing the therapeutic attributes of cannabinoids (LaVigne et al. 2021). Myrcene (**41**), linalool (**49**), and bisabolol (**62**) may enhance cannabis sedative properties and offer potential for treating neuroinflammatory and neurodegenerative diseases (Nuutinen 2018). Recent studies indicate α-pinene (**47**), β-caryophyllene (**59**), and linalool (**49**) may not directly interact with cannabinoid receptors (CB1 or CB2), implying that any synergy may not be receptor-mediated. Linalool (**49**) was found to enhance the effects of analgesics (e.g., morphine), potentially reducing tolerance and dependence (Nuutinen 2018). Besides, linalool (**49**), limonene (**46**), α-pinene (**47**), and β-myrcene (**41**) have shown sedative and anxiolytic effects through multiple mechanisms. β-Caryophyllene (**59**), for instance, provides anxiolytic and antidepressant effects in a CB2 receptor-dependent way, which may help chronic pain patients with co-occurring anxiety or depression. This interaction provides a possible mechanism for its synergy with cannabinoids and a foundation for future research. Although β-caryophyllene (**59**) is one of the more consistent terpene components in cannabis, it likely does not fully explain the strain-specific effects experienced by humans. Investigating the potential synergistic effects of terpenes on human responses to cannabis is a promising area of study, now increasingly feasible in regions with relaxed legal restrictions (Booth and Bohlmann 2019).

Given that pain, anxiety, and depression are often comorbid, the sedative, anxiolytic, and antidepressant effects of terpenes may enhance their therapeutic value, despite potential overlaps in effects that could confound studies focused solely on pain relief (Nuutinen 2018).

The terpenes found in cannabis demonstrate low acute toxicity, with typical LD_{50} values above 5,000 mg/kg, making them safe at therapeutic doses. Many terpenes, such as β-caryophyllene (**59**), limonene (**46**), and nerolidol (**56**), show potent therapeutic effects at low doses, including analgesic, anti-inflammatory, anxiolytic, and neuroprotective properties. Some terpenes, such as β-eudesmol (**66**), can stimulate appetite and aid digestion, while others, such as borneol and isopulegol (**52**), have sedative and anticonvulsive effects. Modifying terpenes, like creating analogs of β-caryophyllene (**59**), has shown promise in enhancing pharmacological properties by combining CB2 receptor activity with enzyme inhibition.

2.2.4 Pharmacokinetics of Cannabis Terpenes and Their Role in Pain Management

Terpenes are generally recognized as safe by the FDA and have shown potential therapeutic benefits, yet their pharmacokinetics (PK) and drug-drug interactions are not fully investigated. Terpenes and phytocannabinoids (e.g., THC, CBD) can affect liver enzymes such as cytochrome P450, thereby altering drug metabolism. β-Pinene (**48**) and terpinolene (**44**) can influence drug transporters, like P-GP (permeability glycoprotein), which affects drug bioavailability and distribution (Liktor-Busa et al. 2021).

Routes of administration influence terpene bioavailability, as terpenes have low water solubility, limiting absorption, with dermal, buccal, and vaporization being common methods. On the other hand, encapsulation methods (e.g., nanoparticles) can improve terpene absorption and brain penetration, which enhances their effectiveness against pain and inflammation.

Limonene (**46**), linalool (**49**), and β-caryophyllene (**59**) have specific PK profiles that reveal challenges in oral bioavailability but highlight increased brain uptake with advanced formulations. Certain terpenes also act as penetration enhancers, aiding other drugs' absorption, making them useful in transdermal applications (Liktor-Busa et al. 2021).

Current terpene PK research suggests that these compounds are primarily metabolized by CYP450 enzymes and excreted by the liver and kidneys. However, further PK studies in the presence of common analgesics are necessary to clarify potential interactions and synergistic effects, particularly in Cannabis formulations (Liktor-Busa et al. 2021).

2.2.5 Clinical Evidence Supporting the Efficacy of Terpenes in Pain Management

While preclinical animal studies support terpenes' potential in pain relief, human clinical evidence remains limited and methodologically constrained. Key challenges include small sample sizes, lack of placebo controls, and variability in terpene formulations (e.g., essential oils with multiple components). In studies using essential oils rich in terpenes, terpenes showed efficacy in reducing pain and anxiety across various patient populations and pain types (e.g., labor pain, burn pain, and migraine). However, inhalation as the main administration route complicates dose standardization.

Studies with defined terpenes and routes (e.g., oral, intravenous) provide additional support. For example, synthetic terpenes like epomediol and sobrerol have been shown to improve chronic pain symptoms in specific conditions, while Rowatinex outperformed ibuprofen for chronic prostatitis pain. Despite promising results, the influence of terpenes' scents may contribute to placebo effects, complicating conclusions about their efficacy (Liktor-Busa et al. 2021).

Overall, rigorous, placebo-controlled, randomized trials are essential to establish the therapeutic potential of defined terpenes in human pain management as a non-opioid, non-cannabinoid alternative.

2.3 Anthraquinones

Anthraquinones and structurally similar molecules have demonstrated antiviral properties. Among them, denbinobin (**71**) (Figure 8), a 1,4-phenanthrenequinone separated from a variety of cannabis, did not interfere with HIV-1 reverse integration or transcription but prevented reactivation in Jurkat T cells stimulated by TNFα, anti-CD3/CD28 antibodies, or PMA (Sánchez-Duffhues et al. 2008). Additionally, denbinobin prohibited HIV-1-LTR transcriptional activity during the elongation phase and TNFα-induced LTR activity. It blocked NF-κB's binding to DNA, prevented phosphorylation and degradation of its inhibitory protein IκBα, and inhibited phosphorylation of the NF-κB p65 subunit in TNFα-stimulated cells (Sánchez-Duffhues et al. 2008). These findings suggest that 1,4-phenanthrenequinones could offer potential leads for alternative AIDS treatments.

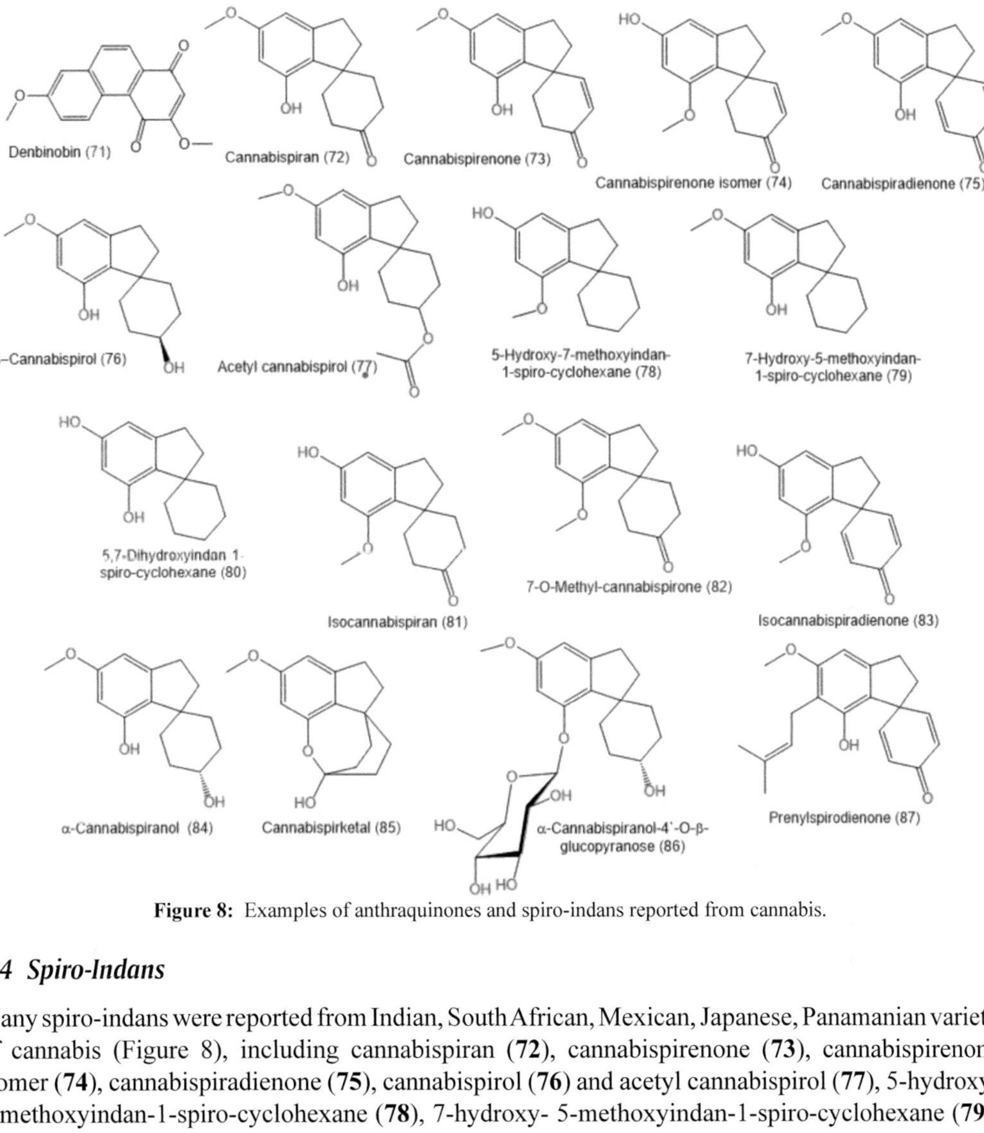

Figure 8: Examples of anthraquinones and spiro-indans reported from cannabis.

2.4 Spiro-Indans

Many spiro-indans were reported from Indian, South African, Mexican, Japanese, Panamanian variety of cannabis (Figure 8), including cannabispiran (**72**), cannabispirenone (**73**), cannabispirenone isomer (**74**), cannabispiradienone (**75**), cannabispirol (**76**) and acetyl cannabispirol (**77**), 5-hydroxy-7-methoxyindan-1-spiro-cyclohexane (**78**), 7-hydroxy- 5-methoxyindan-1-spiro-cyclohexane (**79**), 5,7-dihydroxyindan-1-spiro-cyclohexane (**80**), isocannabispiran (**81**), 7-O-methyl-cannabispirone (**82**), isocannabispiradienone (**83**), *a*-cannabispiranol (**84**), Cannabispirketal (**85**), *a*-cannabispiranol-4*0*-O-β-glucopyranose (**86**), and prenylspirodienone (**87**) (Bercht et al. 1976; Boeren et al. 1977; Cromble et al. 1979; El-Feraly et al. 1986; ElSohly and Turner 1982a, 1982b; Guo et al. 2018; Kettenes-van den Bosch and Salemink 1978; Nalli et al. 2018; Ottersen et al. 1976; Radwan et al. 2008b, Shoyama and Nishioka 1978) using polyamide/silica gel/flash chromatography/C18-HPLC and elucidated by spectral/chemical/X-ray analyses. Unfortunately, only a few studies reported their biological evaluation. Guo et al. (2017) stated that cannabispirketal (**85**) and *a*-cannabispiranol-4`-O-β-glucopyranose (**86**) demonstrated antitumor capacities versus HT-2,9 MCF-7, HepG2, and A549 through promoting apoptosis and inhibiting cell proliferation, whereas spirans' *α*, *β*-unsaturated ketone moiety was found to be crucial for activity (Guo et al. 2018). In 2018, Nalli et al. reported that prenylspirodienone (**87**) (IC_{50} 49.6 μM) exhibited antibacterial potential against *Bacillus thuringiensis* MTCC (Nalli et al. 2018).

2.5 Alkaloids

Alkaloids are nitrogen-containing metabolites renowned for their substantial bioactivities across various plant species. It is noteworthy that alkaloids are less prevalent than terpenoids and flavonoids in cannabis; only a few reports have been published on this plant, with limited evaluation of their biological properties.

Cannabisativine (**88**) and anhydrocannabisativine (**89**), spermidine-type alkaloids, were characterized from *C. sativa* that feature a 13-membered lactam core, forming a ring with a disubstituted tetrahydro-pyridine ring (Figure 9). Cannabisativine (**88**) was the first reported alkaloid from Mexican *Cannabis* roots MeOH extract in 1975, and it was assigned by X-ray analysis (Latter et al. 1975; Ottersen et al. 1976). Also, it was reported that the Thai variant stem and leaves were extracted with EtOH using base/acid partition, SiO_2 CC, TLC, and crystallization from acetone (El Feraly and Turner 1975). The 2nd alkaloid, anhydrocannabisativine (**89**), was separated by Ottersen et al. (1976) and ElSohly et al. (1978) from stems/leaves and roots/leaves of cannabis Mexican variant (ElSohly et al. 1978; Ottersen et al. 1976) through acid/base extraction/ SiO_2 CC, respectively, and characterized by spectral analysis and cannabisativine (**88**) conversion to anhydrocannabisativine (**89**) (ElSohly et al. 1978; Ottersen et al. 1976). Fasakin et al. stated that cannabisativine and anhydrocannabisativine were 410.30 and 218.11 μg/g, respectively (Fasakin et al. 2022).

Yan et al. characterized indole diketopiperazine alkaloids of the echinulin family: (12S,22R)-dihydroxyisoechinulin A (**90**)/(12S,22S)-dihydroxyisoechinulin A (**91**) and (12R)- neoechinulin A (**92**)/(12S)-neoechinulin A (**93**) that are stereoisomers from cannabis seed using spectra/chiral HPLC analyses. Neoechinulin A was found to foster SIRT1 (silent information regulator two homologue-1) in HEK293 cells. SIRT1 is a sirtuin family member that possesses the NAD+-dependent deacetylase function and controls various cellular functions, including aging, energy metabolism, and cell cycle progression. SIRT1-expression promoters are candidates for treating neurodegenerative disorders (Yan et al. 2016).

Other alkaloids, such as choline (**95**), muscarine (**96**), L-(+)-isoleucine betaine (**97**), and neurine (**98**), as well as hexadecamide (**99**), and hordenine (**94**), were identified from *C. sativa* (El Feraly and Turner 1975; Gill et al. 1970; Mechoulam 1989). Neurine and choline's concentration was 0.01% in dried roots (Turner and Mole 1973).

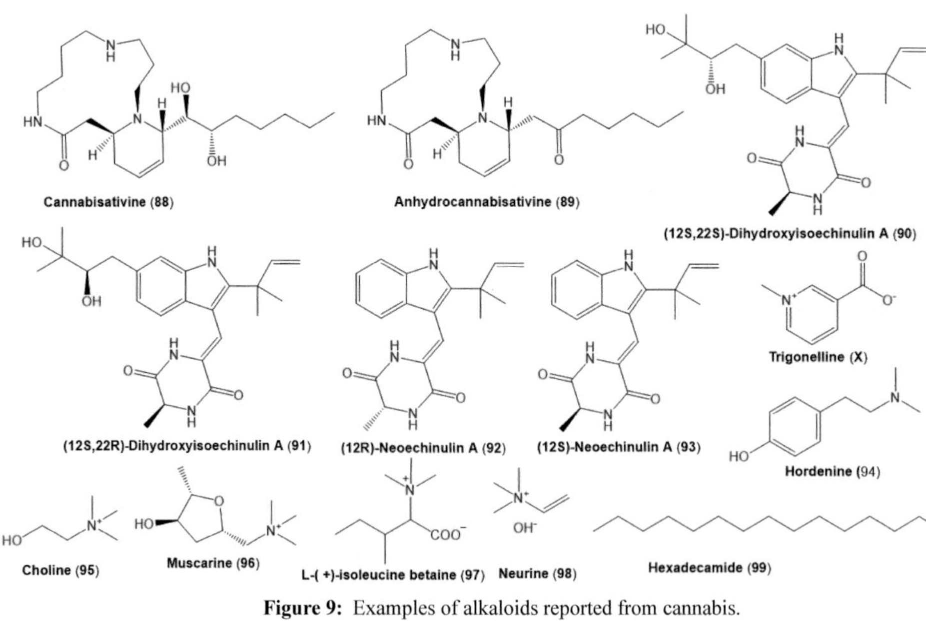

Figure 9: Examples of alkaloids reported from cannabis.

2.6 Fatty Acids

Cannabis seeds contain 30–35% fixed oil, while other parts of the plant contain only about 8–16%. Although cannabis produces some fatty acids, it is not generally regarded as a major dietary source of them. The fatty acids synthesized by cannabis have a unique chemical composition, with shelled seeds containing nearly 50% fat as triglycerides (Babiker et al. 2021). These oils are distinctive among cooking oils due to their low saturated fat content (0.9%) and high polyunsaturated fat content (80%) (Dalli et al. 2023). Commercial cannabis oil includes omega-3 (linolenic, isolinolenic, eicosapentaenoic acids) and omega-6 (linoleic acid), along with other fatty acids like oleic and stearic acids. Key fatty acids include linoleic (54–60%), α-linolenic (18–23%), and oleic acid (7–12%). Cannabis seeds are also nutrient-dense, containing 25% high-quality protein, 35% fat, vitamins (C, E, B1, B2, B6, B12, and folate), minerals (calcium, magnesium, potassium, etc.), and macronutrients (fat, carbs, fiber, and protein) (Farinon et al. 2020; Silver et al. 2021).

3. Conclusion

Abundant non-cannabinoid metabolites have been reported in *Cannabis sativa*, such as phenolics, terpenes, flavonoids, and alkaloids, extending the phytochemical profile of cannabis and adding remarkable depth to its phytochemical profile, beyond the widely studied cannabinoids. These compounds have demonstrated promising pharmacological activities supported by *in vitro* and *in vivo* investigations. Their presence was reported to complement or synergize with the effects of cannabinoids. For instance, β-caryophyllene was reported to have analgesic and anti-inflammatory effects as a selective CB2 receptor agonist in mouse models. Cannflavin A demonstrated anti-inflammatory properties 30 times powerful than aspirin due to its significant suppression of prostaglandin E2 synthesis. Cannflavins are also reported to have significant anti-viral activity *in silico*; however, an *in vitro* investigation will be worthwhile to confirm their validity. Stilbenes are less abundant constituents in cannabis that displayed marked anti-inflammatory and antioxidative potential, whereas alkaloids exhibited anti-aging and neuroprotective properties.

Interestingly, these compounds exerted their activities through different molecular targets other than the endocannabinoid system, including NF-κB signaling pathways, GABA receptors, and TRP channels. Despite their promising reported activities, further studies are needed on their pharmacokinetics, safety, mechanisms of action, and synergistic interactions to validate their therapeutic potential.

The application of omics sciences can aid in numerous aspects of cannabis metabolites research. Proteomic studies would assist a deeper understanding of the environmental impact on the production of specific metabolites and enable the production of metabolites in heterologous hosts for toxicological and pharmacological investigations. Bio-guided fractioning for metabolomics is beneficial for metabolite discovery and pharmacological characterization. Transcriptomic studies would enable the identification of genes and potentially associate metabolomic profiles with specific cultivars or chemotypes.

References

Ahammed, S., Afrin, R., Uddin, N., Al-Amin, Y., Hasan, K., Haque, U. et al. (2021). Acetylcholinesterase inhibitory and antioxidant activity of the compounds isolated from *Vanda roxburghii. Advances in Pharmacological and Pharmaceutical Sciences*, 2021(1): 5569054. https://doi.org/10.1155/2021/5569054

Akhtar, A., Hussain, W., and Rasool, N. (2019). Probing the pharmacological binding properties, and reactivity of selective phytochemicals as potential HIV-1 protease inhibitors. *Universitas Scientiarum*, 24: 441–464. https://revistas.javeriana.edu.co/index.php/scientarium/article/download/22703/22936

Aksorn, N., Losuwannarak, N., Tungsukruthai, S., Roytrakul, S., and Chanvorachote, P. (2021). Analysis of the protein–protein interaction network identifying c-Met as a target of gigantol in the suppression of lung cancer metastasis. *Cancer Genomics & Proteomics*, 18(3): 261–272. https://doi.org/10.21873/CGP.20257

Allegrone, G., Pollastro, F., Magagnini, G., Taglialatela-Scafati, O., Seegers, J., Koeberle, A. et al. (2017). The bibenzyl canniprene inhibits the production of pro-inflammatory eicosanoids and selectively accumulates in some *Cannabis sativa* strains. *Journal of Natural Products*, 80(3): 731–734. https://doi.org/10.1021/ACS.JNATPROD.6B01126/ASSET/IMAGES/LARGE/NP-2016-01126S_0001.JPEG

Ashour, M., Wink, M., and Gershenzon, J. (2010). Biochemistry of terpenoids: Monoterpenes, sesquiterpenes and diterpenes. *Biochemistry of Plant Secondary Metabolism: Second Edition*, 40: 258–303. https://doi.org/10.1002/9781444320503.CH5

Azorín-Ortuño, M., Yáñez-Gascón, M. J., González-Sarrías, A., Larrosa, M., Vallejo, F., Pallarés, F. J. et al. (2012). Effects of long-term consumption of low doses of resveratrol on diet-induced mild hypercholesterolemia in pigs: a transcriptomic approach to disease prevention. *The Journal of Nutritional Biochemistry*, 23(7): 829–837. https://doi.org/10.1016/J.JNUTBIO.2011.04.007

Babiker, E. E., Uslu, N., Al Juhaimi, F., Mohamed Ahmed, I. A., Ghafoor, K., Özcan, M. M. et al. (2021). Effect of roasting on antioxidative properties, polyphenol profile and fatty acids composition of hemp (*Cannabis sativa* L.) seeds. *LWT*, 139: 110537. https://doi.org/10.1016/J.LWT.2020.110537

Barrett, M. L., Gordon, D., and Evans, F. J. (1985). Isolation from *Cannabis sativa* L. of cannflavin—a novel inhibitor of prostaglandin production. *Biochemical Pharmacology*, 34(11): 2019–2024. https://doi.org/10.1016/0006-2952(85)90325-9

Barrett, M. L., Scutt, A. M., and Evans, F. J. (1986). Cannflavin A and B, prenylated flavones from *Cannabis sativa* L. *Experientia*, 42(4): 452–453. https://doi.org/10.1007/BF02118655/METRICS

Basque, A., Nguyen, H. T., Touaibia, M., and Martin, L. J. (2021). Gigantol improves cholesterol metabolism and progesterone biosynthesis in MA-10 leydig cells. *Current Issues in Molecular Biology*, 44(1): 73–93. https://doi.org/10.3390/CIMB44010006

Bercht, C. A. L., van Dongen, J. P. C. M., Heerma, W., Ch. Lousberg, R. J. J., and Küppers, F. J. E. M. (1976). Cannabispirone and cannabispirenone, two naturally occurring spiro-compounds. *Tetrahedron*, 32(23): 2939–2943. https://doi.org/10.1016/0040-4020(76)80149-4

Bhummaphan, N., and Chanvorachote, P. (2015). Gigantol suppresses cancer stem cell-like phenotypes in lung cancer cells. *Evidence-Based Complementary and Alternative Medicine : ECAM*, 2015. https://doi.org/10.1155/2015/836564

Bode, L. M., Bunzel, D., Huch, M., Cho, G. S., Ruhland, D., Bunzel, M. et al. (2013). *In vivo* and *in vitro* metabolism of trans-resveratrol by human gut microbiota. *The American Journal of Clinical Nutrition*, 97(2): 295–309. https://doi.org/10.3945/AJCN.112.049379

Boeren, E. G., ElSohly, M. A., Turner, C. E., and Salemink, C. A. (1977). ß-Cannabispiranol: A new non-cannabinoid phenol from *Cannabis sativa* L. *Experientia*, 33(7): 848. https://doi.org/10.1007/BF01951236/METRICS

Booth, J. K., and Bohlmann, J. (2019). Terpenes in *Cannabis sativa* – From plant genome to humans. *Plant Science*, 284: 67–72. https://doi.org/10.1016/J.PLANTSCI.2019.03.022

Boucher, R., Germain, H., and Desgagné-Penix, I. (2025). Exploring the Lesser-Known Bioactive Natural Products of Plant Species of the Genus *Cannabis* L.: Alkaloids, Phenolic Compounds, and Their Therapeutic Potential. *Plants*, 14: 1372. https://doi.org/10.3390/ plants14091372.

Bourjot, M., Zedet, A., Demange, B., Pudlo, M., and Girard-Thernier, C. (2016). *In vitro* mammalian arginase inhibitory and antioxidant effects of amide derivatives isolated from the hempseed cakes (*Cannabis sativa*). *Planta Medica International Open*, 3(03): e64–e67. https://doi.org/10.1055/S-0042-119400

Brunelli, E., Pinton, G., Bellini, P., Minassi, A., Appendino, G., and Moro, L. (2009). Flavonoid-induced autophagy in hormone sensitive breast cancer cells. *Fitoterapia*, 80(6): 327–332. https://doi.org/10.1016/J.FITOTE.2009.04.002

Byler, K. G., Ogungbe, I. V., and Setzer, W. N. (2016). *In-silico* screening for anti-Zika virus phytochemicals. *Journal of Molecular Graphics and Modelling*, 69: 78–91. https://doi.org/10.1016/J.JMGM.2016.08.011

Caroli, C., Brighenti, V., Cattivelli, A., Salamone, S., Pollastro, F., Tagliazucchi, D., and Pellati, F. (2023). Identification of phenolic compounds from inflorescences of non-psychoactive *Cannabis sativa* L. by UHPLC-HRMS and *in vitro* assessment of the antiproliferative activity against colorectal cancer. *Journal of Pharmaceutical and Biomedical Analysis*, 236: 115723. https://doi.org/10.1016/J.JPBA.2023.115723

Chacon, F. T., Raup-Konsavage, W. M., Vrana, K. E., and Kellogg, J. J. (2022). Secondary terpenes in *Cannabis sativa* L.: Synthesis and synergy. *Biomedicines,10*(12), 3142. https://doi.org/10.3390/BIOMEDICINES10123142

Chen,B.,Cai,G.,Yuan,Y.,Li,T.,He,Q.,andHe,J.(2012).Chemicalconstituentsinhemppectin.*ZhongguoShiyanFangjixue Zazhi*, 18: 98–100. https://scholar.google.com/scholar?hl=en&as_sdt=0%2C5&q=+Chemical+constituents+in+hemp+pectin.+ Zhongguo+Shiyan+Fangjixue+Zazhi+2012%2C+18%2C+98%E2%80%93100.&btnG=

Cheng, L., Kong, D., Hu, G., and Hemp, I. (2008). Chemical constituents from petroleum ether and n-butanol portions of methanol extract. *Zhongguo Yiyao Gongye Zazhi*, 39: 18–21. https://scholar.google.com/scholar?hl=en&as_sdt=0%2C5&q=Cheng%2C+L.%3B+Kong%2C+D.%3B+Hu%2C+G.%3B+Hemp%2C+I.+Chemical+constituents+from+petroleum+ether+and+n-butanol+portions+of+methanol+extract.+Zhongguo+Yiyao+Gongye+Zazhi+2008%2C+39%2C+18%E2%80%9321.&btnG=

Clark, M. N., and Bohm, B. A. (1979). Flavonoid variation in *Cannabis* L. *Botanical Journal of the Linnean Society*, 79(3): 249–257. https://doi.org/10.1111/J.1095-8339.1979.TB01517.X

Crini, G., Lichtfouse, E., Chanet, G., and Morin-Crini, N. (2020). Applications of hemp in textiles, paper industry, insulation and building materials, horticulture, animal nutrition, food and beverages, nutraceuticals, cosmetics and hygiene, medicine, agrochemistry, energy production and environment: a review. *Environmental Chemistry Letters 2020 18:5*, 18(5): 1451–1476. https://doi.org/10.1007/S10311-020-01029-2

Crombie, L., and Crombie, W. M. L. (1982). Natural products of Thailand high Δ1-THC-strain *Cannabis*. The bibenzyl-spiran-dihydrophenanthrene group: relations with cannabinoids and canniflavones. *Journal of the Chemical Society, Perkin Transactions* 1, 0, 1455–1466. https://doi.org/10.1039/P19820001455

Crombie, L., Mary, W., and Crombie, L. (1978). Dihydrostilbenes of Thailand *Cannabis*. *Tetrahedron Letters*, 19(47): 4711–4714. https://doi.org/10.1016/S0040-4039(01)85712-9

Cromble, L., Mary, W., Crombie, L., and Jamieson, S. V. (1979). Isolation of cannabispiradienone and cannabidihydrophenanthrene. biosynthetic relationships between the spirans and dihydrostilbenes of Thailand *Cannabis*. *Tetrahedron Letters*, 20(7): 661–664. https://doi.org/10.1016/S0040-4039(01)86030-5

Curtasu, M. V., Pallesen, B. E., and Norskov, N. P. (2025). Quantitative distribution of polyphenolic compounds during plant development in five varieties of organic Hemp (*Cannabis sativa* L.). *Journal of Agricultural and Food Chemistry*, 73(26): 16359–16369. https://doi.org/10.1021/acs.jafc.5c01299

Dalli, M., Azizi, S. E., Azghar, A., Saddari, A., Benaissa, E., Lahlou, Y. Ben et al. (2023). *Cannabis sativa* L.: A Comprehensive review on legislation, decriminalization, phytochemistry, antimicrobial activity, and safety. *Journal of Food and Drug Analysis*, 31(3): 408–435. https://doi.org/10.38212/2224-6614.3471

Di Giacomo, V., Recinella, L., Chiavaroli, A., Orlando, G., Cataldi, A., Rapino, M. et al. (2021). Metabolomic profile and antioxidant/anti-inflammatory effects of industrial hemp water extract in fibroblasts, Keratinocytes and Isolated Mouse Skin Specimens. *Antioxidants*, 10(1): 44. https://doi.org/10.3390/ANTIOX10010044

Doumar, H., Mostafi, H. E., Elhessni, A., Ebn Touhami, M., and Mesfioui, A. (2025). Exploring the diversity of cannabis cannabinoid and non-cannabinoid compounds and their roles in Alzheimer's disease: A review. *IBRO Neuroscience Reports* 18, 96–119. https://doi.org/10.1016/j.ibneur.2024.12.011

Duggan, P. J. (2021). The chemistry of cannabis and cannabinoids. *Australian Journal of Chemistry*, 74(6): 369–387. https://doi.org/10.1071/CH21006

Eggers, C., Fujitani, M., Kato, R., and Smid, S. (2019). Novel cannabis flavonoid, cannflavin A displays both a hormetic and neuroprotective profile against amyloid β-mediated neurotoxicity in PC12 cells: Comparison with geranylated flavonoids, mimulone and diplacone. *Biochemical Pharmacology*, 169: 113609. https://doi.org/10.1016/J.BCP.2019.08.011

El Feraly, F. S., and Turner, C. E. (1975). Alkaloids of Cannabis sativa leaves. *Phytochemistry*, 14.

El-Feraly, F. S., El-Sherei, M. M., and Al-Muhtadi, F. J. (1986). Spiro-indans from Cannabis sativa. *Phytochemistry*, 25(8): 1992–1994. https://doi.org/10.1016/S0031-9422(00)81194-2

El-Feraly, F. S., ElSohly, M. A., Boeren, E. G., Turner, C. E., Ottersen, T., and Aasen, A. (1977). Crystal and molecular structure of cannabispiran and its correlation to dehydrocannabispiran : Two novel *cannabis* constituents. *Tetrahedron*, 33(18): 2373–2378. https://doi.org/10.1016/0040-4020(77)80249-4

ElSohly, H. N., ElSohly, M. A., Turner, C. E., and Ma, G. E. (1984). Constituents of *Cannabis sativa*, xxv. isolation of two new dihydrostilbenes from a panamanian variant. *Journal of Natural Products*, 47(3): 445–452. https://doi.org/10.1021/NP50033A008/ASSET/NP50033A008.FP.PNG_V03

ElSohly, H. N., and Turner, C. E. (1982a). Constituents of *Cannabis sativa* L. XXII. Isolation of spiro-indan and dihydrostilbene compounds from a Panamanian variant grown in Mississippi, United States of America. *Bulletin on Narcotics*, 34: 51–56. https://www.unodc.org/unodc/en/data-and-analysis/bulletin/bulletin_1982-01-01_2_page005.html

ElSohly, H. N., and Turner, C. E. (1982b). Iso-cannabispiran, a new spiro compound isolated from Panamenian variant of *Cannabis sativa* L. *Experientia*, 38(2): 229. https://doi.org/10.1007/BF01945080/METRICS

ElSohly, M. A., Turner, C. E., Phoebe, C. H., Knapp, J. E., Schiff, P. L., and Slatkin, D. J. (1978). Anhydrocannabisativine, a new alkaloid from *Cannabis sativa* L. *Journal of Pharmaceutical Sciences*, 67(1): 124–124. https://doi.org/10.1002/JPS.2600670135

Farinon, B., Molinari, R., Costantini, L., and Merendino, N. (2020). The Seed of industrial hemp (*Cannabis sativa* L.): Nutritional quality and potential functionality for human health and nutrition. *Nutrients*, 12(7): 1935. https://doi.org/10.3390/NU12071935

Fasakin, O. W., Oboh, G., Ademosun, A. O., and Lawal, A. O. (2022). The modulatory effects of alkaloid extracts of *Cannabis sativa*, *Datura stramonium*, *Nicotiana tabacum* and male *Carica papaya* on neurotransmitter, neurotrophic and neuroinflammatory systems linked to anxiety and depression. *Inflammopharmacology*, 30(6): 2447–2476. https://doi.org/10.1007/S10787-022-01006-X/METRICS

Fei, Y., Zhang, S., Han, S., Qiu, B., Lu, Y., Huang, W. et al. (2022). The Role of Dihydroresveratrol in enhancing the synergistic effect of *Ligilactobacillus salivarius* Li01 and resveratrol in ameliorating colitis in mice. *Research*, https://doi.org/10.34133/2022/9863845

Ferber, S. G., Namdar, D., Hen-Shoval, D., Eger, G., Koltai, H., Shoval, G. et al. (2020). The "Entourage effect": Terpenes coupled with cannabinoids for the treatment of mood disorders and anxiety disorders. *Current Neuropharmacology*, 18(2): 87. https://doi.org/10.2174/1570159X17666190903103923

Fordjour, E., Manful, C. F., Sey, A. A., Javed, R., Pham, T. H., Thomas, R. et al. (2023). *Cannabis*: A multifaceted plant with endless potentials. *Frontiers in Pharmacology*, 14: 1200269. https://doi.org/10.3389/FPHAR.2023.1200269/BIBTEX

Gill, E. W., Paton, W. D. M., and Pertwee, R. G. (1970). Preliminary experiments on the chemistry and pharmacology of *Cannabis*. *Nature*, 228(5267): 134–136. https://doi.org/10.1038/228134a0

Guo, T., Liu, Q., Hou, P., Li, F., Guo, S., Song, W. et al. (2018). Stilbenoids and cannabinoids from the leaves of *Cannabis sativa* f. *sativa* with potential reverse cholesterol transport activity. *Food & Function*, 9(12): 6608–6617. https://doi.org/10.1039/C8FO01896K

Hanuš, L. O., Meyer, S. M., Muñoz, E., Taglialatela-Scafati, O., and Appendino, G. (2016). Phytocannabinoids: a unified critical inventory. *Natural Product Reports*, 33(12): 1357–1392. https://doi.org/10.1039/C6NP00074F

Hendriks, H., Malingré, T. M., Batterman, S., and Bos, R. (1975). Mono- and sesqui-terpene hydrocarbons of the essential oil of *Cannabis sativa*. *Phytochemistry*, 14(3): 814–815. https://doi.org/10.1016/0031-9422(75)83045-7

Hood, L. V. S., Dames, M. E., and Barry, G. T. (1973). Headspace volatiles of marijuana. *Nature*, *242*(5397): 402–403. https://doi.org/10.1038/242402a0

Howes, M. J. R., Quave, C. L., Collemare, J., Tatsis, E. C., Twilley, D., Lulekal, E. et al. (2020). Molecules from nature: Reconciling biodiversity conservation and global healthcare imperatives for sustainable use of medicinal plants and fungi. *Plants, People, Planet*, 2(5): 463–481. https://doi.org/10.1002/PPP3.10138

Huang, J., Liu, C., Duan, S., Lin, J., Luo, Y., Tao, S. et al. (2021). Gigantol inhibits proliferation and enhances DDP-induced apoptosis in breast-cancer cells by downregulating the PI3K/Akt/mTOR signaling pathway. *Life Sciences*, 274: 119354. https://doi.org/10.1016/J.LFS.2021.119354

Ingallina, C., Sobolev, A. P., Circi, S., Spano, M., Fraschetti, C., Filippi, A. et al. (2020). *Cannabis sativa* L. Inflorescences from Monoecious Cultivars Grown in Central Italy: An Untargeted chemical characterization from early flowering to ripening. *Molecules*, 25(8): 1908. https://doi.org/10.3390/MOLECULES25081908

Isidore, E., Karim, H., and Ioannou, I. (2021). Extraction of phenolic compounds and terpenes from *Cannabis sativa* L. By-Products: from conventional to intensified processes. *Antioxidants*, 10(6): 942. https://doi.org/10.3390/ANTIOX10060942

Kaneko, N., Kurata, M., Yamamoto, T., Morikawa, S., and Masumoto, J. (2019). The role of interleukin-1 in general pathology. *Inflammation and Regeneration*, 39(1): 1–16. https://doi.org/10.1186/S41232-019-0101-5

Kang, H., Sun, Y., Hu, X., and Liu, L. (2022). Gigantol inhibits proliferation and enhanced oxidative stress-mediated apoptosis through modulating of Wnt/β-catenin signaling pathway in HeLa cells. *Journal of Biochemical and Molecular Toxicology*, 36(1): e22944. https://doi.org/10.1002/JBT.22944

Kettenes-van den Bosch, J. J., and Salemink, C. A. (1978). Cannabis XIX. Oxygenated 1,2-diphenylethanes from marihuana. *Recueil Des Travaux Chimiques Des Pays-Bas*, 97(7-8): 221–222. https://doi.org/10.1002/RECL.19780970714

Khattab, A. R., and Teleb, M. (2022). *In Silico* Discovery of non-psychoactive scaffolds in *Cannabis* halting SARS-CoV-2 host entry and replication machinery. *Future Virology*, 17(6): 367–386. https://doi.org/10.2217/FVL-2021-0309

Laaboudi, F. Z., Rejdali, M., Amhamdi, H., Salhi, A., Elyoussfi, A., and Ahari, M. 'hamed. (2024). In the weeds: A comprehensive review of cannabis; its chemical complexity, biosynthesis, and healing abilities. *Toxicology Reports*, 13: 101685. https://doi.org/10.1016/J.TOXREP.2024.101685

Latter, H. L., Abraham, D. J., Turner, C. E., Knapp, J. E., Schiff, P. L., and Slatkin, D. J. (1975). Cannabisativine, a new alkaloid from *Cannabis sativa* l. root. *Tetrahedron Letters*, 16(33): 2815–2818. https://doi.org/10.1016/S0040-4039(00)75003-9

LaVigne, J. E., Hecksel, R., Keresztes, A., and Streicher, J. M. (2021). *Cannabis sativa* terpenes are cannabimimetic and selectively enhance cannabinoid activity. *Scientific Reports*, 11(1): 1–15. https://doi.org/10.1038/s41598-021-87740-8

Leinen, Z. J., Mohan, R., Premadasa, L. S., Acharya, A., Mohan, M., and Byrareddy, S. N. (2023). Therapeutic potential of *Cannabis*: A Comprehensive review of current and future applications. *Biomedicines*, 11(10): 2630. https://doi.org/10.3390/BIOMEDICINES11102630

Li, S., Li, H., Yin, D., Xue, X., Chen, X., Li, X. et al. (2022). Effect of gigantol on the proliferation of hepatocellular carcinoma cells tested by a network-based pharmacological approach and experiments. *Frontiers in Bioscience - Landmark*, 27(1): 25. https://doi.org/10.31083/J.FBL2701025/2768-6698-27-1-025/FIG10.JPG

Liktor-Busa, E., Keresztes, A., Lavigne, J., Streicher, J. M., and Largent-Milnes, T. M. (2021). Analgesic potential of terpenes derived from *Cannabis sativa*. *Pharmacological Reviews*, 73(4): 1269–1297. https://doi.org/10.1124/PHARMREV.120.000046

Lin, Z. S., Ku, C. F., Guan, Y. F., Xiao, H. T., Shi, X. K., Wang, H. Q. et al. (2016). Dihydro-resveratrol ameliorates lung injury in rats with cerulein-induced acute pancreatitis. *Phytotherapy Research*, 30(4): 663–670. https://doi.org/10.1002/PTR.5576

Lipson Feder, C., Cohen, O., Shapira, A., Katzir, I., Peer, R., Guberman, O. et al. (2021). Fertilization following pollination predominantly decreases phytocannabinoids accumulation and alters the accumulation of terpenoids in *Cannabis* inflorescences. *Frontiers in Plant Science*, 12: 753847. https://doi.org/10.3389/FPLS.2021.753847/BIBTEX

Liu, Y., Li, S., Shen, M., Guo, F., Li, M., Cai, S. et al. (2025). Integration of transcriptome and metabolome provides insights into metabolites and pathways associated with antiproliferative activity of cannabis flower extracts. *Industrial Crops and Products*, 223: 120239. https://doi.org/10.1016/j.indcrop.2024.120239

Losuwannarak, N., Roytrakul, S., and Chanvorachote, P. (2020). Gigantol targets MYC for ubiquitin-proteasomal degradation and suppresses lung cancer cell growth. *Cancer Genomics & Proteomics*, 17(6): 781–793. https://doi.org/10.21873/CGP.20232

Lowe, H., Steele, B., Bryant, J., Toyang, N., and Ngwa, W. (2021). Non-Cannabinoid metabolites of *Cannabis sativa* L. with therapeutic potential. *Plants*, 10(2): 400. https://doi.org/10.3390/PLANTS10020400

Luo, Q., Yan, X., Bobrovskaya, L., Ji, M., Yuan, H., Lou, H. et al. (2017). Anti-neuroinflammatory effects of grossamide from hemp seed via suppression of TLR-4-mediated NF-κB signaling pathways in lipopolysaccharide-stimulated BV2 microglia cells. *Molecular and Cellular Biochemistry*, 428(1-2): 129–137. https://doi.org/10.1007/S11010-016-2923-7/METRICS

Malingré, T., Hendriks, H., Batterman, S., Bos, R., and Visser, J. (1975). The essential oil of *Cannabis sativa*. *Planta Medica*, 28(1): 56–61. https://doi.org/10.1055/S-0028-1097829/BIB

Mechoulam, R. (1989). Chapter 2 Alkaloids in *Cannabis Sativa* L. *Alkaloids: Chemistry and Pharmacology*, 34(C): 77–93. https://doi.org/10.1016/S0099-9598(08)60227-8

Menghini, L., Ferrante, C., Carradori, S., D'antonio, M., Orlando, G., Cairone, F. et al. (2021). Chemical and bioinformatics analyses of the anti-leishmanial and anti-oxidant activities of hemp essential oil. *Biomolecules*, *11*(2): 272. https://doi.org/10.3390/BIOM11020272

Moreau, M., Ibeh, U., Decosmo, K., Bih, N., Yasmin-Karim, S., Toyang, N. et al. (2019). Flavonoid derivative of cannabis demonstrates therapeutic potential in preclinical models of metastatic pancreatic cancer. *Frontiers in Oncology*, 9: 462635. https://doi.org/10.3389/FONC.2019.00660/BIBTEX

Nalli, Y., Arora, P., Riyaz-Ul-Hassan, S., and Ali, A. (2018). Chemical investigation of *Cannabis sativa* leading to the discovery of a prenylspirodinone with anti-microbial potential. *Tetrahedron Letters*, 59(25): 2470–2472. https://doi.org/10.1016/J.TETLET.2018.05.051

Nigam, M. C., Handa, K. L., Nigam, I. C., and Levi, L. (2011). Essential oils and their constituents: xxix. The essential oil of marihuana: composition of genuine Indian *Cannabis sativa* L. Https://Doi.Org/10.1139/V65-468, 43(12): 3372–3376. https://doi.org/10.1139/V65-468

Nuutinen, T. (2018). Medicinal properties of terpenes found in *Cannabis sativa* and *Humulus lupulus*. *European Journal of Medicinal Chemistry*, 157: 198–228. https://doi.org/10.1016/J.EJMECH.2018.07.076

O'Croinin, C., Garcia Guerra, A., Doschak, M. R., Löbenberg, R., and Davies, N. M. (2023). Therapeutic potential and predictive pharmaceutical modeling of stilbenes in *Cannabis sativa*. *Pharmaceutics*, 15(7): 1941. https://doi.org/10.3390/PHARMACEUTICS15071941

Ogungbe, I. V., Erwin, W. R., and Setzer, W. N. (2014). Antileishmanial phytochemical phenolics: Molecular docking to potential protein targets. *Journal of Molecular Graphics and Modelling*, 48: 105–117. https://doi.org/10.1016/J.JMGM.2013.12.010

Ottersen, T., Aasen, A., El-Feraly, F. S., and Turner, C. E. (1976). X-Ray structure of cannabispiran: a novel *Cannabis* constituent. *Journal of the Chemical Society, Chemical Communications*, 15: 580–581. https://doi.org/10.1039/C39760000580

Pathak, S., Jeyabalan, J. B., Liu, K., Cook, P., Lange, B., Kim, S. et al. (2024). Assessing effects of *Cannabis* on various neuropathologies: A systematic review. *Journal of Ayurveda and Integrative Medicine*, 15(3): 100911. https://doi.org/10.1016/J.JAIM.2024.100911

Pettit, G. R., and Singh, S. B. (2011). Isolation, structure, and synthesis of combretastatin A-2, A-3, and B-2. *Canadian Journal of Chemistry*, 65(10): 2390–2396. https://doi.org/10.1139/V87-399

Pisanti, S., and Bifulco, M. (2019). Medical *Cannabis*: A plurimillennial history of an evergreen. *Journal of Cellular Physiology*, 234(6): 8342–8351. https://doi.org/10.1002/JCP.27725

Powers, C., and Setzer, W. (2016). An *In-Silico* investigation of phytochemicals as antiviral agents against dengue fever. *Combinatorial Chemistry & High Throughput Screening*, 19: 516–536.

Radwan, M. M., Chandra, S., Gul, S., and Elsohly, M. A. (2021). Cannabinoids, phenolics, terpenes and alkaloids of *Cannabis*. *Molecules*, *26*(9): 2774. https://doi.org/10.3390/MOLECULES26092774

Radwan, M. M., ElSohly, M. A., Slade, D., Ahmed, S. A., Wilson, L., El-Alfy, A. T. et al. (2008a). Non-cannabinoid constituents from a high potency *Cannabis sativa* variety. *Phytochemistry*, 69(14): 2627–2633. https://doi.org/10.1016/J.PHYTOCHEM.2008.07.010

Radwan, M. M., Ross, S. A., Slade, D., Ahmed, S. A., Zulfiqar, F., and Elsohly, M. A. (2008b). Isolation and characterization of new *Cannabis* constituents from a high potency variety. *Planta Medica*, 74(3): 267–272. https://doi.org/10.1055/S-2008-1034311/BIB

Rahman, F., Tabrez, S., Ali, R., Akand, S. K., Zahid, M., Alaidarous, M. A. et al. (2021). Virtual screening of natural compounds for potential inhibitors of Sterol C-24 methyltransferase of *Leishmania donovani* to overcome leishmaniasis. *Journal of Cellular Biochemistry*, 122(9): 1216–1228. https://doi.org/10.1002/JCB.29944

Riboulet-Zemouli, K. (2020). 'Cannabis' ontologies I: Conceptual issues with *Cannabis* and cannabinoids terminology. *Drug Science, Policy and Law*, 6. https://doi.org/10.1177/2050324520945797

Rodríguez-Calvo, R., Girona, J., Rodríguez, M., Samino, S., Barroso, E., de Gonzalo-Calvo, D. et al. (2019). Fatty acid binding protein 4 (FABP4) as a potential biomarker reflecting myocardial lipid storage in type 2 diabetes. *Metabolism*, 96: 12–21. https://doi.org/10.1016/J.METABOL.2019.04.007

Romero Salamanca, J. M., and Castañeda Castellanos, B. A. (2019). Modelo de interacción molecular de metabolitos presentes en la especie *Cannabis satival* con la enzima ciclooxigebasa-1 (COX1) y la enzima ciclooxigensa-2 (COX2) de homo sapines. In *Universidad de Ciencias Aplicadas y Ambientales*. https://repository.udca.edu.co/handle/11158/1376

Ross, S. A., and ElSohly, M. A. (1996). The volatile oil composition of fresh and air-dried buds of *Cannabis sativa*. *Journal of Natural Products*, 59(1): 49–51. https://doi.org/10.1021/NP960004A

Ross, S. A., ElSohly, M. A., Sultana, G. N. N., Mehmedic, Z., Hossain, C. F., and Chandra, S. (2005). Flavonoid glycosides and cannabinoids from the pollen of *Cannabis sativa* L. *Phytochemical Analysis*, 16(1): 45–48. https://doi.org/10.1002/PCA.809

Roupe, K. A., Remsberg, C. M., Yanez, J. A., and Davies, N. M. (2008). Pharmacometrics of stilbenes: Seguing towards the clinic. *Current Clinical Pharmacology*, 1(1): 81–101. https://doi.org/10.2174/157488406775268246

Rubin, P., and Mollison, K. W. (2007). Pharmacotherapy of diseases mediated by 5-lipoxygenase pathway eicosanoids. *Prostaglandins & Other Lipid Mediators*, 83(3): 188–197. https://doi.org/10.1016/J.PROSTAGLANDINS.2007.01.005

Salem, M. M., Capers, J., Rito, S., and Werbovetz, K. A. (2011). Antiparasitic Activity of C-geranyl flavonoids from Mimulus bigelovii. *Phytotherapy Research*, 25(8): 1246–1249. https://doi.org/10.1002/PTR.3404

Sánchez-Duffhues, G., Calzado, M. A., de Vinuesa, A. G., Caballero, F. J., Ech-Chahad, A., Appendino, G. et al. (2008). Denbinobin, a naturally occurring 1,4-phenanthrenequinone, inhibits HIV-1 replication through an NF-κB-dependent pathway. *Biochemical Pharmacology*, 76(10): 1240–1250. https://doi.org/10.1016/J.BCP.2008.09.006

Sauer, M. A., Rifka, S. M., Hawks, R. L., Cutler, G. B., and Loriaux, D. L. (1983). Marijuana: interaction with the estrogen receptor. *Journal of Pharmacology and Experimental Therapeutics*, 224(2).

Shakil, S. S. M., Gowan, M., Hughes, K., Azam, M. N. K., and Ahmed, M. N. (2021). A narrative review of the ethnomedicinal usage of *Cannabis sativa* Linnaeus as traditional phytomedicine by folk medicine practitioners of Bangladesh. *Journal of Cannabis Research*, 3(1): 1–12. https://doi.org/10.1186/S42238-021-00063-3/METRICS

Shi, L., Wu, Z., Zhang, Y., Zhang, Z., Fang, W., Wang, Y. et al. (2020). Herbicidal secondary metabolites from *Actinomycetes*: structure diversity, modes of action, and their roles in the development of herbicides. *Journal of Agricultural and Food Chemistry*, 68(1): 17–32. https://doi.org/10.1021/ACS.JAFC.9B06126/ASSET/IMAGES/LARGE/JF9B06126_0010.JPEG

Shoyama, Y., and Nishioka, I. (1978). *Cannabis*. XIII. Two new spiro-compounds, cannabispirol and acetyl cannabispirol. *Chemical and Pharmaceutical Bulletin*, 26(12): 3641–3646. https://doi.org/10.1248/CPB.26.3641

Silver, R., Wakshalg, J., Wynn, S., and Kramer, K. (2021). Nutritional analysis of *Cannabis*. *Cannabis Therapy in Veterinary Medicine*, 271–293. https://doi.org/10.1007/978-3-030-68317-7_11

Simonsen, J. L., and Todd, A. R. (1942). 32. Cannabis indica. Part X. The essential oil from Egyptian hashish. *Journal of the Chemical Society (Resumed)*: 0: 188–191. https://doi.org/10.1039/JR9420000188

Singh, M. K., Singh, S., Mishra, S., Shankar, U., Maurya, A., Sahu, K. S. et al. (2025). Investigating the phytochemical diversity and anti-inflammatory activity of a non-psychoactive genotype of *Cannabis sativa* L. from India. *Microchemical Journal*, 211: 113111.

Smeriglio, A., Galati, E. M., Monforte, M. T., Lanuzza, F., D'Angelo, V., and Circosta, C. (2016). Polyphenolic compounds and antioxidant activity of cold-pressed seed oil from Finola cultivar of *Cannabis sativa* L. *Phytotherapy Research*, 30(8): 1298–1307. https://doi.org/10.1002/PTR.5623

Sorini, C., Cosorich, I., Conte, M. Lo, De Giorgi, L., Facciotti, F., Lucianò, R. et al. (2019). Loss of gut barrier integrity triggers activation of islet-reactive T cells and autoimmune diabetes. *Proceedings of the National Academy of Sciences of the United States of America*, 116(30): 15140–15149. https://doi.org/10.1073/PNAS.1814558116/SUPPL_FILE/PNAS.1814558116.SAPP.PDF

Strömberg, L. (1976). Minor components of cannabis resin : VI. Mass spectrometric data and gas chromatographic retention times of components eluted after cannabinol. *Journal of Chromatography A*, 121(2): 313–322. https://doi.org/10.1016/S0021-9673(00)85028-1

Su, S. Q., Jiang, H., Li, Q. M., Zha, X. Q., and Luo, J. P. (2020). Study on chemical constituents of *Dendrobium huoshanense* stems and their anti-inflammatory activity. *China Journal of Chinese Materia Medica*, 45(14): 3452–3458. https://doi.org/10.19540/J.CNKI.CJCMM.20200423.201

Tanaka, T., Narazaki, M., and Kishimoto, T. (2014). IL-6 in inflammation, immunity, and disease. *Cold Spring Harbor Perspectives in Biology*, 6(10): a016295. https://doi.org/10.1101/CSHPERSPECT.A016295

Tomko, A. M., Whynot, E. G., and Dupré, D. J. (2022). Anti-cancer properties of cannflavin A and potential synergistic effects with gemcitabine, cisplatin, and cannabinoids in bladder cancer. *Journal of Cannabis Research*, 4(1): 1–14. https://doi.org/10.1186/S42238-022-00151-Y/TABLES/2

Tsang, S. W., Guan, Y. F., Wang, J., Bian, Z. X., and Zhang, H. J. (2016). Inhibition of pancreatic oxidative damage by stilbene derivative dihydro-resveratrol: implication for treatment of acute pancreatitis. *Scientific Reports*, *6*(1): 1–15. https://doi.org/10.1038/srep22859

Turner, C. E., Elsohly, M. A., and Boeren, E. G. (1980). Constituents of cannabis sativa l. xvii. a review of the natural constituents. *Journal of Natural Products*, 43(2): 169–234. https://doi.org/10.1021/NP50008A001/ASSET/NP50008A001.FP.PNG_V03

Turner, C. E., and Mole, M. L. (1973). Chemical components of *Cannabis sativa*. *JAMA*, 225(6): 639–639. https://doi.org/10.1001/JAMA.1973.03220330051027

Walsh, K. B., McKinney, A. E., and Holmes, A. E. (2021). Minor Cannabinoids: Biosynthesis, molecular pharmacology and potential therapeutic uses. *Frontiers in Pharmacology*, 12: 777804. https://doi.org/10.3389/FPHAR.2021.777804/BIBTEX

Wang, C., and Kurzer, M. S. (1997). Phytoestrogen concentration determines effects on DNA synthesis in human breast cancer cells. *Nutrition and Cancer*, 28(3): 236–247. https://doi.org/10.1080/01635589709514582

Wang, S., Luo, Q., and Fan, P. (2019). Cannabisin F from hemp (*Cannabis sativa*) seed suppresses lipopolysaccharide-induced inflammatory responses in BV2 Microglia as SIRT1 modulator. *International Journal of Molecular Sciences*, 20(3): 507. https://doi.org/10.3390/IJMS20030507

Werz, O., Seegers, J., Schaible, A. M., Weinigel, C., Barz, D., Koeberle, A. et al. (2014). Cannflavins from hemp sprouts, a novel cannabinoid-free hemp food product, target microsomal prostaglandin E2 synthase-1 and 5-lipoxygenase. *PharmaNutrition*, 2(3): 53–60. https://doi.org/10.1016/J.PHANU.2014.05.001

Wirth, P. W., Murphy, J. C., El-Feraly, F. S., and Turner, C. E. (1981). Constituents of *Cannabis sativa* L. XXI: Estrogenic activity of a non-cannabinoid constituent. *Experientia*, 37(11): 1181–1182. https://doi.org/10.1007/BF01989907/METRICS

Wozniczka, K., Viapiana, A., Roszkowska, A., Plenis, A., Baczek, T., and Konieczynski, P. (2025). Evaluation of commercially available products of *Cannabis sativa* L. Inflorescences to identify their contents of elemental and phenolic compounds. *Foods*, 14: 1208. https://doi.org/10.3390/ foods14071208

Yan, X., Tang, J., Dos Santos Passos, C., Nurisso, A., Simoes-Pires, C. A., Ji, M. et al. (2015). Characterization of lignanamides from hemp (*Cannabis sativa* L.) seed and their antioxidant and acetylcholinesterase inhibitory activities. *Journal of Agricultural and Food Chemistry*, 63(49): 10611–10619. https://doi.org/10.1021/ACS.JAFC.5B05282/SUPPL_FILE/JF5B05282_SI_001.PDF

Yan, X., Zhou, Y., Tang, J., Ji, M., Lou, H., and Fan, P. (2016). Diketopiperazine indole alkaloids from hemp seed. *Phytochemistry Letters*, 18: 77–82. https://doi.org/10.1016/J.PHYTOL.2016.09.001

Zhang, B., Zhang, Y., Liu, X., Yin, J., Li, X., Zhang, X. et al. (2022). differential protective effect of resveratrol and its microbial metabolites on intestinal barrier dysfunction is mediated by the AMPK pathway. *Journal of Agricultural and Food Chemistry*, 70(36): 11301–11313. https://doi.org/10.1021/ACS.JAFC.2C04101/ASSET/IMAGES/LARGE/JF2C04101_0009.JPEG

Zhang, B., Zhang, Y., Liu, X., Zhao, C., Yin, J., Li, X. et al. (2023). Distinctive anti-inflammatory effects of resveratrol, dihydroresveratrol, and 3-(4-hydroxyphenyl)-propionic acid on DSS-induced colitis in pseudo-germ-free mice. *Food Chemistry*, 400: 133904. https://doi.org/10.1016/J.FOODCHEM.2022.133904

Zhang, S., Huang, J., Fu, J., Qin, Y., Zhang, X., Yao, X. et al. (2024). Structurally diverse phenylpropanamides from *Cannabis Fructus* and Their potential neuroprotective effects. *Journal of Agricultural and Food Chemistry*, 72(21): 12100–12118. https://doi.org/10.1021/ACS.JAFC.4C00242/SUPPL_FILE/JF4C00242_SI_001.PDF

Zheljazkov, V. D., and Maggi, F. (2021). Valorization of CBD-hemp through distillation to provide essential oil and improved cannabinoids profile. *Scientific Reports*, 11(1): 1–11. https://doi.org/10.1038/s41598-021-99335-4

Zhou, Y., Wang, S., Ji, J., Lou, H., and Fan, P. (2018). Hemp (*Cannabis sativa* L.) seed phenylpropionamides composition and effects on memory dysfunction and biomarkers of neuroinflammation induced by lipopolysaccharide in mice. *ACS Omega*, 3(11): 15988–15995. https://doi.org/10.1021/ACSOMEGA.8B02250/ASSET/IMAGES/LARGE/AO-2018-022505_0004.JPEG

Zhu, X., Zeng, X., Sun, C., and Chen, S. (2014). Biosynthetic pathway of terpenoid indole alkaloids in *Catharanthus roseus*. *Frontiers of Medicine in China*, 8(3): 285–293. https://doi.org/10.1007/S11684-014-0350-2/METRICS

CHAPTER 7

Impact of Cannabinoids on Sleep

*Estefanía Butassi, Melina Di Liberto, Alan Blanc, Luz Rivero Márquez, Estefanía Cordisco, Maximiliano Sortino** and *Laura Svetaz**

1. Introduction

Sleep is an essential biological process for maintaining physical, cognitive, and emotional health; the disturbance of which is associated with an increased risk of cardiovascular disease, metabolic disorders, and psychiatric disorders (Morin and Benca 2012; Irwin 2015). Sleep disorders, particularly insomnia, affect a substantial proportion of the global population, prompting increasing interest in effective and safe therapeutic alternatives. In this context, cannabis has emerged as a potential therapeutic option for managing various sleep disorders (Babson et al. 2017). The sleep-inducing properties of cannabinoid compounds have been recognized for nearly two centuries (Kesner and Lovinger 2020). In recent years, there has been growing interest in the therapeutic potential of *Cannabis sativa* derivatives and other cannabinoid-based compounds as sleep-promoting agents. This resurgence aligns with a broader revival in research exploring the interplay between cannabis and sleep, with a particular focus on the role of endogenous cannabinoids (endocannabinoids) in regulating both normal and pathological sleep processes. Despite these advances, our understanding of how cannabinoids affect sleep in humans and animal models remains incomplete.

Historically, cannabis has been used across various cultures as a therapeutic agent to induce sleep and alleviate insomnia. Records dating back over 4,000 years in ancient China describe its use for managing pain, reducing anxiety, and promoting restful sleep, and its medicinal value is documented in foundational texts such as the Shennong Bencaojing (Russo 2007; Block 2023). Its sedative and anxiolytic properties were also recognized in ancient Egypt and within the Ayurvedic tradition of India, where it was utilized to enhance sleep quality and treat related ailments (Russo 2005). In the 19th century, European physicians such as William O'Shaughnessy introduced cannabis into Western medicine, recommending it for the treatment of pain and sleep disorders, which led to its inclusion in the pharmacopoeias of the time. However, by the early 20th century, the medical use of cannabis had declined significantly because of issues related to the lack of standardization, difficulties in dosing, and concerns over quality control (Russo 2007; Ranade et al. 2022).

Scientific interest in the therapeutic potential of cannabis for treating sleep disorders has increased significantly in recent years, driven by legislative changes and growing social acceptance. This renewed focus is grounded in the discovery of the endocannabinoid system (ECS). This

Laboratorio de Bioprospección de Productos Antimicrobianos, Facultad de Ciencias Bioquímicas y Farmacéuticas, Universidad Nacional de Rosario, Suipacha 531, S2002LRK, Rosario, Argentina.

* Corresponding authors: sortinomaximiliano@gmail.com; svetaz@rosario-conicet.gov.ar

DOI: 10.1201/9781003668190-9

complex and ubiquitous neuromodulatory network includes cannabinoid receptors type 1 (CB1R) and 2 (CB2R), which regulate numerous biological processes, including the sleep-wake cycle and sleep homeostasis (Murillo-Rodríguez et al. 2011). Cannabinoids primarily interact with CB1R and CB2R, modulating key neurotransmitters that influence sleep latency, architecture, and overall sleep quality (Choi et al. 2020; Suraev et al. 2020).

However, the current scientific evidence remains heterogeneous and at times contradictory. While some studies suggest that cannabis may facilitate sleep onset and enhance deep sleep, others report suppression of rapid eye movement (REM) sleep and highlight the potential adverse effects associated with chronic use (Gates et al. 2014; Suraev et al. 2020; AminiLari et al. 2022). Variations in cannabinoid concentrations, routes of administration, and individual user characteristics further complicate the interpretation of these findings.

This chapter examines the relationship between cannabis and sleep from a multidisciplinary perspective, exploring sleep physiology, the role of the ECS, and the specific effects of major cannabinoids on different stages of sleep. It also addresses the potential therapeutic benefits and risks, as well as the clinical implications of cannabis consumption. The aim is to provide a critical and up-to-date overview to support healthcare professionals, researchers, and readers interested in this evolving field.

2. Sleep Physiology, Architecture, and Cycles

Sleep is a complex and dynamic biological process that plays a critical role in maintaining physical, cognitive, and emotional health (Vanini and Torterolo 2021). It is characterized by cyclical alternation between two major stages: non-rapid eye movement (NREM) sleep and REM sleep.

Electroencephalography (EEG) and electromyography (EMG) are widely accepted as reliable physiological tools for differentiating between the sleep and wake states. EEG records cortical electrical activity, and EMG measures muscle activity. During wakefulness, EEG signals typically exhibit low-amplitude, high-frequency patterns, and EMG shows variable muscle tone, reflecting voluntary and postural activities. In NREM sleep, the EEG shifts toward slower frequencies, with a pronounced increase in delta activity (0.5–4 Hz), accompanied by a notable reduction in muscle tone, as recorded by EMG. In REM sleep, EEG patterns closely resemble those of wakefulness (low amplitude and high frequency), whereas EMG reveals profound muscle atonia and characteristic rapid eye movements. Due to this combination of wake-like cortical activity and muscle paralysis, REM sleep is often referred to as "paradoxical sleep" (Scammell et al. 2017; Vanini and Torterolo 2021).

NREM sleep is not a homogeneous state and accounts for approximately 75–80% of the total sleep time. In humans, it is subdivided into three progressive stages: N1, N2, and N3. The anterior hypothalamus primarily regulates this sleep phase. Stage N1 represents the transition from wakefulness to sleep. During this phase, brain activity begins to slow, the muscles relax, and the individual remains highly susceptible to awakening. This is a brief stage and is considered a light form of sleep. Stage N2 constitutes the largest portion of NREM sleep and is characterized by EEG patterns, including sleep spindles (short synchronized bursts of electrical activity) and K-complexes (large electrical sharp waves). These electrophysiological features are associated with sensory inhibition and memory consolidation. During this phase, both body temperature and heart rate decrease. Stage N3, also known as Slow Wave Sleep (SWS) or deep sleep, represents the most restorative phase of NREM sleep. It is marked by the dominance of high-amplitude, low-frequency delta waves in the brain activity. This stage is essential for physical recovery, energy restoration, hormonal regulation, and consolidation of declarative memory. Deep sleep deprivation has been linked to fatigue, cognitive impairment, and immune system dysfunction (Scammell et al. 2017; Vanini and Torterolo 2021).

REM sleep accounts for approximately 20–25% of the total sleep time. This stage is characterized by vivid, emotionally charged, narrative-like dreams, accompanied by rapid eye

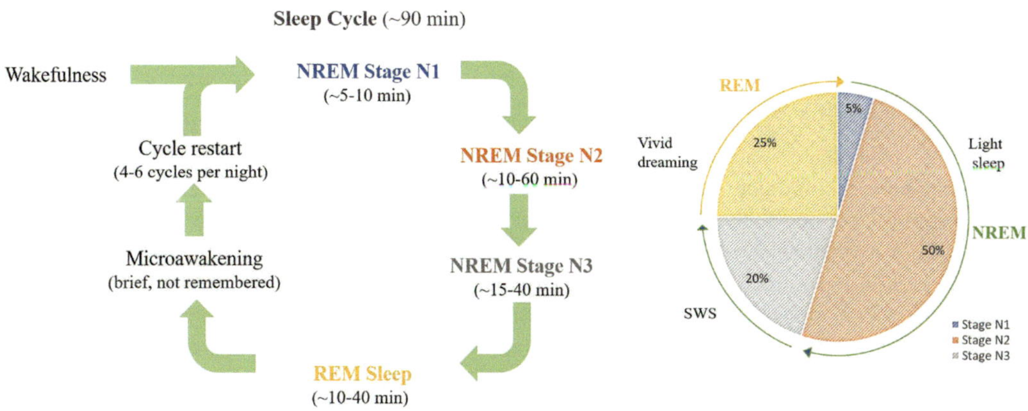

Figure 1: A typical night of sleep comprises four to six cycles of ~90 minutes each, progressing from NREM stages (N1, N2, and N3) to REM sleep.

movements and fluctuations in autonomic functions, such as heart rate and respiration. REM sleep plays a critical role in consolidating emotional and procedural memories, including motor skills and habitual behaviours, as well as regulating mood and promoting synaptic plasticity. During this phase, brain regions involved in emotional processing, such as the amygdala, exhibit heightened activity (Scammell et al. 2017; Vanini and Torterolo 2021).

During a typical night, an individual undergoes approximately four to six complete sleep cycles, each lasting about 90 minutes (Carskadon and Dement 2011). Each cycle follows a structured sequence of stages, beginning with NREM sleep (stages N1, N2, and N3) and culminating in REM sleep (Figure 1). Deep NREM sleep (especially stage N3) predominated in the early sleep cycles (Irwin 2015; Krueger et al. 2016). As the night progresses, the proportion of REM sleep progressively increases in each successive cycle, promoting emotional processing, memory consolidation, and mood regulation. This dynamic architecture ensures that the body receives both the restorative benefits of deep NREM sleep and the cognitive and emotional functions associated with REM sleep (Desai et al. 2024).

3. Neurobiological Regulation of Sleep

Sleep and wakefulness are regulated by multiple, partially redundant neural circuits and signaling molecules distributed throughout the brain and brainstem. Specialized brain regions govern distinct phases of the sleep-wake cycle, each utilizing specific neurotransmitters and neuromodulators to initiate, maintain, and modulate the transitions between states (Vanini and Torterolo 2021; Nir and de Lecea 2023).

3.1 Neurotransmitters in the Regulation of Sleep

The regulation of the sleep-wake cycle is a highly complex process that involves multiple neural circuits and a wide array of endogenous signaling molecules (Murillo-Rodriguez et al. 2011). Wakefulness is maintained through the coordinated activity of various neuroanatomical and neurochemical systems, including those involving acetylcholine, dopamine, serotonin, noradrenaline, histamine, and hypocretin/orexin. In contrast, sleep onset is governed by the interacting forces of the sleep drive, which steadily increases with the duration of waking and circadian fluctuations. Sleep-promoting neurons located in the anterior hypothalamus, particularly within the ventrolateral preoptic nucleus, release gamma-aminobutyric acid (GABA) and inhibit wake-promoting regions in the hypothalamus and brainstem, facilitating the initiation and maintenance of SWS. During REM sleep, brainstem regions that are typically suppressed during wakefulness and SWS become active. In this phase, ascending cholinergic projections from the brainstem stimulate the thalamus, leading to increased cortical neuron firing and characteristic cortical activation during REM sleep (Murillo-Rodriguez et al. 2011).

3.2 ECS and Sleep Modulation

Over the past three decades, experimental evidence has supported the hypothesis that endocannabinoids modulate the regulation of the sleep-wake cycle. The ECS is a complex physiological signaling network that is widely distributed throughout the brain and body. It plays a key role in regulating various biological functions, including food intake, learning and memory, immune responses, motivation, the sleep-wake cycle, and sleep homeostasis (Pacher et al. 2006; Méndez-Díaz et al. 2021; Di Marzo and Piscitelli 2015; Rezende et al. 2023).

The endocannabinoid signaling system consists of (1) at least two well-characterized G protein-coupled receptors (GPCRs) with seven transmembrane domains, known as CB1R and CB2R; (2) the two most extensively studied endogenous ligands, N-arachidonoylethanolamine (anandamide, AEA) and 2-arachidonoylglycerol (2-AG); and (3) a set of biosynthetic and degradative enzymes, along with membrane transporters, that tightly regulate endocannabinoid levels and their activity at cannabinoid receptors (Castillo et al. 2012; Di Marzo and Piscitelli 2015; Pertwee et al. 2015; Rezende et al. 2023).

CB1R is the most abundant GPCR expressed in the brain, although it is also present at much lower levels in various peripheral tissues and cell types (Pacher et al. 2006; Méndez-Díaz et al. 2021). CB1R activation inhibits the release of GABA and glutamate at the presynaptic terminals, modulating neurotransmission. Moreover, it facilitates acetylcholine release and enhances serotonergic system activity (Murillo-Rodriguez et al. 2011). The second cannabinoid GPCR, CB2R, is predominantly expressed in immune and hematopoietic cells; however, more recent studies have also detected its presence in the brain and other peripheral organs (Pacher et al. 2006; Kano et al. 2009; Castillo et al. 2012; Di Marzo and Piscitelli 2015).

The endocannabinoids AEA and 2-AG are endogenous lipid mediators derived from arachidonic acid that act as natural ligands for CB1R and CB2R (Kano et al. 2009; Rezende et al. 2023). In the brain, the basal level of 2-AG is approximately 1,000 times higher than that of AEA. AEA is a high-affinity partial agonist of CB1R and is nearly inactive at CB2R, whereas 2-AG acts as a full agonist at both CB1R and CB2R, albeit with moderate to low affinity. The principal mechanism by which endocannabinoids modulate synaptic transmission is retrograde signaling (Castillo et al. 2012). In response to elevated intracellular calcium levels, AEA and 2-AG are released from the postsynaptic neuron into the synaptic cleft, where they function as retrograde neurotransmitters by binding to cannabinoid receptors located on the presynaptic terminals (Méndez-Díaz et al. 2021). This receptor activation inhibits the further release of excitatory or inhibitory neurotransmitters, contributing to synaptic homeostasis and preventing excessive neuronal activity. These endogenous ligands are synthesized on demand, typically via activity-dependent cleavage of membrane phospholipids, and are released immediately after biosynthesis to act as pro-homeostatic factors through interactions with specific cannabinoid receptors (Rezende et al. 2023).

The synthesis and degradation of endocannabinoids are tightly regulated by specific enzymes that control their local concentration and activity. AEA is primarily synthesized by N-acyl-phosphatidylethanolamine-specific phospholipase D (NAPE-PLD), whereas 2-AG is generated through the action of diacylglycerol lipases α and β (DAGLα and DAGLβ). Conversely, the hydrolytic inactivation of these endocannabinoids is mediated by fatty acid amide hydrolase (FAAH) for AEA and monoacylglycerol lipase (MAGL) for 2-AG, respectively. The activity of these enzymes ensures that endocannabinoid signaling remains transient and spatially restricted, allowing precise control of cannabinoid receptor activation (Kano et al. 2009; Di Marzo and Piscitelli 2015).

The role of the ECS in sleep modulation has been suggested by experimental evidence (Murillo-Rodriguez et al. 2011). The first approach to show the role of CB1R in sleep modulation was achieved by Santucci et al. in 1996. These authors systematically injected the cannabinoid CB1R antagonist SR141716A at varying concentrations into rats, finding a dose-dependent enhancement of wakefulness and reductions in SWS and REM (Santucci et al. 1996). They suggested that an endogenous cannabimimetic system may regulate the organization of the sleep-wake cycle. Two years later, the role of AEA in sleep modulation was investigated. Intracerebroventricular administration of AEA in rats increased both NREM and REM sleep while reducing wakefulness (Murillo-Rodríguez et al. 1998). Subsequent studies have demonstrated that the CB1R antagonist SR141716A blocks AEA-induced sleep enhancement in normal rats, indicating that these effects are mediated by CB1R activation (Murillo-Rodríguez et al. 2001). Additional studies have revealed that AEA promotes sleep, at least in part, by increasing adenosine levels, a neuromodulator known to facilitate sleep (Murillo-Rodríguez et al. 2003). Supporting these findings, Vaughn et al. (2010) reported that AEA concentrations were approximately three times higher immediately after waking than pre-sleep levels. A range of *in vivo* studies has consistently shown that AEA administration enhances SWS and NREM sleep while suppressing wakefulness in rats (Herrera-Solís et al. 2010; Puskar et al. 2021).

Other studies have demonstrated that enhancing 2-AG signaling in the lateral hypothalamus increases REM sleep, an effect blocked by CB1R antagonists such as AM251. Furthermore, inhibition of 2-AG synthesis with DAGL inhibitors prevents this REM-promoting effect, confirming the essential role of 2-AG in this process (Pérez-Morales et al. 2013; 2014). Moreover, Perez-Morales et al. (2012) found that tetrahydrolipstatin, an inhibitor of the 2-AG-synthesizing enzyme DAGL, reduces the activity of melanin-concentrating hormone (MCH)-releasing neurons in the hypothalamus, leading to decreased REM sleep and reduced food intake. This suggests that CB1R may regulate sleep by modulating the activity of MCH neurons, which are predominantly located in the lateral hypothalamus and are active during REM sleep.

Although still limited, experimental evidence suggests that the AEA membrane transporter and the FAAH enzyme are involved in modulating the sleep-wake cycle. For instance, intracerebroventricular administration of the FAAH inhibitor URB597 in rats during the lights-on phase has been shown to increase wakefulness while reducing both SWS and REM. In addition, URB597-treated rats exhibited increased c-Fos immunoreactivity in the hypothalamus and dorsal raphe nucleus, which are associated with arousal regulation. Moreover, URB597 administration elevates extracellular dopamine levels. Collectively, these findings indicate that FAAH inhibition via URB597 promotes wakefulness (Murillo-Rodríguez et al. 2007).

In addition, several lines of evidence support the circadian modulation of the ECS, as endocannabinoid concentrations, receptor expression, and the activity of degradative enzymes exhibit distinct diurnal variations across various tissues, including the brain. This rhythmic regulation suggests that the influence of the ECS on sleep-wake cycles is not static, but varies throughout the 24 h, contributing to time-of-day-dependent regulation of sleep expression (Méndez-Díaz et al. 2021).

Phytocannabinoids, which are cannabinoids derived from *C. sativa*, refer to a group of over 120 compounds primarily found in the glandular trichomes of the plant. Among these, Δ9-tetrahydrocannabinol (Δ9-THC or THC), cannabidiol (CBD), cannabichromene (CBC), and cannabigerol (CBG) are the most abundant and well-studied. These compounds exert their effects in the body by modulating multiple molecular targets, including the ECS. For instance, THC, the primary psychoactive component of cannabis, acts as a partial agonist at CB1R and CB2R (Di Marzo and Piscitelli 2015), thereby mimicking the action of endogenous cannabinoids and influencing the neurotransmitter systems involved in sleep regulation. This interaction can induce sleepiness and alter the sleep architecture (Babson et al. 2017).

In contrast, CBD, the second most abundant phytocannabinoid, has a low affinity for both CB1R and CB2R (Di Marzo and Piscitelli 2015) but indirectly modulates the ECS by inhibiting the enzymatic degradation of endogenous cannabinoids. This mechanism enhances endocannabinoid signaling, improves sleep quality, regulates anxiety and inflammation, and does not produce psychoactive effects (Pacher et al. 2006; Di Marzo and Piscitelli 2015). Although the complex pharmacological properties of phytocannabinoids are not yet fully understood, they have emerged as promising therapeutic agents for the management of sleep disorders (D'Angelo and Steardo 2024).

4. Effects of Cannabis on Sleep

Research on the effects of cannabis on sleep began in the 1970s and included several studies utilizing polysomnography (PSG) to assess sleep architecture objectively. Findings from this early work were mixed: some studies reported reductions in sleep onset latency (SOL) and wake after sleep onset (WASO), while others failed to replicate these effects, instead reporting increases in SWS and decreases in REM sleep. Additional evidence suggests that cannabis may confer short-term benefits on sleep, particularly in facilitating sleep initiation. However, chronic cannabis use appears to be associated with tolerance development, potentially diminishing its sleep-inducing and SWS-enhancing effects over time (Babson 2017).

Since the mid-2000s, there has been a resurgence in research focused on the relationship between cannabis and sleep. In contrast to PSG-based studies of the 1970s, much contemporary research has relied on self-reported sleep measures and has increasingly explored the potential therapeutic applications of cannabinoids for sleep disorders. This resurgence is likely attributable to advancements in scientific understanding of cannabis and its constituent compounds. Recent studies have highlighted that sleep-related outcomes are influenced by multiple factors, including the specific type of cannabinoid, cannabinoid ratio, dosage, timing of administration, and route of delivery (Babson 2017; Maddison et al. 2022).

4.1 Effects of Cannabis on Sleep Quality and Architecture

4.1.1 Effects of THC

Short-term THC use has been associated with enhanced sleep consolidation, reduced SOL, increased total sleep time (TST), and decreased WASO. Acute administration of THC has also been associated with a reduction in REM sleep and an increase in SWS, findings that are consistent with results from preclinical animal studies. However, these effects on SWS and TST do not persist (Kaul et al. 2021; Maddison et al. 2022).

In contrast to the short-term effects, chronic administration of THC has been associated with a reduction in SWS, suggesting the development of tolerance with prolonged use. Unlike the consistent findings for SWS, the effects of chronic THC use on REM sleep are more variable in human and animal studies. Chronic use has also been linked to increased sleep disturbances, including prolonged SOL, increased WASO, and reduced TST. A PSG-based study demonstrated these effects by evaluating objective and subjective sleep parameters in regular cannabis users, revealing that most participants exhibited reduced TST (78%), with increased SOL (> 30 minutes), poor sleep efficiency (< 85%), and increased WASO. Additionally, increased REM sleep latency and a reduced proportion of REM sleep (17.7%) have been reported (Kaul et al. 2021; Maddison et al. 2022).

Cannabis withdrawal is commonly associated with sleep disturbances and vivid dreams. A study evaluating PSG characteristics in former heavy cannabis users reported reduced TST, decreased SWS, and shortened REM sleep latency compared to that in control subjects. This group also exhibited prolonged SOL and poorer sleep efficiency; however, the absence of baseline PSG data in both groups limited the interpretation of these findings. Another study observed an increase in periodic limb movements following the abrupt cessation of heavy cannabis use. Withdrawal-related sleep disturbances tend to be more pronounced in heavy users, typically emerging within 24–72 h after discontinuation and potentially persisting for up to 6–7 weeks (Kaul et al. 2021).

4.1.2 Effects of CBD

Evidence on the effects of CBD on sleep is still emerging and remains unclear. Preclinical studies in rodents have shown that increasing doses of CBD can elevate TST, with dose-dependent effects on REM sleep latency; low doses reduce latency, whereas high doses prolong it. However, these findings have not been consistently replicated in humans. A recent controlled trial found increased subjective sleepiness following the use of CBD-dominant cannabis, although it remains unclear whether this effect was attributable to CBD itself or to residual THC content. Moreover, the long-term effects of CBD on sleep have not yet been systematically explored. Overall, research examining the isolated effects of CBD on sleep architecture is limited and yields inconsistent results (Babson et al. 2017; Kaul et al. 2021; Maddison et al. 2022).

Beyond its direct effects on sleep, CBD has been widely studied for its anxiolytic properties. Clinical studies suggest that CBD can significantly alleviate anxiety symptoms, potentially facilitating sleep initiation and continuity (Blessing et al. 2015; Shannon et al. 2019). An observational study reported a significant reduction in anticipatory anxiety and subjective improvements in sleep quality among patients with anxiety disorders following CBD administration (Shannon et al. 2019). Moreover, in patients with chronic pain, CBD has been shown to improve sleep quality by alleviating both pain and associated anxiety (Vučković et al. 2018).

4.1.3 Effects of Combined THC and CBD

Studies evaluating the combined effects of CBD and THC have demonstrated that CBD exerts alerting properties and may attenuate the sedative effects of THC, particularly at higher doses. This antagonistic interaction was observed in a double-blind, placebo-controlled, four-arm crossover trial employing EEG monitoring. However, the interpretation of findings across studies remains limited due to heterogeneity in study designs, small sample sizes, methodological variability, and differing THC: CBD ratios. In a study, when combined with THC, CBD was observed to reduce SWS (Kaul et al. 2021).

4.1.4 Effects of Other Cannabinoids and Terpenes

Recent preclinical studies have highlighted that CBG, a non-psychoactive cannabinoid, has the potential to enhance deep sleep quality without producing psychoactive effects, thus offering promising therapeutic prospects (Russo et al. 2022; Whibley et al. 2025). Similarly, cannabinol (CBN) has been associated with increased TST and deep sleep; however, clinical evidence in humans remains limited (Arnold et al. 2025). In contrast, tetrahydrocannabivarin (THCV) may promote wakefulness and reduce sleep latency; however, its effects on REM sleep remain unclear and warrant further investigation (Baron et al. 2018).

Additionally, a wide array of terpenes, including β-caryophyllene, myrcene, α-pinene, humulene, linalool, limonene, terpineol, and geraniol, among others, may modulate or enhance cannabinoid activity through synergistic mechanisms. These compounds are believed to influence the overall pharmacological profile of cannabis (Baron 2018). β-caryophyllene, a selective CB2R agonist, has been shown to modulate neuroinflammation and improve emotional and cognitive functions, which are closely linked to sleep quality (Gertsch et al. 2008; Ricardi et al. 2024). Its anti-inflammatory and antioxidant properties suggest promising therapeutic potential for sleep disorders associated with neuroinflammatory conditions. Myrcene, one of the most abundant terpenes in cannabis, exhibits sedative and muscle-relaxant effects that may facilitate sleep onset and enhance the quality of sleep. This compound is thought to potentiate the sedative effects of THC by increasing blood-brain barrier permeability, thereby intensifying cannabinoid activity within the central nervous system (Russo 2011). Additionally, preclinical studies have indicated that myrcene possesses anxiolytic properties and may help reduce stress, an important contributor to sleep disturbances (Baron et al. 2018; Gurgel do Vale et al. 2002).

4.2 Effects of Cannabis on Sleep Disorders

The treatment of poor sleep and sleep disorders is among the most common reasons for the use of medicinal cannabis. This section summarizes the highest-quality clinical evidence currently available regarding the use of medicinal cannabis for the treatment of various sleep disorders, including insomnia, restless legs syndrome, obstructive sleep apnea, nightmare disorder, REM sleep behavior disorder, and narcolepsy (Maddison et al. 2022).

4.2.1 Insomnia

Insomnia disorder is defined as a persistent dissatisfaction with sleep quantity or quality despite adequate opportunities for rest. It typically involves difficulties with sleep initiation, sleep maintenance, and/or early-morning awakenings, occurring at least 3 times per week for at least 3 months. These disturbances must cause clinically significant distress or impairment in social, occupational, or other important areas of functioning (Babson et al. 2017; Vivek et al. 2024).

Cognitive-behavioral therapy is the first-line treatment for chronic insomnia. However, its limited accessibility and variable efficacy have led to increased interest in alternative pharmacological approaches to treat this condition. Cannabinoids are being explored for their anxiolytic and sleep-modulating properties. Historically used as sleep aids, cannabinoids are now being investigated in controlled settings as potential therapeutic agents (Kolla et al. 2022; Velzeboer et al. 2022).

Emerging evidence suggests that the effects of cannabinoids on sleep are dose-dependent and influenced by specific cannabinoid composition and treatment duration (Kaul et al. 2021; Maddison et al. 2022). Randomized controlled trials have demonstrated that THC reduces SOL but has minimal impact on total wake time or the frequency of nighttime awakenings. Higher doses are associated with adverse effects, such as dry mouth, dizziness, impaired concentration, and next-day sedation or hangover-like symptoms. Some users also reported a reduction in dreaming at high THC doses. Nabilone, a synthetic cannabinoid similar to THC, has been shown to improve insomnia severity in patients with chronic pain and perform better than amitriptyline in some studies, although it is associated with a higher incidence of mild adverse effects (Maddison et al. 2022).

In contrast, evidence supporting the use of CBD as a sleep-promoting agent remains limited. In a double-blind, placebo-controlled trial, only the highest dose (160 mg) increased self-reported sleep duration, whereas no significant effects were observed on sleep initiation or maintenance. Interestingly, all CBD doses were associated with reduced dream recall, suggesting a potential effect on REM sleep. CBD was generally well-tolerated, with no major adverse effects and no significant differences in morning alertness or concentration compared with placebo (Maddison et al. 2022).

A more comprehensive formulation combining THC, CBD, and CBN, known as ZTL-101, was evaluated in a double-blind, randomized, placebo-controlled trial involving patients with chronic insomnia. The formulation significantly improved insomnia severity and subjective sleep outcomes, including SOL, WASO, TST, sleep quality, and feeling refreshed upon waking. Actigraphy data confirmed improvements in TST and reduced nocturnal wakefulness in the intervention group. However, PSG measurements did not show significant changes, possibly because of the short assessment duration. Sleep architecture remained largely unchanged, with a slight reduction in the proportion of REM sleep. Adverse events were mild and transient but occurred more frequently in the treatment group (Maddison et al. 2022).

Despite the increasing interest, empirical evidence on the efficacy of cannabinoids in treating insomnia remains limited. Although cannabis is frequently used for managing sleep disturbances, including poorly defined complaints of "poor sleep," controlled clinical trials are scarce. Many existing studies have assessed sleep outcomes as secondary endpoints in populations with comorbid conditions (e.g., chronic pain), limiting their ability to detect meaningful changes in sleep due to a potential ceiling effect (Maddison et al. 2022).

4.2.2 Restless Legs Syndrome

Restless Legs Syndrome (RLS) is a common sensorimotor disorder marked by an irresistible urge to move the legs, worsening with inactivity and improving with movement, primarily in the evening. It impairs sleep quality and quality of life and is often accompanied by periodic limb movements during sleep. Its pathophysiology involves central dopaminergic dysfunction and neurotransmitters such as glutamate, GABA, and endogenous opioids (Kaul et al. 2021; Kolla et al. 2022). Side effects and refractory cases limit standard treatments (dopamine agonists, anticonvulsants, and opioids). Given the ECS's neuromodulatory role and the presence of cannabinoid receptors in pain and motor pathways, cannabinoids are being investigated as potential therapies (Maddison et al. 2022).

Two case series on treatment-resistant RLS patients who used cannabis showed promising results. The first series reported complete symptom resolution in five patients with severe RLS who smoked cannabis and one who used sublingual CBD. In the second series, 12 patients with moderate to severe RLS were included, of whom 66% experienced total remission and three others reported significant symptom relief (60%, 80%, and 90%) with smoked cannabis, while continuing their prescribed RLS medications. Only one patient did not report any improvement. Some patients who had complete relief with cannabis also benefited from CBD alone, although one did not (Kaul et al. 2021; Kolla et al. 2022; Maddison et al. 2022).

The distinct pharmacological actions of phytocannabinoids may explain these findings: THC's CB1 receptor agonism may help reduce discomfort and restlessness, while CBD's anti-inflammatory effects and its modulation of serotonin 5-HT1A receptors could further contribute to symptom relief and improved sleep quality (Kolla et al. 2022; Velzeboer et al. 2022).

4.2.3 Obstructive and Central Sleep Apnea

Obstructive Sleep Apnea (OSA) is a prevalent and increasingly recognized sleep-related breathing disorder characterized by recurrent episodes of complete or partial upper airway collapse during sleep. If left untreated, OSA is associated with a range of adverse outcomes, including an increased risk of cardiovascular and metabolic diseases, neurocognitive impairments, mood disorders such as depression, and a heightened risk of accidents related to excessive daytime sleepiness. Current standard therapies, such as continuous positive airway pressure, oral appliance therapy, and upper airway surgery, primarily address the anatomical component of OSA. Emerging pharmacological approaches represent a promising avenue, either as standalone treatments or adjunctive therapies, particularly for individuals whose OSA is driven by non-anatomical mechanisms or who are intolerant to conventional treatments (Kolla et al. 2022; Maddison et al. 2022).

Preclinical studies in rats have shown that the synthetic THC analog dronabinol reduces apnea frequency by activating CB1R and CB2R, modulating vagal nerve activity, and increasing genioglossus muscle tone to maintain airway patency (Kaul et al. 2021; Maddison et al. 2022; Velzeboer et al. 2022). In human trials, dronabinol has shown modest reductions in the apnea-hypopnea index (AHI) and improvements in daytime sleepiness. However, reductions in AHI did not reach statistical significance compared to baseline. Significant improvements in daytime sleepiness were observed at higher doses, while measures of oxygen saturation and arousal indices remained unchanged. Sleep architecture was largely preserved, with a slight increase in REM sleep. Adverse events, including somnolence, headache, nausea, and dizziness, were commonly reported but generally mild in severity (Kolla et al. 2022; Maddison et al. 2022).

Despite promising preliminary data, the routine use of cannabinoids for OSA is not currently recommended because of limited evidence. Given OSA's heterogeneous pathophysiology, cannabinoids may serve as adjuncts, potentially improving positive airway pressure adherence and suppressing central apneas (Kaul et al. 2021; Velzeboer et al. 2022).

4.2.4 PTSD-Related Nightmare Disorder

Recurring nightmares are a highly distressing and difficult-to-treat symptom of Post-Traumatic Stress Disorder (PTSD), for which current recommended treatments, such as image rehearsal therapy and prazosin, offer only moderate efficacy (Kolla et al. 2022; Maddison et al. 2022).

Nabilone has shown potential benefits in two retrospective case series studies. In one series involving 47 patients with weekly PTSD-related nightmares despite prior treatments, 72% experienced a reduction or cessation of nightmares after nightly nabilone administration, although 28% discontinued early due to side effects such as dizziness and memory difficulties. A small proportion (9%) of patients were able to stop treatment without symptom recurrence after several months. Another case series of 104 inmates reported a significant decrease in nightmare frequency and an increase in sleep duration during an average 11-week treatment period. A more rigorous double-blind, randomized, placebo-controlled trial involving 19 military veterans titrated nabilone daily and found improvements in nightmare frequency, intensity, and overall functioning compared to placebo (Kaul et al. 2021; Velzeboer et al. 2022).

A case series evaluating the use of CBD for insomnia in patients with PTSD reported a reduction in sleep disturbances, as measured using the Pittsburgh Sleep Quality Index (Kaul et al. 2021). Preliminary findings suggest that CBD may improve overall sleep efficiency in this population, although it may paradoxically increase SOL in some cases (Velzeboer et al. 2022).

Cannabinoids likely reduce PTSD symptoms by modulating the ECS and limbic areas (amygdala and hypothalamus) and decreasing hypervigilance and hyperarousal (Maddison et al. 2022).

4.2.5 REM Behavior Disorder

REM Sleep Behavior Disorder (RBD) is a parasomnia characterized by the loss of normal muscle atonia during REM sleep, leading to dream enactment behaviors such as punching, kicking, vocalizations, and even falling out of bed. RBD is commonly associated with neurodegenerative diseases, including Parkinson's disease, Lewy body dementia, and multisystem atrophy (Kaul et al. 2021; Kolla et al. 2022). Current pharmacological treatments mainly involve clonazepam and melatonin, which can reduce symptoms but often have limited long-term efficacy and significant side effects, such as nocturnal confusion, falls, and worsening of obstructive sleep apnea (Maddison et al. 2022).

CBD has been investigated for RBD, with mixed results. A small case series reported that four patients with Parkinson's disease treated with CBD experienced a reduction in RBD event frequency without notable side effects. Three patients reported complete remission of symptoms during treatment, which returned upon treatment cessation (Kolla et al. 2022). However, a subsequent 12-week randomized, placebo-controlled trial involving 33 patients with Parkinson's disease found no significant difference between CBD and placebo in reducing RBD events, despite a transient improvement in self-reported sleep satisfaction in the CBD group between weeks 4 and 8. PSG measures of sleep quality and architecture showed no differences, and adverse events were infrequent and mild (Velzeboer et al. 2022).

4.2.6 Narcolepsy and Idiopathic Hypersomnia

No clinical studies have been published on the use of medical cannabis for central disorders of hypersomnolence, such as narcolepsy and idiopathic hypersomnia. However, preclinical animal studies have suggested potential therapeutic effects. In narcoleptic rats deficient in hypocretin, CBD administration reduced excessive sleepiness, whereas synthetic THC reduced REM sleep (Kolla et al. 2022; Kaul et al. 2021).

Theoretically, the combined REM-suppressing effect of THC and the wake-promoting effect of CBD could be beneficial for narcolepsy patients. THC-induced REM suppression may also alleviate REM sleep disturbances common in narcolepsy, including nightmares, sleep paralysis, REM behavior disorder, hallucinations, and cataplexy (Maddison et al. 2022). Clinical evidence indicates that acute THC use increases SWS and suppresses REM, effects similar to those of sodium oxybate, an effective treatment for narcolepsy (Kolla et al. 2022).

A recent animal study showed that CBD administered at the start of the dark phase blocked excessive sleepiness in orexin-deficient narcoleptic rats, supporting its potential role in managing daytime sleepiness (Kaul et al. 2021).

5. Risks and Adverse Effects of Cannabis on Sleep

Frequent or prolonged cannabis use can negatively impact sleep quality and architecture, with significant consequences for physical, cognitive, and mental health across populations (Volkow et al. 2016; AminiLari et al. 2022). These risks include impairments in memory, attention, processing speed, and emotional regulation, as well as increased vulnerability to psychiatric disorders, such as anxiety, depression, and psychosis (Volkow et al. 2016; Gobbi et al. 2019).

5.1 Tolerance and Dependence

Prolonged and frequent cannabis use can lead to the development of tolerance, a condition in which the effectiveness of THC in inducing sleep and other effects diminishes over time. As tolerance builds, users require progressively higher doses to achieve the desired effects, increasing the risk of cannabis use disorder and reducing its efficacy for managing sleep problems (Babson et al. 2017; NIDA 2024).

Abrupt cessation of cannabis use by habitual users often triggers withdrawal symptoms. Budney et al. (2004) describe cannabis withdrawal syndrome as including insomnia, irritability, anxiety, mood disturbances, and changes in sleep architecture such as increased REM sleep, which may be associated with vivid dreams or nightmares. These symptoms can emerge within the first week of abstinence and contribute to relapse, thus complicating cessation efforts. The United States National Institute on Drug Abuse (NIDA 2024) further emphasizes that withdrawal symptoms reflect neuroadaptations in the ECS caused by chronic THC exposure, and that these symptoms can vary in intensity depending on the duration and frequency of use.

5.2 Alterations in Sleep Architecture

Chronic cannabis use, especially with high THC content, leads to sustained suppression of REM sleep, which is a critical phase for memory consolidation and emotional regulation. Gates et al. (2014) reviewed several studies reporting REM reductions among chronic users, though results vary and the functional implications require further investigation. Babson et al. (2017) similarly highlight that frequent cannabis use disrupts sleep architecture, potentially impairing emotional regulation and increasing vulnerability to anxiety and depression. This disruption may prompt self-medication with cannabis, which can worsen sleep and mental health problems over time.

Despite subjective reports of sedation, cannabis does not necessarily enhance physiological restorative sleep. Althoff et al. (2024) found that cannabis use within 3 h before bedtime increased wakefulness after sleep onset and the proportion of light sleep (stage N1), without improving TST or efficiency. Supporting this, Suraev et al. (2020) concluded that the current evidence is insufficient to recommend cannabinoids for sleep disorders, emphasizing the need for larger, well-controlled trials to clarify their effects and safety. In addition, Pacek et al. (2017) used in-home PSG and self-reports in treatment-seeking cannabis users, revealing widespread sleep disturbances such as fragmented sleep and low efficiency, with notable sex differences.

5.3 Daytime Sleepiness and Cognitive Impairment

High doses of THC are associated with sedation and increased daytime sleepiness, which can impair cognitive functions such as attention, working memory, and executive function, potentially affecting activities that require sustained concentration. Winiger et al. (2021) examined cannabis use and sleep outcomes in a sample of moderate users aged 21 to 70 years. They found that, although many users expect cannabis to improve sleep, frequent use is associated with poorer subjective sleep quality, lower sleep efficiency and duration, and increased daytime sleepiness. By contrast, higher CBD concentrations were associated with improved sleep duration and quality, particularly in older adults, suggesting a modulatory effect of CBD.

CBD may counteract some negative effects of THC. For example, Shannon et al. (2019) reported that adjunctive CBD treatment was well tolerated and was associated with reductions in anxiety and improvements in sleep quality in most patients, although sleep improvements fluctuated over time. Similarly, in patients with Parkinson's disease, short-term administration of low-dose cannabis extracts (THC: CBD) improved cognition and insomnia symptoms, although some patients experienced increased daytime sleepiness, likely due to THC's sedative properties (Ruver-Martins et al. 2025). No serious adverse effects were observed, suggesting that low-dose cannabis extract is a safe and effective option for managing certain non-motor symptoms.

However, heavy or chronic cannabis use raises concerns regarding long-term cognitive health, partly due to its impact on sleep. Pacek et al. (2017) highlighted that the sleep disturbances observed in treatment-seeking heavy cannabis users, such as low sleep efficiency, prolonged sleep latency, and high rates of clinical or subthreshold insomnia, may contribute to daytime cognitive impairment. Women reported greater perceived sleep-related dysfunction despite longer sleep durations.

5.4 Psychiatric Risks

Frequent use of high-potency THC cannabis is linked to an increased risk of psychiatric disorders, especially in vulnerable individuals. Epidemiological and experimental evidence demonstrate a dose-response relationship between cannabis use and the risk of psychotic outcomes, with high-potency cannabis and synthetic cannabinoids carrying the greatest risk. THC primarily acts through CB1R activation, modulating dopaminergic neurotransmission in the limbic and prefrontal brain regions, mechanisms implicated in psychotic symptoms. Experimental administration of THC induces transient psychosis in healthy subjects, an effect that can be mitigated by the co-administration of CBD (Murray et al. 2016).

A comprehensive umbrella review by Groening et al. (2024) synthesized evidence from 32 systematic reviews and meta-analyses, confirming the association between cannabis use and subclinical psychotic experiences and schizotypal traits in the general population. Cannabis use is also linked to an earlier onset and increased risk of clinical psychosis, although evidence regarding the transition to psychosis in high-risk clinical groups is inconclusive. In patients with established psychotic disorders, cannabis use increases the risk of relapse. Although the associations are robust, causality remains unconfirmed. Supporting this, a large multicenter study by Di Forti et al. (2019) showed that daily use of high-potency cannabis (THC $\geq$ 10%) nearly quintupled the odds of psychosis compared to non-users. Complementing this epidemiological evidence, genetic studies have revealed the important role of genetic predisposition in this relationship. Pasman et al. (2018) identified genetic overlap between schizophrenia liability and cannabis use through a large genome-wide association study, showing that genetic risk for schizophrenia causally influences cannabis consumption. Similarly, Power et al. (2014) demonstrated that individuals with a higher burden of schizophrenia risk alleles are more likely to use cannabis and consume it in larger quantities.

Beyond adult populations, accumulating evidence highlights that exposure during sensitive developmental periods confers additional risks. In particular, the adolescent brain cognitive development study has documented that prenatal cannabis exposure is associated with cognitive impairments and a higher risk of psychopathology, including psychotic-like experiences, in children during middle childhood (Paul et al. 2021; NIDA 2024). Moreover, cannabis use during adolescence has been linked to significant mental health risks, including an increased incidence of depression, anxiety, and suicidality among young adults (Gobbi et al. 2019). Sorkhou et al. (2024) reviewed the relationship between cannabis use and mood disorders and reported that cannabis consumption correlates with worsening depressive and manic symptoms and poorer prognosis in major depressive disorder and bipolar disorder. Together, these studies underscore the importance of preventive and educational policies targeting vulnerable populations and critical developmental windows to mitigate the mental health burden associated with cannabis use (Volkow et al. 2016; Hall and Lynskey 2020; Solmi et al. 2022).

Chronic cannabis use disrupts sleep architecture by suppressing REM sleep, a phase essential for emotional regulation (Babson et al. 2017). This disruption, combined with REM rebound following cessation, may exacerbate psychiatric symptoms and elevate the risk of psychiatric disorders (Groening et al. 2024). Consequently, sleep disturbances likely intensify the psychiatric vulnerability associated with cannabis use.

These findings emphasize the need for continued research and informed policy to balance potential therapeutic applications of cannabis with its documented risks.

6. Scientific Gaps in the Study of Cannabis for Sleep Disorders

The scientific evidence regarding the effects of cannabis on sleep remains limited and inconsistent. Most available studies are observational, often with small sample sizes and methodological limitations, which restrict the generalizability of their findings. Amaral et al. (2023) reviewed 40 studies and found that cannabis improved sleep in approximately 21% of cases, worsened it in 48%, and showed mixed or no effects in the remaining cases. This variability, linked to dosage, formulation (THC/CBD ratio), administration route, and user characteristics (age, comorbidities, and consumption patterns), limits the strength of the current conclusions (Babson et al. 2017; NIDA 2024). Suraev et al. (2020) identified a limited number of preclinical and clinical studies on cannabinoids and sleep disorders, many with moderate to high risk of bias. They concluded that the current evidence is insufficient to support the routine use of cannabinoids for treating sleep disorders and called for rigorous, long-term, controlled trials to assess their safety, efficacy, and impact on sleep architecture and specific conditions such as sleep apnea, insomnia, and REM sleep behavior disorder.

Preliminary studies suggest that low doses of THC may facilitate sleep onset, whereas high doses or chronic use can alter sleep architecture, including REM sleep suppression, with possible adverse effects (Gates et al. 2014; Suraev et al. 2020). Some non-psychoactive compounds, such as CBD, have the potential to improve sleep quality and reduce anxiety. Blessing et al. (2015) supported CBD's anxiolytic effects based on preclinical and clinical evidence but emphasized the need for further controlled trials to confirm its long-term benefits and safety in specific clinical populations. Shannon et al. (2019), in a clinical case series, reported that CBD reduced anxiety symptoms in 79% of patients and improved sleep quality in 67% of patients, although sleep effects varied over time. More recently, Bonn-Miller et al. (2024) conducted a double-blind, randomized, placebo-controlled trial to evaluate the safety and efficacy of CBN, alone and in combination with CBD, in adults with poor sleep quality. They found that CBN significantly reduced nighttime awakenings and overall sleep disturbance without affecting daytime fatigue. The addition of CBD did not enhance these effects.

A significant proportion of medical cannabis users reported improvements in sleep quality, especially in the early stages of treatment. However, the persistence of these benefits over the long term is limited and varies (Babson et al. 2017; Maddison et al. 2022). Ried et al. (2023) evaluated a medicinal oil (10 mg/ml THC and 15 mg/ml CBD) in adults with insomnia and found that 60% of the participants no longer met the diagnostic criteria for insomnia after two weeks of treatment, with significant improvements in sleep duration and quality, including increased light sleep and elevated midnight melatonin levels; the treatment was well tolerated.

However, chronic cannabis use has been associated with reduced sleep quality and duration, including insomnia, underscoring the need to evaluate long-term effects and develop strategies to minimize tolerance and dependence on cannabis (Winiger et al. 2021).

Overall, robust, randomized, long-term trials are needed to rigorously assess the efficacy, safety, optimal dosing, and mechanisms of cannabis and its derivatives in managing sleep disorders, especially in vulnerable populations, such as adolescents and individuals with psychiatric conditions (Volkow et al. 2016; Babson et al. 2017; Suraev et al. 2020; AminiLari et al. 2022; NIDA 2024).

7. Medical Supervision and Therapeutic Use

Therapeutic use of cannabis for sleep disorders should always be supervised by qualified healthcare professionals, who must carefully assess individual risks, potential drug interactions, and comorbidities, adjusting doses and formulations to maximize benefits and minimize adverse effects. Recent systematic reviews and meta-analyses confirm that medical cannabis and cannabinoids can provide minor improvements in sleep quality for patients with chronic pain or insomnia, although these effects are modest and often accompanied by side effects such as dizziness, somnolence, and fatigue (AminiLari et al. 2022; Suraev et al. 2024). For example, observational data from the UK Medical Cannabis Registry indicate that patients with insomnia experienced significant and sustained improvements in sleep quality, anxiety symptoms, and overall health-related quality of life after initiating plant-derived cannabis-based medicinal products under medical supervision, with benefits observed at one, three, and six months. Although nearly 46% of adverse events were reported, these were generally mild and non-life-threatening, supporting the relative safety of these treatments in the medium term (Vivek et al. 2024). Similarly, a recent randomized, double-blind, crossover trial in adults with physician-diagnosed insomnia who infrequently use cannabis found that a single evening oral dose of 10 mg THC combined with 200 mg CBD produced no notable next-day impairment in cognitive or psychomotor function, nor in simulated driving performance, despite a slight increase in self-reported sedation (Suraev et al. 2024).

However, recent evidence highlights the critical need for ongoing medical oversight and careful patient selection when using cannabis therapeutically, as unsupervised or inappropriate use can lead to adverse effects, including the development of cannabis use disorder and psychiatric complications. A large patient series reports common but mostly mild adverse events, underscoring the importance of cautious prescribing (Arkell et al. 2023). Surveys of physicians reveal significant gaps in knowledge and variable clinical practices, emphasizing the need for improved education and supervision (Syed et al. 2025). Moreover, longitudinal studies indicate that frequent cannabis use may not improve symptoms such as insomnia or anxiety and is associated with increased risk of dependence (Cooke et al. 2023). Comprehensive evidence maps further stress the necessity for rigorous research and clinical oversight to optimize benefits and minimize harms (Montagner et al. 2024).

8. Responsible Use and Vulnerable Populations

Particular caution is warranted in vulnerable groups, such as adolescents, pregnant or breastfeeding women, and individuals with a history of psychiatric illness. Cannabis use during adolescence represents a significant risk due to the vulnerability of the developing brain and is associated with an increased risk of psychiatric disorders, memory difficulties, lower academic achievement, and risky behaviors (Meier et al. 2012; Silins et al. 2014; Gobbi et al. 2019). The perception among youth that cannabis use is low-risk may contribute to increased consumption, underscoring the need for evidence-based public policies and educational campaigns to prevent early and prolonged use (Terry-McElrath et al. 2025). Prenatal cannabis exposure is linked to adverse neonatal outcomes, such as low birth weight and neurodevelopmental delays (Volkow et al. 2019). Additionally, individuals with psychiatric histories face a higher risk of symptom exacerbation and neuropsychiatric complications (Gobbi et al. 2019; Volkow et al. 2019).

Emerging evidence also indicates increased cardiovascular risk, including stroke and acute coronary events, particularly among frequent users or those with pre-existing cardiovascular conditions (Pasha et al. 2021; Montagner et al. 2024). Given these risks, clinical evaluation must be rigorous and personalized, considering individual patient characteristics to minimize harm and optimize therapeutic outcomes (National Academies of Sciences 2017).

9. Conclusions and Perspectives

Cannabis modulates sleep through its interaction with the ECS, influencing various sleep stages and the overall sleep quality. While cannabinoids, such as THC and CBD, show promise for treating sleep disorders, such as insomnia and PTSD-related nightmares, their effects are dose-dependent and complex. Low doses of THC may reduce sleep latency; however, higher doses and chronic use can disrupt sleep architecture, particularly by suppressing REM sleep, potentially leading to rebound effects upon cessation. In contrast, CBD may improve sleep quality at moderate doses but can cause sedation at higher doses. Additionally, emerging preclinical evidence suggests that minor cannabinoids, such as CBN, may increase total sleep time and sleep stability, highlighting new therapeutic possibilities (Gates et al. 2014; Babson et al. 2017; Suraev et al. 2020; Arnold et al. 2025).

Moreover, chronic or recreational cannabis use has been associated with adverse effects, including tolerance, dependence, psychiatric symptoms, and impaired cognitive and motor functions, which may worsen sleep quality and daytime functioning (Gobbi et al. 2019; Solmi et al. 2022). Vulnerable populations, such as adolescents, older adults, pregnant women, and individuals with psychiatric comorbidities, require special consideration in research and clinical practice.

To safely integrate cannabis into sleep medicine, future research must focus on determining the optimal dosing and cannabinoid ratios, standardizing product quality, and conducting rigorous controlled clinical trials. Additionally, exploring the neuroprotective potential of cannabinoids in aging and neurodegenerative diseases may open new therapeutic avenues for improving sleep in older adults (Fernández-Ruiz et al. 2015; Babson et al. 2017; National Academies of Sciences 2017).

In summary, although cannabis shows promising therapeutic potential for sleep disorders, the current evidence remains insufficient for definitive clinical recommendations. Rigorous multidisciplinary research is essential for the safe and effective integration of cannabis into sleep-related clinical practice.

Acknowledgments

Authors gratefully acknowledge Agencia Nacional de Promoción Científica y Tecnológica (ANPCyT) and Universidad Nacional de Rosario (UNR) for financial support (PICT-2020-SERIEA-02687 and 80020210300027UR). EC, LRM, and AB are also thankful to Consejo Nacional de Investigaciones Científicas y Técnicas (CONICET) for their doctoral and postdoctoral fellowships.

References

Althoff, M. D., Kinney, G. L., Aloia, M. S., Sempio, C., Klawitter, J., and Bowler, R. P. (2024). The impact of cannabis use proximal to sleep and cannabinoid metabolites on sleep architecture. *Journal of Clinical Sleep Medicine*, 20: 1615–1625.

Amaral, C., Carvalho, C., Scaranelo, A., Chapman, K., Chatkin, J., and Ferreira, I. (2023). Cannabis and sleep disorders: Not ready for prime time? A qualitative scoping review. *Journal of Clinical Sleep Medicine*, 19: 975–990.

AminiLari, M., Wang, L., Neumark, S., Adli, T., Couban, R. J., Giangregorio, A. et al. (2022). Medical cannabis and cannabinoids for impaired sleep: a systematic review and meta-analysis of randomized clinical trials. *Sleep*, 45:zsab234.

Arkell, T. R., Downey, L. A., Hayley, A. C., and Roth, S. (2023). Assessment of medical cannabis and health-related quality of life. *JAMA network open*, 6: e2312522-e2312522

Arnold, J. C., Occelli Hanbury-Brown, C. V., Anderson, L. L., Bedoya-Pérez, M. A., Udoh, M., Sharman, L. A. et al. (2025). A sleepy cannabis constituent: cannabinol and its active metabolite influence sleep architecture in rats. *Neuropsychopharmacology*, 50: 586–595.

Babson, K. A., Sottile, J., and Morabito, D. (2017). Cannabis, cannabinoids, and sleep: a review of the literature. *Current Psychiatry Reports*, 19: 23.

Baron, E. P. (2018). Medicinal properties of cannabinoids, terpenes, and flavonoids in cannabis, and benefits in migraine, headache, and pain: An update on current evidence and cannabis science. *Headache*, 58: 1139–1186.

Blessing, E. M., Steenkamp, M. M., Manzanares, J., and Marmar, C. R. (2015). Cannabidiol as a potential treatment for anxiety disorders. *Neurotherapeutics*, 12: 825–836.

Block, J. S. (2023). The history of cannabis: a story of coevolution and human discovery. In: Mahmoud A. ElSohly (Ed.). *Cannabis Chemistry and Biology: Fundamentals*. Walter de Gruyter GmbH, Berlin, Germany

Bonn-Miller, M. O., Feldner, M. T., Bynion, T. M., Eglit, G. M. L., Brunstetter, M., Kalaba, M. et al. (2024). A double-blind, randomized, placebo-controlled study of the safety and effects of cannabinol (CBN) with and without cannabidiol (CBD) on sleep quality. *Experimental and Clinical Psychopharmacology*, 32: 277.

Budney, A. J., Hughes, J. R., Moore, B. A., and Vandrey, R. (2004). Review of the validity and significance of cannabis withdrawal syndrome. *American Journal of Psychiatry*, 161: 1967–1977.

Carskadon, M. A., and Dement, W. C. (2011). Normal human sleep: an overview. In Kryger MH, Roth T, Dement WC (Eds) Principles and Practice of Sleep Medicine (6th ed, pp. 15–24) Elsevier.

Castillo, P. E., Younts, T. J., Chávez, A. E., and Hashimotodani, Y. (2012). Endocannabinoid signaling and synaptic function. *Neuron*, 76: 70–81.

Choi, S., Huang, B. C., and Gamaldo, C. E. (2020). Therapeutic uses of cannabis on sleep disorders and related conditions. *Journal of Clinical Neurophysiology*, 37: 39–49.

Cooke, M. E., Potter, K. W., Jashinski, J., Pascale, M., Schuster, R. M., Tervo-Clemmens, B. et al. (2023). Development of cannabis use disorder in medical cannabis users: A 9-month follow-up of a randomized clinical trial testing effects of medical cannabis card ownership. *Frontiers in psychiatry*, 14: 1083334.

D'Angelo, M., and Steardo, Jr. L. (2024). Cannabinoids and sleep: exploring biological mechanisms and therapeutic potentials. *International Journal of Molecular Sciences*, 25: 3603.

Desai, D., Momin, A., Hirpara, P., Jha, H., Thaker, R., Patel, J. et al. (2024). Exploring the role of circadian rhythms in sleep and recovery: a review article. *Cureus*, 16: e61568.

Di Forti, M., Quattrone, D., Freeman, T. P., Tripoli, G., Gayer-Anderson, C., Quigley, H. et al. (2019). The contribution of cannabis use to variation in the incidence of psychotic disorder across Europe (EU-GEI): a multicentre case-control study. *The Lancet Psychiatry*, 6: 427–436.

Di Marzo, V., and Piscitelli, F. (2015). The endocannabinoid system and its modulation by phytocannabinoids. *Neurotherapeutics*, 12: 692–698.

Fernández-Ruiz, J., Moro, M. A., and Martínez-Orgado, J. (2015). Cannabinoids in neurodegenerative disorders and stroke/brain trauma: from preclinical models to clinical applications. *Neurotherapeutics*, 12: 793–806.

Gates, P. J., Albertella, L., and Copeland, J. (2014). The effects of cannabinoid administration on sleep: a systematic review of human studies. *Sleep Medicine Reviews*, 18: 477–487.

Gertsch, J., Leonti, M., Raduner, S., Racz, I., Chen, J. Z., Xie, X. Q. et al. (2008). Beta-caryophyllene as a dietary cannabinoid. *Proceedings of the National Academy of Sciences*, 121: e2301234119.

Gobbi, G., Atkin, T., Zytynski, T., Wang, S., Askari, S., Boruff, J., Ware, M. et al. (2019). Association of cannabis use in adolescence and risk of depression, anxiety, and suicidality in young adulthood: a systematic review and meta-analysis. *JAMA Psychiatry*, 76: 426–434.

Groening, J. M., Denton, E., Parvaiz, R., Brunet, D. L., Von Daniken, A., Shi, Y. et al.(2024). A systematic evidence map of the association between cannabis use and psychosis-related outcomes across the psychosis continuum: An umbrella review of systematic reviews and meta-analyses. *Psychiatry Research*, 331: 115626.

Gurgel do Vale, T. G., Furtado, E. C., Santos, Jr. J. G., and Viana, G. S. B. (2002). Central effects of citral, myrcene and limonene, constituents of essential oils from *Lippia alba* chemotypes. *Phytomedicine*, 9: 254–258.

Hall, W., and Lynskey, M. (2020). Assessing the public health impacts of legalizing recreational cannabis use: the US experience. *World Psychiatry*, 19: 179–186.

Herrera-Solís, A., Vásquez, K. G., and Prospéro-García, O. (2010). Acute and subchronic administration of anandamide or oleamide increases REM sleep in rats. *Pharmacology Biochemistry and Behavior*, 95: 106–112.

Irwin, M. R. (2015). Why sleep is important for health: a psychoneuroimmunology perspective. *Annual Review of Psychology*, 66: 143–172.

Kano, M., Ohno-Shosaku, T., Hashimotodani, Y., Uchigashima, M., and Watanabe, M. (2009). Endocannabinoid-mediated control of synaptic transmission. *Physiological Reviews*, 89: 309–380.

Kaul, M., Zee, P. C., and Sahni, A. S. (2021). Effects of cannabinoids on sleep and their therapeutic potential for sleep disorders. *Neurotherapeutics*, 18: 217–227.

Kesner, P., and Lovinger, D. M. (2020). Cannabinoids, endocannabinoids and sleep. *Frontiers in Molecular Neuroscience*, 13: 125.

Kolla, B. P., Hayes, L., Cox, C., Eatwell, L., Deyo-Svendsen, M., and Mansukhani, M. P. (2022). The effects of cannabinoids on sleep. *Journal of Primary Care & Community Health*, 13: 21501319221081277.

Krueger, J. M., Frank, M. G., Wisor, J. P., and Roy, S. (2016). Sleep function: Toward elucidating an enigma. *Sleep Medicine Reviews*, 28: 46–54.

Maddison, K., Kosky, C., and Walsh, J. H. (2022). Is there a place for medicinal cannabis in treating patients with sleep disorders? What we know so far. *Nature and Science of Sleep*, 14: 957–968.

Meier, M. H., Caspi, A., Ambler, A., Harrington, H., Houts, R., Keefe, R. S. et al. (2012). Persistent cannabis users show neuropsychological decline from childhood to midlife. *Proceedings of the National Academy of Sciences*, 109: E2657–E2664.

Méndez-Díaz, M., Ruiz-Contreras, A. E., Cortés-Morelos, J., and Prospéro-García, O. (2021). Cannabinoids and Sleep/Wake Control. pp. 83–96. *In*: Monti, J. M., Pandi-Perumal, S. R., and Murillo-Rodríguez, E. (Eds.). *Cannabinoids and Sleep: Molecular, Functional and Clinical Aspects*. Springer.

Montagner, P., de Salas Quiroga, A., Ferreira, A. S., Duarte da Luz, B. M., Ruppelt, B. M., Schlechta Portella, C. F. et al. (2024). Charting the therapeutic landscape: a comprehensive evidence map on medical cannabis for health outcomes. *Frontiers in Pharmacology*, 15: 1494492.

Morin, C. M., and Benca, R. (2012). Chronic insomnia. *The Lancet*, 379: 1129–1141.

Murillo-Rodriguez, E., Blanco-Centurion, C., Sanchez, C., Daniele, P., and Shiromani, P. J. (2003). Anandamide enhances extracellular levels of adenosine and induces sleep: an in vivo microdialysis study. *Sleep*, 26: 943–947.

Murillo-Rodriguez, E., Cabeza, R., Méndez-Díaz, M., Navarro, L., and Prospéro-García, O. (2001). Anandamide-induced sleep is blocked by SR141716A, a CB1 receptor antagonist and by U73122, a phospholipase C inhibitor. *Neuroreport*, 12: 2131–2136.

Murillo-Rodríguez, E., Poot-Aké, A., Arias-Carrión, O., Pacheco-Pantoja, E., de la Fuente-Ortegón, A., and Arankowsky-Sandoval, G. (2011). The emerging role of the endocannabinoid system in the sleep–wake cycle modulation. *Current Neuropharmacology*, 9: 448–457.

Murillo-Rodriguez, E., Sánchez-Alavez, M., Navarro, L., Martınez-Gonzalez, D., Drucker-Colın, R., and Prospero-Garcıa, O. (1998). Anandamide modulates sleep and memory in rats. *Brain Research*, 812: 270–274.

Murillo-Rodríguez, E., Vázquez, E., Millán-Aldaco, D., Palomero-Rivero, M., and Drucker-Colin, R. (2007). Effects of the fatty acid amide hydrolase inhibitor URB597 on the sleep-wake cycle, c-Fos expression and dopamine levels of the rat. *European Journal of Pharmacology*, 562: 82–91.

Murray, R. M., Quigley, H., Quattrone, D., Englund, A., and Di Forti, M (2016). Traditional marijuana, high-potency cannabis and synthetic cannabinoids: increasing risk for psychosis. *World Psychiatry*, 15: 195–204.

National Academies of Sciences, Medicine, Medicine Division, Board on Population Health, Public Health Practice, Committee on the Health Effects of Marijuana: An Evidence Review and Research Agenda (2017). The health effects of cannabis and cannabinoids: the current state of evidence and recommendations for research.

NIDA (National Institute on Drug Abuse) (2024) Cannabis (Marihuana). Retrieved from https://nida.nih.gov/research-topics/cannabis-marijuana.

Nir, Y., and de Lecea, L. (2023). Sleep and vigilance states: Embracing spatiotemporal dynamics. *Neuron*, 111: 1998–2011.

Pacek, L. R., Herrmann, E. S., Smith, M. T., and Vandrey, R. (2017). Sleep continuity, architecture and quality among treatment-seeking cannabis users: An in-home, unattended polysomnographic study. *Experimental and Clinical Psychopharmacology*, 25: 295–303.

Pacher, P., Bátkai, S., and Kunos, G. (2006). The endocannabinoid system as an emerging target of pharmacotherapy. *Pharmacological Reviews*, 58: 389–462.

Pasha, A. K., Clements, C. Y., Reynolds, C. A., Lopez, M. K., Lugo, C. A., Gonzalez, Y. et al. (2021). Cardiovascular effects of medical marijuana: a systematic review. *The American Journal of Medicine*, 134: 182–193.

Pasman, J. A., Verweij, K. J., Gerring, Z., Stringer, S., Sanchez-Roige, S., Treur, J. L. et al. (2018). GWAS of lifetime cannabis use reveals new risk loci, genetic overlap with psychiatric traits, and a causal effect of schizophrenia liability. *Nature Neuroscience*, 21: 1161–1170.

Paul, S. E., Hatoum, A. S., Fine, J. D., Johnson, E. C., Hansen, I., Karcher, N. R., Moreau, A. L. et al. (2021) Associations between prenatal cannabis exposure and childhood outcomes: Results from the ABCD Study. *JAMA Psychiatry*, 78: 64–76.

Pérez-Morales, M., Alberto, K., Méndez-Díaz, M., Ruiz-Contreras, A. E., Drucker-Colín, R., and Prospéro-García, O. (2013). 2-AG into the lateral hypothalamus increases REM sleep and cFos expression in melanin concentrating hormone neurons in rats. *Pharmacology Biochemistry and Behavior*, 108: 1–7.

Pérez-Morales, M., Alvarado-Capuleño, I., López-Colomé, A. M., Méndez-Díaz, M., Ruiz-Contreras, A. E. et al. (2012). Activation of PAR1 in the lateral hypothalamus of rats enhances food intake and REMS through CB1R. *Neuroreport*, 23: 814–818.

Pérez-Morales, M., Fajardo-Valdez, A., Méndez-Díaz, M., Ruiz-Contreras, A. E., and Prospéro-García, O. (2014). 2-Arachidonoylglycerol into the lateral hypothalamus improves reduced sleep in adult rats subjected to maternal separation. *NeuroReport*, 25: 1437–1441.

Pertwee, R. G. (2015). Endocannabinoids and their pharmacological actions. In *Handbook of Experimental Pharmacology* (Vol 231, pp. 1–37) Springer.

Power, R. A., Verweij, K. J. H., Zuhair, M., Montgomery, G. W., Henders, A. K., Heath, A. C. et al. (2014). Genetic predisposition to schizophrenia associated with increased use of cannabis. *Molecular Psychiatry*, 19: 1201–1204.

Puskar, P., Sengupta, T., Sharma, B., Nath, S. S., Mallick, H., and Akhtar, N. (2021). Changes in sleep-wake cycle after microinjection of agonist and antagonist of endocannabinoid receptors at the medial septum of rats. *Physiology & Behavior*, 237: 113448.

Ranade, A., Tavhare, S. D., Acharya, R., and Pawar, S. D. (2022). Cannabis (*Bhanga*) in classical text of Ayurveda: an evidence-based rationale. *In*: Agrawal, D. C., Kumar, R., and Dhanasekaran, M. (Eds.). *Cannabis/Marijuana for Healthcare*. Springer, Singapore.

Rezende, B., Alencar, A. K. N., de Bem, G. F., Fontes-Dantas, F. L., and Montes, G. C. (2023) Endocannabinoid system: chemical characteristics and biological activity. *Pharmaceuticals*, 16: 148.

Ricardi, C., Barachini, S., Consoli, G., Marazziti, D., Polini, B., and Chiellini, G. (2024). Beta-caryophyllene, a cannabinoid receptor type 2 selective agonist, in emotional and cognitive disorders. *International Journal of Molecular Sciences*, 25: 3203.

Ried, K., Tamanna, T., Matthews, S., and Sali, A. (2023). Medicinal cannabis improves sleep in adults with insomnia: a randomised double-blind placebo-controlled crossover study. *Journal of Sleep Research*, 32: e13793.

Russo, E. B. (2005). History of cannabis and its preparations in saga, science, and sobriquet. *Chemistry & Biodiversity*, 4: 1614–1648.

Russo, E. B. (2011). Taming THC: potential cannabis synergy and phytocannabinoid-terpenoid entourage effects. *British Journal of Pharmacology*, 163: 1344–1364.

Russo, E. B., Cuttler, C., Cooper, Z. D., Stueber, A., Whiteley, V. L., and Sexton, M. (2022). Survey of patients employing cannabigerol-predominant cannabis preparations: Perceived medical effects, adverse events, and withdrawal symptoms. *Cannabis and Cannabinoid Research*, 7: 706–716.

Ruver-Martins, A. C., Martinez, I. A. R., Holla, V. G., Souza, B. L. D., Silva, E. G. D., Novoa, D. M. A., Souza-Silva, E. et al. (2025). Low doses of cannabis extract ameliorate non-motor symptoms of Parkinson's disease patients: a case series. *Frontiers in Human Neuroscience*, 18: 1466438.

Santucci, V., Storme, J. J., Soubrié, P., and Le Fur, G. (1996). Arousal-enhancing properties of the CB1 cannabinoid receptor antagonist SR 141716A in rats as assessed by electroencephalographic spectral and sleep-waking cycle analysis. *Life Sciences*, 58: PL103–PL110.

Scammell, T. E., Arrigoni, E., and Lipton, J. O. (2017). Neural circuitry of wakefulness and sleep. *Neuron*, 93: 747–765.

Shannon S, Lewis N, Lee H, Hughes S (2019). Cannabidiol in anxiety and sleep: a large case series. *The Permanente Journal*, 23: 18–041.

Silins, E., Horwood, L. J., Patton, G. C., Fergusson, D. M., Olsson, C. A., Hutchinson, D. M. et al. (2014). Young adult sequelae of adolescent cannabis use: an integrative analysis. *The Lancet Psychiatry*, 1: 286–293.

Solmi, M., Radua, J., Olivola, M., Croce, E., Soardo, L., Salazar de Pablo, G. et al. (2022) Age at onset of mental disorders worldwide: large-scale meta-analysis of 192 epidemiological studies. *Molecular Psychiatry*, 27: 281–295.

Sorkhou, M., Dent, E. L., and George, T. P. (2024). Cannabis use and mood disorders: a systematic review. *Frontiers in Public Health*, 12: 1346207.

Suraev, A., McCartney, D., Marshall, N. S., Irwin, C., Vandrey, R., Grunstein, R. R., D'Rozario, A. L. e al. (2024). Evaluating possible 'next day' impairment in insomnia patients administered an oral medicinal cannabis product by night: a pilot randomized controlled trial. *Psychopharmacology*, 241: 1815–1825.

Suraev, A. S., Marshall, N. S., Vandrey, R., McCartney, D., Benson, M. J., McGregor, I. S. et al. (2020). Cannabinoid therapies in the management of sleep disorders: A systematic review of preclinical and clinical studies. *Sleep Medicine Reviews*, 53: 101339.

Syed, S. A., Singh, J., Elkholy, H., Rojnić Palavra, I., Tomicevic, M., Eric, A. P. et al. (2025). International perspectives on physician knowledge, attitudes, and practices related to medical cannabis. *Frontiers in Public Health*, 13: 1463871.

Terry-McElrath, Y. M., Pang, Y. C., and Patrick, M. E. (2025). Historical change in associations between perceived risk, disapproval, and use of cannabis among young adults ages 19–30: 2011–2022. *Addictive Behaviors*, 160: 108185.

Vanini, G., and Torterolo, P. (2021). Sleep-wake neurobiology. pp. 65–82. *In*: Monti, J. M., Pandi-Perumal, S. R., and Murillo-Rodríguez, E. (Eds.). *Cannabinoids and Sleep: Molecular, Functional and Clinical Aspects*. Springer

Vaughn, L. K., Denning, G., Stuhr, K. L., de Wit, H., Hill, M. N., and Hillard, C. J. (2010). Endocannabinoid signalling: has it got rhythm? *British Journal of Pharmacology*, 160: 530–543.

Velzeboer, R., Malas, A., Boerkoel, P., Cullen, K., Hawkins, M., Roesler, J. et al. (2022). Cannabis dosing and administration for sleep: a systematic review. *Sleep*, 45:zsac218.

Vivek, K., Karagozlu, Z., Erridge, S., Holvey, C., Coomber, R., Rucker, J. J. et al. (2024). UK Medical Cannabis Registry: Assessment of clinical outcomes in patients with insomnia. *Brain and Behavior*, 14: e3410.

Volkow, N. D., Han, B., Compton, W. M., and McCance-Katz, E. F. (2019). Self-reported medical and nonmedical cannabis use among pregnant women in the United States. *JAMA*, 322: 167–169.

Volkow, N. D., Swanson, J. M., Evins, A. E., DeLisi, L. E., Meier, M. H., Gonzalez, R. et al. (2016). Effects of cannabis use on human behavior, including cognition, motivation, and psychosis: A review. *JAMA Psychiatry*, 73: 292–297.

Vučković, S., Srebro, D., Vujović, K. S., Vučetić, Č., and Prostran, M. (2018). Cannabinoids and Pain: New Insights From Old Molecules. *Frontiers in Pharmacology*, 9: 1259.

Whibley, D., Braley, T. J., Kratz, A. L., and Boehnke, K. F. (2025). Cannabinoids for treating sleep. *Current Addiction Reports*, 12: 24.

Winiger, E. A., Hitchcock, L. N., Bryan, A. D., and Bidwell, L. C. (2021). Cannabis use and sleep: Expectations, outcomes, and the role of age. *Addictive Behaviors*, 112:106642.

Chapter 8

Cannabis as Medicine

Clinical Trials and Applications

Renata da Silva Carneiro, Felipe Alves Batista, Michelle Vicente Torres, José Zilton Lima Verde Santos and *Anderson Nogueira Mendes**

1. Introduction

The use of *Cannabis* spp. in drug formulations has grown globally in recent years (Manning et al. 2024). Rich in phytocannabinoids such as delta-9-tetrahydrocannabinol (THC) and cannabidiol (CBD), medicinal cannabis has been used to treat chronic pain, anxiety disorders, and depression, and to relieve symptoms associated with inflammatory conditions. The therapeutic efficacy of products derived from medicinal cannabis is associated with the analgesic, anxiolytic, and anti-inflammatory activities present in its chemical constituents (Burstein 2015; Orrin et al. 2025a). The use of cannabis for therapeutic purposes is reported in Chinese pharmacopoeias from the 2nd century BC (Aldrich 1997), and plants of this genus stand out as some of the oldest cultivated for human use (Friedman and Sirven 2017). Over the years, however, clinical use and research involving this group of plants have encountered ethical, legal, and cultural issues. These economic and social issues have been reviewed, given the scientific evidence on the efficacy and safety of products based on the phytoconstituents of this plant (Pisanti and Bifulco 2017). The elucidation of the chemical components of cannabis and the discovery of the mechanisms of action of these active ingredients with the endocannabinoid system date back to the 1960s and 1990s, respectively, and since then, therapeutic strategies involving products based on medicinal cannabis have gained ground in the treatment of various pathologies (Clarke and Merlin 2013; Friedman and Sirven 2017).

Countries such as Germany, Australia, Canada, the Netherlands, Israel, and Italy stand out as pioneers in the legalization of medicinal cannabis, and their legislation and regulatory regimes for prescribing and dispensing cannabis-based medicines influence other actions (de Souza and Limberger 2022; Schlag 2020). Currently, several countries have greater acceptance and legalization of medicinal cannabis for the treatment of epilepsy (Mukhtar et al. 2025), other neural disorders, and chronic pain (Lopera et al. 2024).

Patients with chronic pain report facing difficulties in alleviating symptoms with the use of usual medications alone and demonstrate interest in adopting strategies that involve the use of medicinal cannabis. However, these patients face barriers such as the cost of legal cannabis-based

Laboratory of Science in Innovation and Technology - LACITEC, Department of Biophysics and Physiology, Federal University of Piauí, 64049-550, Teresina, Piauí, Brazil.
* Corresponding author: anderson.mendes@ufpi.edu.br

DOI: 10.1201/9781003668190-10

products, social and family stigmas, as well as the difficulty in receiving adequate information and indications from health professionals (Sinclair et al. 2023).

The barriers faced by the advancement of clinical use and the conduct of research with medicinal cannabis may be closely associated with the widespread stigma and complex pharmacology of these plant species (Banerjee et al. 2022). In this perspective, randomized clinical trials should be prioritized to provide information that helps establish clinical practices associated with the use of cannabis-derived products.

In this chapter, we present recent and relevant clinical trials with medicinal cannabis, highlighting the main medical conditions treated and the mechanisms of action of cannabinoids such as THC and CBD in the endocannabinoid system. The methods of administration of cannabis-derived products and their possible adverse effects are also discussed in this section, which ends with the proposal of future perspectives related to the medical use of cannabis.

2. Clinical Trials With Medicinal Cannabis

Cannabis spp., a complex mixture of phytocannabinoids such as CBD and THC, has a long and challenging history associated with recreational and medicinal use (Fordjour et al. 2023). With the recent major advances in legalization and regulatory laws regarding cannabis for medicinal purposes in several countries, clinical trials are necessary to investigate the therapeutic benefits of medicines based on these plants and their phytoconstituents (Thu et al. 2025).

Several clinical studies have been carried out to investigate the action of cannabis-based preparations in the treatment of epilepsy (Baratta et al. 2022). A study developed by Mitelpunkt et al. (2019) analyzed the effect of PTL-101, an oral formulation of purified CBD, in children with treatment-resistant epilepsy (Mitelpunkt et al. 2019). In this prospective phase II clinical trial, pediatric patients were treated for 12 weeks with oral doses of 13.6 to 25 mg/kg of the phytocannabinoid-based medication, and at the end of the study, there was a reduction in the seizure frequency and severity in the treated patients. The results of this open-label clinical trial suggest that cannabis-based medications have potential action in the treatment of neurological diseases such as epilepsy.

The effects of drugs containing purified CBD can be influenced by their bioavailability. In PTL-101, the formulation of the phytocannabinoid incorporated into a gelatinous matrix maintains a constant gastrointestinal transit time (Mitelpunkt et al. 2019). In another open-label study using capsules containing 99% CBD, it was found that higher-fat diets significantly increased the maximum concentration of the active ingredient of this medication, improving its absorption in patients undergoing treatment for epilepsy (Birnbaum et al. 2019).

The treatment of chronic pain in adults using medicinal cannabis is also the subject of investigation based on clinical trials. A randomized study conducted by Almog et al. (2020) analyzed the analgesic action of inhaled doses of 0.5 and 1.0 mg of delta-9-tetrahydrocannabinol in patients with chronic pain (Almog et al. 2020). The results of this controlled study showed a reduction in pain intensity in patients undergoing treatment with THC in the time interval investigated, with the 1.0 mg dose presenting a significant difference when compared to the placebo group. The experimental evidence from this study suggests that the pharmacokinetics of THC vary depending on its route of administration and dose, requiring additional studies to allow the development of standardized pharmaceutical formulations, aiming at a safe and effective analgesic effect.

The analgesic effect of medicinal cannabis was evaluated in a single-center, crossover observational study with patients with low back pain associated with fibromyalgia (Yassin et al. 2019). In this study, adults undergoing conventional analgesia treatment were exposed to 20 mg of cannabis via smoke inhalation for 3–6 months. Observational results indicate a significant improvement in lumbar range of motion and in all patient reports during the treatment periods. Further randomized studies will be needed, however, to indicate the generalizability of these observations to other patients with fibromyalgia and chronic pain (Yassin et al. 2019).

The efficacy of cannabis-based products in the treatment of symptoms of Alzheimer's disease (AD) has also been investigated by randomized trials. In a randomized double-blind crossover trial, researchers analyzed the action of 1–2 mg per day doses of nabilone, a synthetic molecule analogous to THC, in the treatment of agitation in patients with moderate to severe AD (Herrmann et al. 2019). The results of this study indicate that the cannabinoid nabilone acts with potential benefits on neuropsychiatric symptoms, helping to control agitation in AD patients. The randomized study, however, indicates that nabilone may have side effects such as sedation and cognitive decline in the conditions analyzed.

An oral THC: CBD extract was evaluated in the prevention of nausea and vomiting induced by refractory chemotherapy in a randomized, multicenter, double-blind, placebo-controlled study (Grimison et al. 2020). Patients undergoing intravenous chemotherapy received oral doses of THC 2.5 mg/CBD 2.5 mg for 5 days, followed by placebo doses, and presented, at the end of the study, with less nausea and vomiting when they associated the cannabis-based medication with other traditional emetic medications. In this study, moderate adverse events, including sedation, dizziness, and disorientation, were reported. Similar results were found by Sukpiriyagul et al. (2023).

Clinical trials are also important to indicate results where medicinal cannabis-based formulations are not effective for some therapeutic conditions. A randomized clinical study conducted by Bonn-Miller et al. (2021) showed that there was no significant difference in the improvement of post-traumatic stress disorder symptoms in military veterans treated with different active concentrations of smoked cannabis (THC and CBD) and placebo (Bonn-Miller et al. 2021). Another clinical study using a single oral dose of THC/CBD in patients with indolent B-cell leukemic lymphoma showed that, under the conditions investigated, cannabinoids do not contribute to the treatment of indolent lymphomas because their use did not affect the apoptosis and proliferation of malignant cells (Melén et al. 2022).

Figure 1 illustrates the typical steps in a clinical trial with medicinal cannabis-derived products, from the design phase through publication of results, in the various countries where cannabis is legalized for therapeutic purposes.

Clinical studies involving cannabis-based products begin with approval from the ethics committee, ensuring that the research protocol complies with fundamental ethical principles. This step is accompanied by the adoption of the Declaration of Helsinki, a central document for the protection of human participants in clinical studies. The study must then be duly registered in an online clinical trials database, promoting transparency and traceability of the research.

After these preparatory steps, participants provide voluntary consent, followed by screening and patient recruitment. Once selected, individuals receive the cannabis-based product in accordance with all safety and quality standards for the input. In the subsequent step, participants are randomized

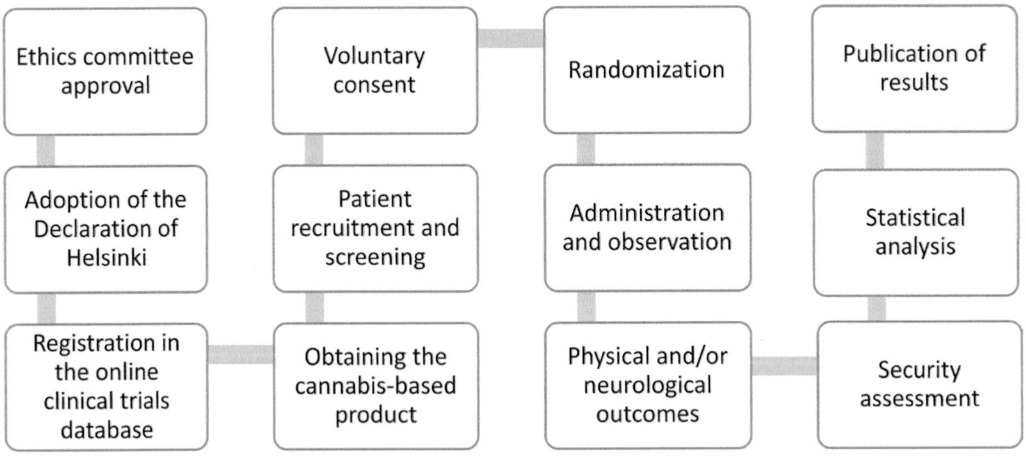

Figure 1: Stages of the cannabis clinical research process

to ensure an equitable distribution of individuals between the intervention and control groups, reducing bias. Next, the product is administered, and clinical observation is conducted, with strict monitoring of the patient's physiological and behavioral responses. Physical and/or neurological outcomes are then evaluated, representing the main parameters of treatment efficacy.

Once data collection is complete, statistical analysis is performed to allow for objective interpretation of the results. In parallel, a safety assessment is performed to ensure that adverse effects are documented and understood. Finally, the findings are organized for publication, contributing scientific evidence for the therapeutic use of cannabis and enabling future meta-analyses and systematic reviews. This flowchart exemplifies a rigorous, ethical, and structured approach to conducting clinical research with cannabis, ensuring the safety of participants and the validity of the data obtained.

3. Therapeutic Actions of Medicinal Cannabis

Medicinal cannabis has been widely studied as a therapeutic option for several medical conditions, including cases of chronic pain, epilepsy, multiple sclerosis, anxiety disorders and depression, chemotherapy-induced nausea and vomiting, and inflammatory conditions such as arthritis (Borowicz-Reutt et al. 2024; Cummings et al. 2024; Kelly et al. 2024; Melén et al. 2022; Murphy et al. 2024). In chronic pain, medicinal cannabis has proven to be a relevant therapeutic option for its management, especially in patients who do not respond adequately to conventional treatments (Cummings et al. 2024; Häuser et al. 2018; Nutt et al. 2021). Studies by Häuser et al. (2018) and Nutt et al. (2022) indicate that cannabinoids can reduce pain intensity by approximately 30% to 50% compared with placebo (Häuser et al. 2018; Nutt et al. 2021). This effect occurs through the interaction of active compounds, such as tetrahydrocannabinol (THC) and cannabidiol (CBD), with the endocannabinoid receptors CB1 and CB2, controlling the perception of pain and reducing inflammation. According to Abrams et al. (2011), patients reported improvements in quality of life, with an average increase of 20% in functionality scores. Adverse events such as dizziness and drowsiness were observed in 8% to 12% of participants in these studies.

In the treatment of epilepsy, cannabidiol (CBD) has demonstrated significant efficacy, reducing seizure frequency by up to 50% in patients with Dravet syndrome (Devinsky et al. 2017) and by 42–44% in those with Lennox-Gastaut syndrome (Thiele et al. 2018; Devinsky et al. 2014). Studies such as those by Perucca (2017) and Rosenberg et al. (2015 and 2017) also indicate that approximately 40% to 50% of patients responded to treatment with a significant reduction in seizures, while 5% achieved complete absence of seizures (Perucca 2017; Rosenberg et al. 2017; Rosenberg et al. 2015). Adverse effects, such as fatigue and diarrhea, occurred in approximately 10% to 15% of cases, but were considered manageable.

In cases of chemotherapy-induced nausea and vomiting (CINV), especially in cases refractory to conventional antiemetics, studies indicate that THC reduces the frequency of vomiting episodes in up to 70% of cases (Duran et al. 2010) and improves symptom control in 47% to 80% of patients compared to placebo (Tramèr et al. 2001). Parker et al. 2011 demonstrated that these effects are attributed to the interaction of THC with CB1 receptors located in the central nervous system (Parker et al. 2011). Reported adverse effects, such as dizziness and drowsiness, occurred in approximately 5% to 10% of participants.

In the treatment of anxiety disorders and depression, medicinal cannabis has a promising therapeutic profile, as CBD has been shown to significantly reduce anxiety scores by up to 50% in clinical assessments (Scott et al. 2019) and increase sleep quality in 66% of patients (Blessing et al. 2015). Moreno-Sanz et al. (2022) reported that there are differences in prescription and clinical effects between men and women, suggesting that sexual factors may influence therapeutic outcomes (Moreno-Sanz et al. 2022). The mechanism of action involves interaction with serotonin (5-HT1A) receptors, promoting anxiolytic and antidepressant effects. Adverse effects were reported by fewer than 10% of participants and were of low severity.

Medical cannabis has also been shown to be effective in treating inflammatory conditions such as rheumatoid arthritis and osteoarthritis. In a randomized study, the use of a cannabis spray based on THC and CBD resulted in a 20% reduction in pain intensity and a 22% reduction in morning stiffness, with a 30% improvement in sleep quality (Blake et al. 2006). THC and CBD modulate the release of pro-inflammatory cytokines, thereby promoting anti-inflammatory effects (Malfait et al. 2000). Serious adverse events were rare, with overall tolerability being good in 90% of cases. Data from the UK Medical Cannabis Registry indicate significant improvement in symptoms in patients in palliative care with the use of medicinal cannabis (Nimalan et al. 2022).

Table 1 summarizes the clinical evidence, mechanisms of action, and impacts on quality of life associated with the use of medicinal cannabis. Figure 2 then presents statistics on medical conditions treated with cannabis-based medicines.

The use of medicinal cannabis in the treatment of various clinical conditions has gained increasing attention in the scientific and medical community. This trend is driven by evidence demonstrating significant benefits in patients with diseases refractory to conventional treatments.

Table 1: Overview of the use of medicinal cannabis in various medical conditions.

Medical Condition	Clinical Evidence	Mechanism of Action	Impacts on Quality of Life	Quantitative Data	References
Chronic Pain	Significant pain reduction in patients refractory to conventional treatments.	Modulation of CB1 and CB2 receptors reduces the perception of pain and inflammation.	Increased functionality, better pain control, and general well-being.	64% reported a significant reduction in pain intensity.	Abrams et al. (2005); Häuser et al. (2018); Nutt et al. (2022)
Epilepsy	Reduction of up to 50% in the frequency of seizures in refractory syndromes such as Lennox-Gastaut and Dravet.	Modulation of ion channels and GABA receptors, to reduce neuronal hyperexcitability.	Improved seizure frequency, greater patient safety, and relief for caregivers.	40–50% of patients had a significant reduction.	Devinsky et al. (2017); Thiele et al. (2018); Rosenberg et al. (2015, 2017)
Nausea and Vomiting Induced by Chemotherapy	Effective control in cases refractory to conventional antiemetics, with mild adverse events.	Action on CB1 receptors in the CNS regulates the vomiting reflex.	Reduced symptoms of nausea and vomiting, allowing greater adherence and tolerance to chemotherapy treatment.	Reduced nausea in 71% of patients receiving medical cannabis compared to 22% of the control group.	Duran et al. (2010); Tramèr et al. (2001); Parker et al. (2011).
Anxiety and Depression Disorders	Reduction of symptoms such as insomnia and emotional tension, with a good safety profile.	Modulation of serotonin receptors (5-HT1A), promoting anxiolytic and antidepressant effects.	Improved sleep, reduced anxiety, and greater emotional well-being.	79% showed a decrease in anxiety levels within 3 months	Shannon et al. (2019); Blessing et al. (2015). Moreno-Sanz et al. (2022)
Inflammatory Conditions (Arthritis)	Reduction of pain and inflammation in patients with rheumatoid arthritis and osteoarthritis, with good tolerance.	Modulation of the release of pro-inflammatory cytokines and reduction of nociceptive sensitivity.	Improved mobility, relief of stiffness, and increased functional quality of life.	A 50% reduction in reported pain in 58% of arthritis patients after 5 weeks of medical cannabis use.	Blake et al. (2006); Malfait et al. (2000); Nimalan et al. (2022).

The action of phytocannabinoids, such as tetrahydrocannabinol (THC) and cannabidiol (CBD), on the receptors of the endocannabinoid system enables a wide range of therapeutic effects, including analgesic, anticonvulsant, antiemetic, anxiolytic, and anti-inflammatory properties.

One of the most consolidated fields of application of medicinal cannabis is the treatment of chronic pain. Clinical studies indicate that approximately 64% of patients refractory to traditional analgesics reported significant pain relief after using cannabis derivatives. This effect occurs through modulation of CB1 and CB2 receptors, which interfere with pain perception and inflammatory processes (Abrams et al. 2011; Häuser et al. 2018; Nutt et al. 2021). As a result, there is an improvement in patient functionality, with an increased capacity for daily activities and a greater sense of general well-being.

In the field of neurology, the effectiveness of cannabidiol in controlling epileptic seizures in refractory syndromes, such as Lennox-Gastaut and Dravet, stands out. In these cases, cannabis acts to modulate ion channels and GABAergic receptors, reducing neuronal excitability and, consequently, the frequency and intensity of seizures. Studies show that between 40% and 50% of patients have a significant reduction in seizure activity (Orrin et al. 2025b; Rosenberg et al. 2017, 2015; Thiele et al. 2018). In addition to clinical control, there are positive effects on the quality of life of patients and their caregivers, resulting in greater safety and autonomy.

Another widely documented use refers to the management of chemotherapy-induced nausea and vomiting. Patients who do not respond to conventional antiemetics have benefited from the action of THC on CB1 receptors in the central nervous system, which modulate the gag reflex. In comparative studies, 71% of patients who used medicinal cannabis reported significant improvement in symptoms, compared to only 22% in the control group (Duran et al. 2010; Parker et al. 2011; Tramèr et al. 2001). This positive response has contributed to adherence to cancer treatment, providing greater comfort and tolerability to patients during chemotherapy.

In the field of mental health, cannabidiol has also shown potential in the treatment of anxiety disorders and depression. Through the modulation of serotonin receptors (5-HT1A), CBD promotes anxiolytic and antidepressant effects, reducing symptoms such as insomnia, irritability, and emotional tension. In observational studies, 79% of patients reported improvements in anxiety levels after 3 months of treatment (Blessing et al. 2015; Melas et al. 2021; Moreno-Sanz et al. 2022). This result highlights the potential of medicinal cannabis as a safe alternative for the management of emotional disorders, especially in patients who present adverse effects to conventional psychotropic drugs.

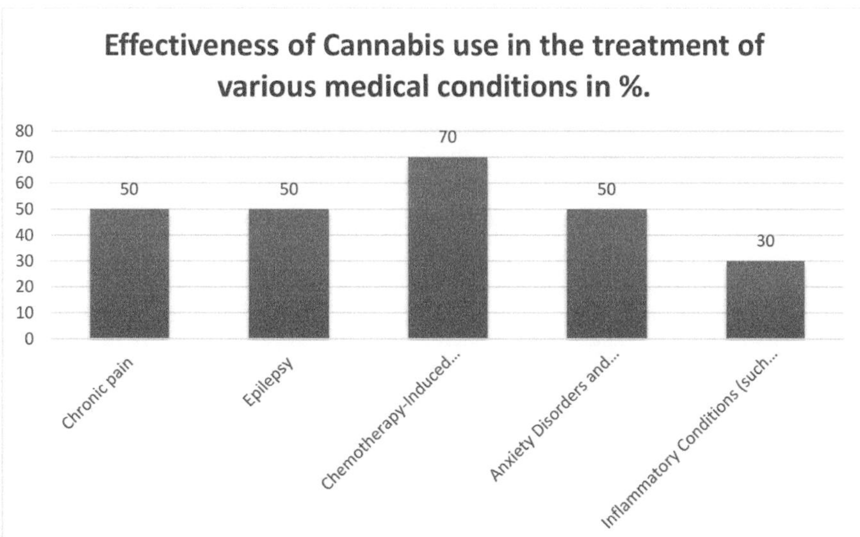

Figure 2: Efficacy of Cannabis in Medical Conditions: Results of Clinical Trials.

Finally, in inflammatory conditions such as rheumatoid arthritis and osteoarthritis, cannabis has shown good results in reducing pain and joint inflammation. Cannabinoids regulate the immune response by inhibiting the release of pro-inflammatory cytokines and decreasing nociceptive sensitivity. This leads to improved mobility and relief from stiffness, with 58% of patients reporting a reduction of up to 50% in pain after five weeks of use (Blake et al. 2006; Malfait et al. 2000; Nimalan et al. 2022). These effects directly improve the functional quality of life of patients with rheumatological diseases.

Given this evidence, it is possible to conclude that medicinal cannabis represents a viable and safe therapeutic alternative for the treatment of several clinical conditions. Its positive effects on symptom reduction and good tolerability indicate a significant potential for clinical application. However, controlled, long-term clinical studies are still needed to standardize doses, formulations, and therapeutic protocols. Ethical and scientific regulation of cannabis use is essential to ensure responsible and evidence-based access, consolidating its role as a complementary tool in health care.

Figure 2 illustrates the effectiveness of medicinal cannabis use in the treatment of different clinical conditions, expressed as a percentage. It can be seen that the highest effectiveness rate was recorded in patients with chemotherapy-induced nausea and vomiting, with a 70% positive response to treatment, reinforcing its use as an alternative in cases refractory to conventional antiemetics. Next, conditions such as chronic pain, epilepsy, and anxiety and depression disorders showed similar effectiveness, around 50%, which demonstrates the therapeutic potential of cannabis in modulating pain, neuronal activity, and mood-related neurotransmitters. Finally, inflammatory conditions, such as arthritis, showed the lowest effectiveness rate (30%), although they still represent a clinically relevant response, considering the chronic and resistant nature of these pathologies. These data suggest that, although the therapeutic effects of cannabis vary according to the condition treated, its use may be promising as a complementary therapy, as long as it is supported by scientific evidence and safe clinical protocols.

4. Mechanisms of Action of the Constituents of Medicinal Cannabis

Before beginning our discussion of the mechanisms of interaction between the main cannabinoid substances and their molecular receptors, CB1 and CB2, we must understand which class these proteins belong to and their relationship to the main signaling pathways in our body.

Currently, an important class of proteins has been the target of several studies on the actions of molecules as potential drugs, as they play an important role in mediating signals in the human body. Approximately 88% of the drugs approved by the FDA, the North American regulatory agency, target G-protein coupled receptors (GPCRs) (Downey and Peralta-Yahya 2024). These receptors are cell membrane proteins with dynamic functions that can trigger signal transduction pathways involved in various biological processes. The question then arises: What stimuli can trigger these events in the cell? The main ones are interactions with photons, ions, lipid molecules, neurotransmitters, hormones, peptides, odorants, etc. (Zhang et al. 2024).

A good approach to understanding the various interactions with GPCRs is to examine their chemical structures and the main effects they produce. GPCR proteins, in simple terms, have an extracellular amino group, an intracellular carboxyl group, and seven α-helical domains that are subdivided into intra- and extracellular loops (3 each), in addition to a domain linked to the intracellular G protein, which is formed by three subunits α, β, and γ. Figure 3 below illustrates the basic structure of the GPCR (Dahlgren et al. 2023).

The CB1 and CB2 receptors are representatives of the GPCR class, both of which are responsible for mediating endocannabinoid signaling processes in humans. CB1 is the most widely expressed G-protein-coupled receptor in the brain and is predominantly found in the central nervous system (CNS). However, it can also be located in peripheral regions, such as the liver, reproductive tissues, gastrointestinal tract, cardiovascular system, and skeletal muscle. As for CB2, it was originally described as a peripheral receptor, since it was not found in the CNS. This receptor is distributed

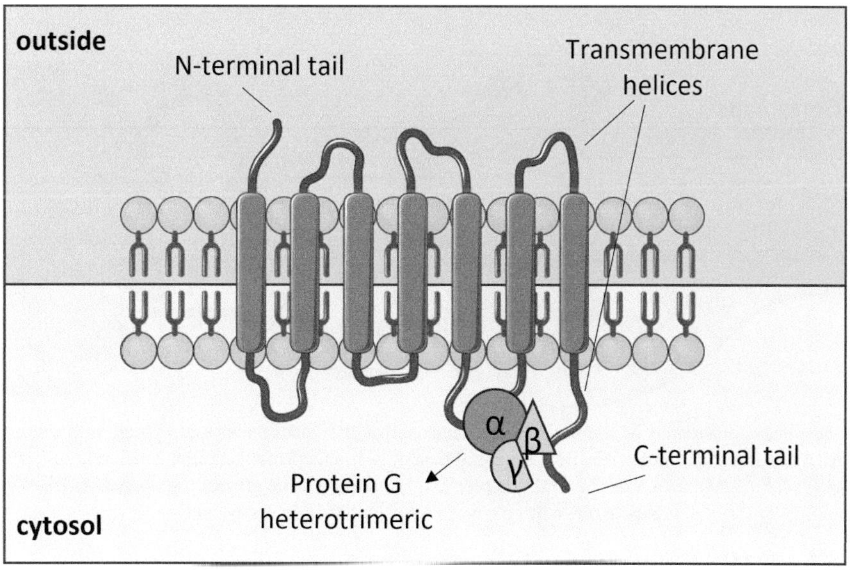

Figure 3: Schematic description of GPCR showing the interaction of a ligand with the binding site available on the cell surface and the G-coupled signal domain facing the cytosol.

throughout cells of our immune system and is an important target for processes involving pain and inflammation (Brust et al. 2023).

How important are these receptors for the health of our body? The endocannabinoid system is responsible for most of our body's functioning, regulating and controlling of many critical functions, such as learning, memory, emotions, sleep, temperature, pain, inflammatory and immunological responses, and feeding (Kayser et al. 2020).

In the brain, CB1 receptors are more numerous than any other type of receptor, and they act by controlling the levels and activity of many neurotransmitters. In this way, there is the so-called "immediate regulation of things," a kind of "biological thermostat" that signals the increase or decrease of any system that needs adjustment (Wu 2019).

Sleep is a good example of this; studies show that ingesting low doses of cannabidiol (CBD), 1–1.5 h before bed, leads to significantly better sleep quality. It is believed that the sedative effect of CBD is due to a process of central downregulation of the corticotropin-releasing hormone gene, resulting in a decrease in systemic cortisol, which in turn is mediated by CB1 receptor expression (Kisiolek et al. 2023). The two main components of Cannabis sativa, Δ-9-tetrahydrocannabinol (THC) and CBD, are molecules that interact effectively with the endocannabinoid system, thereby promoting the production of important biomolecules in our body (Pagano et al. 2023).

THC is a partial agonist at both CB1 and CB2; that is, it is an activating ligand with attenuated effects when compared to the original endogenous ligand. CBD, on the other hand, acts as an antagonist of these two receptors; that is, it inhibits their active sites (Boggs et al. 2016).

Endogenous ligands are molecules naturally produced by the body that have affinity for specific receptors. The ligands that are part of the endocannabinoid system are the molecules arachidonoyl ethanolamine (AEA or anandamine), 2-arachidonoyl glycerol (2-AG), palmitoyl ethanolamine (PEA), and oleoyl ethanolamine (OEA). With AEA and 2-AG playing more prominent roles in presynaptic and postsynaptic effects, Figure 4 presents a schematic representation of the simplified endocannabinoid system mechanism (Khoury et al. 2022).

The metabolism of endocannabinoids, AEA and 2-AG, is carried out by the enzymes fatty acid amide hydrolase (FAAH) and monoacylglycerol lipase (MAGL), respectively. The production of these two biomolecules occurs on demand, that is, they require an "external stimulus" that can be

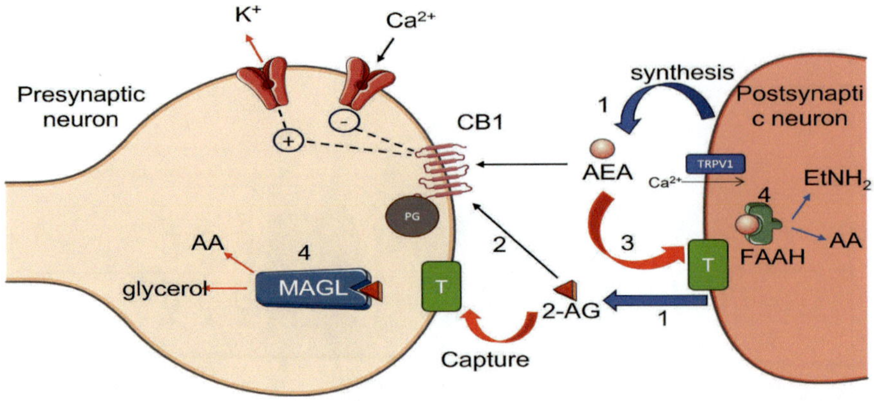

Figure 4: Schematic illustration of the simplified mechanism of the endocannabinoid system with emphasis on CB1 receptors. AEA and 2-AG are synthesized from the membrane of postsynaptic neurons after calcium influx. (1) Propagation to the synaptic cleft (2) and action on the CB1 receptor (3). Limitation of the process via uptake (4) AEA and 2-AG are broken down by enzymes FAAH and MAGL, respectively.

induced by changes in the concentration of ions (Ca2+ and K+) or other specific molecules, such as THC, CBD, and other similar structures (Fabrício et al. 2010).

AEA and 2-AG are rapidly hydrolyzed; FAAH and MAGL also act in the degradation mechanisms of other molecules of biological importance. For example, MAGL functions as an enzyme that limits the rate of arachidonic acid production, which is the precursor of AEA and 2-AG, and is also the main component of the cell wall. Thus, MAGL inhibitors can exert antinociceptive and anti-inflammatory effects by increasing the levels of 2-AG, stimulating cannabinoid receptors, and decreasing the levels of arachidonic acid and its pro-inflammatory metabolites (Donvito et al. 2018).

These endocannabinoid ligands participate in natural and drug reward mechanisms by interacting with the dopaminergic system, which regulates dopamine release. For example, the use of the substance THC triggers transient peaks of dopamine, a rapid and explosive effect; the rate of this effect is controlled by the A10 neuron (dopamine) and by dependent interaction with the CB1 receptor. The interaction of the drug with the endocannabinoid receptor induces a "firing of dopaminergic neurons and an increase in intracellular calcium levels, which activates some structures present in the cell, mainly diacylglycerol lipase (DAGL), which is responsible for the synthesis of 2-AG. Then, 2-AG begins to act retrogradely, inhibiting presynaptic GABA neurons, causing disinhibition and suppression of dopaminergic neurons; that is, this change in stimuli (activation and inhibition) is what causes the search for reward and search stimuli (Spanagel 2020).

Therefore, since the interaction with endocannabinoid receptors and the levels of endocannabinoid ligands, AEA and 2-AG, play important roles in many functions and stimuli in our body, the current approach to developing new drugs has been the search for substances with affinity and agonist or antagonist activity at CB1 and CB2 receptors. Another approach to enhance the effects of drugs would be to inhibit the catabolism of endocannabinoids; for this purpose, developing molecules that inhibit the action of the FAAH and MAGL enzymes.

5. Clinical Applications of Medicinal Cannabis

Several cannabinoid-based medicines have been approved by the United States Food and Drug Administration (FDA), the European Medicines Agency (EMA), the Australian Therapeutic Goods Administration (TGA), and other regulatory agencies worldwide. The forms of application/administration of these drugs involve different routes, such as oral (capsules, tablets), sublingual, oromucosal (spray), dermal, transdermal, subcutaneous, intramuscular, rectal, intravenous, and inhalation (smoking and vaporization) (Hossain et al. 2023; Pagano et al. 2023; Vinette et al. 2022).

The choice therapeutic administration form will depend on several factors, such as clinical indications and scientific evidence for each form. Pharmacokinetic factors, such as the bioavailability of cannabinoids, vary depending on the route of administration, which can impact the onset of drug action, the duration of its effect, and its efficacy (Fraguas-Sánchez and Torres-Suárez 2018; Sirichai 2021).

5.1 Therapeutic Actions of Medicinal Cannabis

The inhalation route of administration, via vaporization and smoking, has a faster onset and better bioavailability than the oral route, although these effects are less long-lasting (Huestis 2007). When administered by smoking, the effects last approximately 2 to 3 hours, while when administered orally, they last for 4 to 12 hours (MacCallum and Russo 2018). Its indications include analgesia for sensory neuropathy in patients with human immunodeficiency virus, and neuropathic pain in patients with spinal cord injury, peripheral neuropathy, complex regional pain syndrome, and nerve injury, among others (Fraguas-Sánchez and Torres-Suárez 2018).

Cannabinoids administered by inhalation have similar pharmacokinetics to those administered intravenously. For this route of administration, peak plasma concentrations of THC and CBD are reached rapidly (within 3–10 min), and peak concentrations are higher than those achieved with oral ingestion (Newmeyer et al. 2016).

The bioavailability of THC after inhalation ranges from 10% to 35%, depending on the characteristics of this form of administration, such as the number, duration, and interval of puffs, breath-hold time, inhalation volume, and inhaler device, size of inhaled particles, and site of deposition in the respiratory system. Inhaled CBD has an average systemic bioavailability of 31% and a plasma concentration-time profile similar to that of THC (Grotenhermen 2003; Sholler et. al. 2021).

When inhaled, the onset of action is rapid (3–5 min), maximum effects are achieved in 30–60 min, and euphoria is intense and can last 2–4 h. Regarding inhaled CBD, its plasma concentration-time profile is similar to that of THC (Sirichai 2021). After inhalation, THC and its metabolites enter the bloodstream rapidly through the lungs, with peak levels reached within 6–10 minutes (Grotenhermen 2003).

It is important to note that the inhalation route, whether for recreational or medicinal use, impacts the risk of lung injury. Studies show that inhaled use can lead to bronchitis and is associated with changes in lung function (Gracie and Hancox 2021; Mishra et al. 2018).

The inhaled forms of cannabis are smoking and vaporization. The first, which involves combustion, and produces toxic metabolites, tar, polycyclic aromatic hydrocarbons, carbon monoxide, and ammonia, is not acceptable for therapeutic purposes. The second, however, does not offer the toxic characteristics (MacCallum and Russo 2018). The plant's inflorescence is the commercial form used for vaporization (Eyal et al. 2022). Among the options available on the market, TILRAY Flor Seca THC 18 stands out, an extract containing both THC and CBD (McCoy et al. 2018).

5.2 Administration by the Oromucosal Route

The oromucosal route of administration is rapidly absorbed and avoids the high plasma levels of THC that are observed in herbal inhalation, thus avoiding psychoactive effects. In addition, it has a bioavailability of 10 to 25%, and it is most evaluated in multiple sclerosis. However, despite this advantage of this route, offered in the form of an oral spray, it is necessary to point out that part of the dose can be swallowed and absorbed orally, which can reduce its bioavailability through the inhalation route, since part of the drug concentration is significantly reduced by the liver before reaching the systemic circulation (Überall 2020).

For this route of administration, naxibimol is available, a generic name for the preparation of a whole extract of the *Cannabis sativa* plant, including mainly Δ9-THC and CBD in a 1:1 ratio. Each 100-microliter spray contains 2.7 mg of THC and 2.5 mg of CBD. The brand names for the drug are Sativex® (United Kingdom, Canada, New Zealand, Germany, Netherlands, and Australia) and Mevatyl® (Brazil) and its effects apply mainly to spasticity in multiple sclerosis, neuropathic pain and pain in patients with advanced cancer (Fraguas-Sánchez and Torres-Suárez 2018; Mücke et al. 2018).

The onset time of naxibimol's effect, which varies from person to person, can be 30 to 60 minutes. This rapid onset of action makes this presentation a favorable choice in cases where relatively rapid relief of symptoms such as spasticity and neuropathic pain is needed, especially in patients with multiple sclerosis. The duration of the effect is 4 to 6 hours, which depends on individual factors such as the dose administered and the patient's response to treatment (Lessa et al. 2016).

5.3 Oral Administration

The oral route is one of the most widely used for the therapeutic use of cannabinoids. It involves using capsules, oils, tinctures, solutions, tablets, and edibles. Regarding the pharmacokinetic aspects of *Cannabis sativa* and its use by this route, studies show that Δ9-THC exhibits slow, unpredictable oral absorption with peak plasma levels occurring 1–5 h after the dose. After absorption, it is metabolized by liver enzymes in its inactive form, with a bioavailability of 6%. CBD also has a similar absorption and oral bioavailability profile. More generally, more than 95% of ingested cannabinoids are degraded by first-pass hepatic metabolism.

In addition, its instability under the influence of gastric pH and temperature is a likely explanation for its low oral bioavailability (Fraguas-Sánchez and Torres-Suárez 2018; Tijani et al. 2021). Intestinal lymphatic transport is an important factor to consider when ingesting highly lipophilic compounds, such as cannabinoids. Fatty acids generated by the lipolysis of medium and long-chain triglycerides undergo several different processes. It is known that long-chain fatty acids are associated with chylomicrons that are secreted into the lymphatic system and not via the portal vein. Thus, THC and CBD, when combinaed with long-chain triglycerides, can bypass the liver, reducing potential pre-systemic metabolism, and can reach 22% bioavailability (Zgair et al. 2016).

In general, due to the high lipophilicity of cannabinoids, encapsulation in customized nanosystems can potentially achieve several objectives, such as gradual release, taste masking, superior oral bioavailability, and greater physical stability than conventional formulations (O'Sullivan et al. 2024). The oral route of administration, despite the loss of availability cited in the literature, overcomes many of the disadvantages of inhalation. Tablets contain purified extracts or synthesized molecules of known dosage, and serum concentrations remain relatively stable (Legare et al. 2022).

The metabolism of THC involves the production of hydroxytetrahydrocannabinol (11-OH-THC), a psychoactive metabolite that readily crosses the blood-brain barrier and is more potent than Δ9-THC, appearing in the blood in higher amounts when Δ9-THC is ingested than when it is inhaled. This factor may be responsible for the stronger and longer-lasting drug effect of oral use compared with comparable doses of inhaled cannabis (Barrus et al. 2016).

5.3.1 Synthetic and Semi-Synthetic Capsules

The oral supply of cannabinoid drugs in capsule form is represented by dronabinol, nabilone and herbal extracts. Dronabinol, ((-)-trans-Δ9-THC), is a synthetic, water-insoluble compound formulated in sesame oil. It is commercially known as Marinol® (in the United Kingdom, Ireland, the USA, and Canada) or Dronabinol®, and its gelatin capsules (2.5, 5, and 10mg) are almost completely absorbed

(90% to 95%) after single oral doses (ElSohly et al. 2001; Gaisey and Narouze 2021; O'Donnell et al. 2025). Despite this, due to the combined effects of first-pass hepatic metabolism and its high lipid solubility, only 10% to 20% of the dose reaches the systemic circulation. It is indicated especially for cases of anorexia in patients with HIV, nausea and vomiting induced by chemotherapy, as well as analgesia (Parikhet al. 2016; Stella et al. 2021).

After oral administration, dronabinol has an onset of action of approximately 0.5 to 1 hour and a peak effect in 2 to 4 hours. The duration of action for psychoactive effects is 4 to 6 hours, but the appetite-stimulating effect of dronabinol may continue for 24 hours or more after administration (Gaisey and Narouze 2021).

The cannabinoid nabilone, also a synthetic (Δ9-THC analogue), is indicated as an antiemetic and analgesic in neuropathic pain. It is traded under the names Cesamet® (the UK, Ireland, the USA, and Canada) and Canemes® (Germany and Austria) (Abuhasira et al. 2018; Harrison and Simpson 2021). Each capsule contains 1 mg (2.7 μmol) of nabilone. The amount of 1 mg of nabilone has approximately the same effect as 7 to 8 mg of Dronabinol (Bedi et al. 2013; Calhoun et al. 1998; Haney et al. 2013). Thus, despite being structurally distinct from THC, nabilone mimics its structure and pharmacological activity through weak partial agonist activity at CB1R and CB2R receptors, but is considered twice as active as Δ^9-THC.

When administered as gelatin capsules, nabilone is completely absorbed from the human gastrointestinal tract when taken orally, and is indicated for the treatment of nausea and vomiting associated with chemotherapy in patients who have not responded adequately to conventional antiemetic treatments (Schussel et al. 2018). The onset time of action of this compound is variable, and can occur from 1 to 2 hours after administration, and the effects can last from 6 to 8 hours, longer than when using cannabis via inhalation. The onset of action of nabilone is slower than that of dronabinol, with peak action reached more slowly and with greater dependence on dose effects. The synthetic also has a bioavailability of 60% (Ben Amar 2006).

5.3.2 Extract Capsules

An example of a drug presented in capsules with herbal extract of Cannabis sativa is Cannador® (Society for Clinical Research, Germany, and Weleda, Trademark AG, Switzerland), which comes from a crude (whole) extract of Δ9-THC and CBD, usually in a 2:1 ratio, extracted from the plant, administered orally through capsules (Lessa et al. 2016). It is indicated for patients with changes in spasticity in multiple sclerosis, having shown a slight reduction in postoperative pain. However, adverse effects such as sedation and psychoactive changes were evident (Newmeyer et al. 2016; Penha et al. 2019). Other lesser-known medications are Bedrocan®, developed in the Netherlands, which has more than 20% THC in its original formula, in addition to its variations with different percentages of this substance, such as Bedica® and Bediol®, with 14% and 6.5% THC, respectively (Penha et al. 2019).

5.3.3 Oral Solutions

Dronabinol can also be available on the market as an oral solution, with Syndros® (Dronabinol oral solution 5 mg) being the best known. In this presentation, dronabinol is almost completely absorbed (90% to 95%) after a single oral dose. However, due to the combined effects of first-pass hepatic metabolism and high lipid solubility, only 10% to 20% of the administered dose reaches the systemic circulation (Lyu et al. 2023; Pickle 2018). The other characteristics of onset and duration of effects are similar to those of the capsule presentation. The first pharmaceutical-grade, purified, plant-derived cannabidiol (CBD) drug is marketed under the name Epidyolex®, administered in the form of a 100 mg/mL oral solution, and has been authorized for therapeutic use in countries of the European Union and the USA (Buxeraud and Faure 2023; Müller et al. 2024). It is especially indicated as an adjuvant therapy in the treatment of seizures associated with Lennox-Gastaut syndrome or Dravet syndrome in patients aged 2 years or older (Abu-Sawwa and Stehling 2019).

The low oral bioavailability of CBD (13 to 19%) remains a major limiting factor in its therapeutic efficacy (Millar et al. 2018). Although the oral route is the most common for CBD administration, its hydrophobic substance limits its absorption, and the fraction absorbed is subject to first-pass metabolism by the liver, which explains its low bioavailability. In addition, the delayed onset of action, ranging from 30 to 120 min (Baban et al. 2021). Therefore, studies suggest that oral consumption of CBD with high-fat foods, or even in a lipid solution, can increase its bioavailability (Itin et al. 2020). In patients, a high-fat meal has also been shown to increase the bioavailability of cannabidiol (three-fold).

A variety of techniques have been used to improve the drug's dissolution profile, reduce its degradation, and promote and control its site-specific release, thereby enhancing CBD bioavailability. One such approach involves incorporating or complexing CBD with advanced carriers to formulate amorphous solid dispersions, polymer-based CBD inclusion complexes, lipid-based formulations, and/or nanoformulations, which are administered via different routes and demonstrating improved bioavailability (K. R. Hossain et al. 2023; Stella et al. 2021).

There are other offerings of oral solutions obtained by the extraction of substances from the *Cannabis sativa* plant (extract), available in different proportions of CBD and Δ9-THC. One example is Tilray THC 5: CBD 20® Oral Solution, which contains 5 mg/ml of Δ9-THC and 20 mg/ml of cannabidiol (CBD), using medium-chain triglyceride oil as an excipient. It is approved in Canada, South America, Australia, New Zealand, and Europe (Arkell et al. 2019; Kirilov et al. 2020; McCoy et al. 2018b; Mersiades et al. 2023).

The indications for these oral solutions, similar to the other options on offer, are for adjuvant therapy of spasticity associated with multiple sclerosis or spinal cord injuries, nausea and vomiting resulting from chemotherapy, radiotherapy, and combination therapy for HIV and hepatitis C medication. It is also prescribed for appetite stimulation in palliative care for patients undergoing cancer treatments or with HIV, chronic pain (associated with cancer or the nervous system), Gilles de la Tourette syndrome, and therapy-resistant glaucoma (Vinette et al. 2022). Like the drug mentioned, there are other oral solutions obtained with varying proportions of THC and CBD, legalized for commercial use and with similar indications. The effects may begin within approximately 40–60 minutes after administration and may last for several hours, depending on variables such as the dose, the amount ingested, whether food was ingested, the type of food ingested at the time of administration, and the individual response of each person. Adverse effects include changes already mentioned for other drugs based on oral cannabis.

5.3.4 Edible Products Based on Cannabis Sativa

Cannabis-derived edibles are food products infused with cannabis extract. They come in many forms, including baked goods, candies, gummies, chocolates, lozenges, and beverages, and can be homemade or commercially prepared for dispensaries (Barrus et al. 2016). Despite their popularity, edibles have significant restrictions for medicinal use. A major challenge is the low level of oversight of the cannabis industry in several countries, resulting in products that are sometimes inconsistent in terms of potency and safety (K. R. Hossain et al. 2023). Given the scarcity of studies analyzing edibles, it is estimated that, although the onset of their psychoactive effects is felt later, from 30 to 90 minutes, this is more prolonged, with a peak of 2 to 4 hours after ingestion (Grotenhermen 2003). However, variability in bioavailability and uncertainty regarding the onset of action make edibles a less predictable option for rigorous therapeutic use.

Another challenge is that the delayed action of cannabinoids after oral ingestion can lead to overdose. This is because unnecessary additional doses may be ingested due to anxiety for relief before waiting for the initial therapeutic effects, often resulting in accidental intoxication and adverse effects related to high doses, especially of THC. In addition, edibles may be ingested unintentionally in amounts of Δ9-THCthat are larger than intended, which makes it very difficult to titrate the dose of these products (Zipursky et al. 2020).

It is also necessary to consider that the dose of Δ9-THC in homemade products depends on the concentration of THCA in the plant from which it is extracted or on the concentration of Δ9-THC in the purchased oil. However, when Δ9-THC is obtained through an extraction process, cannabinoid extraction is often incomplete, complicating dosage estimates in the resulting cannabis-infused oil. Consequently, Δ9-THC concentrations may not be available for products made with homemade oils or they may be inaccurate if a purchased oil is mislabeled (Barrus et al. 2016).

5.4 Sublingual Route

Sublingual administration allows direct absorption of cannabinoids through the oral mucosa into the bloodstream, partially avoiding first-pass hepatic metabolism. This route results in a faster onset of action and higher plasma concentrations than the oral route, for example, with capsules or solution. It is usually done with oils and tinctures (Huestis 2007).

Oils containing cannabinoids, in their different proportions of Δ9-THC and CBD concentrations, if administered orally, take about 1 to 2 hours to take effect and remain in the metabolism for 6 to 8 hours. One should always be aware of the dose of THC, which, even if low, may eventually cause some undesirable adverse effects (Briques et al. 2023). When administered sublingually, hyperconcentrated CBD/CBG/THC oils can have an onset of action of 15–45 min and a duration of action of 6–8 h (MacCallum and Russo 2018). Non-pharmaceutical cannabis oils are readily available for purchase in health stores and online. These products are not classified as medicinal products and are not licensed. They may contain varying levels of cannabis, contain impurities because they are not pharmaceutical grade, and because they tend to have minimal amounts of CBD, it is unclear how effective they are and what side effects they may have (Serrano et al. 2023).

5.5 Topical and Transdermal Routes

The topical and intradermal routes emerge as the most effective therapeutic administration possibilities for cannabis, given that they may represent more acceptable routes for users, bypassing the effects of the first hepatic pass, preventing the degradation of compounds by intestinal enzymes, and avoiding exposure to gastric pH. In addition, it offers easier withdrawal in case of toxicity, better dosage control, and a non-invasive route (Aziz et al. 2024).

Topical administration of cannabinoids is developed for local application in the layers of the skin, aiming to treat dermatological conditions, and transdermal administration provides sustained systemic administrationfor weeks in chronic cases and other situations that require long-term treatment (Scholfield et al. 2022).

The most commonly used transdermal systems are patches and gels. Patches are developed in various forms, includingmatrix-type, reservoir-type, single-layer drug-in-adhesive or multiple-layer drug-in-adhesive. Given the highly lipophilic nature of cannabinoids, they tend to concentrate in the outermost layer of the skin (stratum corneum), which can hinder their access to deeper layers, where blood vessels are concentrated, and also hinder the passive diffusion of the drug into the systemic circulation. To this end, research indicates the need to use chemical penetration enhancers, volatile oils, alcohols, and solubilizers to optimize delivery (Tijani et al. 2021). Topical use of cannabinoids is promising for the treatment of diseases such as acne vulgaris, allergic contact dermatitis, asteatotic dermatitis, atopic dermatitis, hidradenitis suppurativa, Kaposi's sarcoma, pain, pruritus, psoriasis, skin pigmentation disorders, and skin cancer, in addition to improving skin protection, barrier function, and wound healing results (Lapteva et al. 2024). In the case of the transdermal route, the indications are promising for chronic pain, spasticity, anorexia, nausea, and epilepsy (Tijani et al. 2021).

In view of the information provided here on the topical and transdermal routes, data on bioavailability, onset time, and duration of effects, according to the literature presented, are still variable and depend crucially on factors such as skin integrity, application site, dose, and frequency of application. Furthermore, concentrations and types of cannabinoids influence these variables (Lapteva et al. 2024; Lefebvre et al. 2024; Sheriff et al. 2020; Varadi et al. 2023). Despite the wide availability of cannabinoid-based products (oils, creams, lotions, tinctures, and ointments), there are serious potential risks to their use due to the lack of clinical evidence and, consequently, the lack of approval by regulatory agencies.

5.6 Other Routes of Administration

In addition to the aforementioned routes of administration, other routes such as rectal, vaginal, ophthalmic, intravenous, and some parenteral routes have also been considered for the development of cannabis-based products. However, studies involving these routes are scarcer and provide less robust evidence of clinical efficacy, which is still insufficient and inconclusive (ANVISA 2023; Bell et al. 2023; Bridgeman and Abazia 2017; Bruni et al. 2018; Russell et al. 2018; Wolowich et al. 2019). Table 2 presents the main routes of clinical administration of cannabinoids.

6. Safety Considerations and Side Effects

One of the major challenges associated with the adoption of cannabis-based medicines in official health systems and their acceptance by patients is knowledge about the safety of these formulations and the possible side effects related to their use. Several clinical studies that attest to the efficacy of medicinal cannabis also present information about its common and rare side effects. A randomized, double-blind, placebo-controlled study investigated the effects of CannEpil®, a medicinal cannabis oil containing 100 mg of CBD and 5 mg of THC, on the neurocognitive performance of adults who consumed 1 mL sublingual doses. The results of the clinical experiment indicate that this cannabinoid-based medicine impairs selected aspects of working memory, including the visualization and manipulation of spatial information, and negatively influences pattern recognition (Manning et al. 2024).

The safety and preliminary pharmacokinetics of a pharmaceutical formulation of purified CBD were evaluated in children with Dravet syndrome in a randomized study that revealed that daily doses of this drug at concentrations of 5, 10, or 20 mg/kg during the exposure time evaluated can result in adverse effects such as fever, drowsiness, decreased appetite, sedation, vomiting, and ataxia (Devinsky et al. 2018).

In addition to cannabis-based pharmaceutical drugs, such as sativex, nabilone and dronabinol, other herbal medicinal cannabis products are marketed and for these drugs, there is still not much safety information reported in the literature (MacCallum et al. 2021). In this context, more clinical studies are needed to provide information to health professionals and patients on the safe use of these formulations, considering particularities such as contraindications and drug interactions (Alsherbiny and Li 2019).

Table 2 summarizes the main side effects observed with formulations with cannabinoids in their composition. The adverse effects listed for the various types of applications have been reported in many randomized clinical studies and are considered tolerable compared to other traditional medicines. An overview of the safety of a given medicinal cannabis-based medicine must therefore take into account the data provided by clinical studies, the profile of the patient candidate for consumption, and the possibility of drug interactions (Hossain and Chae 2024).

Table 2: Methods of clinical administration of Cannabis sativa: comparison of characteristics.

Method of Application	Cannabinoid Component	Route	Start of Action	Effect Duration	Most Common Side Effects
Vaporization andsmoke	Cannabis flower for vaporization, handmade cigarettes from the dried plant.	Inhalation	3 to 5 min	2 to 4 hours	Tiredness or drowsiness, nausea, changes in appetite, dry mouth, muscle weakness, mood swings, a general feeling of discomfort, blurred vision, anxiety, mental confusion, impaired memory or concentration, lack of balance, or falls.
Spray bucal	Naxibimois (Δ^9-THC and CBD)	Oromucosal	30 to 60 min	4 to 6h	Drowsiness, dizziness, xerostomia, changes in appetite, mood swings, and nausea.
Capsule	Nabilone - Δ^9-THC analog, synthetic (Cesamet)	Oral	1 to 2h	8 to 12h	Mood swings, decreases in cognitive performance and memory, a decreased ability to control impulses and drives, and changes in the experience of reality, psychosis, dry mouth, and hypotension.
	Dronabinol - (-)-trans-Δ^9THC, synthetic (Marinol)	Oral	30 to 60 min	4 to 6 h	Mood swings, decreases in cognitive performance and memory, tachycardia, changes in the experience of reality, nervousness and anxiety, depression, and confusion.
	Crude extract of *Cannabis sativa* (Cannador)	Oral	Variable	up to 6 hours	Paranoia, hallucinations, tachycardia, hypotension, vertigo, dizziness or fainting, seizures, depression or thoughts of suicide, tiredness or drowsiness, nausea, changes in appetite, dry mouth, muscle weakness, mood swings, a general feeling of discomfort, blurred vision, anxiety, mental confusion, memory or concentration problems, lack of balance or falls.
Oral solution	Syndros (Dronabinol-Δ^9-THC analog)	Oral	30 to 60 min	4 to 6 h	Abdominal pain, dizziness, euphoria, nausea, paranoid reaction, drowsiness, abnormal thinking, and vomiting.
	Cannabidiol (Epidolex)	Oral	30 to 120 min	6 hours or more (varies with individual dose in mL)	Dizziness or drowsiness, diarrhea, decreased appetite, fever, vomiting, feeling tired.
	CBD + THC (variable concentrations) (Tilray oral solution)	Oral	40 to 60 min	4 hours or more	Paranoia, hallucination, tachycardia, hypotension, if associated with vertigo, dizziness, or fainting, convulsion, depression, or suicidal thoughts.
Oil	*Cannabis sativa* extract hyperconcentrates	Oral	1 to Sublingual2 hours	6 to 8h	Tiredness or drowsiness, nausea, changes in appetite, dry mouth, muscle weakness, mood swings, a general feeling of discomfort, blurred vision, anxiety, mental confusion, impaired memory or concentration, lack of balance, or falls.
Edibles (baked goods, sweets, gums, chocolates, pastilles, and drinks)	CBD and Δ^9-THC Variable	Oral	30 to 90min		Cognitive and motor impairment, extreme sedation, agitation, anxiety, cardiac stress, and vomiting, transient psychotic effects symptoms such as hallucinations, delusions, and anxiety.
Oil, dye	Cannabis extract hyperconcentrates.	Sublingual	15 to 45 min	6 to 8h	Tiredness or drowsiness, nausea, changes in appetite, dry mouth, muscle weakness, mood swings, a general feeling of discomfort, blurred vision, anxiety, mental confusion, impaired memory or concentration, lack of balance, or falls.
Oils, creams, lotions, tinctures, and ointments	CBD and Δ^9-THC Variable	Topic	Variable	Variable	Skin irritation and allergies

7. Conclusion and Perspectives

Medicinal cannabis has emerged as a promising therapeutic alternative for various clinical conditions, particularly those refractory to conventional treatments. Clinical trials and observational studies have consistently demonstrated the efficacy of cannabis-based formulations in managing chronic pain, epilepsy, chemotherapy-induced nausea and vomiting, anxiety disorders, and inflammatory diseases. The mechanisms of action of phytocannabinoids—particularly THC and CBD—via CB1 and CB2 receptors within the endocannabinoid system explain much of their broad pharmacological potential.

Despite the growing body of scientific evidence, the incorporation of cannabis-derived medicines into public health systems still faces numerous challenges, including legal barriers, social stigma, and a need for greater standardization in formulation, dosage, and administration routes. While synthetic and semi-synthetic options such as dronabinol, nabilone, and nabiximols offer more precise dosing, variability in bioavailability and individual patient response remains a critical issue.

From a safety perspective, most adverse effects are mild to moderate and tolerable, especially when compared with traditional pharmacological treatments. However, reports of cognitive impairment, sedation, and gastrointestinal symptoms underscore the importance of continued pharmacovigilance and patient-specific risk assessments.

Future perspectives for medicinal cannabis lie in the development of more refined drug delivery systems that enhance bioavailability and therapeutic efficacy while minimizing adverse effects. Advances in nanotechnology, transdermal systems, and targeted receptor agonists or enzyme inhibitors offer exciting potential for innovation in cannabis-based pharmacotherapy. Furthermore, long-term, multicenter randomized controlled trials are essential to solidify cannabis's role in modern medicine, define evidence-based treatment protocols, and ensure regulatory approval with scientific rigor.

Ultimately, medicinal cannabis represents not only a new pharmacological tool but also a shift in the paradigm of integrative and personalized medicine. Responsible integration into clinical practice will depend on continuous research, professional education, regulatory evolution, and the active engagement of patients and health systems in this emerging field.

References

Abrams, D. I., Couey, P., Shade, S. B., Kelly, M. E., and Benowitz, N. L. (2011). Cannabinoid–Opioid Interaction in Chronic Pain. *Clinical Pharmacology and Therapeutics*, 90(6): 844–851. https://doi.org/https://doi.org/10.1038/clpt.2011.188

Abuhasira, R., Shbiro, L., and Landschaft, Y. (2018). Medical use of cannabis and cannabinoids containing products–Regulations in Europe and North America. *European Journal of Internal Medicine*, 49: 2–6. https://doi.org/https://doi.org/10.1016/j.ejim.2018.01.001

Abu-Sawwa, R., and Stehling, C. (2019). Epidiolex (Cannabidiol) Primer: Frequently Asked Questions for Patients and Caregivers. *The Journal of Pediatric Pharmacology and Therapeutics*, 25(1): 75–77. https://doi.org/10.5863/1551-6776-25.1.75

Almog, S., Aharon-Peretz, J., Vulfsons, S., Ogintz, M., Abalia, H., Lupo, T. et al. (2020). The pharmacokinetics, efficacy, and safety of a novel selective-dose cannabis inhaler in patients with chronic pain: A randomized, double-blinded, placebo-controlled trial. *European Journal of Pain*, 24(8): 1505–1516. https://doi.org/https://doi.org/10.1002/ejp.1605

Alsherbiny, M. A., and Li, C. G. (2019). Medicinal Cannabis—Potential Drug Interactions. *Medicines*, 6(1). https://doi.org/10.3390/medicines6010003

ANVISA. (2023). *Relatório De Análise De Impacto Regulatório Sobre Produtos De Cannabis Para Fins Medicinais*. Retrieved from https://www.gov.br/anvisa/pt-br/assuntos/regulamentacao/air/analises-de-impacto-regulatorio/2024/arquivos-relatorios-de-air-2024/relatorio_air_produtos_cannabis_dicol_15052024.pdf

Arkell, T. R., Kevin, R. C., Stuart, J., Lintzeris, N., Haber, P. S., Ramaekers, J. G. et al. (2019). Detection of Δ9 THC in oral fluid following vaporized cannabis with varied cannabidiol (CBD) content: An evaluation of two point-of-collection testing devices. *Drug Testing and Analysis*, 11(10): 1486–1497. https://doi.org/https://doi.org/10.1002/dta.2687

Aziz, A. F. A., Beh, Y. Q., Farahiyah, I. I., Azmir, S. S., Kee, P. E., Uddin, A. B. M. H. et al. (2024). A Review on the mechanisms, applications, and clinical trials of advanced technologies in the transdermal drug delivery system. *Current Pharmaceutical Biotechnology*. https://doi.org/10.2174/0113892010318519240813053106

Baban, B., Khodadadi, H., Salles, É. L., Costigliola, V., Morgan, J. C., Hess, D. C. et al. (2021). Inflammaging and Cannabinoids. *Ageing Research Reviews*, 72: 101487. https://doi.org/https://doi.org/10.1016/j.arr.2021.101487

Banerjee, R., Erridge, S., Salazar, O., Mangal, N., Couch, D., Pacchetti, B., and Sodergren, M. H. (2022). Real world evidence in medical cannabis research. *Therapeutic Innovation and Regulatory Science*, 56(1): 8–14. https://doi.org/10.1007/s43441-021-00346-0

Baratta, F., Pignata, I., Ravetto Enri, L., and Brusa, P. (2022). Cannabis for medical use: analysis of recent clinical trials in view of current legislation. *Frontiers in Pharmacology*, 13. https://doi.org/10.3389/fphar.2022.888903

Barrus, D. G., Capogrossi, K. L., Cates, S. C., Gourdet, C. K., Peiper, N. C., Novak, S. P. et al. (2016). Tasty THC: Promises and Challenges of Cannabis Edibles. *Methods Report (RTI Press)*, 2016. https://doi.org/10.3768/rtipress.2016.op.0035.1611

Bedi, G., Cooper, Z. D., and Haney, M. (2013). Subjective, cognitive and cardiovascular dose-effect profile of nabilone and dronabinol in marijuana smokers. *Addiction Biology*, 18(5): 872–881. https://doi.org/https://doi.org/10.1111/j.1369-1600.2011.00427.x

Bell, A. D., MacCallum, C., Margolese, S., Walsh, Z., Wright, P., Daeninck, P. J. et al. (2023). Clinical practice guidelines for cannabis and cannabinoid-based medicines in the management of chronic pain and co-occurring conditions. *Cannabis and Cannabinoid Research*, 9(2): 669–687. https://doi.org/10.1089/can.2021.0156

Ben Amar, M. (2006). Cannabinoids in medicine: A review of their therapeutic potential. *Journal of Ethnopharmacology*, 105(1): 1–25. https://doi.org/https://doi.org/10.1016/j.jep.2006.02.001

Birnbaum, A. K., Karanam, A., Marino, S. E., Barkley, C. M., Remmel, R. P., Roslawski, M. et al. (2019). Food effect on pharmacokinetics of cannabidiol oral capsules in adult patients with refractory epilepsy. *Epilepsia*, 60(8): 1586–1592. https://doi.org/https://doi.org/10.1111/epi.16093

Blake, D. R., Robson, P., Ho, M., Jubb, R. W., and McCabe, C. S. (2006). Preliminary assessment of the efficacy, tolerability and safety of a cannabis-based medicine (Sativex) in the treatment of pain caused by rheumatoid arthritis. *Rheumatology*, 45(1): 50–52. https://doi.org/10.1093/rheumatology/kei183

Blessing, E. M., Steenkamp, M. M., Manzanares, J., and Marmar, C. R. (2015). Cannabidiol as a potential treatment for anxiety disorders. *Neurotherapeutics*, 12(4): 825–836. https://doi.org/10.1007/s13311-015-0387-1

Boggs, D. L., Peckham, A., Boggs, A. A., and Ranganathan, M. (2016). Delta-9-tetrahydrocannabinol and cannabidiol: Separating the chemicals from the "weed," a pharmacodynamic discussion. *Mental Health Clinician*, 6(6): 277–284. https://doi.org/10.9740/mhc.2016.11.277

Bonn-Miller, M. O., Sisley, S., Riggs, P., Yazar-Klosinski, B., Wang, J. B., Loflin, M. J. E. et al. (2021). The short-term impact of 3 smoked cannabis preparations versus placebo on PTSD symptoms: A randomized cross-over clinical trial. *PLoS ONE*, 16(3 March). https://doi.org/10.1371/journal.pone.0246990

Borowicz-Reutt, K., Czernia, J., and Krawczyk, M. (2024). CBD in the Treatment of Epilepsy. *Molecules*, 29(9). https://doi.org/10.3390/molecules29091981

Bridgeman, M. B., and Abazia, D. T. (2017). Medicinal Cannabis: History, pharmacology, and implications for the acute care setting. *Brazilian Journal of Pain*, 42(3): S114–S119.

Briques, W., Pereira, C. L., and Feliz, P. S. (2023). Practical aspects of the use of medicinal cannabis in chronic pain. *Brazilian Journal Of Pain*, 6(Supl.2). https://doi.org/10.5935/2595-0118.20230056-en

Bruni, N., Pepa, C. Della, Oliaro-Bosso, S., Pessione, E., Gastaldi, D., and Dosio, F. (2018, September 27). Cannabinoid delivery systems for pain and inflammation treatment. *Molecules*, Vol. 23. MDPI AG. https://doi.org/10.3390/molecules23102478

Brust, C. A., Swanson, M. A., and Bohn, L. M. (2023). Structural and functional insights into the G protein-coupled receptors: CB1 and CB2. *Biochemical Society Transactions*, 51(4): 1533–1543. https://doi.org/10.1042/BST20221316

Burstein, S. (2015). Cannabidiol (CBD) and its analogs: a review of their effects on inflammation. *Bioorganic and Medicinal Chemistry*, 23(7): 1377–1385. https://doi.org/https://doi.org/10.1016/j.bmc.2015.01.059

Buxeraud, J., and Faure, S. (2023). Le cannabidiol (Epidyolex®), un antiépileptique. *Actualités Pharmaceutiques*, 62(627): 12–13. https://doi.org/https://doi.org/10.1016/j.actpha.2023.03.038

Calhoun, S. R., Gantt P., G., and and Smith, D. E. (1998). Abuse Potential of Dronabinol (Marinol®). *Journal of Psychoactive Drugs*, 30(2): 187–196. https://doi.org/10.1080/02791072.1998.10399689

Clarke, R. C., and Merlin, M. D. (2013). *Evolution and Ethnobotany* (1st ed.). University of California Press. Retrieved from http://www.jstor.org/stable/10.1525/j.ctt3fh2f8

Cummings, H., Moizza Zia, U. H., Amne, D., Nauman, S., Jason, W. B., Andrea, J. D. et al. (2024). Individuals' Values and Preferences Regarding Medical Cannabis for Chronic Pain: A Descriptive Qualitative Study. *Journal of Pain Research*, 17(null), 21–34. https://doi.org/10.2147/JPR.S432823

Dahlgren, C., Lind, S., Mårtensson, J., Björkman, L., Wu, Y., Sundqvist, M. et al. (2023). G protein coupled pattern recognition receptors expressed in neutrophils: Recognition, activation/modulation, signaling and receptor regulated functions. *Immunological Reviews*, 314(1): 69–92. https://doi.org/https://doi.org/10.1111/imr.13151

de Fátima dos Santos Sampaio, M., de Paiva, Y. B., Sampaio, T. B., Pereira, M. G., and Coimbra, N. C. (2024). Therapeutic applicability of cannabidiol and other phytocannabinoids in epilepsy, multiple sclerosis and Parkinson's disease and in comorbidity with psychiatric disorders. *Basic and Clinical Pharmacology and Toxicology*, 134(5): 574–601. https://doi.org/https://doi.org/10.1111/bcpt.13997

de Souza, M. R., Henriques, A. T., and Limberger, R. P. (2022). Medical cannabis regulation: an overview of models around the world with emphasis on the Brazilian scenario. *Journal of Cannabis Research*, 4(1): 33. https://doi.org/10.1186/s42238-022-00142-z

Devinsky, O., Cilio, M. R., Cross, H., Fernandez-Ruiz, J., French, J., Hill, C. et al. (2014). Cannabidiol: Pharmacology and potential therapeutic role in epilepsy and other neuropsychiatric disorders. *Epilepsia*, 55(6): 791–802. https://doi.org/https://doi.org/10.1111/epi.12631

Devinsky, O., Patel, A. D., Thiele, E. A., Wong, M. H., Appleton, R., Harden, C. L. et al (2018). Randomized, dose-ranging safety trial of cannabidiol in Dravet syndrome. *Neurology*, 90(14): e1204–e1211. https://doi.org/10.1212/WNL.0000000000005254

Donvito, G., Nass, S. R., Wilkerson, J. L., Curry, Z. A., Schurman, L. D., Kinsey, S. G. et al. (2018). The Endogenous Cannabinoid System: A Budding Source of Targets for Treating Inflammatory and Neuropathic Pain. *Neuropsychopharmacology*, 43(1): 52–79. https://doi.org/10.1038/npp.2017.204

Downey, M. L., and Peralta-Yahya, P. (2024). Technologies for the discovery of G protein–coupled receptor–targeting biologics. *Current Opinion in Biotechnology*, 87: 103138. https://doi.org/https://doi.org/10.1016/j.copbio.2024.103138

Duran, M., Pérez, E., Abanades, S., Vidal, X., Saura, C., Majem, M. et al. (2010). Preliminary efficacy and safety of an oromucosal standardized cannabis extract in chemotherapy-induced nausea and vomiting. *British Journal of Clinical Pharmacology*, 70(5): 656–663. https://doi.org/https://doi.org/10.1111/j.1365-2125.2010.03743.x

ElSohly, M. A., deWit, H., Wachtel, S. R., Feng, S., and Murphy, T. P. (2001). Δ9-Tetrahydrocannabivarin as a Marker for the Ingestion of Marijuana versus Marinol®: Results of a Clinical Study. *Journal of Analytical Toxicology*, 25(7): 565–571. https://doi.org/10.1093/jat/25.7.565

Eyal, A. M., Berneman Zeitouni, D., Tal, D., Schlesinger, D., Davidson, E. M., and Raz, N. (2022). Vapor Pressure, Vaping, and Corrections to Misconceptions Related to Medical Cannabis' Active Pharmaceutical Ingredients' Physical Properties and Compositions. *Cannabis and Cannabinoid Research*, 8(3): 414–425. https://doi.org/10.1089/can.2021.0173

Fabrício Moreira, C. A., Saito, V. M., Wotjak, C. T., and Moreira, F. A. (2010). Pharmacological exploitation of the endocannabinoid system: new perspectives for the treatment of depression and anxiety disorders? *Revista Brasileira de Psiquiatria*, 32: S7–S14.

Fordjour, E., Manful, C. F., Sey, A. A., Javed, R., Pham, T. H., Thomas, R. et al. (2023). Cannabis: a multifaceted plant with endless potentials. *Frontiers in Pharmacology*, Vol. 14. Frontiers Media SA. https://doi.org/10.3389/fphar.2023.1200269

Fraguas-Sánchez, A. I., and Torres-Suárez, A. I. (2018). Medical Use of Cannabinoids. *Drugs*, 78(16): 1665–1703. https://doi.org/10.1007/s40265-018-0996-1

Friedman, D., and Sirven, J. I. (2017). Historical perspective on the medical use of cannabis for epilepsy: Ancient times to the 1980s. *Epilepsy and Behavior*, 70: 298–301. https://doi.org/https://doi.org/10.1016/j.yebeh.2016.11.033

Gaisey, J., and Narouze, S. N. (2021). Dronabinol (Marinol®). In S. N. Narouze (Ed.), *Cannabinoids and Pain* (pp. 105–107). Cham: Springer International Publishing. https://doi.org/10.1007/978-3-030-69186-8_14

Gracie, K., and Hancox, R. J. (2021). Cannabis use disorder and the lungs. *Addiction*, 116(1): 182–190. https://doi.org/https://doi.org/10.1111/add.15075

Grimison, P., Mersiades, A., Kirby, A., Lintzeris, N., Morton, R., Haber, P. et al. (2020). Oral THC:CBD cannabis extract for refractory chemotherapy-induced nausea and vomiting: a randomised, placebo-controlled, phase II crossover trial. *Annals of Oncology*, 31(11): 1553–1560. https://doi.org/https://doi.org/10.1016/j.annonc.2020.07.020

Grotenhermen, F. (2003). Pharmacokinetics and Pharmacodynamics of Cannabinoids. *Clinical Pharmacokinetics*, 42(4): 327–360. https://doi.org/10.2165/00003088-200342040-00003

Haney, M., Cooper, Z. D., Bedi, G., Vosburg, S. K., Comer, S. D., and Foltin, R. W. (2013). Nabilone Decreases Marijuana Withdrawal and a Laboratory Measure of Marijuana Relapse. *Neuropsychopharmacology*, 38(8): 1557–1565. https://doi.org/10.1038/npp.2013.54

Harrison, N. J., and Simpson, H. (2021). Nabilone (Cesamet). pp. 109–112. *In*: Narouze, S. N. (Ed.). *Cannabinoids and Pain*. Cham: Springer International Publishing. https://doi.org/10.1007/978-3-030-69186-8_15

Häuser, W., Petzke, F., and Fitzcharles, M. A. (2018). Efficacy, tolerability and safety of cannabis-based medicines for chronic pain management – An overview of systematic reviews. *European Journal of Pain*, 22(3): 455–470. https://doi.org/https://doi.org/10.1002/ejp.1118

Herrmann, N., Ruthirakuhan, M., Gallagher, D., Verhoeff, N. P. L. G., Kiss, A., Black, S. E. et al. (2019). Randomized placebo-controlled trial of nabilone for agitation in alzheimer's disease. *The American Journal of Geriatric Psychiatry*, 27(11): 1161–1173. https://doi.org/https://doi.org/10.1016/j.jagp.2019.05.002

Hossain, K. R., Alghalayini, A., and Valenzuela, S. M. (2023). Current Challenges and Opportunities for Improved Cannabidiol Solubility. *International Journal of Molecular Sciences*, 24(19). https://doi.org/10.3390/ijms241914514

Hossain, M. K., and Chae, H. J. (2024). Medical cannabis: From research breakthroughs to shifting public perceptions and ensuring safe use. *Integrative Medicine Research*, 13(4): 101094. https://doi.org/https://doi.org/10.1016/j.imr.2024.101094

Huestis, M. A. (2007). Human Cannabinoid Pharmacokinetics. *Chemistry and Biodiversity*, 4(8): 1770–1804. https://doi.org/https://doi.org/10.1002/cbdv.200790152

Itin, C., Barasch, D., Domb, A. J., and Hoffman, A. (2020). Prolonged oral transmucosal delivery of highly lipophilic drug cannabidiol. *International Journal of Pharmaceutics*, 581: 119276. https://doi.org/https://doi.org/10.1016/j.ijpharm.2020.119276

Kayser, R. R., Haney, M., Raskin, M., Arout, C., and Simpson, H. B. (2020). Acute effects of cannabinoids on symptoms of obsessive-compulsive disorder: A human laboratory study. *Depression and Anxiety*, 37(8): 801–811. https://doi.org/https://doi.org/10.1002/da.23032

Kelly, L. E., Rieder, M. J., and Finkelstein, Y. (2024). Medical cannabis for children: Evidence and recommendations. *Paediatrics and Child Health*, 29(2): 104–112. https://doi.org/10.1093/pch/pxad078

Khoury, M., Cohen, I., and Bar-Sela, G. (2022, February 1). "The Two Sides of the Same Coin"—Medical Cannabis, Cannabinoids and Immunity: Pros and Cons Explained. *Pharmaceutics*, Vol. 14. MDPI. https://doi.org/10.3390/pharmaceutics14020389

Kirilov, B., Margarita, Z., Elina, P.-G., and and Momekov, G. (2020). Regulation and marketing of cannabidiol-containing products in European countries. Pharmacists' knowledge in Bulgaria. *Biotechnology and Biotechnological Equipment*, 34(1): 1158–1165. https://doi.org/10.1080/13102818.2020.1824620

Kisiolek, J. N., Flores, V. A., Ramani, A., Butler, B., Haughian, J. M., and Stewart, L. K. (2023). Eight Weeks of Daily Cannabidiol Supplementation Improves Sleep Quality and Immune Cell Cytotoxicity. *Nutrients*, 15(19). https://doi.org/10.3390/nu15194173

Lapteva, M., Faro Barros, J., and Kalia, Y. N. (2024). Cutaneous Delivery and Biodistribution of Cannabidiol in Human Skin after Topical Application of Colloidal Formulations. *Pharmaceutics*, 16(2). https://doi.org/10.3390/pharmaceutics16020202

Lefebvre, È., Tawil, N., and Yahia, L. (2024). Transdermal Delivery of Cannabidiol for the Management of Acute Inflammatory Pain: A Comprehensive Review of the Literature. *International Journal of Molecular Sciences*, 25(11). https://doi.org/10.3390/ijms25115858

Legare, C. A., Raup-Konsavage, W. M., and Vrana, K. E. (2022). Therapeutic Potential of Cannabis, Cannabidiol, and Cannabinoid-Based Pharmaceuticals. *Pharmacology*, 107(3-4): 131–149. https://doi.org/10.1159/000521683

Lessa, M. A., Cavalcanti, I. L., and Figueiredo, N. V. (2016). Cannabinoid derivatives and the pharmacological management of pain. *Revista Dor*, 17(1). https://doi.org/10.5935/1806-0013.20160012

Lopera, V., Restrepo, J. C., and Amariles, P. (2024). Effectiveness and safety of cannabis-based products for medical use in patients with fibromyalgia syndrome: A systematic review. *Exploratory Research in Clinical and Social Pharmacy*, 16: 100524. https://doi.org/https://doi.org/10.1016/j.rcsop.2024.100524

Lyu, X., Illamola, S. M., Marino, S. E., Leppik, I. E., Dahmer, S., Lehfeldt, P. et al. (2023). Medical cannabis received by patients according to qualifying condition in a US State cannabis program: product choice, dosing, and age-related trends. *Current Therapeutic Research*, 99: 100709. https://doi.org/https://doi.org/10.1016/j.curtheres.2023.100709

MacCallum, C. A., Lo, L. A., and Boivin, M. (2021). Is medical cannabis safe for my patients? A practical review of cannabis safety considerations. *European Journal of Internal Medicine*, 89: 10–18. https://doi.org/https://doi.org/10.1016/j.ejim.2021.05.002

MacCallum, C. A., and Russo, E. B. (2018). Practical considerations in medical cannabis administration and dosing. *European Journal of Internal Medicine*, 49: 12–19. https://doi.org/https://doi.org/10.1016/j.ejim.2018.01.004

Malfait, A., Gallily, R., Sumariwalla, P., Malik, A., Andreakos, E., Mechoulam, R. et al. (2000). The nonpsychoactive cannabis constituent cannabidiol is an oral anti-arthritic therapeutic in murine collagen-induced arthritis. *Proceedings of the National Academy of Sciences of the United States of America*, 97(17): 9561–9566.

Manning, B., Hayley, A. C., Catchlove, S., Stough, C., and Downey, L. A. (2024). A randomised, placebo-controlled, double blind, crossover trial on the effect of a 20:1 cannabidiol: Δ9-tetrahydrocannabinol medical cannabis product on neurocognition, attention, and mood. *European Neuropsychopharmacology*, 82: 35–43. https://doi.org/https://doi.org/10.1016/j.euroneuro.2024.02.002

McCoy, B., Wang, L., Zak, M., Al-Mehmadi, S., Kabir, N., Alhadid, K. et al. (2018a). A prospective open-label trial of a CBD/THC cannabis oil in dravet syndrome. *Annals of Clinical and Translational Neurology*, 5(9): 1077–1088. https://doi.org/https://doi.org/10.1002/acn3.621

McCoy, B., Wang, L., Zak, M., Al-Mehmadi, S., Kabir, N., Alhadid, K. et al. (2018b). A prospective open-label trial of a CBD/THC cannabis oil in dravet syndrome. *Annals of Clinical and Translational Neurology*, 5(9): 1077–1088. https://doi.org/https://doi.org/10.1002/acn3.621

Melas, P. A., Scherma, M., Fratta, W., Cifani, C., and Fadda, P. (2021). Cannabidiol as a potential treatment for anxiety and mood disorders: molecular targets and epigenetic insights from preclinical research. *International Journal of Molecular Sciences*, 22(4). https://doi.org/10.3390/ijms22041863

Melén, C. M., Magali, M., Agata M., W., Georgios, P., Olof, B., Kristina, S. et al. (2022). Clinical effects of a single dose of cannabinoids to patients with chronic lymphocytic leukemia. *Leukemia and Lymphoma*, 63(6): 1387–1397. https://doi.org/10.1080/10428194.2021.2020776

Mersiades, A., Kirby, A., Stockler, M. R., Tognela, A., Olver, I. N., Morton, R. L. et al. (2023). Cannabis extract for secondary prevention of chemotherapy-induced nausea and vomiting: Results of a phase II/III, placebo-controlled, randomised trial. *Journal of Clinical Oncology*, 41(16_suppl), 12019. https://doi.org/10.1200/JCO.2023.41.16_suppl.12019

Millar, S. A., Stone, N. L., Yates, A. S., and O'Sullivan, S. E. (2018, November 26). A systematic review on the pharmacokinetics of cannabidiol in humans. *Frontiers in Pharmacology*, Vol. 9. Frontiers Media S.A. https://doi.org/10.3389/fphar.2018.01365

Mishra, V., Desai, J., and Patel, K. I. (2018). (UV/Oxidative) dual curing polyurethane dispersion from cardanol based polyol: Synthesis and characterization. *Industrial Crops and Products*, 111: 165–178. https://doi.org/https://doi.org/10.1016/j.indcrop.2017.10.015

Mitelpunkt, A., Kramer, U., Hausman Kedem, M., Zilbershot Fink, E., Orbach, R., Chernuha, V. et al. (2019). The safety, tolerability, and effectiveness of PTL-101, an oral cannabidiol formulation, in pediatric intractable epilepsy: A phase II, open-label, single-center study. *Epilepsy and Behavior*, 98: 233–237. https://doi.org/https://doi.org/10.1016/j.yebeh.2019.07.007

Moreno-Sanz, G., Madiedo, A., Hernandez, P., Kratz, J., Aizpurua-Olaizola, O., Brown, M. R. D. et al. (2022). Sex-Dependent Prescription Patterns and Clinical Outcomes Associated With the Use of Two Oral Cannabis Formulations in the Multimodal Management of Chronic Pain Patients in Colombia. *Frontiers in Pain Research*, 3. https://doi.org/10.3389/fpain.2022.854795

Mücke, M., Phillips, T., Radbruch, L., Petzke, F., and Häuser, W. (2018). Cannabis-based medicines for chronic neuropathic pain in adults. *Cochrane Database of Systematic Reviews*, (3). https://doi.org/10.1002/14651858.CD012182.pub2

Mukhtar, Mohd. S. A., Gupta, R., and Balpande, R. (2025). Assessing the neuroprotective benefits of Cannabis sativa in epilepsy management. *Brain Disorders*, 17: 100180. https://doi.org/https://doi.org/10.1016/j.dscb.2024.100180

Müller, A. R., den Hollander, B., van de Ven, P. M., Roes, K. C. B., Geertjens, L., Bruining, H. et al. (2024). Cannabidiol (Epidyolex®) for severe behavioral manifestations in patients with tuberous sclerosis complex, mucopolysaccharidosis type III and fragile X syndrome: protocol for a series of randomized, placebo-controlled N-of-1 trials. *BMC Psychiatry*, 24(1): 23. https://doi.org/10.1186/s12888-023-05422-3

Murphy, M., Kaur, V., Bui, H. L., Yang, T., Erridge, S., Holvey, C. et al. (2024). Clinical outcome analysis of patients with multiple sclerosis – Analysis from the UK Medical Cannabis Registry. *Multiple Sclerosis and Related Disorders*, 87: 105665. https://doi.org/https://doi.org/10.1016/j.msard.2024.105665

Newmeyer, M. N., Swortwood, M. J., Barnes, A. J., Abulseoud, O. A., Scheidweiler, K. B., and Huestis, M. A. (2016). Free and glucuronide whole blood cannabinoids' pharmacokinetics after controlled smoked, vaporized, and oral cannabis administration in frequent and occasional cannabis users: Identification of recent cannabis intake. *Clinical Chemistry*, 62(12): 1579–1592. https://doi.org/10.1373/clinchem.2016.263475

Nimalan, D., Kawka, M., Erridge, S., Ergisi, M., Harris, M., Salazar, O. et al. (2022). UK Medical Cannabis Registry palliative care patients cohort: initial experience and outcomes. *Journal of Cannabis Research*, 4(1): 3. https://doi.org/10.1186/s42238-021-00114-9

Nutt, D. J., Phillips, L. D., Barnes, M. P., Brander, B., Curran, H. V., Fayaz, A. et al. (2021). A multicriteria decision analysis comparing pharmacotherapy for chronic neuropathic pain, including cannabinoids and cannabis-based medical products. *Cannabis and Cannabinoid Research*, 7(4): 482–500. https://doi.org/10.1089/can.2020.0129

O'Donnell, B., Meissner, H., and Gupta, V. (2025). *Dronabinol*. StatPearls Publishing, Treasure Island (FL). Retrieved from http://europepmc.org/abstract/MED/32491463

Orrin, D., Helen, C. J., Linda, L., Eric, M., Ian, M., Rima, N. et al. (2025a). Trial of Cannabidiol for Drug-Resistant Seizures in the Dravet Syndrome. *New England Journal of Medicine*, 376(21): 2011–2020. https://doi.org/10.1056/NEJMoa1611618

Orrin, D., Helen, C. J., Linda, L., Eric, M., Ian, M., Rima, N. et al. (2025b). Trial of Cannabidiol for Drug-Resistant Seizures in the Dravet Syndrome. *New England Journal of Medicine*, 376(21): 2011–2020. https://doi.org/10.1056/NEJMoa1611618

O'Sullivan, S. E., Jensen, S. S., Kolli, A. R., Nikolajsen, G. N., Bruun, H. Z., and Hoeng, J. (2024). Strategies to Improve Cannabidiol Bioavailability and Drug Delivery. *Pharmaceuticals*, 17(2). https://doi.org/10.3390/ph17020244

Pagano, C., Savarese, B., Coppola, L., Navarra, G., Avilia, G., Laezza, C. et al. (2023, February 1). Cannabinoids in the Modulation of Oxidative Signaling. *International Journal of Molecular Sciences*, Vol. 24. MDPI. https://doi.org/10.3390/ijms24032513

Parikh, N., Kramer, W. G., Khurana, V., Cognata Smith, C., and Vetticaden, S. (2016). Bioavailability study of dronabinol oral solution versus dronabinol capsules in healthy volunteers. *Clinical Pharmacology: Advances and Applications*, 8: 155–162. https://doi.org/10.2147/CPAA.S115679

Parker, L. A., Rock, E. M., and Limebeer, C. L. (2011). Regulation of nausea and vomiting by cannabinoids. *British Journal of Pharmacology*, 163(7): 1411–1422. https://doi.org/https://doi.org/10.1111/j.1476-5381.2010.01176.x

Penha, E. M., Cardoso, D. D. e S., Coelho, L. P., and Bueno, A. M. (2019). A Regulamentação de Medicamentos Derivados da Cannabis sativa no Brasil. *Brazilian Journal of Forensic Sciences, Medical Law and Bioethics*, 9(1): 125–145. https://doi.org/10.17063/bjfs9(1)y2019125

Perucca, E. (2017). Cannabinoids in the Treatment of Epilepsy: Hard Evidence at Last? *J. Epilepsy Res.*, 7(2): 61–76. https://doi.org/10.14581/jer.17012

Pickle, K. (2018). Big Pharma Takes On Marijuana Legalization: The Synthetic Marijuana vs. Botanical Marijuana Paradox, 5 Emory Corp. In *Governance and Accountability Rev. Perspectives* (Vol. 127).

Pisanti, S., and Bifulco, M. (2017). Modern History of Medical <em>Cannabis:</em> From Widespread Use to Prohibitionism and Back. *Trends in Pharmacological Sciences*, 38(3): 195–198. https://doi.org/10.1016/j.tips.2016.12.002

Rosenberg, E. C., Patra, P. H., and Whalley, B. J. (2017). Therapeutic effects of cannabinoids in animal models of seizures, epilepsy, epileptogenesis, and epilepsy-related neuroprotection. *Epilepsy and Behavior*, 70: 319–327. https://doi.org/https://doi.org/10.1016/j.yebeh.2016.11.006

Rosenberg, E. C., Tsien, R. W., Whalley, B. J., and Devinsky, O. (2015). Cannabinoids and Epilepsy. *Neurotherapeutics*, 12(4): 747–768. https://doi.org/10.1007/s13311-015-0375-5

Russell, C., Rueda, S., Room, R., Tyndall, M., and Fischer, B. (2018). Routes of administration for cannabis use – basic prevalence and related health outcomes: A scoping review and synthesis. *International Journal of Drug Policy*, 52: 87–96. https://doi.org/https://doi.org/10.1016/j.drugpo.2017.11.008

Schlag, A. K. (2020). An Evaluation of Regulatory Regimes of Medical Cannabis: What Lessons Can Be Learned for the UK? *Medical Cannabis and Cannabinoids*, 3(1): 25–60. https://doi.org/10.1159/000505028

Scholfield, C. N., Waranuch, N., and Kongkaew, C. (2022). Systematic Review on Transdermal/Topical Cannabidiol Trials: A Reconsidered Way Forward. *Cannabis and Cannabinoid Research*, 8(4): 589–602. https://doi.org/10.1089/can.2021.0154

Schussel, V., Kenzo, L., Santos, A., Bueno, J., Yoshimura, E., de Oliveira Cruz Latorraca, C. et al. (2018). Cannabinoids for nausea and vomiting related to chemotherapy: Overview of systematic reviews. *Phytotherapy Research*, 32(4): 567–576. https://doi.org/https://doi.org/10.1002/ptr.5975

Scott, S., Nicole, L., Heather, L., and Shannon, H. (2019). Cannabidiol in Anxiety and Sleep: A Large Case Series. *The Permanente Journal*, 23(1): 18–041. https://doi.org/10.7812/TPP/18-041

Serrano, S. C., Campos, F. G. de, and Tanaka, V. O. P. (2023). Pediatric patients and medical cannabis: new trends. *Brazilian Journal Of Pain*, 6(Supl.2). https://doi.org/10.5935/2595-0118.20230059-en

Sheriff, T., Lin, M. J., Dubin, D., and Khorasani, H. (2020, November 16). The potential role of cannabinoids in dermatology. *Journal of Dermatological Treatment*, 31: 839–845. Taylor and Francis Ltd. https://doi.org/10.1080/09546634.2019.1675854

Sholler, D. J., Strickland, J. C., Spindle, T. R., Weerts, E. M., and Vandrey, R. (2021). Sex differences in the acute effects of oral and vaporized cannabis among healthy adults. *Addiction Biology*, 26(4): e12968. https://doi.org/https://doi.org/10.1111/adb.12968

Sinclair, J., Abbott, J., Mikocka-Walus, A., Ng, C., Sarris, J., Evans, S., and Armour, M. (2023). 'A glimmer of hope': perceptions, barriers, and drivers for medicinal cannabis use amongst Australian and New Zealand people with endometriosis – a qualitative study. *Reproduction and Fertility*, 4(4): e230049. https://doi.org/10.1530/RAF-23-0049

Sirichai, C. (2021). Mechanisms of Action and Pharmacokinetics of Cannabis. *The Permanente Journal*, 25(1): 1–3. https://doi.org/10.7812/TPP/19.200

Spanagel, R. (2020). Cannabinoids and the endocannabinoid system in reward processing and addiction: from mechanisms to interventions. *Dialogues in Clinical Neuroscience*, 22(3): 241–250. https://doi.org/10.31887/DCNS.2020.22.3/rspanagel

Stella, B., Baratta, F., Della Pepa, C., Arpicco, S., Gastaldi, D., and Dosio, F. (2021). Cannabinoid formulations and delivery systems: current and future options to treat pain. *Drugs*, 81(13): 1513–1557. https://doi.org/10.1007/s40265-021-01579-x

Sukpiriyagul, A., Chartchaiyarerk, R., Tabtipwon, P., Smanchat, B., Prommas, S., Bhamarapravatana, K. et al. (2023). Oral Tetrahydrocannabinol (THC):Cannabinoid (CBD) Cannabis Extract Adjuvant for Reducing Chemotherapy-Induced Nausea and Vomiting (CINV): A Randomized, Double-Blinded, Placebo-Controlled, Crossover Trial. *International Journal of Women's Health, 15*, 1345–1352. https://doi.org/10.2147/IJWH.S401938

Thiele, E. A., Marsh, E. D., French, J. A., Mazurkiewicz-Beldzinska, M., Benbadis, S. R., Joshi, C. et al. (2018). Cannabidiol in patients with seizures associated with Lennox-Gastaut syndrome (GWPCARE4): a randomised, double-blind, placebo-controlled phase 3 trial. *The Lancet*, 391(10125): 1085–1096. https://doi.org/https://doi.org/10.1016/S0140-6736(18)30136-3

Thu, M. S., Campbell, B. J., Hirankarn, N., Nopsopon, T., Ondee, T., Hall, S. R. et al. (2025). Cannabis and cannabinoid-microbiome interactions in varied clinical contexts: A comprehensive systematic review. *Biomedicine and Pharmacotherapy*, 182: 117764. https://doi.org/https://doi.org/10.1016/j.biopha.2024.117764

Tijani, A. O., Thakur, D., Mishra, D., Frempong, D., Chukwunyere, U. I., and Puri, A. (2021). Delivering therapeutic cannabinoids via skin: Current state and future perspectives. *Journal of Controlled Release*, 334: 427–451. https://doi.org/https://doi.org/10.1016/j.jconrel.2021.05.005

Tramèr, M. R., Carroll, D., Campbell, F. A., Reynolds, D. J. M., Moore, R. A., and McQuay, H. J. (2001). Cannabinoids for control of chemotherapy induced nausea and vomiting: Quantitative systematic review. *British Medical Journal*, 323(7303): 16–21. https://doi.org/10.1136/bmj.323.7303.16

Überall, M. A. (2020). A review of scientific evidence for THC:CBD oromucosal spray (nabiximols) in the management of chronic pain. *Journal of Pain Research*,13: 399–410. Dove Medical Press Ltd. https://doi.org/10.2147/JPR.S240011

Varadi, G., Zhu, Z., Crowley, H. D., Moulin, M., Dey, R., Lewis, E. D. et al. (2023). Examining the Systemic Bioavailability of Cannabidiol and Tetrahydrocannabinol from a Novel Transdermal Delivery System in Healthy Adults: A Single-Arm, Open-Label, Exploratory Study. *Advances in Therapy*, 40(1): 282–293. https://doi.org/10.1007/s12325-022-02345-5

Vinette, B., Côté, J., El-Akhras, A., Mrad, H., Chicoine, G., and Bilodeau, K. (2022). Routes of administration, reasons for use, and approved indications of medical cannabis in oncology: a scoping review. *BMC Cancer*, 22(1): 319. https://doi.org/10.1186/s12885-022-09378-7

Wolowich, W. R., Greif, R., Kleine-Brueggeney, M., Bernhard, W., and Theiler, L. (2019). Minimal Physiologically Based Pharmacokinetic Model of Intravenously and Orally Administered Delta-9-Tetrahydrocannabinol in Healthy Volunteers. *European Journal of Drug Metabolism and Pharmacokinetics*, 44(5): 691–711. https://doi.org/10.1007/s13318-019-00559-7

Wu, J. (2019). Cannabis, cannabinoid receptors, and endocannabinoid system: yesterday, today, and tomorrow. *Acta Pharmacologica Sinica*, 40(3): 297–299. https://doi.org/10.1038/s41401-019-0210-3

Yassin, M., Oron, A., and Robinson, D. (2019). Effect of adding medical cannabis to analgesic treatment in patients with low back pain related to fibromyalgia: an observational cross-over single centre study. In *Clin. Exp. Rheumatol.* (Vol. 37).

Zgair, A., Wong, J. C., Lee, J. B., Mistry, J., Sivak, O., Wasan, K. M. et al. (2016). Dietary fats and pharmaceutical lipid excipients increase systemic exposure to orally administered cannabis and cannabis-based medicines. In *Am. J. Transl. Res.* (Vol. 8). Retrieved from www.ajtr.org

Zhang, M., Chen, T., Lu, X., Lan, X., Chen, Z., and Lu, S. (2024). G protein-coupled receptors (GPCRs): advances in structures, mechanisms and drug discovery. *Signal Transduction and Targeted Therapy*, 9(1): 88. https://doi.org/10.1038/s41392-024-01803-6

Zipursky, J. S., Bogler, O. D., and Stall, N. M. (2020). Edible cannabis. *Canadian Medical Association Journal*, 92(7): E162.

Chapter 9

Action of Cannabis Constituents in the Modulation of Oxidative Stress and Inflammation

Lívia Alves Figueiras, Mateus Henrique de Almeida da Costa, Francisco das Chagas Pereira de Andrade, Maria Hillana Nunes and *Anderson Nogueira Mendes**

1. Introduction

Cannabis sativa contains 566 identified and isolated compounds, spanning more than 18 classes of secondary metabolites primarily found in the plant's flowers and leaves (Hosu and Oyedeji 2022). Among these, 125 are cannabinoids, 198 are non-cannabinoids, and 120 are terpenes, accounting for a total of 443 substances. Additional compounds identified in 2021 include 2 alkaloids, 34 flavonoids, 42 phenols, and 3 sterols (dos Santos and Romão 2023; Fordjour et al. 2023; Muhsien et al. 2022).

Cannabis sativa has been used for medicinal purposes for more than 6,000 years. To date, over 100 plant-derived cannabinoids, also known as phytocannabinoids, have been documented. One of the most prominent is tetrahydrocannabinol (THC), a psychoactive compound associated with several key processes in sepsis, including immune modulation, inflammation, and redox regulation (Ben Amar 2006; Daniel Lafreniere and Lehmann 2017).

The THC derivative Δ9-THC exhibits psychoactive, analgesic (antinociceptive), anti-inflammatory, euphoric, antioxidant, and antiemetic properties. Cannabidiol (CBD) and its derivatives are recognized for their anxiolytic, antipsychotic, antinociceptive, antispasmodic, anti-inflammatory, and antioxidant effects (Bartkowiak-Wieczorek et al. 2024). When combined, Δ9-THC and CBD enhance the biosynthesis of inflammatory mediators, thereby reducing the overall inflammatory profile.

The Endocannabinoid System (ECS) is a highly complex and widely distributed biological system involved in numerous physiological and pathological processes (Charytoniuk et al. 2022). This neuronal system regulates functions such as attention, anxiety, mood, memory, appetite, reward mechanisms, and immune responses. Interactions mediate the effects of cannabinoid ligands and various neurotransmitter systems, including dopamine, serotonin, glutamate, norepinephrine, opioids, and GABA (Brunt and Bossong 2022).

Laboratory of Science in Innovation and Technology – LACITEC, Department of Biophysics and Physiology, Federal University of Piauí, 64049-550, Teresina, Piauí, Brazil.
* Corresponding author: anderson.mendes@ufpi.edu.br

DOI: 10.1201/9781003668190-11

The two primary endogenous cannabinoids—anandamide and 2-arachidonoylglycerol—are small molecules derived from arachidonic acid that act on a class of G-protein-coupled receptors. Among them, the CB1 receptor is densely distributed in brain regions involved in motor control, cognition, emotional processing, motivated behavior, and homeostasis (de Fonseca et al. 2004).

There are two major cannabinoid receptors. CB1 is predominantly located in the brain and central nervous system (CNS) (Kendall and Yudowski 2017), while CB2 is mainly found in the spleen and immune cells, with lower expression in peripheral tissues under normal physiological conditions (Hashiesh et al. 2023). CB1 is responsible for the psychotropic effects of THC and regulates neurotransmitter release through retrograde signaling by inhibiting presynaptic calcium channels (Augustin and Lovinger 2022; Palmer 2006). Figure 1 shows the chemical structures of the two main phytocannabinoids extracted from the Cannabis sativa plant: Δ^9-tetrahydrocannabinol (THC) and cannabidiol (CBD). Both are compounds with the same molecular formula ($C_{21}H_{30}O_2$), but exhibit important structural differences that result in distinct pharmacological properties. This relationship between chemical structure and biological activity is a classic example of the importance of molecular conformation in the pharmacodynamics of bioactive compounds.

CB2 receptors, in contrast, are most abundantly expressed in immune cells. Their activation modulates immune responses by lowering cyclic adenosine monophosphate (cAMP) levels and altering signaling pathways, including p38 and NF-κB. This results in predominantly anti-inflammatory effects (Atalay Ekiner et al. 2022a; Chen et al. 2023; Zachut et al. 2025). Several studies have demonstrated that cannabinoids can reduce oxidative stress at both the mitochondrial and cellular levels. These effects involve the activation of specific endocannabinoid receptors, such as CB1 and CB2, which, in turn, modulate the expression of microRNAs that regulate immune cell function (Carvalho et al. 2024; Rahn and Hohmann 2009).

Both THC and CBD activate the CB1 and CB2 cannabinoid receptors (Bartkowiak-Wieczorek et al. 2024; Cabral et al. 2015) and exhibit a wide range of biological activities, including modulation of appetite, pain, and immune function (Carvalho et al. 2024; dos Santos and Romão 2023; Pantoja-Ruiz et al. 2022). They also possess potent antioxidant properties, such as reducing reactive oxygen species (ROS) (Pagano et al. 2023; Raja et al. 2020), anti-inflammatory effects, and immune modulation mediated by CB2 receptors (Cabral and Griffin-Thomas 2009; Rahaman and Ganguly 2021; Zhu et al. 2000).

Although CBD has lower affinity for CB1 and CB2 receptors (Etemad et al. 2022; Peng et al. 2022; Vučkovic et al. 2018), it interacts with other molecular targets, including TRPV1, PPAR-γ, and 5-HT1A receptors, which are involved in antioxidant activity and pain modulation (Alexander et al. 2025; Martinez Naya et al. 2023; Peng et al. 2022). CBD also exhibits direct antioxidant action (Kletkiewicz et al. 2024; Martinelli et al. 2022; Szőke et al. 2023) and promotes antioxidant defense by inducing enzymes such as HO-1 (Bravo Iniguez et al. 2024; Martinelli et al. 2022), SOD, and GPx (Chen et al. 2023; Jîtcă et al. 2023; Martinez Naya et al. 2023). Furthermore, it has prominent anti-inflammatory properties, reducing pro-inflammatory cytokines such as IL-6, IL-1β, IL-17, and TNF-α (Aswad et al. 2022; Bravo Iniguez et al. 2024; Henshaw et al. 2021b), and inhibiting the activation of the transcription factor NF-κB (Atalay Ekiner et al. 2022a; Chen et al. 2023).

Cannabis-derived terpenes and flavonoids are increasingly recognized in the literature as promising bioactive compounds due to their diverse therapeutic effects. Terpenes interact directly

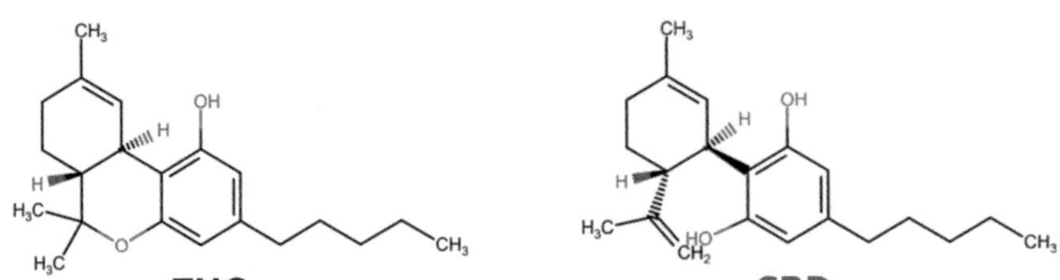

Figure 1: Molecular Structures of Cannabinoids THC and CBD.

with cellular receptors such as TRPV1 and GABA, modulating both neuronal and inflammatory responses (Araújo et al. 2023; Jansen et al. 2019). They also enhance the actions of cannabinoids through the "entourage effect" (André et al. 2024; Ferber et al. 2019; LaVigne et al. 2021). Their antioxidant effects are reflected in their ability to neutralize lipid peroxidation (Del Prado-Audelo et al. 2021; Rocha et al. 2020), and they also inhibit pro-inflammatory cytokines and enzymes, including COX-2 (Liktor-Busa et al. 2021; Wang et al. 2023).

Cannabis flavonoids also exhibit strong antioxidant potential by neutralizing free radicals (Cásedas et al. 2022; Cui et al. 2023; Tumilaar et al. 2023) and boosting the activity of antioxidant enzymes such as glutathione (Cásedas et al. 2022; Stasiłowicz-Krzemień et al. 2023; Vitorović et al. 2021). Moreover, they regulate key signaling pathways, such as MAPK, which are involved in inflammatory responses and cellular stress (Faiz et al. 2024; Iqbal and Matsabisa 2024; Tomko et al. 2020). Notably, certain flavonoids, such as cannflavins A and B, are effective at inhibiting prostaglandin production and the COX-2 enzyme, thereby playing a significant role in reducing inflammation (Bautista et al. 2021; Eggers et al. 2019). These characteristics make terpenes and flavonoids attractive targets for research and the development of new therapeutic agents derived from Cannabis sativa.

As summarized in Table 1, in addition to their affinity for CB1 and CB2 receptors and their analgesic potential, THC and CBD also display anti-inflammatory and antioxidant properties.

Table 1: Mechanisms of Action and Effects of Cannabinoids, Terpenes, and Flavonoids.

Compound	Mechanism of Action	Oxidative Stress Modulation	Anti-Inflammatory Effects
THC	- Activates CB1 and CB2 receptors (Bartkowiak-Wieczorek et al. 2024; Cabral et al. 2015); - Modulates appetite, pain, and immune function (Carvalho et al. 2024; Nayak et al. 2023; Pantoja-Ruiz et al. 2022).	- Reduces reactive oxygen species (ROS) (Pagano et al. 2023; Raja et al. 2020).	- Modulates the immune system via CB2 receptor (Cabral and Griffin-Thomas 2009; Rahaman and Ganguly 2021; Zhu et al. 2000).
CBD	- Lower affinity for CB1 and CB2 (Etemad et al. 2022; Peng et al. 2022; Vučkovic et al. 2018); - Acts on TRPV1, PPAR-γ, and 5-HT1A receptors (Alexander et al. 2025; Martinez Naya et al. 2023; Peng et al. 2022).	- Direct antioxidant activity (Kletkiewicz et al. 2024; Martinelli et al. 2022; Szőke et al. 2023). - Induces antioxidant enzymes such as HO-1 (Bravo Iniguez et al. 2024; Martinelli et al. 2022). - Stimulates enzymes such as SOD and GPx (Bryś et al. 2025; Jîtcă et al. 2023; Martinez Naya et al. 2023).	- Reduces pro-inflammatory cytokines IL-6, IL-1β, IL-17, TNF-α (Aswad et al. 2022; Bravo Iniguez et al. 2024; Henshaw et al. 2021b); - Inhibits NF-κB activation (Atalay Ekiner et al. 2022a; Chen et al. 2023).
Terpenes	- Enhance the effects of cannabinoids – the "entourage effect" (André et al. 2024; Ferber et al. 2019; LaVigne et al. 2021); - Act on TRPV1 and GABA receptors (Araújo et al. 2023; Jansen et al. 2019).	- Neutralize lipid peroxidation (Del Prado-Audelo et al. 2021; Rocha et al. 2020).	- Inhibit pro-inflammatory cytokines and enzymes such as COX-2 (Liktor-Busa et al. 2021; Wang et al. 2023).
Flavonoids	- Neutralize free radicals (Cásedas et al. 2022; Cui et al. 2023; Tumilaar et al. 2023); - Regulate signaling pathways such as MAPK (Faiz et al. 2024; Iqbal and Matsabisa 2024; Tomko et al. 2020).	- Increase antioxidant enzymes such as glutathione (Cásedas et al. 2022; Stasiłowicz-Krzemień et al. 2023; Vitorović et al. 2021).	- Inhibit prostaglandins and COX-2. Example: Cannflavins A and B reduce inflammatory processes (Bautista et al. 2021; Eggers et al. 2019).

Moreover, the combination of these cannabinoids with terpenes and flavonoids from Cannabis sativa produces synergistic effects across multiple pathways, including neuroprotection and tissue repair, maintenance of redox balance, protection against oxidative damage, and the reduction of chronic inflammation.

2. Anti-Inflammatory and Antioxidant Effects: Review of Studies on Cannabis in Reducing Oxidative Stress and Modulating Inflammation. Discussion of Experimental Models Used

Cannabinoids such as cannabidiol (CBD) and tetrahydrocannabinol (THC) have attracted growing therapeutic interest in recent years due to their antioxidant and anti-inflammatory properties. Studies by Dos-Santos-Pereira et al. (2020) revealed that CBD exerts a significant anti-inflammatory effect in microglial cells by inhibiting the release of pro-inflammatory cytokines such as TNF-α and IL-1β, primarily through receptor-independent mechanisms.

In the same study, CBD was also shown to prevent microglial inflammation by inhibiting glucose consumption and glucose-dependent synthesis of NADPH, a crucial cofactor required for the generation of reactive oxygen species (ROS) by NADPH oxidase (Dos-Santos-Pereira et al. 2020). This dual mechanism—direct intrinsic antioxidant action and suppression of NADPH production—enhances the compound's anti-inflammatory effects.

In both *in vivo* and *in vitro* experimental models, CBD and THC have demonstrated the ability to modulate key signaling pathways associated with oxidative stress reduction, both under baseline conditions and in response to tissue injury—particularly when applied at appropriate concentrations (Atalay et al. 2019). This modulation enhances cellular defense mechanisms against oxidative stress and reduces inflammation. These effects are closely associated with regulatory pathways such as Nrf2, a master regulator of antioxidant responses (Atalay Ekiner et al. 2022b).

In recent studies, both CBD and THC have been shown to modulate and regulate the expression of key cytokines involved in the inflammatory response (Figure 2). Henshaw et al. (2021a) report that, in *in vivo* models, cannabinoids can reduce levels of pro-inflammatory cytokines such as IL-6, as well as chemokines critical for immune cell migration. Research using systemic inflammation models suggests that cannabis, through compounds such as CBD, may modulate immune signaling pathways—thereby decreasing the release of pro-inflammatory mediators while simultaneously promoting controlled immunosuppressive effects (Peyravian et al. 2020).

In intestinal inflammation models, CBD was shown to reduce ROS levels under both baseline and oxidative stress conditions (Cocetta et al. 2021). Moreover, CBD preserved the integrity of intestinal epithelial tight junctions under inflammatory conditions, indicating its potential as an adjuvant therapy for inflammatory bowel diseases.

Liu et al. (2020) demonstrated that the NLRP3 inflammasome—an essential component of the inflammatory process—can be inhibited by CBD in human monocytes, resulting in reduced IL-1β production and consequent mitigation of tissue damage. This represents another key anti-inflammatory mechanism through which CBD exerts its effects. Additionally, recent studies indicate that, when used at appropriate doses and in specific contexts, CBD may help regulate immune responses and protect against pro-inflammatory cytokines (Henshaw et al. 2021a; Cocetta et al. 2021). Table 2 summarizes the main molecular mechanisms and signaling pathways modulated by cannabinoids (CBD and THC) in *in vitro* and *in vivo* studies.

In models of arthritis and other systemic inflammatory conditions, cannabinoids have been shown to modulate innate and adaptive immune responses (Malfait et al., 2000). CBD, in particular, has been shown to reduce chronic inflammation across various experimental contexts. The anti-inflammatory and antioxidant mechanisms of cannabis are complex and involve multiple cellular signaling pathways. The ability of cannabinoids to simultaneously modulate different

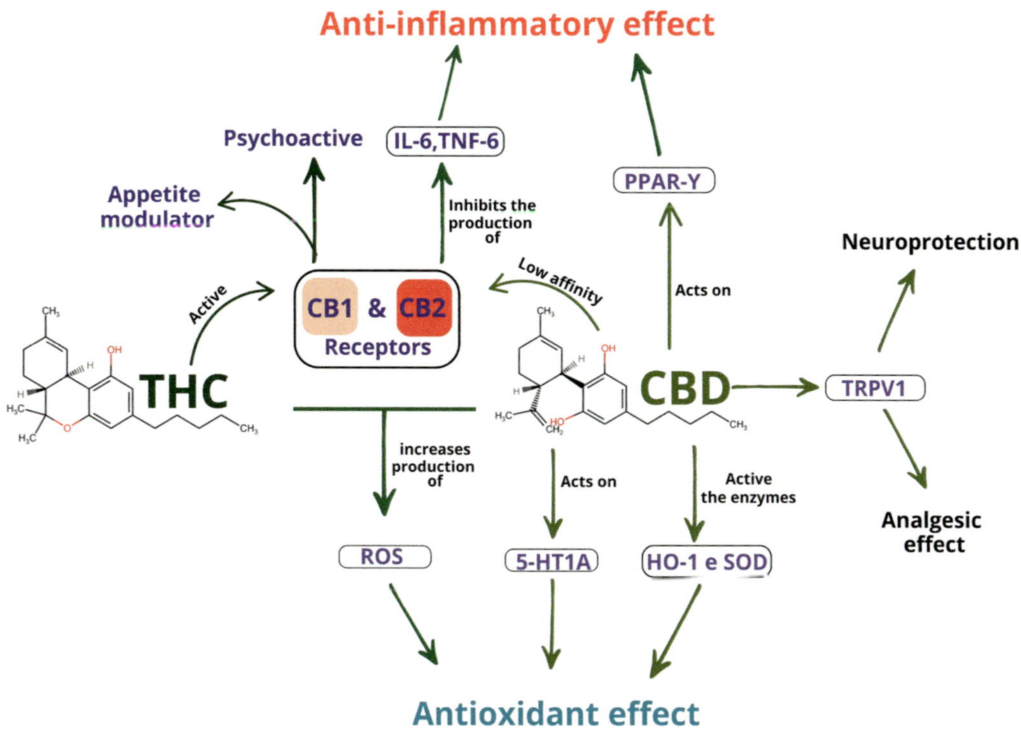

Figure 2: Key anti-inflammatory and antioxidant mechanisms of THC and CBD.

aspects of the inflammatory response and oxidative stress suggests their therapeutic potential in conditions where these processes are prominent, although further studies are needed to optimize their clinical use. Figure 3 outlines the main effects of modulation exerted by THC and CBD as anti-inflammatory agents.

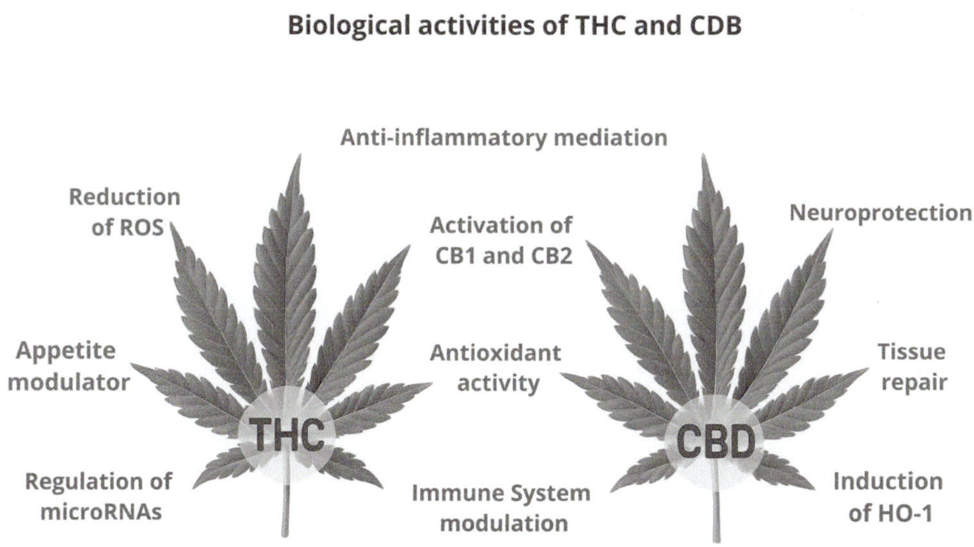

Figure 3: Anti-Inflammatory Mediation.

Table 2: Overview of the main molecular mechanisms and signaling pathways modulated by cannabinoids (CBD and THC) in *in vitro* and *in vivo* studies, highlighting their effects on inflammatory processes and oxidative stress.

Cannabinoid(s)	Pathway/Mechanism	Study Model	Main Effects	References
CBD	NF-κB/ROS/NLRP3	BV-2 microglial cells	1. Reduction in ROS production; 2. Decrease in TNF-α and IL-1β; 3. Inhibition of microglial activation; 4. Modulation of glucose metabolism.	(dos-Santos-Pereira et al. 2020)
CBD	Nrf2/NF-κB	Human endothelial cells	1. Increase in antioxidant enzymes; 2. Reduction in oxidative stress; 3. Elevation of HO-1 and NQO1; 4. Modulation of antioxidant response.	(Atalay Ekiner et al. 2022)
CBD + THC	STAT3/TYK2/IL-6	THP-1 macrophages	1. Inhibition of cytokine storm; 2. Reduction of IL-6 and IL-1β; 3. Decrease in NLRP3 activation; 4. Regulation of innate immune response.	(Liu et al. 2020)
CBD	Adenosine A2A	Mouse model of lung injury	1. Reduction in neutrophils; 2. Decrease in TNF-α and IL-6; 3. Improvement in lung function; 4. Protection of lung tissue.	(Ribeiro et al. 2012)
THC	CB1/CB2/TLR4	Primary microglial cells	1. Inhibition of NF-κB; 2. Reduction of COX-2; 3. Decrease in iNOS; 4. Modulation of microglial activation.	(Kozela et al. 2010)
CBD	PPARγ/NF-κB	Mouse model of colitis	1. Reduction of intestinal inflammation; 2. Decrease in TNF-α; 3. Strengthening of intestinal barrier; 4. Protection of mucosa.	(Borrelli et al. 2009)
CBD	Wnt/β-catenin	Alzheimer's model	1. Reduction of neuroinflammation; 2. Decrease in oxidative stress; 3. Increase in neuroprotection; 4. Modulation of synaptic plasticity.	(Vallée et al. 2017)
THC + CBD	mTOR/AMPK	Tumor cells	1. Inhibition of cell proliferation; 2. Increase in autophagy; 3. Reduction in ROS; 4. Modulation of energy metabolism.	(Massi et al. 2013)
CBD	JAK/STAT	T helper cells	1. Inhibition of Th17 differentiation; 2. Decrease in IL-17; 3. Increase in regulatory T cells; 4. Modulation of adaptive response.	(Kozela et al. 2010)
CBD	MAPK/ERK	Cortical neurons	1. Increase in neuroprotection; 2. Reduction of apoptosis; 3. Elevation of BDNF; 4. Modulation of neuronal survival.	(Campos et al. 2016)
THC	CB2/PI3K/Akt	RAW264.7 macrophages	1. Decrease in inflammation; 2. Reduction in NO; 3. Decrease in COX-2; 4. Modulation of macrophage activation.	(Nichols and Kaplan 2020)
CBD	PPAR/NF-κB	Endothelial cells	1. Reduction in leukocyte adhesion; 2. Decrease in VCAM-1; 3. Reduction in ICAM-1; 4. Endothelial protection.	(Rajesh et al. 2010)
CBD + THC	TLR3/TLR4	Dendritic cells	1. Reduction in pro-inflammatory cytokines; 2. Increase in IL-10; 3. Decrease in CD80/CD86; 4. Modulation of antigen presentation.	(Juknat et al. 2012)
CBD	Keap1/Nrf2/ARE	Fibroblasts	1. Increase in GSH; 2. Elevation of NQO1; 3. Increase in HO-1; 4. Activation of antioxidant response.	(Juknat et al. 2012)
THC	CB1/mTOR	Neuronal cells	1. Reduction in excitotoxicity; 2. Increase in autophagy; 3. Decrease in intracellular Ca^{2+}; 4. Protection against neuronal death.	(Blázquez et al. 2015)

Legend:↑: Increase/Activation.↓: Decrease/Inhibition.NF-κB: Nuclear Factor kappa B.ROS: Reactive Oxygen Species.NLRP3: NOD-like Receptor Protein 3.Nrf2: Erythroid Nuclear Factor 2. STAT3: Signal Transducer and Activator of Transcription 3.TYK2: Tyrosine Kinase 2.PPARγ: Peroxisome Proliferator-Activated Receptor gamma.mTOR: Mammalian Target of Rapamycin. MAPK: Mitogen-Activated Protein Kinase.PI3K: Phosphoinositide 3-Kinase.ARE: Antioxidant Response Element.HO-1: Heme Oxygenase-1.NQO1: NAD(P)H Quinone Dehydrogenase 1. GSH: Glutathione. iNOS: Inducible Nitric Oxide Synthase. COX-2: Cyclooxygenase 2.

3. Therapeutic Potential of Cannabis in Inflammatory Diseases

In recent years, Cannabis sativa and its derivatives have been extensively studied for their therapeutic potential in inflammatory and neurodegenerative diseases. Cannabidiol (CBD) and tetrahydrocannabinol (THC) exhibit anti-inflammatory and neuroprotective properties and are considered potential allies in modulating inflammation and oxidative stress in various pathological conditions (Almeida et al. 2024). Recent studies suggest that activating the endocannabinoid system can reduce cellular damage, promote neurogenesis, and improve the quality of life of patients with inflammatory and neurodegenerative diseases (Cardoso et al. 2025).

Oxidative stress is a key factor in the progression of chronic inflammatory and neurodegenerative diseases, as it contributes to programmed cell death and perpetuates the inflammatory response. The imbalance between the production of reactive oxygen species (ROS) and the body's antioxidant capacity has been linked to diseases such as multiple sclerosis, Parkinson's disease, and Alzheimer's disease (De Souza et al. 2023). CBD has demonstrated significant antioxidant effects, reducing ROS levels and modulating the inflammatory response, thereby slowing the progression of these diseases and minimizing cellular damage (Gavioli et al. 2024).

Cannabinoid modulation of inflammation occurs through interaction with the CB1 and CB2 receptors of the endocannabinoid system, which play a crucial role in immune and neural homeostasis. Research indicates that CBD may reduce the production of pro-inflammatory cytokines, such as TNF-α and IL-6, which are essential for controlling inflammatory diseases like rheumatoid arthritis and multiple sclerosis (Campos and Schwingel 2023). Furthermore, CBD's action on microglia, the immune cells of the central nervous system, may reduce neuroinflammation in neurodegenerative diseases such as Alzheimer's disease (Leandro et al. 2023).

CBD use has also been investigated in the management of chronic pain associated with inflammatory diseases. Studies indicate that its action on vanilloid receptors (TRPV1) can reduce pain hypersensitivity and modulate nociceptive response in patients with fibromyalgia and inflammatory neuropathies (Cardoso et al. 2025). Additionally, its interaction with serotonin receptors may improve mood and sleep quality, both of which are essential for patients with chronic diseases (Salustiano and Bortoli 2022).

In the context of neurodegenerative diseases, the neuroprotective action of cannabinoids has been widely explored. Studies suggest that CBD may reduce glutamate-mediated excitotoxicity and prevent neuronal death in diseases such as amyotrophic lateral sclerosis (ALS) (De Almeida et al. 2024). Moreover, its anxiolytic effect may benefit patients with neurodegenerative disorders, reducing symptoms of anxiety and depression frequently associated with these conditions (Lopes et al. 2023).

Emerging research also indicates that cannabis may play a relevant role in modulating the immune response. In experimental models of multiple sclerosis, CBD has been shown to reduce the infiltration of inflammatory cells in the central nervous system, decreasing the severity of motor symptoms and promoting neuroprotection (Teixeira 2023). These findings strengthen the therapeutic potential of cannabinoids as a complementary approach for inflammatory and neurodegenerative diseases.

The impact of cannabis on the treatment of inflammatory and neurodegenerative diseases has been widely studied in the scientific literature. Chronic inflammatory diseases such as rheumatoid arthritis, inflammatory bowel disease, and autoimmune diseases are associated with increased oxidative stress and immune system dysfunction. In this perspective, cannabinoids, especially cannabidiol (CBD), have demonstrated a significant role in modulating the inflammatory response and reducing cellular damage caused by oxidative stress (Almeida et al. 2024).

In addition to rheumatoid arthritis, cannabis compounds have shown efficacy in controlling gastrointestinal inflammation. According to Sampaio et al. (2021), studies indicate that cannabinoids can reduce inflammation in inflammatory bowel diseases such as Crohn's disease and ulcerative colitis. CBD has been identified as a promising therapeutic alternative due to its ability to modulate immune function and reduce symptoms associated with these diseases.

In autoimmune diseases, cannabinoids can reduce autoimmunity by minimizing the immune response against the body's own tissues. In multiple sclerosis, for example, where myelin is destroyed by the immune system, cannabinoids show potential to reduce inflammation and slow the progression of neuronal destruction. These effects appear to be mediated by the activation of cannabinoid receptors in the central nervous system and immune cells (Sampaio et al. 2021; Cardoso et al. 2025).

Neurodegenerative diseases such as Alzheimer's, Parkinson's, and multiple sclerosis are strongly linked to inflammatory processes and oxidative stress. Damage caused by reactive oxygen species (ROS) in the central nervous system can accelerate neuronal degeneration, impairing cognitive and motor functions. The therapeutic use of cannabis has been explored as an alternative to mitigate these processes and offer new treatment pathways for these diseases (De Souza et al. 2023; Gavioli et al. 2024).

According to De Souza et al. (2023), modulation of the endocannabinoid system by CBD has the potential to reduce brain inflammation and mitigate the production of free radicals. These effects are particularly relevant in the treatment of Alzheimer's disease, where neuroinflammation and oxidative stress are key factors in disease progression. Additionally, CBD has neuroprotective properties, which may contribute to the preservation of cognitive functions in patients with neurodegenerative diseases (Leandro et al. 2023).

In multiple sclerosis, a study by De Almeida et al. (2024) found that cannabinoid use reduces muscle spasticity, relieves pain, and improves motor function. These effects are attributed to the anti-inflammatory and antioxidant actions of cannabinoids, which promote a better quality of life for patients.

In Parkinson's disease, tetrahydrocannabinol (THC) has shown benefits in treating neurological symptoms such as tremors and dystonia. The combination of THC and CBD has been shown to improve mobility and reduce pain, allowing patients to perform their daily activities with greater autonomy. The neuroprotective effect of these compounds may be associated with modulation of the inflammatory response in the central nervous system and a reduction in ROS-induced damage to dopaminergic neurons (De Almeida et al. 2024; Cardoso 2019).

Although cannabinoids, especially CBD, have demonstrated benefits in controlling oxidative stress and inflammation, it is essential to consider their potential adverse effects. The therapeutic use of cannabis may result in side effects such as drowsiness, changes in appetite, and mood alterations. Furthermore, drug interactions should be closely monitored, as cannabinoids may interfere with drug metabolism, altering their efficacy (De Almeida et al. 2024; Lopes et al 2023).

Medical supervision is essential to ensure the safety and effectiveness of cannabis treatment. Dosage and administration methods should be adjusted to individual patient needs, taking into account factors such as age, comorbidities, and disease type. The choice of cannabinoid type (CBD or THC) and the administration route (oils, capsules, and vaporization) should be personalized according to the clinical condition and therapeutic goals (Salustiano and Bortoli 2022).

Cannabis and its derivatives, especially CBD, have shown great therapeutic potential in treating inflammatory and neurodegenerative diseases. Its role in reducing oxidative stress and modulating the inflammatory response opens new possibilities for managing chronic conditions such as rheumatoid arthritis, inflammatory bowel disease, and neurodegenerative diseases (Alves et al. 2022; Florio 2024).

Research indicates that the use of cannabinoids may represent a promising alternative for patients suffering from inflammatory and neurodegenerative diseases, highlighting the anti-inflammatory and antioxidant properties of these compounds. CBD, in particular, has been shown to modulate the endocannabinoid system, providing relief for inflammatory and neurological conditions. By directly acting on inflammatory pathways, CBD reduces the production of pro-inflammatory cytokines, helping control diseases such as rheumatoid arthritis, Crohn's disease, and multiple sclerosis (Teixeira 2023).

Furthermore, CBD's antioxidant effect may protect against cellular damage caused by oxidative stress, a common factor in many chronic diseases. The use of cannabis has also proven effective in reducing symptoms associated with neurological disorders, such as Parkinson's and Alzheimer's, by modulating the inflammatory response in the central nervous system and reducing the impact of reactive oxygen species (De Almeida et al. 2024; Gavioli et al. 2024).

Despite the therapeutic potential of cannabis, more clinical studies are needed to deepen the understanding of its mechanisms of action and long-term effects. Additionally, the regulation of medicinal cannabis use must progress to ensure greater safety for patients and healthcare professionals. The clinical application of cannabis requires a careful approach, based on robust scientific evidence, to ensure its use is safe and effective (Cardoso 2019; Da Silva et al. 2022).

Thus, medicinal cannabis presents itself as a promising therapeutic strategy for inflammatory and neurodegenerative diseases, provided it is used under medical supervision and supported by scientific studies. Ongoing research may provide new approaches to treating these conditions, significantly improving patients' quality of life.

4. Challenges and Opportunities: Limitations of Current Research. Future Opportunities for Clinical and Preclinical Studies

The current challenges surrounding the use of cannabis in clinical research are complex and multifactorial. One of the main challenges is the divergence in federal and state regulations across different countries. This makes it difficult to standardize studies and compare results between different research centers (Cooper et al. 2021). In addition, variability in chemical composition, mainly driven by different cultivation methods, the lack of standardization in extraction methods, and other factors that hinder assay reproducibility, are limiting factors for the development of more robust studies (Goodin et al. 2023).

Different formulations, extraction methods, and administration routes yield products with varied chemical and pharmacokinetic profiles, making direct comparisons between studies difficult. This heterogeneity compromises the reproducibility of results and the ability to establish clear therapeutic guidelines, limiting the clinical application of cannabis in the treatment of inflammatory diseases (Chandra et al. 2019).

Regulatory and legal barriers also play a critical role in limiting the advancement of research and access to pharmaceutical-grade products. In many countries, cannabis is still classified as a controlled substance, which restricts its availability for scientific and medical purposes. The absence of clear and unified regulations makes it difficult to conduct clinical studies and produce standardized medications, perpetuating a scenario of uncertainty regarding their therapeutic potential (The Health Effects of Cannabis and Cannabinoids 2017).

Another significant challenge is the scarcity of robust, randomized, placebo-controlled, long-term clinical trials. Most available studies have methodological limitations, such as small sample sizes and short intervention periods, which compromise the validity of the results. The lack of consistent data on the long-term safety and efficacy of cannabis makes it difficult to create reliable clinical guidelines and adopt this therapy on a large scale (Volkow et al. 2014).

The variability in cannabis composition also represents a complex challenge. The plant contains hundreds of compounds, including cannabinoids, terpenes, and flavonoids, that interact with each other through the so-called "entourage effect." While this interaction may enhance therapeutic effects, it also makes it difficult to isolate the components responsible for specific benefits. An incomplete understanding of these mechanisms of action limits the development of evidence-based treatments and the optimization of formulations for specific conditions, such as inflammatory diseases (Russo 2011).

On the other hand, it is important to highlight that future opportunities for clinical and preclinical studies involving cannabis and its derivatives are promising. The growing acceptance of medicinal cannabis has stimulated the development of new research methods and brought new investments in analytical technologies. The 2024 Cannabis Clinical Outcomes Research Conference (CCORC) showed significant and promising advances in this regard (Goodin et al. 2024).

There is increasing interest in the development of new formulations containing cannabis derivatives, the investigation of new cannabinoids, and the study of the endocannabinoid system. Integrated with technological advances, such as artificial intelligence and Big Data analysis, and with the expansion of international research networks, more comprehensive therapeutic protocols have accelerated the development of high-quality, multicenter clinical trials with cannabis (Campos et al. 2016).

5. Conclusion and Perspectives

The growing body of research on Cannabis sativa and its bioactive compounds underscores their significant therapeutic potential in modulating oxidative stress and inflammation, key pathological processes in numerous chronic and degenerative diseases. The synergistic action of cannabinoids such as THC and CBD, along with terpenes and flavonoids, demonstrates a multifaceted mechanism of action that targets the endocannabinoid system (ECS) and other molecular pathways. These interactions result in reduced production of pro-inflammatory cytokines, enhanced antioxidant defenses, and neuroprotective effects, offering promising applications in conditions ranging from autoimmune disorders to neurodegenerative diseases.

However, translating these findings into clinical practice faces considerable challenges. The inherent variability in cannabis composition due to differences in cultivation, extraction methods, and strain specificity complicates the standardization of therapeutic formulations. Moreover, the legal and regulatory landscape surrounding cannabis research remains fragmented, limiting the scope and reproducibility of studies. While preclinical evidence is compelling, the lack of large-scale, long-term clinical trials hinders the establishment of definitive dosing guidelines and safety profiles. Addressing these limitations requires a concerted effort to harmonize research methodologies, expand clinical investigations, and develop evidence-based regulatory frameworks that facilitate access to medical cannabis while ensuring patient safety.

Looking ahead, the future of cannabis-based medicine lies in deepening our understanding of the pharmacodynamics of its constituents, particularly the entourage effect, which could unlock new therapeutic synergies. Advances in biotechnology and data science may further refine extraction techniques and personalize treatment approaches. As societal acceptance grows and scientific rigor strengthens, Cannabis sativa is poised to become an integral component of integrative medicine, offering novel solutions for managing inflammation and oxidative stress-related disorders. The path forward demands interdisciplinary collaboration, robust clinical validation, and progressive policymaking to fully realize the therapeutic promise of this ancient yet increasingly relevant medicinal plant.

References

Alexander, C., Jeon, J., Nickerson, K., Hassler, S., and Vasefi, M. (2025). CBD and the 5-HT1A receptor: A medicinal and pharmacological review. *Biochemical Pharmacology*, 233: 116742. https://doi.org/https://doi.org/10.1016/j.bcp.2025.116742

André, R., Gomes, A. P., Pereira-Leite, C., Marques-da-Costa, A., Monteiro Rodrigues, L., Sassano, M. et al. (2024). The entourage effect in cannabis medicinal products: A comprehensive review. *Pharmaceuticals*, 17(11). https://doi.org/10.3390/ph17111543

Araújo, M., Almeida, M. B., and Araújo, L. L. N. (2023). The cannabinoids mechanism of action: an overview. *Brazilian Journal Of Pain*, 6(Suppl 2): 109–113. https://doi.org/10.5935/2595-0118.20230028-en

Aswad, M., Hamza, H., Pechkovsky, A., Zikrach, A., Popov, T., Zohar, Y. et al. (2022). High-CBD Extract (CBD-X) Downregulates Cytokine Storm Systemically and Locally in Inflamed Lungs. *Frontiers in Immunology*, 13(May): 1–14. https://doi.org/10.3389/fimmu.2022.875546

Atalay Ekiner, S., Gęgotek, A., and Skrzydlewska, E. (2022a). The molecular activity of cannabidiol in the regulation of Nrf2 system interacting with NF-κB pathway under oxidative stress. *Redox Biology*, 57: 102489. https://doi.org/https://doi.org/10.1016/j.redox.2022.102489

Atalay Ekiner, S., Gęgotek, A., and Skrzydlewska, E. (2022b). The molecular activity of cannabidiol in the regulation of Nrf2 system interacting with NF-κB pathway under oxidative stress. *In Redox Biology* (Vol. 57). Elsevier B.V. https://doi.org/10.1016/j.redox.2022.102489

Atalay Ekiner, S., Gęgotek, A., and Skrzydlewska, E. (2022c). The molecular activity of cannabidiol in the regulation of Nrf2 system interacting with NF-κB pathway under oxidative stress. *Redox Biology*, 57: 102489. https://doi.org/10.1016/j.redox.2022.102489

Atalay, S., Jarocka-Karpowicz, I., and Skrzydlewska, E. (2019). Antioxidative and Anti-Inflammatory Properties of Cannabidiol. *Antioxidants*, 9(1): 21. https://doi.org/10.3390/antiox9010021

Augustin, S. M., and Lovinger, D. M. (2022). Synaptic changes induced by cannabinoid drugs and cannabis use disorder. *Neurobiology of Disease*, 167: 105670. https://doi.org/https://doi.org/10.1016/j.nbd.2022.105670

Bartkowiak-wieczorek, J., Bienert, A., Czora-poczwardowska, K., Kujawski, R., Szulc, M., Mikołajczak, P. et al. (2024). *Cannabis sativa* L . Extract Alleviates Neuropathic Pain and Modulates CB1 and CB2 Receptor Expression in Rat. *Biomolecules*, 14: 1–22.

Bautista, J. L., Yu, S., and Tian, L. (2021). Flavonoids in Cannabis sativa: Biosynthesis, Bioactivities, and Biotechnology. *ACS Omega*, 6(8): 5119 5123. https://doi.org/10.1021/acsomega.1c00318

Ben Amar, M. (2006). Cannabinoids in medicine: A review of their therapeutic potential. *Journal of Ethnopharmacology*, 105(1): 1–25. https://doi.org/https://doi.org/10.1016/j.jep.2006.02.001

Blázquez, C., Chiarlone, A., Bellocchio, L., Resel, E., Pruunsild, P., García-Rincón, D., Sendtner, M., Timmusk, T., Lutz, B., Galve-Roperh, I., and Guzmán, M. (2015). The CB1 cannabinoid receptor signals striatal neuroprotection via a PI3K/Akt/mTORC1/BDNF pathway. *Cell Death and Differentiation*, 22(10): 1618–1629. https://doi.org/10.1038/cdd.2015.11

Borrelli, F., Aviello, G., Romano, B., Orlando, P., Capasso, R., Maiello, F. et al. (2009). Cannabidiol, a safe and non-psychotropic ingredient of the marijuana plant Cannabis sativa, is protective in a murine model of colitis. *Journal of Molecular Medicine*, 87(11): 1111–1121. https://doi.org/10.1007/s00109-009-0512-x

Bravo Iniguez, A., Sun, Q., Cui, Q., Du, M., and Zhu, M. J. (2024). Cannabidiol enhances mitochondrial metabolism and antioxidant defenses in human intestinal epithelial Caco-2 Cells. *Nutrients*, 16(22): 1–12. https://doi.org/10.3390/nu16223843

Brunt, T. M., and Bossong, M. G. (2022). The neuropharmacology of cannabinoid receptor ligands in central signaling pathways. *European Journal of Neuroscience*, 55(4): 909–921. https://doi.org/10.1111/ejn.14982

Bryś, M. S., Olszewski, K., Bartoń, M., and Strachecka, A. (2025). Changes in the activities of antioxidant enzymes in the fat body and hemolymph of *Apis mellifera* L. Due to Pollen Monodiets. *Antioxidants*, 14(1): 1–21. https://doi.org/10.3390/antiox14010069

Cabral, G. A., and Griffin-Thomas, L. T. (2009). Emerging role of the cannabinoid receptor CB 2 in immune regulation: Therapeutic prospects for neuroinflammation. *Expert Reviews in Molecular Medicine*, 11(January), 1–25. https://doi.org/10.1017/S1462399409000957

Cabral, G. A., Rogers, T. J., and Lichtman, A. H. (2015). Turning over a new leaf: cannabinoid and endocannabinoid modulation of immune function. *Journal of Neuroimmune Pharmacology*, 10(2): 193–203. https://doi.org/10.1007/s11481-015-9615-z

Campos, A. C., Fogaça, M. V., Sonego, A. B., and Guimarães, F. S. (2016). Cannabidiol, neuroprotection and neuropsychiatric disorders. *Pharmacological Research*, 112: 119–127. https://doi.org/10.1016/j.phrs.2016.01.033

Carvalho, R. de O., Lopes, H. M., Nogueira, M. A., Alves, M. C., Cano, A. C. S., Soares, V. C. et al. (2024). Nutrological modulation of cannabidiol in the inflammatory processes of athletes: a systematic review. *International Journal of Nutrology*, 17(S3). https://doi.org/10.54448/ijn24s301

Cásedas, G., Moliner, C., Maggi, F., Mazzara, E., and López, V. (2022). Evaluation of two different *Cannabis sativa* L. extracts as antioxidant and neuroprotective agents. *Frontiers in Pharmacology*, 13(September), 1–11. https://doi.org/10.3389/fphar.2022.1009868

Charytoniuk, T., Zywno, H., Berk, K., Bzdega, W., Kolakowski, A., Chabowski, A., and Konstantynowicz-Nowicka, K. (2022). The endocannabinoid system and physical activity—a robust duo in the novel therapeutic approach against metabolic disorders. *International Journal of Molecular Sciences*, 23(6). https://doi.org/10.3390/ijms23063083

Chen, H., Liu, Y., Yu, S., Li, C., Gao, B., and Zhou, X. (2023). Cannabidiol attenuates periodontal inflammation through inhibiting TLR4/NF-κB pathway. *Journal of Periodontal Research*, 58(4): 697–707. https://doi.org/10.1111/jre.13118

Cocetta, V., Governa, P., Borgonetti, V., Tinazzi, M., Peron, G., Catanzaro, D. et al. (2021). Cannabidiol Isolated From *Cannabis sativa* L. Protects intestinal barrier from *in vitro* inflammation and oxidative stress. *Frontiers in Pharmacology*, 12. https://doi.org/10.3389/fphar.2021.641210

Cui, Q., Li, J., and Yu, C. (2023). Extraction and purification of total flavonoids from Cannabis sativa fibers and their evaluation for antioxidant and antibacterial activities. *Textile Research Journal*, 93(1-2): 56–69. https://doi.org/10.1177/00405175221114929

Daniel Lafreniere, J., and Lehmann, C. (2017). Parameters of the endocannabinoid system as novel biomarkers in sepsis and septic shock. *Metabolites*, 7(4). https://doi.org/10.3390/metabo7040055

de Fonseca, F., Del Arco, I., Bermudez-Silva, F. J., Bilbao, A., Cippitelli, A., and Navarro, M. (2004). The endocannabinoid system: physiology and pharmacology. *Alcohol and Alcoholism*, 40(1): 2–14. https://doi.org/10.1093/alcalc/agh110

Del Prado-Audelo, M. L., Cortés, H., Caballero-Florán, I. H., González-Torres, M., Escutia-Guadarrama, L., Bernal-Chávez, S. A. et al. (2021). Therapeutic Applications of Terpenes on Inflammatory Diseases. *Frontiers in Pharmacology*, 12(August), 1–7. https://doi.org/10.3389/fphar.2021.704197

dos Santos, N. A., and Romão, W. (2023). Cannabis–A state of the art about the millenary plant: Part I. *Forensic Chemistry*, 32: 100470.

dos-Santos-Pereira, M., Guimarães, F. S., Del-Bel, E., Raisman-Vozari, R., and Michel, P. P. (2020). Cannabidiol prevents LPS-induced microglial inflammation by inhibiting ROS/NF-κB-dependent signaling and glucose consumption. *GLIA*, 68(3): 561–573. https://doi.org/10.1002/glia.23738

Eggers, C., Fujitani, M., Kato, R., and Smid, S. (2019). Novel cannabis flavonoid, cannflavin A displays both a hormetic and neuroprotective profile against amyloid β-mediated neurotoxicity in PC12 cells: Comparison with geranylated flavonoids, mimulone and diplacone. *Biochemical Pharmacology*, 169: 113609. https://doi.org/https://doi.org/10.1016/j.bcp.2019.08.011

Etemad, L., Karimi, G., Alavi, M. S., and Roohbakhsh, A. (2022). Pharmacological effects of cannabidiol by transient receptor potential channels. *Life Sciences*, 300: 120582. https://doi.org/https://doi.org/10.1016/j.lfs.2022.120582

Faiz, M. B., Naeem, F., Irfan, M., Aslam, M. A., Estevinho, L. M., Ateşşahin, D. A. et al. (2024). Exploring the therapeutic potential of cannabinoids in cancer by modulating signaling pathways and addressing clinical challenges. *Discover Oncology*, 15(1). https://doi.org/10.1007/s12672-024-01356-8

Ferber, S. G., Namdar, D., Hen-Shoval, D., Eger, G., Koltai, H., Shoval, G. et al. (2019). The "Entourage Effect": terpenes coupled with cannabinoids for the treatment of mood disorders and anxiety disorders. *Current Neuropharmacology*, 18(2): 87–96. https://doi.org/10.2174/1570159x17666190903103923

Fordjour, E., Manful, C. F., Sey, A. A., Javed, R., Pham, T. H., Thomas, R. et al. (2023). Cannabis : a multifaceted plant with endless potentials. *Frontiers in Pharmacology*, June, 1–36. https://doi.org/10.3389/fphar.2023.1200269

Hashiesh, H. M., Jha, N. K., Thomas, S. D., Sadek, B., Kumar, S., Adeghate, E. et al. (2023). Targeting the CB (2) receptor to delay progression of cardiovascular diseases. pp. 171–182. *In*: Preedy, V. R., Patel, V. B., and Martin, C. R. (Eds.). Medicinal Usage of Cannabis and Cannabinoids. Academic Press. https://doi.org/https://doi.org/10.1016/B978-0-323-90036-2.00036-3

Henshaw, F. R., Dewsbury, L. S., Lim, C. K., and Steiner, G. Z. (2021a). The effects of cannabinoids on pro- and anti-inflammatory cytokines: a systematic review of *in vivo* studies. *Cannabis and Cannabinoid Research*, 6(3): 177–195. https://doi.org/10.1089/can.2020.0105

Henshaw, F. R., Dewsbury, L. S., Lim, C. K., and Steiner, G. Z. (2021b). The effects of cannabinoids on pro-and anti-inflammatory cytokines: a systematic review of *in vivo* studies. *Cannabis and Cannabinoid Research*, 6(3): 177–195. https://doi.org/10.1089/can.2020.0105

Hosu, Y. S., and Oyedeji, A. O. (2022). The Medicinal Natural Products of Cannabis sativa Linn .: A Review. Molecules, 1–23.

Iqbal, S., and Matsabisa, M. (2024). In silico investigation of cannabinoids from Cannabis sativa leaves as a potential anticancer drug to inhibit MAPK-ERK signaling pathway and EMT induction. *In Silico Pharmacology*, 12(1). https://doi.org/10.1007/s40203-024-00213-4

Jansen, C., Shimoda, L. M. N., Kawakami, J. K., Ang, L., Bacani, A. J., Baker, J. D. et al. (2019). Myrcene and terpene regulation of TRPV1. *Channels*, 13(1), 344–366. https://doi.org/10.1080/19336950.2019.1654347

Jîtcă, G., Ősz, B. E., Vari, C. E., Rusz, C. M., Tero-Vescan, A., and Puşcaş, A. (2023). Cannabidiol: Bridge between Antioxidant Effect, Cellular Protection, and Cognitive and Physical Performance. *Antioxidants*, 12(2): 1–25. https://doi.org/10.3390/antiox12020485

Juknat, A., Rimmerman, N., Levy, R., Vogel, Z., and Kozela, E. (2012). Cannabidiol affects the expression of genes involved in zinc homeostasis in BV-2 microglial cells. *Neurochemistry International*, 61(6): 923–930. https://doi.org/10.1016/j.neuint.2011.12.002

Kendall, D. A., and Yudowski, G. A. (2017). Cannabinoid receptors in the central nervous system: Their signaling and roles in disease. *Frontiers in Cellular Neuroscience*, 10(January), 1–10. https://doi.org/10.3389/fncel.2016.00294

Kletkiewicz, H., Wojciechowski, M. S., and Rogalska, J. (2024). Cannabidiol effectively prevents oxidative stress and stabilizes hypoxia-inducible factor-1 alpha (HIF-1α) in an animal model of global hypoxia. *Scientific Reports*, 14(1): 1–9. https://doi.org/10.1038/s41598-024-66599-5

Kozela, E., Pietr, M., Juknat, A., Rimmerman, N., Levy, R., and Vogel, Z. (2010). Cannabinoids Δ9-tetrahydrocannabinol and cannabidiol differentially inhibit the lipopolysaccharide-activated NF-κB and interferon-β/STAT proinflammatory pathways in BV-2 microglial cells. *Journal of Biological Chemistry*, 285(3): 1616–1626. https://doi.org/10.1074/jbc.M109.069294

LaVigne, J. E., Hecksel, R., Keresztes, A., and Streicher, J. M. (2021). Cannabis sativa terpenes are cannabimimetic and selectively enhance cannabinoid activity. *Scientific Reports*, 11(1): 1–15. https://doi.org/10.1038/s41598-021-87740-8

Liktor-Busa, E., Keresztes, A., Lavigne, J., Streicher, J. M., and Largent-Milnes, T. M. (2021). Analgesic potential of terpenes derived from *Cannabis sativa*. Pharmacological Reviews, 73(4): 1270–1297. https://doi.org/10.1124/pharmrev.120.000046

Liu, C., Ma, H., Slitt, A. L., and Seeram, N. P. (2020). Inhibitory effect of cannabidiol on the activation of NLRP3 inflammasome is associated with its modulation of the P2X7 receptor in human monocytes. *Journal of Natural Products*, 83(6): 2025–2029. https://doi.org/10.1021/acs.jnatprod.0c00138

Malfait, A. M., Gallily, R., Sumariwalla, P. F., Malik, A. S., Andreakos, E., Mechoulam, R. et al. (2000). The nonpsychoactive cannabis constituent cannabidiol is an oral anti-arthritic therapeutic in murine collagen-induced arthritis. *Proceedings of the National Academy of Sciences*, 97(17): 9561–9566. https://doi.org/10.1073/pnas.160105897

Martinelli, G., Magnavacca, A., Fumagalli, M., Dell'Agli, M., Piazza, S., and Sangiovanni, E. (2022). *Cannabis sativa* and Skin Health: Dissecting the Role of Phytocannabinoids. *Planta Medica*, 88(7): 492–506. https://doi.org/10.1055/a-1420-5780

Martinez Naya, N., Kelly, J., Corna, G., Golino, M., Abbate, A., and Toldo, S. (2023). Molecular and cellular mechanisms of action of cannabidiol. *Molecules*, 28(16), 1–24. https://doi.org/10.3390/molecules28165980

Massi, P., Solinas, M., Cinquina, V., and Parolaro, D. (2013). Cannabidiol as potential anticancer drug. *British Journal of Clinical Pharmacology*, 75(2): 303–312. https://doi.org/10.1111/j.1365-2125.2012.04298.x

Muhsien, H., Al, S., Bhuyan, D. J., Alsherbiny, M. A., Basu, A., and Vuong, Q. V. (2022). A comprehensive review on the techniques for extraction of bioactive compounds from medicinal cannabis. *Molecules*, 1–18.

Nayak, A. P., Loblundo, C., and Bielory, L. (2023). Immunomodulatory actions of cannabinoids: clinical correlates and therapeutic opportunities for allergic inflammation. *The Journal of Allergy and Clinical Immunology: In Practice*, 11(2), 449–457. https://doi.org/https://doi.org/10.1016/j.jaip.2022.10.009

Nichols, J. M., and Kaplan, B. L. F. (2020). Immune responses regulated by cannabidiol. *Cannabis and Cannabinoid Research*, 5(1), 12–31. https://doi.org/10.1089/can.2018.0073

Pagano, C., Savarese, B., Coppola, L., Navarra, G., Avilia, G., Laezza, C. et al. (2023). Cannabinoids in the modulation of oxidative signaling. *International Journal of Molecular Sciences*, 24(3): 1–15. https://doi.org/10.3390/ijms24032513

Palmer, J. (2006). The central nervous system. Fundamentals of Surgical Practice, Second Edition, 415–439. https://doi.org/10.1017/CBO9780511545740.022

Pantoja-Ruiz, C., Restrepo-Jimenez, P., Castañeda-Cardona, C., Ferreirós, A., and Rosselli, D. (2022). Cannabis and pain: a scoping review. Brazilian Journal of Anesthesiology (English Edition), 72(1): 142–151. https://doi.org/10.1016/j.bjane.2021.06.018

Peng, J., Fan, M., An, C., Ni, F., Huang, W., and Luo, J. (2022). A narrative review of molecular mechanism and therapeutic effect of cannabidiol (CBD). *Basic and Clinical Pharmacology and Toxicology*, 130(4): 439–456. https://doi.org/10.1111/bcpt.13710

Peyravian, N., Deo, S., Daunert, S., and Jimenez, J. J. (2020). Cannabidiol as a novel therapeutic for immune modulation. *ImmunoTargets and Therapy*, 9: 131–140. https://doi.org/10.2147/ITT.S263690

Rahaman, O., and Ganguly, D. (2021). Endocannabinoids in immune regulation and immunopathologies. Immunology, 164(2): 242–252. https://doi.org/10.1111/imm.13378

Rahn, E. J., and Hohmann, A. G. (2009). Cannabinoids as Pharmacotherapies for Neuropathic Pain : From the Bench to the Bedside. *The Journal of the American Society for Experimental NeuroTherapeutics*, 6(October): 713–737.

Raja, A., Ahmadi, S., de Costa, F., Li, N., and Kerman, K. (2020). Attenuation of oxidative stress by cannabinoids and cannabis extracts in differentiated neuronal cells. *Pharmaceuticals*, 13(11): 1–16. https://doi.org/10.3390/ph13110328

Rajesh, M., Mukhopadhyay, P., Bátkai, S., Patel, V., Saito, K., Matsumoto, S. et al. (2010). Cannabidiol attenuates cardiac dysfunction, oxidative stress, fibrosis, and inflammatory and cell death signaling pathways in diabetic cardiomyopathy. *Journal of the American College of Cardiology*, 56(25): 2115–2125. https://doi.org/10.1016/j.jacc.2010.07.033

Ribeiro, A., Ferraz-de-Paula, V., Pinheiro, M. L., Vitoretti, L. B., Mariano-Souza, D. P., Quinteiro-Filho, W. M. et al. (2012). Cannabidiol, a non-psychotropic plant-derived cannabinoid, decreases inflammation in a murine model of acute lung injury: Role for the adenosine A2A receptor. *European Journal of Pharmacology*, 678(1–3): 78–85. https://doi.org/10.1016/j.ejphar.2011.12.043

Rocha, E. D., Silva, V. E. A., Pereira, F. C. S., Jean, V. M., Costa Souza, F. L., Baratto, L. C. et al. (2020). Qualitative terpene profiling of Cannabis varieties cultivated for medical purposes. *Rodriguesia*, 7. https://doi.org/10.1590/2175-7860202071040

Stasiłowicz-Krzemień, A., Sip, S., Szulc, P., and Cielecka-Piontek, J. (2023). Determining antioxidant activity of cannabis leaves extracts from different varieties—unveiling nature's treasure trove. *Antioxidants*, 12(7). https://doi.org/10.3390/antiox12071390

Szőke, K., Kajtár, R., Gyöngyösi, A., Czompa, A., Fésüs, A., Lőrincz, E. B. et al. (2023). Pharmacological evaluation of newly synthesized Cannabidiol Derivates on H9c2 Cells. *Antioxidants*, 12(9). https://doi.org/10.3390/antiox12091714

Tomko, A. M., Whynot, E. G., Ellis, L. D., and Dupré, D. J. (2020). Anti-cancer potential of cannabinoids, terpenes, and flavonoids present in cannabis. *Cancers*, 12(7): 1–81. https://doi.org/10.3390/cancers12071985

Tumilaar, S. G., Hardianto, A., Dohi, H., and Kurnia, D. (2023). A comprehensive review of free radicals, oxidative stress, and antioxidants: overview, clinical applications, global perspectives, future directions, and mechanisms of antioxidant activity of flavonoid compounds. *Journal of Chemistry*, 2024. https://doi.org/10.1155/2024/5594386

Vallée, A., Lecarpentier, Y., Guillevin, R., and Vallée, J.-N. (2017). Effects of cannabidiol interactions with Wnt/andamp;beta;-catenin pathway and PPARandamp;gamma; on oxidative stress and neuroinflammation in Alzheimer's disease. *Acta Biochimica et Biophysica Sinica*, 49(10): 853–866. https://doi.org/10.1093/abbs/gmx073

Vitorović, J., Joković, N., Radulović, N., Mihajilov-Krstev, T., Cvetković, V. J., Jovanović, N. et al. (2021). Antioxidant activity of hemp (*Cannabis sativa* l.) seed oil in drosophila melanogaster larvae under non-stress and h2o2-induced oxidative stress conditions. *Antioxidants*, 10(6). https://doi.org/10.3390/antiox10060830

Vučkovic, S., Srebro, D., Vujovic, K. S., Vučetic, Č., and Prostran, M. (2018). Cannabinoids and pain: New insights from old molecules. *Frontiers in Pharmacology*, 9(NOV), 1–19. https://doi.org/10.3389/fphar.2018.01259

Wang, B., Li, D., Fiselier, A., Kovalchuk, I., and Kovalchuk, O. (2023). High-CBD cannabis extracts inhibit the expression of proinflammatory factors via miRNA-mediated silencing in human small intestinal epithelial cells. *Heliyon*, 9(8): e18817. https://doi.org/https://doi.org/10.1016/j.heliyon.2023.e18817

Zachut, M., Butenko, Y., and dos Santos Silva, P. (2025). International symposium on ruminant physiology: The involvement of the endocannabinoid system in metabolic and inflammatory responses in dairy cows during negative energy balance. *Journal of Dairy Science*. https://doi.org/https://doi.org/10.3168/jds.2024-25772

Zhu, L. X., Sharma, S., Stolina, M., Gardner, B., Roth, M. D., Tashkin, D. P. et al. (2000). Δ-9-Tetrahydrocannabinol Inhibits Antitumor Immunity by a CB2 Receptor-Mediated, Cytokine-Dependent Pathway. *The Journal of Immunology*, 165(1): 373–380. https://doi.org/10.4049/jimmunol.165.1.373

CHAPTER 10

Unlocking the Hidden Power

Chemical and Biological Insights Into *Cannabis sativa* Roots

*Melina Di Liberto, Estefanía Butassi, Alan Blanc, Luz Rivero Márquez, Estefanía Cordisco, Laura Svetaz** and *Maximiliano Sortino**

1. Introduction

For centuries, *Cannabis sativa* has been recognized for its remarkable versatility, serving as both a medicinal resource and a source of industrial materials. Historically, scientific and medical research has focused predominantly on the aerial parts of the plant-flowers, leaves, and stems-owing to their rich content of cannabinoids and their established uses in pharmacology, pain management, and as raw materials for textiles, paper, and construction (Bukowska 2024). This emphasis has led to significant advances in our understanding of the plant's chemical diversity and therapeutic potential, particularly with respect to compounds such as Δ9-tetrahydrocannabinol (Δ9-THC) and cannabidiol (CBD), which are present in the roots at trace or undetectable concentrations (Ryz et al. 2017).

In contrast, the roots of *C. sativa* have remained largely overlooked in modern research, despite historical records indicating that they were traditionally used as natural remedies for a wide range of ailments. They were primarily valued for their anti-inflammatory properties in the treatment of joint diseases such as gout, rheumatism, and arthritis, as well as for their antimicrobial effects against conditions like erysipelas, fever, and malaria. Additionally, cannabis roots were employed to address gastrointestinal issues, including dysentery and constipation, and were used both to reduce vomiting and, conversely, to induce it when necessary. In the context of women's health, the roots were utilized to control postpartum hemorrhage, facilitate placental expulsion, and manage menstrual disorders. Other traditional applications included the treatment of burns, attention disorders, and tumors, highlighting the remarkable versatility of cannabis roots in ancient medicinal practices (Ryz et al. 2017; Elhendawy et al. 2019; Gagné et al. 2024).

Only recently have comprehensive studies begun to reveal the unique chemical profile of cannabis roots, which includes triterpenoids, alkaloids, sterols, and phenolic compounds not typically found in significant quantities in other parts of the plant (Elhendawy et al. 2019, Ryz et al. 2017, Gagné et al. 2024). These discoveries are uncovering new possibilities for therapeutic

Laboratorio de Bioprospección de Productos Antimicrobianos, Facultad de Ciencias Bioquímicas y Farmacéuticas, Universidad Nacional de Rosario Suipacha 531, Rosario, Argentina.
* Corresponding authors: svetaz@rosario-conicet.gov.ar; sortinomaximiliano@gmail.com

DOI: 10.1201/9781003668190-12

applications, including antioxidant, anti-inflammatory, and antimicrobial effects, and are beginning to validate the roots' traditional medicinal uses (Ryz et al. 2017; Gagné et al. 2024).

This chapter aims to shed light on the hidden potential of *C. sativa* roots, exploring their distinct chemical constituents and biological activities, and highlighting their emerging significance in both scientific research and therapeutic innovation.

2. Phytochemical Characterization

Initial phytochemical investigations into cannabis root composition, conducted by Slatkin et al. (1971), revealed the presence of the triterpenes friedelin **1** and epifriedelanol **2** in an ethanolic extract. Subsequent analysis by the same research group identified the steroidal compounds β-sitosterol **3**, campesterol **4**, and stigmasterol **5** (Slatkin et al. 1975). Expanding upon these findings, Sethi et al. (1977) confirmed the presence of friedelin **1**, epifriedelanol **2**, and β-sitosterol **3**, while also reporting the detection of the monoterpenes carvone **6** and dihydrocarvone **7** (Figure 1). Furthermore, they noted the presence of unidentified alkaloidal compounds, albeit at concentrations too low for precise characterization. Latter et al. (1975) pioneered the isolation and structural characterization of the alkaloid canabisativine **8**, while Elsohly et al. (1978) later identified anhydrocannabisativine **9**, significantly advancing the understanding of Cannabis roots' alkaloid composition (Figure 1).

To date, cannabis roots have not been considered a significant source of cannabinoids, with earlier studies failing to detect these compounds in measurable quantities. Farag et al. (2015) demonstrated that cannabinoid production could be induced in *C. sativa* hairy root cultures through auxin treatment, specifically using indole-3-acetic acid (IAA) and indole-3-butyric acid (IBA). Their analysis by HPLC and LC-MS/MS revealed trace amounts of Δ9-tetrahydrocannabinolic acid (Δ9-THCA) **10**, Δ9-THC **11**, and cannabidiolic acid (CBDA) **12** (Figure 2), though concentrations remained extremely low. In a landmark study, Gul et al. 2018 employed a validated LC-MS/MS method to quantify 10 major cannabinoids in root extracts of three varieties: high-CBD, intermediate [Δ9-THC-CBD], and high-Δ9-THC. Using acetonitrile:methanol (80:20, v/v) extraction, they detected: Δ9-THCA **10**, Δ9-THC **11**, CBDA **12**, CBD **13**, cannabigerolic acid (CBGA) **14**, cannabigerol (CBG) **15**, cannabichromene (CBC) **16**, tetrahydrocannabivarin **17**, cannabinol (CBN) **18**, and Δ8-tetrahydrocannabinol (Δ8-THC) **19** (Figure 2). Results showed that CBD **13**, CBG **14**, and CBGA **12** were present in all varieties, with the highest values in the high-Δ9-THC chemovar. CBDA **12** and Δ9-THCA **10** concentrations were directly correlated with their decarboxylated forms, and Δ8-THC **19** levels positively correlated with Δ9-THC **11**.

In 2019, Elhendawy et al. performed a detailed phytochemical analysis of Cannabis root extracts, using a sequential solvent extraction protocol (hexane, dichloromethane, ethyl acetate, and methanol) followed by high-performance liquid chromatography (HPLC) analysis. This rigorous approach led to the purification and unambiguous structural elucidation of ten compounds, achieved through comprehensive 1D and 2D nuclear magnetic resonance (NMR) spectroscopy and mass spectrometry. The identified compounds comprised the triterpenes friedelin **1** and epifriedelanol **2**; the phytosterols β-sitosterol **3**, ergost-5-en-3-ol **20**, and β-sitosterol-β-D-glucoside **21**; the fatty acids pentadecanoic acid **22** and 10E-hexadecenoic acid **23**; along with methyl hexadecanoate **24** (Figure 1).

Jin et al. (2020) conducted a comprehensive investigation into the chemical profiles of various cannabis plant parts, analyzing two Δ9-THC-dominant chemovars ("Indica" varieties, Grand Doggy Purps and Granddaddy Purple), and an intermediate chemovar ("Sativa" variety, CBD Mango Haze, with a Δ9-THC:CBD ratio of 1:2). Employing liquid chromatography-mass spectrometry (LC-MS) for cannabinoids, liquid chromatography-ultraviolet-mass spectrometry (LC-UV-MS) for flavonoids, and gas chromatography-mass spectrometry (GC-MS) for terpenoids and sterols. Results indicated low cannabinoid concentrations in the roots of all chemovars, with flavonoids, monoterpenes, and sesquiterpenes being undetectable. β-sitosterol **3** was identified as the predominant sterol in roots, exhibiting significant variation among chemovars, while campesterol **4** and stigmasterol **5**

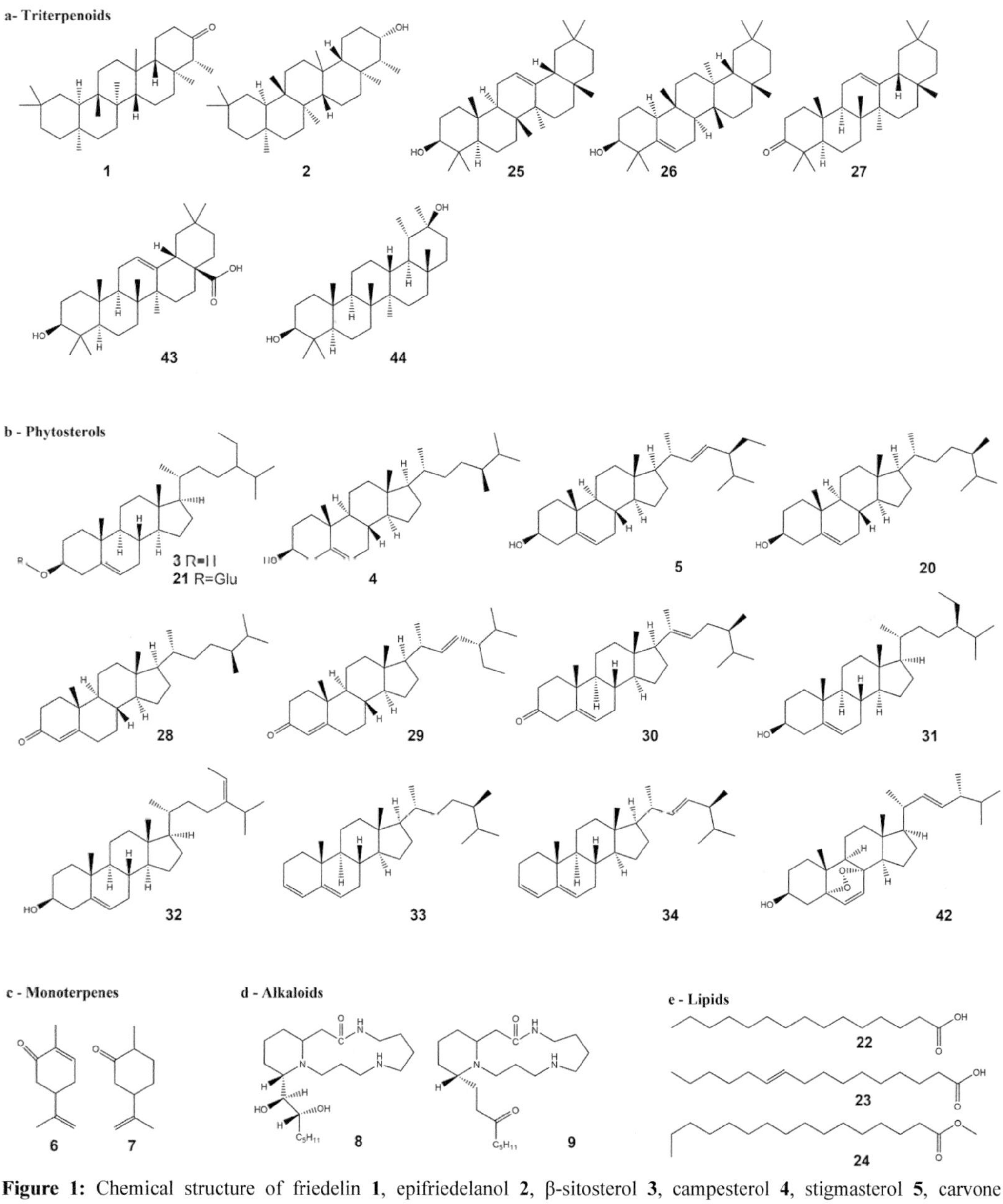

Figure 1: Chemical structure of friedelin **1**, epifriedelanol **2**, β-sitosterol **3**, campesterol **4**, stigmasterol **5**, carvone **6**, dihydrocarvone **7**, canabisativine **8**, anhydrocannabisativine **9**, ergost-5-en-3-ol **20**, β-sitosterol-β-d-glucoside **21**, pentadecanoic acid **22**, 10e-hexadecenoic acid **23**, methyl hexadecanoate **24**, β-amyrin **25**, glutinol **26**, β-amyrone **27**, 4-campesten-3-one **28**, stigmasta-4,22-dien-3-one **29**, stigmast-4-en-3-one **30**, stigmastanol **31**, fucosterol **32**, stigmasta-3,5-diene **33**, stigmasta-3,5,22-triene **34**, 5α,8α-epidioxy-(22E,24R)-ergosta-6,22-dien-3β-ol, **42**, (+)-oleanolic acid **43**, epipseudotaraxastanediol **44**.

were present at low concentrations (Figure 1). Notably, roots displayed the highest triterpenoid concentrations, particularly friedelin **1**, with Chemovar III showing significantly elevated levels of friedelin **1**, epifriedelanol **2**, and β-amyrin **25** in roots and stem barks compared to Chemovars I and II. Conversely, β-amyrin **25** concentrations were higher in leaves than in stem barks or roots (Jin et al. 2020).

Building on these findings, Jin et al. (2021) further explored metabolite distribution across organs of 82 cannabis plants, representing 21 commercially available strains categorized as CBD-

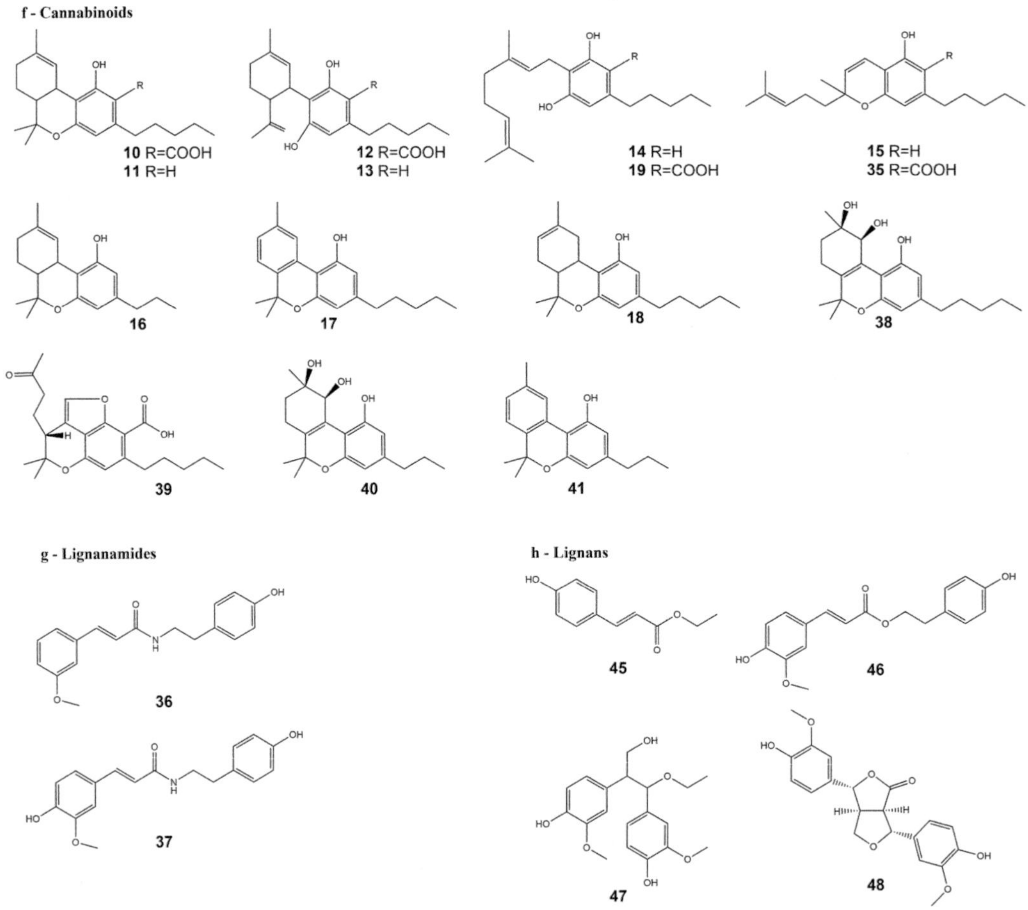

Figure 2: Chemical structure of tetrahydrocannabinolic acid (THCA) **10**, Δ9-tetrahydrocannabinol (Δ9-THC) **11**, cannabidiolic acid (CBDA) **12**, cannabidiol (CBD) **13**, cannabigerolic acid (CBGA) **14**, cannabigerol (CBG) **15**, cannabichromene (CBC) **16**, tetrahydrocannabivarin **17**, cannabinol (CBN) **18**, Δ8-tetrahydrocannabinol (Δ8-THC) **19**, cannabichromenic acid **35**, p-coumaroyltyramine **36**, feruoylyramine **37**, (9R,10S)-6,6,9-trimethyl-3-pentyl-7,8,9,10-tetrahydro-6H-benzo[c]chromene-1,9,10-triol **38**, (-)-7R-cannabicoumarononic acid A **39**, (9R,10S)-6,6,9-trimethyl-3-propyl-7,8,9,10-tetrahydro-6H-benzo[c]chromene-1,9,10-triol **40**, cannabivarin **41**, 3-(4-hydroxyphenyl)-2-propenoic acid ethyl ester **45**, 4-hydroxyphenethyl trans-ferulate **46**, 1,2-diguaiacyl-1-ethoxy-3-propanol **47**, and (+)-4-ketopinoresinol **48**.

dominant, intermediate, and Δ9-THC-dominant. This comparative analysis revealed that roots consistently exhibited the lowest average total content of cannabinoids, flavonoids, monoterpenes, and sesquiterpenes. Conversely, roots displayed the highest total sterol content, specifically the sum of β-sitosterol **3**, campesterol **4**, and stigmasterol **5**, with significantly higher levels in CBD-dominant strains compared to Δ9-THC-dominant strains. Similarly, total triterpenoid content, encompassing friedelin **1**, epifriedelanol **2**, and β-amyrin **25** (Figure 1), was highest in roots. However, the epifriedelanol **2** to friedelin **1** ratio varied, with epifriedelanol **2** being more prevalent in CBD-dominant strains and friedelin **1** in Δ9-THC-dominant strains, further elucidating the chemotypic variations in root composition (Jin et al. 2021).

Ferrini et al. (2021) conducted a comparative chemical characterization of ethyl acetate extracts from Cannabis roots of aeroponically propagated (AP), aeroponically induced (AEP), and soil-grown (SP) plants, employing GC-MS and Gas Chromatography-Flame Ionization Detection (GC-FID) to analyze the phytosterols β-sitosterol **3**, campesterol **4** and stigmasterol **5**, and the triterpenoids friedelin **1** and epifriedelanol **2**. Results showed that aeroponic cultivation significantly enhanced plant growth, resulting in AP and AEP plants exhibiting a considerably greater height than

SP plants. Analysis of root bioactives revealed distinct compositional differences across cultivation methods. When considering absolute amounts, SP roots exhibited higher levels of bioactives than AP and AEP ones, specifically demonstrating significantly greater concentrations of epifriedelanol **2** and friedelin **1**. Conversely, β-sitosterol **3** content was elevated in AP and AEP roots. However, examining the relative composition revealed a contrasting trend: friedelin **1** and epifriedelanol **2** were the predominant compounds in SP roots, while β-sitosterol **3** dominated in AP and AEP roots. Furthermore, a comparative analysis of AP and AEP roots indicated a decrease in β-sitosterol **3** and an increase in epifriedelanol **2** within the AEP samples.

Kornpointner et al. (2021) conducted a study to explore the potential utilization of hemp roots for the extraction and identification of previously undescribed secondary metabolites. This research analyzed the roots of three type III *C. sativa* L. chemovars: Futura 75, Felina 32, and Uso 31. Extractions were performed using conventional methods (hexane and ethanol) and supercritical carbon dioxide, with subsequent analysis by GC-MS and GC-FID. Known triterpenes such as friedelin **1**, epifriedelanol **2**, and β-amyrin **25** were detected, the presence of the pentacyclic triterpenoid glutinol **26** was reported, and another triterpenoid based on the oleanane skeleton, β-amyrone **27**, was discovered for the first time (Figure 1). Regarding sterols, β-sitosterol **3**, campesterol **4**, and stigmasterol **5** were identified, as well as the steroidal ketones 4-campesten-3-one **28**, stigmasta-4,22-dien-3-one **29**, and stigmast-4-en-3-one **30** (Figure 1). In addition, two phytosterols not yet described in the roots, stigmastanol **31** and fucosterol **32**, and two steroidal hydrocarbons, stigmasta-3,5-diene **33** and stigmasta-3,5,22-triene **34**, were extracted (Figure 1).

To explore the therapeutic properties of cannabis roots, several studies have focused on the detailed analysis of their chemical composition. Lima et al. (2021) employed liquid chromatography-mass spectrometry (LC-MS) to analyze the chemical composition of aqueous extracts obtained via decoction from *C. sativa* roots. Samples, originating from a Brazilian cultivation site, revealed the presence of the alkaloids cannabisativine **8** and anhydrocannabisativine **9**, as well as cannabichromenic acid **35** (Figure 2), among other identified compounds. Subsequently, the same research group expanded their investigations in two later studies, consistently identifying the presence of Δ9-THC **11** and the lignanamides p-coumaroyltyramine **36** and feruloyltyramine **37** (Figures 1–2) in aqueous extracts of *C. sativa* roots (Menezes et al. 2021; Menezes et al. 2022). These findings further support the chemical complexity of cannabis roots and provide a foundation for correlating specific compounds with their pharmacological effects.

Furthermore, Huang et al. (2023) prepared ethanolic extracts, from which thirty-two compounds were subsequently isolated and purified using a combination of chromatographic techniques, including silica gel, Sephadex LH-20, thin-layer chromatography (TLC), and semi-preparative high-performance liquid chromatography (HPLC). This process yielded a compound library that included cannabinoids: cannabinol **18**; (9R,10S)-6,6,9-trimethyl-3-pentyl-7,8,9,10-tetrahydro-6H-benzo[c]chromene-1,9,10-triol **27**, (-)-7R-cannabicoumarononic acid A **38**, (9R,10S)-6,6,9-trimethyl-3-propyl-7,8,9,10-tetrahydro-6H-benzo[c]chromene-1,9,10-triol **39**, cannabivarin **41**, and CBD **13**; phytosterols: β-sitosterol **3**, and stigmast-4-en-3-one **20** and 5α,8α-epidioxy-(22E,24R)-ergosta-6,22-dien-3β-ol **42**; triterpenoids: friedelin **1**, epifriedelinol **2**, (+)-oleanolic acid **43** and epipseudotaraxastanediol **44**, and lignans: 3-(4-hydroxyphenyl)-2-propenoic acid ethyl ester **45**, 4-hydroxyphenethyl trans-ferulate **46**, 1,2-diguaiacyl-1-ethoxy-3-propanol **47** and (+)-4-ketopinoresinol **48** (Figures 1–2).

Gagné et al. (2024) investigated the chemical composition of cannabis root extracts using three distinct extraction methods: aqueous decoction, continuous alcoholic extraction (Soxhlet), and acid-base extraction. Ultra-performance liquid chromatography-quadrupole time-of-flight mass spectrometry (UPLC-QTOF-MS) analysis revealed a total of 533 detected ion masses, with a slightly higher count in positive ion mode compared to negative ion mode. Putative compound identities were assigned to these detected masses. Notably, phenolic compounds were identified as the most abundant metabolite class. Furthermore, various terpenoids, including monoterpenes, diterpenoids, and triterpenoids, were detected. Cannabinoids, amino acids, and carbohydrates were found in relatively lower numbers. Additionally, nitrogen-containing compounds, such as alkaloids and lignanamides, were identified.

3. Biological Activity Studies

The cannabis root system contains a diverse array of bioactive compounds with promising therapeutic potential. Recent research has explored its biological activities, including their antioxidant, anti-inflammatory, spasmolytic, antimicrobial, anticholinesterase, and toxicological profiles, as well as the pharmacological relevance of specific isolated compounds. This comprehensive overview highlights the multifaceted nature of Cannabis root bioactivity and emphasizes its relevance as a source of novel therapeutic agents.

3.1 Antioxidant Activity

The root of *C. sativa* has gained attention as a source of bioactive compounds exhibiting antioxidant potential. Recent studies have evaluated the antioxidant properties of root extracts from different chemovars and cultivation systems, employing a wide range of *in vitro* and *in vivo* assays that elucidate their various antioxidant mechanisms. These assays include the Ferric Reducing Antioxidant Power (FRAP), which quantifies the reduction of Fe^{3+} to Fe^{2+} by measuring the formation of a colored complex with maximum absorption at 593 nm; the ABTS (2,2′-azino-bis(3-ethylbenzothiazoline-6-sulfonic acid)) radical scavenging assay; and the inhibition of membrane lipid peroxidation by measuring conjugated diene formation at 234 nm after oxidative stress induction with AAPH in linoleic acid micelles. The total phenolic content (TPC) of the extracts was determined spectrophotometrically using the Folin-Ciocalteu colorimetric method, which quantifies polyphenols by measuring the formation of a blue complex at 765 nm. Furthermore, antioxidant activity was assessed *in vivo* using *Saccharomyces cerevisiae* yeast and THP-1 cells as model systems, with intracellular oxidation evaluated using fluorometric probes such as 2′,7′-dichlorofluorescin (H_2DCF) and MitoPerOx.

Kornpointner et al. (2021) reported moderate antioxidant activity in ethanolic extracts from the roots of three *C. sativa* chemovars, with the findings exhibiting variability based on the specific chemovar and parameters such as harvest time. FRAP values, expressed as Vitamin C Equivalent Antioxidant Capacity (VCE), ranged from 20.6 to 97.1 mg VCE/100 g dry weight, while ABTS results ranged from 22.9 to 89.1 mg VCE/100 g dry weight. Intracellular oxidation in yeast ranged from 0.809 to 1.024, with values below 1 indicating greater antioxidant activity compared to the control (Slatnar et al. 2012). Although the triterpenoids friedelin **1** and epifriedelanol **2** were identified and considered as possible contributors to the antioxidant activity, no significant correlation was found between their content and the results from FRAP ($r^2 = 0.04$), ABTS ($r^2 = 0.001$), or intracellular oxidation assays ($r^2 = 0.006$). These findings suggest that other compounds, such as phytosterols, may play a more prominent role in the observed antioxidant effects.

Gagné et al. (2024) expanded this investigation by analyzing the antioxidant activity of root extracts obtained using different solvents (aqueous, ethanolic, and acid-base) from plants cultivated in both soil and hydroponic systems, all derived from the same mother plant. The ethanolic extracts consistently showed the highest polyphenol concentration, followed by aqueous and acid-base extracts. Soil-grown plants yielded higher phenolic content across all extraction methods than hydroponic plants, with increases of 54% (ethanol), 30% (aqueous), and 35% (acid-base). In ABTS and FRAP assays—expressed as Trolox and Gallic Acid equivalents, respectively—ethanolic soil extracts and aqueous hydroponic extracts exhibited the greatest radical neutralization capacity, while acid-base extracts showed the lowest activity, reflecting their polyphenol content. Additionally, acid-base extracts failed to inhibit lipid peroxidation on linoleic acid micelles, whereas ethanolic extracts were the most effective, followed by aqueous extracts. Intracellular oxidative stress was assessed in THP-1 cells using the MitoPerOx probe. Notably, the ethanolic extract from hydroponically grown roots and the aqueous extract from soil-grown roots significantly reduced mitochondrial oxidative stress by 86% and 72%, respectively, compared to the solvent control, with the ethanolic hydroponic extract even surpassing the Trolox standard.

Overall, both studies underscore the potential of *C. sativa* root extracts, particularly those obtained using ethanol and water, as sources of natural antioxidants. The antioxidant activity appears to be largely influenced by phenolic content, solvent polarity, and cultivation conditions. While acid-base extracts showed limited activity, ethanolic and aqueous extracts from both soil and hydroponically grown plants demonstrated notable protective effects across several antioxidant assays.

3.2 Anti-Inflammatory Activity

The anti-inflammatory potential of *C. sativa* root extracts has been assessed using both *in vivo* and *in vitro* models targeting distinct mechanisms of inflammation. Among *in vivo* methods in murine models, the carrageenan-induced leukocyte migration assay and the carrageenan- and histamine-induced paw edema models have been widely employed to evaluate acute inflammatory responses. These assays measure the infiltration of inflammatory cells and vascular extravasation after an inflammatory stimulus. *In vitro*, inflammation can be modeled using differentiated THP-1 human monocyte-derived macrophages stimulated with lipopolysaccharide (LPS), a bacterial endotoxin that triggers a strong inflammatory response. One key marker of this response is interleukin-6 (IL-6), a pro-inflammatory cytokine that plays a central role in acute-phase reactions and immune regulation.

Lima et al. (2021) evaluated the *in vivo* anti-inflammatory activity of decocted aqueous *C. sativa* root extracts using the carrageenan-induced leukocyte migration assay and models of carrageenan- and histamine-induced paw edema in mice. The extract demonstrated significant inhibitory effects on leukocyte migration at doses of 25, 50, and 100 mg/kg, and it reduced edema formation in a dose-dependent manner at 12.5, 25, 50, and 100 mg/kg following carrageenan injection. Notably, even the lowest dose (12.5 mg/kg) prevented edema formation after histamine administration. These findings suggest that the aqueous root extract mitigates inflammation primarily by reducing vascular permeability and leukocyte recruitment, without affecting the central nervous system.

Complementing these results, Gagné et al. (2024) investigated the anti-inflammatory activity of aqueous, ethanolic, and acid-base Cannabis root extracts obtained from soil-cultivated plants and hydroponic systems by quantifying *in vitro* IL-6 production in LPS-stimulated THP-1 cells. Extracts derived from soil-grown plants, particularly the acid-base and aqueous preparations, significantly decreased IL-6 levels compared to the control, indicating a marked anti-inflammatory effect. Conversely, the ethanolic extract from soil-grown roots did not significantly affect IL-6 levels. Interestingly, none of the extracts obtained from hydroponically cultivated roots demonstrated significant anti-inflammatory activity, suggesting that both the extraction method and cultivation conditions critically influence the bioactivity of the final extract.

Together, these studies highlight the potential of *C. sativa* root extracts—especially aqueous and acid-base extracts from soil-grown plants—as promising candidates for anti-inflammatory applications. Their activity appears closely related to their ability to modulate key inflammatory mediators and suppress cellular infiltration at inflammation sites.

3.3 Antinociceptive Activity

The antinociceptive properties of aqueous cannabis root extract were investigated by Menezes et al. (2021) using three well-established murine models: the acetic acid-induced writhing test, the formalin-induced nociception test, and the hot plate test. These complementary models are commonly used to evaluate both peripheral and central mechanisms involved in pain modulation.

In the acetic acid-induced writhing test, mice pretreated orally with aqueous Cannabis root extract at doses of 12.5, 25, and 50 mg/kg exhibited a significant reduction in the number of abdominal writhes compared to control animals receiving 0.9% NaCl. Writhing behavior, characterized by abdominal constriction followed by trunk rotation and hind limb extension, is triggered by reflex responses to the peritoneal irritation caused by acetic acid injection (Whittle 1964; Yin et al. 2016). The antinociceptive effect of aqueous cannabis root extract was comparable to that of the reference drugs indomethacin and morphine (10 mg/kg, intraperitoneally). These results suggest a dose-dependent peripheral analgesic effect of the extract in response to chemically induced visceral pain.

The formalin-induced nociception test is a biphasic model that allows differentiation between neurogenic pain (first phase) and inflammatory pain (second phase). In this assay, mice were treated with 0.9% NaCl (p.o.), indomethacin, morphine (10 mg/kg, i.p.), or aqueous Cannabis root extract (12.5, 25, and 50 mg/kg, p.o.) one hour before receiving a 2.5% formalin solution injected into the hind paw. Nociceptive responses—licking, biting, or shaking of the affected paw—were recorded during both phases. Aqueous Cannabis root extract at doses of 12.5 and 50 mg/kg significantly reduced nociceptive behaviors during the first phase, whereas doses of 12.5 and 25 mg/kg were effective during the second phase. These findings indicate that aqueous cannabis root extract exerts both central and peripheral antinociceptive effects, with notable activity against inflammatory pain (Menezes et al. 2021).

The hot plate test was used to assess centrally mediated thermal nociception. Mice were placed on a heated surface (55 ± 0.5 °C) at 30, 60, 90, and 120 minutes after treatment with 0.9% NaCl (p.o.), morphine (10 mg/kg, i.p.), or aqueous cannabis root extract (12.5, 25, and 50 mg/kg, p.o.). Latency to a nociceptive response (paw licking or lifting) was measured, with a maximum exposure time of 20 seconds to prevent tissue damage (Franzotti et al. 2000; Deng et al. 2021). Aqueous cannabis root extract produced significant antinociceptive effects at all tested doses, with the lowest dose (12.5 mg/kg) showing prolonged analgesic activity at 60, 90, and 120 minutes, indicating sustained central antinociceptive action.

Taken together, these results demonstrate that aqueous cannabis root extract exhibits strong antinociceptive activity through both peripheral and central mechanisms, supporting its therapeutic potential for the management of pain-related conditions.

3.4 Antipyretic Activity

The antipyretic potential of aqueous cannabis root extract was evaluated by Menezes et al. (2021) using a murine model of yeast-induced pyrexia. Fever was induced via intraperitoneal injection of a suspension of *S. cerevisiae* prepared in sterile 0.9% NaCl solution. Control animals in the basal group received only 0.9% NaCl without yeast. Four hours after induction, animals were treated orally with 0.9% NaCl, aqueous Cannabis root extract at doses of 12.5, 25, or 50 mg/kg, or intraperitoneally with dipyrone (120 mg/kg) as a reference antipyretic drug.

Rectal temperature was recorded hourly over a 12-hour observation period. Aqueous Cannabis root extract at doses of 12.5 and 50 mg/kg produced a statistically significant reduction in body temperature ($p < 0.05$), but only during the final hour of evaluation. However, this late and isolated effect was inconsistent across doses or time points and is unlikely to reflect an actual antipyretic action. Taken together, these results suggest that aqueous Cannabis root extract does not exert meaningful antipyretic activity under the conditions tested.

3.5 Spasmolytic Activity

The spasmolytic activity of plant extracts is commonly evaluated through *in vitro* assays using isolated smooth muscle tissues, such as tracheal rings, in organ bath systems. This approach allows for precise measurement of changes in muscle tone following the application of contractile agents and test compounds. Agents like carbachol (a cholinergic agonist) and potassium chloride (KCl, which induces depolarization) are typically used to precontract the tissue, and a spasmolytic effect is indicated by the ability of a compound to induce relaxation under these conditions.

Lima et al. (2021) investigated the spasmolytic potential of decocted aqueous *C. sativa* root extract using isolated tracheal rings from mice maintained in an organ bath. The tracheal rings were precontracted with either carbachol or potassium chloride to simulate smooth muscle constriction. Upon administration of the aqueous root extract at a concentration of 729 μg/mL, no relaxation response was observed in either condition.

These findings were later corroborated by Menezes et al. (2021), who employed a similar *ex vivo* methodology using tracheal rings from mice under identical physiological conditions. The tissues were maintained in Krebs–Ringer bicarbonate solution at 37°C and continuously aerated with a carbogenic gas mixture (95% O_2 and 5% CO_2). Despite the standardized experimental setup and the use of the same maximum extract concentration (729 μg/mL), no spasmolytic effect was detected in response to the aqueous extract following precontraction with carbachol or KCl.

Together, these results indicate that the aqueous root extract of *C. sativa* does not exhibit a spasmolytic effect on airway smooth muscle and is unlikely to contribute to bronchodilatory activity via direct smooth muscle relaxation.

3.6 Antimicrobial Activity

The antimicrobial activity of plant extracts is typically assessed using *in vitro* assays that measure microbial viability in the presence of test substances. A common method uses colorimetric indicators such as p-iodonitrophenyltetrazolium (INT), which is reduced by metabolically active microorganisms to a colored formazan product, allowing for visual quantification of growth. This assay can be coupled with agar plating to distinguish between growth inhibition (bacteriostatic/fungistatic) and microbicidal effects. Minimum inhibitory concentrations (MICs) and minimum bactericidal or fungicidal concentrations (MBCs/MFCs) are then determined based on extract concentration ranges that inhibit or eliminate microbial growth.

In 2024, Gagné et al. evaluated the antimicrobial properties of aqueous, ethanolic, and acid-base solvent extracts of *C. sativa* roots obtained from both soil-grown and hydroponically cultivated plants. The extracts were tested against *Escherichia coli* (Gram-negative), *Staphylococcus aureus* (Gram-positive), and *Candida albicans* (fungus) using the INT colorimetric assay. Following incubation with the extracts, wells were assessed for color change upon INT addition; absence of color was further analyzed via agar plating to confirm inhibitory versus microbicidal effects.

The extracts showed no activity against *E. coli*, indicating limited efficacy against Gram-negative bacteria. However, they showed inhibitory activity against *S. aureus*, with the most potent response observed for the acid-base extract from hydroponically grown roots at a MIC of 0.89 mg/mL. Bactericidal activity was confirmed at 1.33 mg/mL with both acid-base extracts, suggesting selective efficacy against Gram-positive bacteria.

All tested extracts exhibited notable antifungal activity against *C. albicans*, with growth inhibition occurring at concentrations ranging from 0.12 to 0.89 mg/mL. Fungicidal activity was recorded at 0.89 mg/mL for the ethanolic extract of soil-grown roots, while other extracts required higher concentrations (1.33-3 mg/mL) to achieve complete fungal eradication. These findings underscore the potential of Cannabis root extracts, particularly ethanolic and acid-base preparations, as sources of antimicrobial agents effective against certain fungal and Gram-positive bacterial pathogens.

3.7 Anticholinesterase Activity

The inhibition of cholinesterase enzymes—acetylcholinesterase (AChE) and butyrylcholinesterase (BChE)—is a widely used approach to assess the neuroprotective potential of plant-derived compounds, particularly for applications in neurodegenerative diseases such as Alzheimer's. *In vitro* enzymatic assays typically measure the hydrolysis of synthetic substrates, such as acetylthiocholine iodide, and monitor the reaction rate by colorimetric or spectrophotometric detection. Inhibitory activity is compared to known standards, such as galantamine, a clinically approved cholinesterase inhibitor.

Gagné et al. (2024) investigated the anticholinesterase activity of aqueous, ethanolic, and acid-base extracts from *C. sativa* roots grown in soil and hydroponic systems. The catalytic activities of AChE and BChE toward acetylthiocholine iodide were assessed in the presence of each extract, using galantamine as the positive control.

In assays targeting AChE, five out of six extracts exhibited substantial inhibition, ranging from 45% to 85%, surpassing the inhibitory effect of galantamine. In contrast, the extracts demonstrated only moderate inhibition of BChE, with values ranging from 8% to 20%, comparable to galantamine's activity (18%). Notably, extracts obtained from soil-grown plants showed greater inhibitory activity than those derived from hydroponic cultivation.

These findings suggest the presence of anticholinesterase-active compounds in Cannabis root extracts, likely in variable concentrations and with differing affinities for AChE and BChE. The observed activity may be partially attributed to alkaloids such as cannabisativine **8**, previously identified in cannabis roots. These results point to the therapeutic potential of cannabis root extracts in modulating cholinesterase activity, warranting further investigation into their possible application in the management of cholinergic dysfunction-related disorders.

3.8 Antiasthmatic Activity

The antiasthmatic potential of aqueous Cannabis root extract was evaluated by Menezes et al. (2021) using an ovalbumin (OVA)-induced asthma model in mice, complemented by cellular and histological analyses. This model mimics key features of human allergic asthma, including leukocyte infiltration, eosinophilia, and mucus hypersecretion.

To induce the allergic response, mice were immunized intraperitoneally (days 0–14) with OVA and aluminum potassium sulfate in phosphate-buffered saline (PBS). A control group received isotonic NaCl. From days 21 to 25, the mice were treated once daily with aqueous Cannabis root extract (12.5, 25, or 50 mg/kg, p.o.), dexamethasone (2 mg/kg, i.p., as a positive control), or 0.9% NaCl (p.o.). Thirty minutes after treatment, all groups except the negative control were exposed to an aerosolized OVA solution (10% w/v) for 30 minutes in a glass inhalation chamber.

On day 26, 24 hours after the final challenge, the animals were anesthetized for the collection of blood samples and bronchoalveolar lavage fluid (BALF). Total and differential leukocyte counts were performed, and lung tissues were collected for histological examination using hematoxylin and eosin (H&E) and periodic acid–Schiff (PAS) staining.

Aqueous cannabis root extract demonstrated notable anti-inflammatory effects in this asthma model. Specifically, the 25 mg/kg dose significantly reduced total leukocyte counts in BALF, and all tested doses (12.5, 25, and 50 mg/kg) significantly decreased eosinophil infiltration, a hallmark of allergic asthma. Histopathological analysis of lung sections revealed a dose-dependent reduction in perivascular and peribronchial inflammatory cell accumulation, along with decreased mucus production, as indicated by reduced PAS staining.

These results suggest that aqueous cannabis root extract exerts antiasthmatic effects, likely by suppressing eosinophilic inflammation and mucus hypersecretion, supporting its potential as an adjunct treatment for allergic airway diseases.

3.9 Toxicity

The toxicological evaluation of plant-derived extracts typically involves *in vivo* assays that assess both acute and sub-chronic effects, providing insight into the safety profile of a compound following single or repeated exposure. Key parameters include clinical observations, hematological and biochemical analyses, histopathological examinations, and behavioral assessments such as motor coordination and spontaneous activity. These methods are essential for determining potential adverse effects and establishing safe dosage ranges for future therapeutic applications.

Lima et al. (2021) conducted a comprehensive toxicological assessment of the decocted aqueous root extract of *C. sativa* in mice, including both single-dose (acute) and repeated-dose (sub-chronic) studies over 28 days. In the acute toxicity assay, oral administration of 1,000 mg/kg did not produce clinical signs of toxicity, indicating that the median lethal dose (LD_{50}) exceeds 1,000 mg/kg. In the repeated-dose study, daily oral administration of 25 mg/kg or 100 mg/kg for 28 days did not cause significant alterations in hematological profiles, serum biochemical parameters, or histological architecture of major organs. These results demonstrate a low oral toxicity profile for the aqueous root extract under both acute and sub-chronic exposure conditions.

Behavioral toxicity was also investigated using the rotarod test to assess motor coordination and the open field test to evaluate locomotor activity. At the highest tested dose (100 mg/kg), no significant differences were observed between extract-treated mice and controls, further supporting the extract's lack of neurotoxic effects. Collectively, these findings suggest that the aqueous root extract of *C. sativa* is well tolerated *in vivo* and may be considered safe within the tested dosage range.

3.10 Biological Activity of Isolated Compounds

The investigation of isolated phytochemicals from *C. sativa* roots provides key insights into the specific molecules responsible for the pharmacological properties observed in crude extracts, as well as potential activities not yet studied in these extracts.. Among all the compounds studied, a brief description is provided of those related to the triterpenes friedelin **1** and epifriedelanol **2**.

Friedelin **1** has been associated with a wide range of biological activities, including antiviral effects against SARS-CoV-2 (Radi et al. 2023; Mosquera-Yuqui et al. 2022; Jamiu et al. 2021; Kar et al. 2021) and it has demonstrated analgesic, antipyretic, and anti-inflammatory properties in various *in vitro* and *in vivo* models (Antonisamy et al. 2011; Noufou et al. 2012; Ouedraogo et al. 2017; Tian et al. 2021; Nunes et al. 2021; Shi et al. 2021; Toukam et al. 2018; Ding et al. 2010; Kumari et al. 2011).

Regarding its antimicrobial activity, friedelin **1** has shown significant antimycobacterial activity, suggesting potential as a therapeutic agent for tuberculosis (Chinsembu 2016). Although it has not exhibited antimicrobial activity against *Cryptococcus neoformans* or *Escherichia coli* (Elhendawy et al. 2019), a recent study reported its efficacy in treating MRSA-infected wounds, where it promoted angiogenesis and accelerated wound healing (El-Shiekh et al. 2025). Its wound-healing potential had previously been demonstrated *in vitro* using human keratinocyte models, where friedelin **1** significantly reduced wound size and enhanced cell migration, effects attributed to its anti-inflammatory action (Somwong et al. 2022).

Moreover, friedelin has been shown to induce apoptosis and inhibit the proliferation of tumor cell lines such as MCF-7 (human breast cancer) and AML-196 (human leukemia), while maintaining a favorable toxicity profile (Chang et al. 2020; Subash-Babu et al. 2017; Shi et al. 2021). Additional *in vivo* studies have reported its hypoglycemic (Sunil et al. 2021), hypolipidemic (Duraipandiyan et al. 2016), and estrogenic activities (Aswar et al. 2010). Other documented pharmacological effects include gastroprotective and anti-ulcerogenic properties (Antonisamy et al. 2015), as well as a potential antihypertensive effect likely related to vasodilatory mechanisms (Jiao et al. 2007).

Epifriedelanol **2** has demonstrated anti-inflammatory (Dae et al. 2005) and anticancer (Kundu et al. 2000; Yang et al. 2017; Perumal et al. 2016) properties. Yang et al. (2011) showed that epifriedelanol reduces cellular senescence in human primary cells, thereby controlling tissue aging or aging-associated disorders. Cai et al. (2015) reported that epifriedelanol 2 inhibits protein tyrosine phosphatase 1B (PTP–1B) inhibition, which could be associated with antidiabetic activity and antiobesity properties.

Taken together, these findings highlight the pharmacological relevance of individual compounds in cannabis root, with triterpenoids contributing to anti-inflammatory, antitumor, and antiviral effects. However, the absence of antimicrobial activity for major triterpenes suggests that other constituents, such as lignans, may play a more prominent role in antimicrobial efficacy.

4. Conclusion

This chapter has unveiled the remarkable phytochemical richness of *C. sativa* roots, moving beyond the well-trodden path of flowers and leaves. The investigations specifically highlighted the predominance of triterpenoids and phytosterols, metabolites widely recognized for their diverse biological activities. Furthermore, the systematic identification of other significant compound classes, including alkaloids, cannabinoids, and lignans, painted a more complete picture of the root's intricate chemical profile. This comprehensive analysis sets the stage for understanding the root's therapeutic potential.

Through rigorous biological activity studies, various root extracts demonstrated a compelling array of beneficial properties. Notably, significant antioxidant effects were observed, crucial for combating oxidative stress and cellular damage, alongside potent anti-inflammatory actions, providing insights into their potential to manage inflammatory conditions. The observed spasmolytic effects suggest applications in conditions involving muscle spasms, while their antimicrobial properties indicate a role in combating various pathogens. Moreover, the detection of anticholinesterase effects opens avenues for research into neurodegenerative disorders. Crucially, these extracts consistently exhibited favorable, low toxicity profiles, a critical factor for any potential therapeutic agent, underlining their safety for further development.

These robust findings provide significant scientific validation for numerous traditional uses of cannabis roots, many of which have been passed down through generations without formal scientific backing. More importantly, they underscore the immense and largely untapped potential of these roots as a novel source of therapeutic agents. Given that this integral part of the cannabis plant has historically been largely overlooked and underutilized in research and commercial applications, these results emphatically emphasize the critical importance of continued and in-depth research into cannabis roots. Further exploration will not only profoundly deepen the scientific understanding of their unique chemical compositions and biological properties but also actively promote a more sustainable and comprehensive utilization of *C. sativa*. By unlocking the full potential of its roots, the path can be paved for innovative pharmaceutical and medicinal applications, moving towards a future where no part of this valuable plant remains unexamined or undervalued.

Acknowledgments

Authors gratefully acknowledge Agencia Nacional de Promoción Científica y Tecnológica (ANPCyT) and Universidad Nacional de Rosario (UNR) for financial support (PICT-2020-SERIEA-02687 and 80020210300027UR). EC, LRM, and AB are also thankful to Consejo Nacional de Investigaciones Científicas y Técnicas (CONICET) for their doctoral and postdoctoral fellowships.

References

Antonisamy, P., Duraipandiyan, V., Aravinthan, A., Al-Dhabi, N. A., Ignacimuthu, S., Choi, K. C. et al. (2015). Protective effects of friedelin isolated from *Azima tetracantha* Lam. against ethanol-induced gastric ulcer in rats and possible underlying mechanisms. *European Journal of Pharmacology*, 750: 167–175.

Antonisamy, P., Duraipandiyan, V., and Ignacimuthu, S. (2011). Anti-inflammatory, analgesic and antipyretic effects of friedelin isolated from *Azima tetracantha* Lam. in mouse and rat models. *Journal of Pharmacy and Pharmacology*, 63: 1070–1077.

Aswar, U. M., Bhaskaran, S., Mohan, V., and Bodhankar, S. L. (2010). Estrogenic activity of friedelin rich fraction (IND-HE) separated from *Cissus quadrangularis* and its effect on female sexual function. *Pharmacognosy Research*, 2: 138–144.

Bukowska, B. (2024). Current and potential use of biologically active compounds derived from *Cannabis sativa* L. in the treatment of selected diseases. *International Journal of Molecular Sciences*, 25: 12738.

Cai, J., Zhao, L., and Tao, W. (2015). Potent protein tyrosine phosphatase 1B (PTP1B) inhibiting constituents from *Anoectochilus chapaensis* and molecular docking studies. *Pharmaceutical Biology*, 53: 1030–1034.

Chang, W., Wang, J., and Xiao, Y. (2020). Friedelin inhibits the growth and metastasis of human leukemia cells via modulation of MEK/ERK and PI3K/AKT signalling pathways. *Journal of BUON*, 25: 1594–1599.

Chinsembu, K. C. (2016). Tuberculosis and nature's pharmacy of putative anti-tuberculosis agents. *Acta Tropica*, 153: 46–56.

Dae, K. K., Jong, P. L., Jin, W. K., Hee, W. P., and Jae, S. E. (2005). Antitumor and antiinflammatory constituents from *Celtis sinensis. Archives of Pharmacal Research*, 28: 399–403.

Ding, Y., Liang, C., Kim, J. H., Lee, Y. M., Hyun, J. H., Kang, H. K. et al. (2010). Triterpene compounds isolated from *Acer mandshuricum* and their anti-inflammatory activity. *Bioorganic & Medicinal Chemistry Letters*, 20: 1528–1531.

Duraipandiyan, V., Al-Dhabi, N. A., Irudayaraj, S. S., and Sunil, C. (2016). Hypolipidemic activity of friedelin isolated from *Azima tetracantha* in hyperlipidemic rats. *Revista Brasileira de Farmacognosia*, 26: 89–93.

Elhendawy, M. A., Wanas, A. S., Radwan, M. M., Azzaz, N. A., Toson, E. S., and ElSohly, M. A. (2019). Chemical and biological studies of *Cannabis sativa* roots. *Medical Cannabis and Cannabinoids*, 1: 104–111.

El-Shiekh, R. A., Radi, M. H., Elshimy, R., Abdel-Sattar, E., El-Halawany, A. M., Ibrahim, M. A. et al. (2025). Friedelin: A natural compound exhibited potent antibacterial, anti-inflammatory, and wound healing properties against MRSA-infected wounds. *Naunyn-Schmiedeberg's Archives of Pharmacology*, 1–11.

Elsohly, M. A., Turner, C. E., Phoebe, C. H. Jr., Knapp, J. E., Schiff, P. L., and Slatkin, D. J. (1978). Anhydrocannabisativine, a new alkaloid from *Cannabis sativa* L. *Journal of Pharmaceutical Sciences*, 67: 124–124.

Farag, S., and Kayser, O. (2015). Cannabinoid production by hairy root cultures of *Cannabis sativa* L. *American Journal of Plant Sciences*, 6: 1874-1884.

Ferrini, F., Fraternale, D., Donati Zeppa, S., Verardo, G., Gorassini, A., Carrabs, V. et al. (2021). Yield, characterization, and possible exploitation of *Cannabis sativa* L. roots grown under aeroponics cultivation. *Molecules*, 26:4889.

Gagné, V., Merindol, N., Boucher, R., Boucher, N., and DesGagné-Penix, I. (2024). Rooted in therapeutics: Comprehensive analyses of *Cannabis sativa* root extracts reveal potent antioxidant, anti-inflammatory, and bactericidal properties. *Frontiers in Pharmacology*, 15: 1465136.

Gul, W., Gul, S. W., Chandra, S., Lata, H., Ibrahim, E. A., and ElSohly, M. A. (2018). Detection and quantification of cannabinoids in extracts of cannabis sativa roots using LC-MS/MS. *Planta Medica*, 84: 267–271.

Huang, S., Li, H., Xu, J., Zhou, H., Seeram, N. P., Ma, H. et al. (2023). Chemical constituents of industrial hemp roots and their anti-inflammatory activities. *Journal of Cannabis Research*, 5: 1.

Jamiu, A. T., Pohl, C. H., Bello, S., Adedoja, T., and Sabiu, S. (2021) A review on molecular docking analysis of phytocompounds against SARS-CoV-2 druggable targets. *All Life*, 14: 1100–1128.

Jiao, J., Zhang, Y., Lou, D., Wu, X., and Zhang, Y. (2007). Antihyperlipidemic and antihypertensive effect of a triterpenoid-rich extract from bamboo shavings and vasodilator effect of friedelin on phenylephrine-induced vasoconstriction in thoracic aortas of rats. *Phytotherapy Research*, 21: 1135–1141.

Jin, D., Dai, K., Xie, Z., and Chen, J. (2020). Secondary metabolites profiled in Cannabis inflorescences, leaves, stem barks, and roots for medicinal purposes. *Scientific Reports*, 10: 3309.

Jin, D., Henry, P., Shan, J., and Chen, J. (2021). Identification of chemotypic markers in three chemotype categories of Cannabis using secondary metabolites profiled in inflorescences, leaves, stem bark, and roots. *Frontiers in Plant Science*, 12: 699530.

Kar, P., Sharma, N. R., Singh, B., Sen, A., and Roy, A. (2021). Natural compounds from *Clerodendrum* spp. as possible therapeutic candidates against SARS-CoV-2: an *in silico* investigation. *Journal of Biomolecular Structure and Dynamics*, 39: 4774–4785.

Kornpointner, C., Martinez, A. S., Marinovic, S., Haselmair-Gosch, C., Jamnik, P., Schröder, K. et al. (2021). Chemical composition and antioxidant potential of *Cannabis sativa* L. roots. *Industrial Crops and Products*, 165: 113422.

Kumar, D., Kumar, S., Gupta, J., Arya, R., and Gupta, A. (2011). A review on chemical and biological properties of *Cayratia trifolia* Linn. (Vitaceae). *Pharmacognosy Reviews*, 5: 184–190.

Kumari, R., Meyyappan, A., Selvamani, P., Mukherjee, J., and Jaisankar, P. (2011). Lipoxygenase inhibitory activity of crude bark extracts and isolated compounds from *Commiphora berryi*. *Journal of Ethnopharmacology*, 138: 256–259.

Kundu, J. K., Rouf, A. S. S., Nazmul Hossain, M., Hasan, C. M., and Rashid, M. A. (2000). Antitumor activity of epifriedelanol from *Vitis trifolia. Fitoterapia*, 71: 580–582.

Latter, H. L., Abraham, D. J., Turner, C. E., Knapp, J. E., Schiff, P. L. Jr., and Slatkin, D. J. (1975). Cannabisativine, a new alkaloid from *Cannabis sativa* L. root. *Tetrahedron Letters*, 16: 2815–2818.

Lima, K. S. B., da Cruz Silva, M. E. G., de Lima Araújo, T. C., da Fonseca Silva, C. P., Santos, B. L. et al. (2021). Cannabis roots: Pharmacological and toxicological studies in mice. *Journal of Ethnopharmacology*, 271: 113868.

Menezes, P. M. N., de Lima Araújo, T. C., Pereira, E. C. V., Neto, J. A., Silva, D. S., Brito, M. C. et al. (2021). Investigation of antinociceptive, antipyretic, antiasthmatic, and spasmolytic activities of Brazilian *Cannabis sativa* L. roots in rodents. *Journal of Ethnopharmacology*, 278: 114259.

Menezes, P. M. N., Pereira, E. C. V., Lima, K. S. B., da Silva B. A. O., Brito, M. C., de Lima Araújo, T. C. et al. (2022). Chemical analysis by LC-MS of *Cannabis sativa* root samples from Northeast Brazil and evaluation of antitussive and expectorant activities. *Planta Medica*, 88: 1223–1232.

Mosquera-Yuqui, F., Lopez-Guerra, N., and Moncayo-Palacio, E. A. (2022). Targeting the 3CLpro and RdRp of SARS-CoV-2 with phytochemicals from medicinal plants of the Andean Region: molecular docking and molecular dynamics simulations. *Journal of Biomolecular Structure and Dynamics*, 40: 2010–2023.

Noufou, O., Wamtinga, S. R., André, T., Christine, B., Marius, L., Emmanuelle, H. A., Jean, K. et al. (2012). Pharmacological properties and related constituents of stem bark of *Pterocarpus erinaceus* Poir. (Fabaceae). *Asian Pacific Journal of Tropical Medicine*, 5: 46–51.

Nunes, R., Broering, M. F., De Faveri, R., Goldoni, F. C., Mariano, L. N., Mafessoli, P. C. et al. (2021). Effect of the metanolic extract from the leaves of *Garcinia humilis* Vahl (Clusiaceae) on acute inflammation. *Inflammopharmacology*, 29: 423–438.

Ouedraogo, N., Hay, A. E., Ouedraogo, J. C., Sawadogo, W. R., Tibiri, A., Lompo, M. et al. (2017). Biological and phytochemical investigations of extracts from *Pterocarpus erinaceus* Poir (Fabaceae) root barks. African *Journal of Traditional, Complementary and Alternative Medicines*, 14: 187–195.

Perumal, P. C., Sowmya, S., Velmurugan, D., Sivaraman, T., and Gopalakrishnan, V. K. (2016). Assessment of dual inhibitory activity of epifriedelanol isolated from *Cayratia trifolia* against ovarian cancer. *Bangladesh Journal of Pharmacology*, 11: 389–395.

Radi, M. H., El-Shiekh, R. A., El-Halawany, A. M., and Abdel-Sattar, E. (2023). Friedelin and 3β-friedelinol: pharmacological activities. *Revista Brasileira de Farmacognosia*, 33: 886–900.

Ryz, N. R., Remillard, D. J., Nascimento Meneze, P., Gama Silva, M., Martins Lavor, E., Souza Silva, F. et al. (2017). Cannabis roots: A traditional therapy with future potential for treating inflammation and pain. *Cannabis and Cannabinoid Research*, 2: 210–216.

Sethi, V. K., Jain, M. P., and Thakur, R. S. (1977). Chemical investigation of wild *Cannabis sativa* L. roots. *Planta Medica*, 32: 378–379.

Shi, B., Liu, S., Huang, A., Zhou, M., Sun, B., and Cao, H. (2021). Revealing the mechanism of friedelin in the treatment of ulcerative colitis based on network pharmacology and experimental verification. *Evidence-Based Complementary and Alternative Medicine*, 2021: 4451779.

Slatkin, D. J., Doorenbos, N. J., Harris, L. S., Masoud, A. N., Quimby, M. W., and Schiff, P. L. (1971). Chemical constituents of *Cannabis sativa* L. root. *Journal of Pharmaceutical Sciences*, 60: 1891–1892.

Slatkin, D. J., Knapp, J. E., Schiff, P. L., Turner, C. E., and Mole, M. L. Jr. (1975). Steroids of *Cannabis sativa* root. *Phytochemistry*, 14: 1442–1443.

Slatnar, A., Jakopic, J., Stampar, F., Veberic, R., and Jamnik, P. (2012). The effect of bioactive compounds on *in vitro* and *in vivo* antioxidant activity of different berry juices. *PLoS ONE*, 7: e47880.

Somwong, K., Lertpatipanpong, P., Nimlamool, W., Panya, A., Tragoolpua, Y., Yongsawas, R. et al. (2022). Effect of *Holoptelea integrifolia* (Roxb.) Planch. *n*-Hexane Extract and Its Bioactive Compounds on Wound Healing and AntiInflammatory Activity. *Molecules*, 27: 8540.

Subash-Babu, P., Li, D. K., and Alshatwi, A. A. (2017). *In vitro* cytotoxic potential of friedelin in human MCF-7 breast cancer cell: Regulate early expression of Cdkn2a and PRb1, neutralize Mdm2-p53 amalgamation and functional stabilization of p53. *Experimental and Toxicologic Pathology*, 69: 253–260.

Sunil, C., Duraipandiyan, V., Ignacimuthu, S., and Al-Dhabi, N. A. (2013). Antioxidant, free radical scavenging and liver protective effects of friedelin isolated from *Azima tetracantha* Lam. leaves. *Food Chemistry*, 139: 1582–1589.

Sunil, C., Irudayaraj, S. S., Duraipandiyan, V., Alrashood, S. T., Alharbi, S. A., and Ignacimuthu, S. (2021). Friedelin exhibits antidiabetic effect in diabetic rats via modulation of glucose metabolism in liver and muscle. *Journal of Ethnopharmacology*, 268: 113670.

Tian, J., Han, T., and Pan, M. (2021). Friedelin protects against alveolar epitelial cells apoptosis in LPS-induced acute pneumonia in neonatal rats by suppressing NF-κB activation. *Current Topics in Nutraceutical Research*, 19: 58–63.

Toukam, P. D., Tagatsing, M. F., Yamthe, L. R., Baishya, G., Barua, N. C., Tchinda, A. T. et al. (2018). Novel saponin and benzofuran isoflavonoid with *in vitro* anti-inflammatory and free radical scavenging activities from the stem bark of *Pterocarpus erinaceus* (Poir). *Phytochemistry Letters*, 28:69–75.

Whittle, B. A. (1964). Release of a kinin by intraperitoneal injection of chemical agents in mice. *International Journal of Neuropharmacology*, 3: 369–378.

Yang, H. H., Son, J. K., Jung, B., Zheng, M., and Kim, J. R. (2011). Epifriedelanol from the root bark of *Ulmus davidiana* inhibits cellular senescence in human primary cells. *Planta Medica*, 77: 441–447.

Yang, J., Fa, J., and Li, B. (2017). Apoptosis induction of epifriedelinol on the human cervical cancer cell line. *African Journal of Traditional, Complementary and Alternative Medicines*, 14: 1–7.

Yin, Z. Y., Li, L., Chu, S. S., Sun, Q., Ma, Z. L., and Gu, X. P. (2016) Antinociceptive effects of dehydrocorydaline in mouse models of inflammatory pain involve the opioid receptor and inflammatory cytokines. *Scientific Reports*, 6: 27129.

Chapter 11

Metabolic Health and the Therapeutic Potential of *Cannabis sativa*

Insights Into Obesity, Diabetes, Dyslipidemia, and Hypertension

Lucas Rannier Ribeiro Antonino Carvalho,[1] *Débora Gonçalves Paiva,*[2] *Januse Míllia Dantas de Araújo*[3,4] and *Jailane de Souza Aquino*[3,4,*]

1. Introduction

Cannabis, a plant of the *Cannabaceae* family, has been used for millennia by various cultures around the world, both for its resistant fibers, used in the manufacture of fabrics, ropes, and paper, and for its medicinal compounds in traditional practices to relieve pain, treat inflammation, and combat nausea. The two main subspecies of the plant—*sativa* and *indica*—are widely used, and distinguished by their therapeutic properties (Viana et al. 2024).

Cannabis contains a wide range of chemical compounds that interact uniquely with the human body. With more than 500 components, including terpenes, flavonoids, amino acids, and vitamins (Sánchez et al. 2015), it also stands out for around 100 unique cannabinoids, such as tetrahydrocannabinol (THC), responsible for the psychoactive effect, and cannabidiol (CBD), which does not produce a psychoactive effect (Viana et al. 2024). These compounds have analgesic, antiemetic, anticonvulsant, and anxiolytic functions, among others.

The compounds in this plant interact with the endocannabinoid system, an endogenous mammalian cell-signaling system comprising receptors, enzymes, and endocannabinoids (produced by the body). Receptors are proteins in cells that respond to substances by altering metabolic functions. The main receptors, CB1 and CB2, are concentrated in the central nervous system (CNS) and the immune system, respectively (Honório et al. 2006). CB1 receptors are recognized for their effects on cognition, memory, motor function, and especially pain. CB2 receptors are distributed in

[1] Department of Physiology and Pharmacology, Karolinska Institutet, Stockholm, Sweden.
[2] Centro Universitário de João Pessoa, Unipê, João Pessoa, Brazil.
[3] Department of Nutrition, Federal University of Paraíba, João Pessoa, Brazil.
[4] Postgraduate Program in Nutrition Sciences, Federal University of Paraíba, João Pessoa, Brazil.
* Corresponding author: jailane.aquino@academico.ufpb.br

DOI: 10.1201/9781003668190-13

the pancreas, liver, and immune system cells, including the spleen, thymus, bone marrow, lymph nodes, tonsils, and white blood cells (Small 2017). THC, for example, acts on the CB1 receptor, culminating in the plant's known psychoactive effects.

Endocannabinoids, such as anandamide and 2-AG, are signaling lipids that activate endocannabinoid receptors and function as extracellular retrograde messengers, being released from the postsynaptic neuron to act on presynaptic CB1 in an autocrine and paracrine manner and are responsible for regulating important functions, such as appetite and sleep (Costa et al. 2011).

The effects of receptor interactions are mediated by a signal transduction cascade that includes interactions with calcium and potassium channels, protein kinases, and extracellular signaling molecules that bind and undergo conformational changes to induce intracellular responses through G-protein coupling (Duggan 2021), the type of molecule that is normally bound but detaches when the receptor is stimulated, initiating a chain of biochemical events (Small 2017).

Signaling occurs through two steps: transport of endocannabinoids into cells and hydrolysis by specific enzymes. Unlike most neurotransmitters, such as acetylcholine, dopamine, and serotonin, endocannabinoids are not stored in vesicles; instead, they are synthesized as needed and, after exerting a local and temporary effect, their biological activity is terminated by enzymes such as fatty acid amide hydrolase (FAAH) and monoacylglycerol lipase (Duggan 2021).

Englund et al. (2012) described THC dosages of 5 mg for inhalation and 10 mg orally, resulting in mild effects, with doses higher than 20 mg by inhalation or 70 mg orally potentially resulting in very intense effects. As for CBD, the study obtained doses, between inhalation and oral, ranging from low doses 2.5–10 mg, medium doses 15–25 mg, and high doses 27.5–40 mg, with doses of 400 mg to 600 mg of CBD being used orally for the treatment of anxiety and epilepsy, and to reduce the adverse effects produced by THC.

According to Peyraube et al. (2015), the inhalation route is the most efficient, achieving a THC bioavailability of between 10 and 35%, with the effects beginning between seconds and minutes after inhalation and reaching a maximum effect after 20 minutes, lasting between 2 and 3 hours. Absorption in oral administration, however, is slow, and the same effect cannot be guaranteed in all doses. These effects begin between 30 minutes and 2 hours, with a maximum effect between 2 and 4 hours, and can persist for 5 to 6 hours. Low bioavailability is due to hepatic metabolism.

The use of medicinal Cannabis sativa has become increasingly widespread for the treatment of various diseases and conditions, such as obesity, hypertension, diabetes, dyslipidemia, chronic pain, epilepsy, multiple sclerosis, Alzheimer's, Autism Spectrum Disorder (ASD), anxiety, and stress. Cannabis can be administered in a variety of ways: flowers, vaporizers, added to food, capsules, dermatological creams, and, most commonly, oils. Each of these uses varies in terms of the speed of action and the duration of the effects.

Most commonly used in treatments, the oily extract is also the best way to consume cannabis, as it is lipophilic. Cannabis contains fatty acids, mainly polyunsaturated ones, such as linoleic acid or omega-6 (50% to 60% of the total fatty acids) and alpha-linolenic acid or omega-3 (20% to 25% of the total fatty acids), and is therefore considered to have high nutritional value, since both substances are obtained only through diet and are essential for maintaining human health. In addition, cannabis contains Vitamin E (0.1%) and proteins (25% to 30%) such as arginine and albumin, carbohydrates (20% to 30%), fiber (10% to 15%), and minerals (4% to 6%), mainly calcium, iron, magnesium, phosphorus, and zinc (Small 2017). THC and CBD easily cross the blood-brain and placental barriers and can also accumulate in breast milk. Their elimination is slow due to high binding to fats, their high binding to plasma proteins, and enterohepatic circulation. Most THC appears as metabolites, which are mainly eliminated through feces (68%) or urine (12%), although it is also eliminated through hair, saliva, and sweat (Grotenhermen 2003).

This chapter will describe the interactions and therapeutic possibilities of extracts of isolated or full-spectrum compounds of *Cannabis sativa* in the context of obesity, diabetes, dyslipidemia, and hypertension, correlating clinical and preclinical studies with nutrient absorption and the pathophysiology of metabolic diseases.

2. Cannabis and Obesity

Obesity is recognized as a chronic and multifactorial disease, characterized by excessive accumulation of body fat that compromises health and increases the risk of various comorbidities, such as type 2 diabetes, cardiovascular diseases, and certain types of cancer. Currently, the condition is diagnosed based on body mass index (BMI), with individuals classified as obese when their BMI is 30 kg/m^2 or higher (Rubino et al. 2025; World Health Organization 2024).

Obesity represents one of the major global public health challenges, with over 1 billion people affected in 2022. Among adults, 2.5 billion were overweight, of which 890 million were living with obesity. In children and adolescents aged 5 to 19 years, approximately 160 million were diagnosed with obesity, reflecting a significant increase over the past decades. Projections indicate that by 2035, the number of adults with obesity is expected to reach 1.53 billion, with 79% of affected adults and 88% of affected children primarily from low- and middle-income countries (World Health Organization 2024; World Obesity Federation 2024).

Several studies have established an association between *Cannabis sativa* use and a reduced risk of obesity and metabolic diseases (Alshaarawy and Anthony 2019; Adejumo et al. 2017). Moreover, certain compounds present in cannabis, as well as whole-plant cannabis extracts, have demonstrated anti-obesity potential in animal model experiments (Cluny et al. 2015; Franco-Arroyo et al. 2022; Eitan et al. 2024).

The *Cannabis sativa* plant has been widely used over the years as a therapeutic agent in some disorders. This species is rich in natural compounds, with more than 100 phytocannabinoids identified to date (Amin and Ali 2019), among which cannabidiol (CBD) and Δ9-tetrahydrocannabinol (THC) are the most prominent. In recent years, there has been a significant increase in the use of cannabinoids and medical cannabis, particularly in the form of whole-plant extracts, which contain a wide range of metabolites with potential therapeutic effects, including phytocannabinoids, terpenes, and flavonoids (Poyatos et al. 2020; Bautista et al. 2021), which have been tested mainly in preclinical studies.

2.1 Preclinical and Clinical Studies

Research evaluated the effects of administering organic cannabis extract on pancreatic cell function and tissue alterations in the pancreas of rats with high-fat diet (HFD)-induced obesity. The rats were treated by subcutaneous injection of cannabis extract for 28 days. During the first 5 days of treatment, a dose equivalent to 5 mg THC/kg of body weight (BW) was administered, followed by a dose equivalent to 2.5 mg THC/kg BW for the remaining treatments. The study results showed that the treatment reduced weight gain, improved glucose tolerance, and promoted the regulation of Cannabinoid Receptor Type 1 (CB1), Glucose Transporter Type (GLUT2), Uncoupling Protein 2 (UCP2), and Protein Kinase B (PKB) genes, indicating a protective action on pancreatic β-cells in the obesity model (Levendal et al. 2012).

Research led by Assa-Glazer et al. (2020) investigated the effects of administering cannabis extracts with different cannabinoid profiles in mice with metabolic syndrome induced by a high-fat/high-cholesterol diet (HFCD). The mice were randomized into different treatment groups. Mice in group CN1 received CBD-rich extracts, group CN2 received THC-rich extracts, and group CN6 received extracts containing similar amounts of THC and CBD. All groups received a dose of 5 mg/kg body weight via oral administration every 3 days for 6 months. The data showed that mice in group CN2 exhibited improved glucose tolerance, increased gut microbiota diversity, and reductions in liver enzymes Serum Glutamic-Oxaloacetic Transaminase (SGOT) and Serum Glutamic-Pyruvic Transaminase (SGPT), as well as hepatic inflammatory gene expression. Mice in group CN1 showed increased expression of inflammatory genes in the liver, elevated fasting glucose levels, and reduced gut microbiota diversity, while group CN6 showed intermediate effects with few significant changes. Thus, administration of THC-rich extracts stood out in minimizing changes caused by diet-induced metabolic syndrome in mice.

A study conducted by Eitan et al. (2024) investigated the effects of oil-based cannabis extracts enriched with THC and CBD in mice fed a high-fat diet. The extracts were administered orally in three consecutive phases with an escalating dosing regimen: (1) 10 μL of THC or CBD three times per week; (2) 10 mg/kg of THC or CBD for 5 weeks; and (3) 30 mg/kg for an additional 5 weeks. The results showed that the THC-rich extract prevented HFD-induced weight gain and attenuated hepatic steatosis, whereas the CBD-rich extract failed to prevent weight gain and further exacerbated hepatic steatosis. The study demonstrated that the THC-enriched cannabis extract exhibited greater anti-obesity potential.

In contrast to these findings, a prior study by Ignatowska-Jankowska et al. (2011) investigated the effects of cannabidiol (CBD) on body weight gain in rats and its relationship with type 2 cannabinoid receptors (CB2). Male Wistar rats received intraperitoneal injections of CBD at doses of 2.5 and 5 mg/kg/day for 14 consecutive days. The study demonstrated that CBD can modulate both body weight gain and food intake in these animals. This modulation may be attributed to the activation of CB2 receptors, which have been identified in immune cells, lymphoid organs, the gastrointestinal tract, adipose tissue, and hypothalamic brain regions involved in the regulation of food intake. These receptors have been associated with reduced food consumption and anti-obesogenic effects. These findings suggest that CBD may have therapeutic potential for treating metabolic disorders related to weight gain (Lowe et al. 2021). Some preclinical studies using *Cannabis sativa* in obesity models are summarized in Table 1.

Literature reports indicate that cannabis and its main bioactive compounds, such as THC and CBD, exert complex and multifaceted effects on metabolism. These effects involve the regulation of cannabinoid receptors, modulation of inflammatory pathways, behavioral changes, and influence on

Table 1: Preclinical studies in animal models on the therapeutic potential of *Cannabis sativa* for obesity.

Plant part/ Product	**Animal Model**	**Dose/Method**	**Effects**	**References**
Cannabis organic extract	Male *Wistar* rats fed a high-fat diet (HFD)	The treatment was administered by subcutaneous injection of cannabis extract on alternate days for 28 days. During the first 5 treatments, the dose was 5 mg of THC/kg of BW, and subsequently, the dose was 2.5 mg of THC/kg of BW.	Reduction in weight gain; improvement in glucose tolerance; protective effect on pancreatic β-cells.	Levendal et al. (2012)
Cannabis extracts rich in CBD and/or THC	C57BL/6 male mice fed with a high-fat/ cholesterol diet (HFCD)	The treatment was administered orally every 3 days for 6 weeks. **CN1 Group** –Treated with 5 mg/ kg BW of CBD-rich extract. **CN2 Group** – Treated with 5 mg/ kg BW of THC-rich extract. **CN6 Group** –Treated with 5 mg/ kg BW of CBD and THC-rich extract.	The THC-rich extract (CN2) improved glycemic parameters, liver function, and gut microbiota; the CBD-rich (CN1) extract worsened liver inflammation and fasting blood glucose levels, and reduced gut microbiota diversity.	Assa-Glazer et al. (2020)
Oil-based cannabis extracts enriched with THC or CBD	C57BL/6 male mice fed with HFD	The treatment was administered orally in three consecutive phases with increasing doses: (1) 10 μL of THC or CBD three times per week; (2) 10 mg/kg of THC or CBD for 5 weeks; (3) 30 mg/kg for an additional 5 weeks.	The treatment with THC-enriched extract prevented weight gain and reduced hepatic steatosis.	Eitan et al. (2024)

BW: Body Weight. CBD: Cannabidiol. HFCD: High-Fat/Colesterol Diet. HFD: High-Fat Diet. THC: Δ9-tetrahydrocannabinol.

weight gain associated with obesity (Ignatowska-Jankowska et al. 2020; Eitan et al. 2024). However, there is heterogeneity in the data and a limitation of more robust clinical studies. Therefore, further research is needed to clarify the mechanisms by which cannabis and its metabolites, including CBD and THC, induce metabolic changes that influence the pathophysiological parameters of diseases such as obesity.

3. Cannabis and Diabetes

Diabetes mellitus is a complex chronic metabolic condition characterized by persistently elevated blood glucose levels due to impairments in insulin secretion, insulin action, or both. This glycemic dysregulation leads, over time, to significant disturbances in carbohydrate, lipid, and protein metabolism, resulting in progressive damage to organs and systems, including the eyes, kidneys, peripheral nerves, heart, and blood vessels (American Diabetes Association 2024).

Diagnosis is based on specific laboratory parameters, including fasting plasma glucose, postprandial glucose, an oral glucose tolerance test, or elevated glycated hemoglobin (A1C). Diabetes is classified into four main categories: type 1, type 2, gestational diabetes, and other specific forms associated with defined causes, including genetic defects, exocrine pancreatic diseases, and the use of diabetogenic medications (Yameny 2024; American Diabetes Association 2024).

According to the International Diabetes Federation (2024), approximately 589 million adults aged 20 to 79 years worldwide have diabetes, and this number is expected to increase to approximately 853 million by 2050. The global prevalence of diabetes among adults has risen from 7% in 1990 to 14% in 2022. Most diabetes cases are found in low- and middle-income countries, where the rates of the disease have grown significantly, while access to adequate treatment remains limited.

Considering the complexity and the high global prevalence of diabetes, alternative treatments have been increasingly explored. Among these, plants rich in unsaturated fatty acids, bioactive, and antioxidant compounds have gained attention (García-Gurrola et al. 2024).

C. sativa exhibits potential antidiabetic effects attributed to its composition rich in bioactive compounds, including amino acids, particularly arginine, which contributes to metabolic regulation and the attenuation of type 2 diabetes symptoms (Szlas et al. 2022). Additionally, the oil contains gamma-linolenic acid (GLA), a fatty acid known for its anti-inflammatory and antioxidant properties, which play a role in mitigating diabetes-related complications (Won et al. 2020). The balanced composition of essential fatty acids in hemp oil, such as alpha-linolenic acid (ALA) and linoleic acid (LA), also exerts beneficial effects, as diets rich in ALA have demonstrated potential to improve insulin resistance by upregulating the expression of glucose transporter type 4 (GLUT4) in cells (Moran et al. 2014; Belury et al. 2018).

In this regard, various parts and derivatives of *C. sativa* have been the focus of numerous research studies aimed at exploring their effects and elucidating their mechanisms of action in the context of diabetes. These investigations seek to assess the potential of the plant's bioactive compounds in modulating the pathological mechanisms involved in the disease, including insulin resistance, glycemic control, and the prevention of associated metabolic complications.

3.1 Preclinical and Clinical Studies

A study conducted by Munteanu et al. (2023) investigated the effects of *Cannabis sativa* seed administration in *Wistar* rats with streptozotocin-induced diabetes. The findings demonstrated that a hemp seed-based diet significantly reduced blood glucose and total cholesterol levels compared to the untreated diabetic group. These beneficial effects were attributed to the seeds' nutritional composition, which is rich in proteins, polyunsaturated fatty acids, phenolic compounds, and other antioxidants, suggesting potential hypoglycemic, hypolipidemic, and anti-inflammatory properties.

A study conducted by Oliveira Carvalho et al. (2024) evaluated the effects of *C. sativa* oil on symptoms and biochemical parameters in rats with streptozotocin-induced diabetes. After induction of diabetes, the animals that received treatment were randomized into two groups: treated with CSO (400 mg/kg) or NCS (200 mg/kg) via oral administration for 30 days. The treatments with CSO and NCS promoted a reduction in the symptoms of polydipsia, polyuria, and alleviated body weight loss. A significant reduction in blood and urine glucose levels was observed, along with an elevation in insulin concentrations. Furthermore, the treatments increased the number of cells in the islets of Langerhans, with indications of cellular regeneration.

Another study that investigated the antidiabetic potential of the hydroethanolic extract of cannabis seeds (CSSE) in rats with diabetes induced by alloxan monohydrate solution demonstrated that treatment with the extract at a dose of 300 mg/kg administered orally for 28 days was able to significantly reduce fasting blood glucose, improve the lipid profile by lowering total cholesterol, LDL, and triglyceride levels, and exhibited hepatoprotective and nephroprotective effects, evidenced by the normalization of Aspartate Aminotransferase (AST), Alanine Aminotransferase (ALT), urea, and creatinine levels (El-Mernissi et al. 2024). Table 2 lists preclinical studies evaluating the effects of *C. sativa* in animal models of diabetes.

A randomized clinical trial evaluated the effects of cannabidiol (CBD) and tetrahydrocannabivarin (THCV) on glycemic and lipid parameters in patients with type 2 diabetes not receiving insulin. Participants were randomized into four groups for a 13-week treatment: CBD (100 mg twice daily), THCV (5 mg twice daily), a 1:1 combination of CBD and THCV (5 mg/5 mg twice daily), and a 20:1 combination of CBD and THCV (100 mg/5 mg twice daily). Treatment with THCV resulted in reduced fasting glucose levels, increased adiponectin and apolipoprotein A concentrations, and improved pancreatic β-cell function. Treatment with CBD reduced resistin levels and increased glucose-dependent insulinotropic peptide (GIP), while the combinations of CBD and THCV showed no significant effects (Zheng et al. 2023).

Research suggests that cannabis and its bioactive compounds may contribute to blood glucose regulation, improved insulin sensitivity, regeneration of pancreatic islet cells, and reduction of inflammation associated with diabetes. Although results from preclinical models are promising, thorough clinical studies are needed to validate the safety and efficacy of cannabis in diabetes treatment.

Table 2: Preclinical studies in animal models on the therapeutic potential of *Cannabis sativa* for diabetes.

Plant Part/Product	Animal Model	Dose/Method	Effects	References
Cannabis sativa seeds	Male *Wistar* rats with diabetes induced by intraperitoneal (i.p.) administration of STZ.	Cannabis seeds were offered ad libitum as part of the diet for 5 weeks.	Reduction of blood glucose and total cholesterol levels.	Munteanu et al. (2023)
Cannabis sativa seed oil (CSO) and oil nanoemulsion of *C. sativa* oil (NCS)	Male *Wistar* rats with diabetes induced by intraperitoneal (i.p.) administration of STZ.	Treatment administered orally for 30 days. **CSO Group** –Treated with 400 mg/kg of CSO. **NCS Group** –Treated with 200 mg/kg of NCS.	Reduction of blood glucose levels. Elevation of the number of cells in the islets of Langerhans. Increase in insulin levels.	de Oliveira Carvalho et al. (2024)
Hydro-ethanolic extract of *C. sativa L.* Seeds (CSSE)	Male Wistar rats with diabetes induced by alloxan monohydrate solution	Treatment with a dose of 300 mg/kg BW of CSSE was administered orally for 28 days.	Reduction of blood glucose. Improvement of lipid profile. Hepatoprotective and nephroprotective activity.	El-Mernissi et al. (2024)

BW: Body Weight. STZ: Streptozotocin.

4. Cannabis and Dyslipidemia

Dyslipidemia is a disorder of lipid metabolism, characterized by elevated levels of triglycerides (TG), total cholesterol (TC), and low-density lipoprotein cholesterol (LDL-C), along with reduced levels of high-density lipoprotein cholesterol (HDL-C) (Dakal et al. 2025). Dyslipidemia is considered a relevant and complex public health issue, as it is commonly linked to an increased risk and prevalence of cardiovascular diseases, which are the leading cause of death worldwide (Liu et al. 2022).

Elevated LDL-C reduces HDL-C and increases TG levels, disrupting lipid homeostasis, a key factor in the development of atherosclerotic cardiovascular disease (ASCVD) and cardiometabolic disorders (Liu et al. 2022). More specifically, dyslipidemia promotes endothelial dysfunction, persistent low-level inflammation, the formation of atherosclerotic plaques, and reduced insulin sensitivity, all of which collectively heighten the likelihood of developing cardiovascular and metabolic conditions (Rhee et al. 2024).

A recent study showed an increase in the prevalence of dyslipidemia from 41.3% to 48.4% between 2005 and 2022. Despite the rise in health interventions and treatment adherence, only 31.8% of individuals diagnosed with dyslipidemia achieved adequate lipid control (Lee et al. 2025). The increasing global prevalence of dyslipidemia has made this disorder a significant focus of scientific research aimed at identifying novel therapeutic strategies to reduce associated morbidity and mortality (Brunham et al. 2024; Pirillo et al. 2021).

In this context, medicinal plants have emerged as a prominent area of investigation due to their potential as alternative treatment sources. Among these, bioactive compounds and product derivatives from cannabis species have demonstrated promising effects in the management of dyslipidemia (De Oliveira Carvalho et al. 2024).

Cannabis seed oil has a high content of unsaturated fatty acids (UFAs), which constitute approximately 80 % of its total fatty acid composition. Among these, linoleic and linolenic acids are present at concentrations considered adequate to meet nutritional requirements. Studies investigating the effects of UFAs on lipid metabolism have demonstrated their potential to improve lipid profiles, as well as their cardioprotective properties and beneficial effects on the vascular endothelium (Kaushal et al. 2020a).

Furthermore, compounds derived from *Cannabis sativa*, particularly the cannabinoids CBD and THC, have shown therapeutic potential in various metabolic disorders. These cannabinoids can modulate hepatic metabolism and reduce oxidative stress in the organism. Their effects may be enhanced by terpenes, aromatic compounds found in cannabis. Some terpenes exhibit anti-inflammatory, antioxidant, and hepatoprotective properties that may synergize with cannabinoid activity (Pagano et al. 2023; Nuutinen 2018; Pattnaik et al. 2022).

In this context, preclinical and clinical studies have investigated the effects and mechanisms of action of various parts and derivatives of *C. sativa* on the pathophysiological processes underlying metabolic disorders and diseases.

4.1 Preclinical and Clinical Studies

Research conducted by Kaushal et al. (2020b) evaluated the effects of hempseed (*C. sativa*) supplementation in rats with diet-induced hypercholesterolemia. The rats were fed a high-fat diet containing 10% hempseed in its composition for 1 month. The results demonstrated that supplementation normalized the lipid profile by lowering cholesterol and triglyceride levels, attenuated cyclooxygenase-2 (COX-2)-mediated inflammation, and ameliorated tissue redox balance. Furthermore, it preserved vascular integrity and improved functional cardiovascular parameters in the treated animals. These findings suggest that the hypocholesterolemic effects of hempseed are mediated by modulation of inflammatory pathways involved in prostaglandin biosynthesis, regulated by redox-sensitive mechanisms.

Another study investigated the therapeutic potential of hempseed (*Cannabis sativa*) in rats with hypercholesterolemia, comparing its effects to those of statins. The treatment consisted of adding 10% hempseed to the rats' diet, which was offered for 1 month. The treatment with hempseed significantly reduced total cholesterol, triglycerides, and LDL-C, while increasing HDL-C levels. Additionally, hempseed powder decreased inflammatory markers and oxidative stress, lowered hepatic enzymes (AST and ALT), and reduced the expression of apolipoproteins Apo B and Apo E, which are essential in the regulation of lipid metabolism, as they are part of lipoproteins and play a role in the transport and metabolism of lipids in the body. These findings support the antihypercholesterolemic potential of *C. sativa* seeds (Kaur et al. 2021).

A study conducted by de Oliveira Carvalho et al. (2024) evaluated the effects of *C. sativa* seed oil (CSO) and a *C. sativa* oil nanoemulsion (NCS) in a rat model of dyslipidemia induced by intraperitoneal administration of Triton WR1339. The rats were treated orally with CSO (400 mg/kg) and NCS (200 mg/kg) for 10 days. Both treatments significantly reduced triglyceride, total cholesterol, and LDL-C levels, while increasing HDL-C levels in the rats. Some preclinical studies with *C. sativa* conducted in animal models with dyslipidemia are detailed in Table 3.

A study conducted by Brown et al. (2024) evaluated the influence of CBD on the activation of the pregnane X receptor (PXR) and its relationship with the risk of dyslipidemia. Mice were treated via oral gavage with a dose of 10 mg/kg/day of CBD for seven days. The findings showed

Table 3: Preclinical studies in animal models on the therapeutic potential of *Cannabis sativa* for dyslipidemia.

Plant Part/Product	Animal Model	Dose/Method	Effects	References
Cannabis sativa seeds (Hempseed)	Female *Wistar* rats fed a high-fat diet (HFD),	HFD supplemented with a 10% hempseed for 1 month,	Reduction of fat accumulation in the liver. Normalization of the lipid profile. Anti-inflammatory activity. Improved the redox status in the tissues.	Kaushal et al. (2020b).
Cannabis sativa seeds (Hempseed)	Female *Wistar* rats were fed a high-fat diet (HFD).	HFD supplemented with a 10% hempseed for 1 month.	Reduction of liver enzymes AST and ALT. Reduction of triglyceride, total cholesterol, and LDL-C and increased HDL-C levels. Decreased pro-inflammatory markers. Suppressed the expression of Apo B and Apo E. Attenuated oxidative stress markers.	Kaur et al. (2021)
Cannabis sativa seed oil (CSO) and oil nanoemulsion of *C. sativa* oil (NCS)	Male *Wistar* rats with dyslipidemia induced by intraperitoneal (i.p.) administration of Triton WR-1339.	Treatment administered orally for 10 days. CSO Group –Treated with 400 mg/kg of CSO. **NCS Group** –Treated with 200 mg/kg of NCS.	Reduction of triglyceride, total cholesterol, and LDL-C and increased HDL-C levels in rats.	de Oliveira Carvalho et al. (2024)
Cannabidiol	C57BL/6 male mice fed with HFD.	Treatment with a dose of 10 mg/kg BW of cannabidiol was administered orally for 7 days.	CDB increased plasma levels of cholesterol, LDL, and VLDL, as well as intestinal cholesterol uptake.	Brown et al. (2024)

ALT: Alanine Transaminase. AST: Aspartate Transaminase. BW: Body Weight. CBD: Cannabidiol. HDL-C: High-Density Lipoprotein Cholesterol. HFD: High-Fat Diet. LDL-C: Low-Density Lipoprotein Cholesterol. VLDL: Very Low-Density Lipoprotein.

that CBD increased plasma levels of total cholesterol, VLDL, and LDL, as well as upregulated the expression of cholesterol transporter genes Niemann-Pick C1-Like (NPC1L1), Microsomal Triglyceride Transfer Protein (MTP), and Cluster of Differentiation 36 (CD36) and PXR target genes Cytochrome P450 (CYP3A11) and Multidrug Resistance 1a (MDR1a). These effects were observed only in the group treated with CBD alone, but not in those receiving the combination of CBD and resveratrol. These results suggest that CBD negatively affected lipid metabolism in the animals.

To date, there is a lack of robust clinical studies directly investigating the therapeutic use of cannabis in humans with dyslipidemia. However, some preclinical studies have explored the effects of cannabinoid compounds such as cannabidiol (CBD) and tetrahydrocannabivarin (THCV) on related metabolic parameters related to dyslipidemia. Nevertheless, the effects and mechanisms influenced by cannabis and its derivatives remain poorly understood.

5. Cannabis and Hypertension

According to the World Health Organization (WHO), for the purpose of monitoring population health, hypertension is defined as having systolic blood pressure (SPB) greater than or equal to 140 mmHg or diastolic blood pressure (DPB) greater than or equal to 90 mmHg or taking medication for hypertension (Martin et al. 2025).

This is one of the most prevalent diseases and a major cause of premature death worldwide. It is estimated that 1.3 billion adults aged 30–79 years worldwide have hypertension, most (two-thirds) living in low- and middle-income countries. Another key factor about this condition is that less than half of adults (42%) with hypertension are diagnosed and treated, which leads to issues of social education and monitoring as pillars in the control, prevention, and treatment of hypertension worldwide (WHO 2023).

Regarding the pathophysiological pathways of hypertension, blood pressure (BP) under is normally regulated by the balance of several cardiovascular mechanisms, such as circulating blood volume and cardiac output—that is, the amount of blood pumped by the heart each minute. In addition, the balance of arterial tone, influenced by both intravascular volume and neurohumoral mechanisms, also plays a fundamental role. It is important to highlight that maintaining BP at physiological levels depends on a complex interaction among multiple factors within an integrated neurohumoral system, which includes the renin-angiotensin-aldosterone system (RAAS), natriuretic peptides, vascular endothelium, the sympathetic nervous system (SNS), and the immune system (Boron and Boulpaep 2020).

Pathological increase in blood pressure is also a multifactorial condition associated with metabolic disorders and changes in target organs, often aggravated by factors such as dyslipidemia, obesity, and diabetes mellitus (discussed above in this chapter). The development of the disease is related to age, sex, family history, race/color, diet (when rich in sodium or other food components), excessive alcohol consumption, and certain medications (Leopoldino et al. 2025).

Hypertension is often asymptomatic, with most individuals unaware of elevated blood pressure until it is measured. However, severely elevated blood pressure levels, typically above 180/120 mmHg, can manifest with symptoms such as severe headaches, chest pain, dizziness, dyspnea, nausea, vomiting, visual disturbances, including blurred vision, anxiety, confusion, tinnitus, epistaxis, and arrhythmias. Routine blood pressure monitoring is essential for early detection, as untreated hypertension significantly increases the risk of serious complications, including chronic kidney disease, cardiovascular disease, and stroke (WHO 2023; Martin et al. 2025).

Given the current scenario of hypertension in the world, new control and prevention strategies are important. In this context, multimodal strategies are often recommended, such as lifestyle improvements, a balanced diet, and regular physical exercise. Regarding these strategies, possible interactions with the endocannabinoid system have recently been discussed as an alternative for controlling cardiovascular changes (Mensah et al. 2022).

The endocannabinoid system (ECS) plays a crucial role in cardiovascular control by modulating cannabinoid receptors CB1 and CB2, which are distributed throughout the heart and blood vessels. Activation of the CB1 receptor, present mainly in cardiomyocytes and endothelial cells, promotes acute vasodilation and reduced cardiac contractility, but its chronic stimulation can contribute to vascular dysfunction, increased oxidative stress, and hypertension. On the other hand, the CB2 receptor, expressed mainly in immune system cells and in vessels under inflammatory conditions, exerts protective effects by attenuating inflammatory processes, reducing cell proliferation, and preventing vascular remodeling, playing an important role in protecting against cardiovascular diseases and controlling hypertension (Dziemitko et al. 2023; Rorabaugh et al. 2023). Thus, the balance between signaling via CB1 and CB2 is fundamental for cardiovascular homeostasis and constitutes a promising therapeutic avenue for interventions in cardiac and vascular diseases.

Currently, cannabinoids, that is, the molecules that act on the ECS, are classified into three large groups according to their origin: (i) phytocannabinoids, such as Δ^9-tetrahydrocannabinol (THC) and cannabidiol (CBD), derived mainly from the *Cannabis sativa* plant — although other plants, such as those of the Radula and Helichrysum genera, also contain cannabinoid compounds; (ii) endocannabinoids, such as anandamide (AEA) and 2-arachidonoylglycerol (2-AG), which are naturally produced by the mammalian body and act as endogenous messengers in the ECS; and (iii) synthetic cannabinoids, such as CP 55,940 and WIN 55,212-2, laboratory-created molecules that mimic or modulate the action of natural cannabinoids in the ECS, being important tools for research and potential therapeutic agents (Mensah et al. 2022).

In this topic, we will focus on the interactions of phytocannabinoids derived from *Cannabis sativa* in cardiovascular control and hypertension. More than 500 active compounds have been identified in different parts of the plant, but THC and CBD are the most relevant for modulating cardiovascular function by acting on different receptors of the ECS. THC predominantly activates the CB1 receptor, causing acute effects such as vasodilation and hypotension. However, it is worth noting that chronic use can result in adverse cardiovascular changes, such as hypertension. On the other hand, CBD acts indirectly, modulating the CB2 receptor and other pathways, promoting anti-inflammatory and antioxidant effects that help protect the cardiovascular system and control blood pressure (Dziemitko et al. 2023).

5.1 *Preclinical and Clinical Studies*

Most scientific research on this topic, as well as on other pathological conditions, explores the therapeutic potential of CBD extract, and to a lesser extent, full-spectrum extracts or combined extracts of CBD and THC. In cardiovascular pharmacology and research on hypertension, it is no different; CBD extract presents promising therapeutic properties in several clinical conditions, reducing blood pressure, directly influencing oxidative stress and redox balance of the vascular endothelium and sympathetic tone, all mechanisms directly involved in the control of heart activity and blood pressure (Harasim-Symbor et al. 2024).

To better understand the correlation between CBD and hypertension, Harasim-Symbor et al. (2024) investigated the influence of CBD on the myocardial lipid environment under hypertensive conditions in rats with spontaneous hypertension. The animals were divided into four groups: hypertensive rats, CBD-treated hypertensive rats, control normotensive rats, and control normotensive rats treated with CBD. The animals received 10 mg/kg of CBD for 14 days. The parameters (body weight, hemodynamic parameters, cardiac hypertrophy, systolic blood pressure, and heart rate) were measured on days 0, 7, and 14. The plasma fatty acid composition in normotensive rats remained the same after 14 days of CBD treatment. CBD treatment for 14 days resulted in a small improvement in the plasma lipid profile in hypertensive rats, accompanied by decreases in saturated fatty acids (–33.4%) and monounsaturated fatty acids (–55.9%). Polyunsaturated fatty acids were significantly lower in rats compared to control rats.

Another study conducted by Baranowska-Kuczko et al. (2021) examined the protective effects of CBD administration (10 mg/kg, once daily, for 2 weeks) on the (vascular) endothelium in aortas and small mesenteric arteries (G3) isolated from deoxycorticosterone-induced hypertensive rats (DOCA-salt) and spontaneously hypertensive rats (SHR). CBD reduced hypertrophy and improved vasodilation in both groups. CBD was shown to have vasoprotective effects regardless of vessel size and hypertension model (whether primary or secondary).

Krzyżewska and collaborators (2023) investigated whether CBD has antifibrotic potential in the right ventricle of rats with hypertension induced by monocrotaline at a dose of 60 mg/kg (administered once). Rats that received CBD at a dose of 10 mg/kg for 21 days had a 20% reduction in the amount of NT-proBNP (plasma B-type natriuretic peptide, considered one of the most important and useful indicators in the diagnosis of right ventricular failure resulting from hypertension), cardiomyocyte width (which had been increased by 75% and was decreased by around 10%), fibrosis area, and the expression of fibronectin and fibroblasts (the interstitial area of fibrosis of the right ventricle decreased by approximately 70% and the perivascular area of fibrosis of the right ventricle decreased by approximately 60%). The same authors demonstrated significant changes in the expression of TGF-β1 (transforming growth factor beta 1), Gal-3 (galectin 3, a marker of myocardial fibrosis in patients with heart failure), and SMAD2 and pSMAD2 (markers of the TGF-β pathway). Such factors are important because persistent overload, accompanied by concomitant inflammation leads to pathological remodeling and fibrosis of the heart (Krzyżewska et al. 2023).

Unlike studies using isolated CBD extracts, Khamseekaew and collaborators (2025) investigated the cardiovascular protective effects of *Cannabis sativa* L. leaf oil (known as full-spectrum) in Sprague Dawley rats with nitric oxide inhibitor-induced hypertension. During the experimental period, the rats developed a significant increase in blood pressure (184.75 ± 4.06 mmHg) compared with control rats (116.38 ± 1.02 mmHg). Hypertensive rats treated with *Cannabis sativa* L. leaf oil at doses of 1.0 and 1.5 mL/kg/day showed a significant reduction in the gradual increase in blood pressure (151.38 ± 3.34 and 147.38 ± 3.04 mmHg, respectively) compared to the hypertensive group (Khamseekaew et al. 2025).

Using a full-spectrum extract in a different animal model, Pereyra et al. (2025) investigated the effect of cannabis oil treatment on hypertrophy and mitochondrial status in the hearts of spontaneously hypertensive rats. The oil was administered for 1 month at a dose of 10 mg/kg per day. Echocardiographic analysis, performed at the beginning and end of the treatment period, demonstrated a significant reduction in the left ventricular mass index and diastolic wall thickness in the treated animals. There was preservation of systolic and diastolic ventricular diameters, while a significant increase in systolic ventricular diameter and a tendency towards an increase in diastolic ventricular diameter were observed on day 30 in the control group.

In addition, the treatment preserved ejection fraction, corroborating its beneficial impact on myocardial contractility, since the reduction in cardiac mass observed in this group was not accompanied by normalization of hemodynamic overload. Regarding blood pressure, no statistical difference was found between the groups (Pereyra et al. 2025). Some preclinical studies with *C. sativa* conducted in animal models with hypertension are detailed in Table 4.

Overall, the effects of *Cannabis sativa* are associated with improvements in glucose and lipid metabolism, modulation of redox balance, and antioxidant and anti-inflammatory activities. The main mechanisms underlying its potential therapeutic effects on obesity, diabetes, dyslipidemia, and hypertension are summarized in Figure 1.

Table 4: Preclinical studies in animal models on the therapeutic potential of *Cannabis sativa* for hypertension.

Plant Part/ Product	Animal Model	Dose/Method	Effects	References
CBD extract	Deoxycorticosterone-salt-induced hypertensive rats and spontaneously hypertensive rats.	10 mg/kg once daily for 2 weeks.	Reduced hypertrophy and improved the endothelium-dependent vasodilation in response to acetylcholine in the aortas and G3.	Baranowska-Kuczko et al. (2021)
CBD extract	Male *Wistar* rats	The treatment was administered by subcutaneous injection of CBD extract for 21 days.	Reduction in NT-proBNP, TGF-β1, Gal-3, SMAD2, and pSMAD2 markers. Increase in VE-cahderin.	Krzyżewska et al. 2023
CBD extract	Male spontaneously hypertensive rats and normotensive Wistar-Kyoto control rats.	The rats were injected intraperitoneally (i.p.) with CBD in a dose of 10 mg/kg once a day for 14 days.	SFAs (-33.4%), MUFAs (-55.9%), and PUFAs were significantly decreased in hypertensive rats compared to the normotensive controls.	Harasim-Symbor et al. 2024
Hemp (*Cannabis sativa* L.) leaf oil (HLO)	Sprague Dawley rats.	The rats were treated with HLO at doses of 1.0 and 1.5 mL/kg/day.	Significant reduction in the gradual increase in SBP (151.38 ± 3.34 and 147.38 ± 3.04 mmHg, respectively) compared to that in the hypertensive rats group.	Khamseekaew et al. 2025
Cannabis Oil (CBD+THC)	Male spontaneously hypertensive rats (SHR)	The daily dose of Cannabis oil used was 10 mg/kg/day for 1 month.	Significant reduction in the left ventricular mass index (LVMI) and diastolic wall thickness. Treatment also preserved both systolic and diastolic ventricular diameters.	Pereyra et al. 2025

SFAs: Saturated Fatty Acids. MUFAs: Monounsaturated Fatty Acids. PUFAs: Polyunsaturated Fatty Acids. SBP: Systolic Blood Pressure.

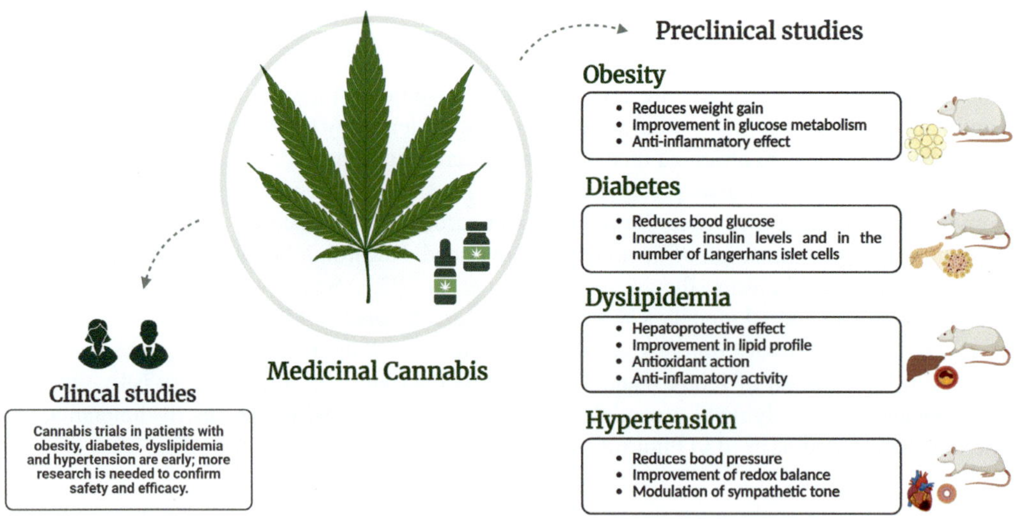

Figure 1: Mechanisms of the potential therapeutic effects of *Cannabis sativa* in obesity, diabetes, dyslipidemia, and hypertension. Source: Elaborated by the authors.

6. Conclusions and Perspectives

Cannabis sativa has shown significant therapeutic potential in the context of metabolic disorders, particularly through its major cannabinoids, THC and CBD. Preclinical and clinical studies suggest benefits in conditions such as obesity, diabetes, dyslipidemia, and hypertension, including improvements in glucose and lipid metabolism, anti-inflammatory effects, and cardiovascular protection, as shown in the graphical abstract.

While THC-enriched extracts have demonstrated anti-obesity and hepatoprotective effects, CBD shows promise for its vasodilatory and antifibrotic properties. However, isolated CBD may exert adverse effects on lipid metabolism, underscoring the importance of evaluating compound combinations, dosages, and the critical role of prescribing physicians in monitoring and managing treatment.

To translate these findings into clinical practice, robust randomized trials are needed to establish efficacy, safety, and optimal therapeutic protocols. Future research should also consider individual variability, drug interactions, and standardized production of cannabis-based formulations. With appropriate scientific and regulatory advances, *Cannabis sativa* may become a valuable tool in the management of metabolic and cardiovascular diseases.

References

Abrahamowicz, A. A., Ebinger, J., Whelton, S. P., Mensah, Y. C., and Yang, E. (2023). Racial and ethnic disparities in hypertension: Barriers and opportunities to improve blood pressure control. *Current Cardiology Reports*, 25(1): 17–27. https://doi.org/10.1007/s11886-022-01826-x

Adejumo, A. C., Alliu, S., Ajayi, T. O., Adejumo, K. L., Adegbala, O. M., Onyeakusi, N. E. et al. (2017). Cannabis use is associated with reduced prevalence of non-alcoholic fatty liver disease: A cross-sectional study. *PloS one*, 12(4): e0176416.

Alshaarawy, O., and Anthony, J. C. (2019). Cannabis use among women of reproductive age in the United States: 2002–2017. *Addictive behaviors*, 99: 106082.

American Diabetes Association. (2024). Diagnosis and classification of diabetes: Standards of care in diabetes—2024. *Diabetes Care,* 47(Suppl 1): S20–S42.

Amin, M. R., and Ali, D. W. (2019). Pharmacology of medical cannabis. *Recent advances in cannabinoid physiology and pathology*, 151–165.

Assa-Glazer, T., Gorelick, J., Sela, N., Nyska, A., Bernstein, N., and Madar, Z. (2020). Cannabis extracts affected metabolic syndrome parameters in mice fed high-fat/cholesterol diet. *Cannabis and Cannabinoid Research*, 5(3): 202–214.

Baranowska-Kuczko, M., Kozłowska, H., Kloza, M., Kusaczuk, M., Harasim-Symbor, E., Biernacki, M. et al. (2021). Vasoprotective endothelial effects of chronic cannabidiol treatment and its influence on the endocannabinoid system in rats with primary and secondary hypertension. *Pharmaceuticals*, 14: 1120. https://doi.org/10.3390/ph14111120.

Bautista, J. L., Yu, S., and Tian, L. (2021). Flavonoids in *Cannabis sativa*: Biosynthesis, bioactivities, and biotechnology. *ACS omega*, 6(8): 5119–5123.

Belury, M. A., Cole, R. M., Snoke, D. B., Banh, T., and Angelotti, A. (2018). Linoleic acid, glycemic control, and Type 2 diabetes. Prostaglandins, Leukotrienes, and Essential Fatty Acids, 132: 30–33.

Boron, W. F., and Boulpaep, E. L. (2020). *Medical physiology* (5th ed.). Elsevier.

Brown, C., Kariuki, W., Zhong, H. A., Kippes, A., and Sui, Y. (2024). Cannabidiol promotes intestinal cholesterol uptake mediated by Pregnane X receptor. *Frontiers in Endocrinology*, 15: 1398462.

Brunham, L. R., Lonn, E., and Mehta, S. R. (2024). Dyslipidemia and the current state of cardiovascular disease: epidemiology, risk factors, and effect of lipid lowering. *Canadian Journal of Cardiology*, 40(8): S4-S12.

Cluny, N. L., Keenan, C. M., Reimer, R. A., Le Foll, B., and Sharkey, K. A. (2015). Prevention of diet-induced obesity effects on body weight and gut microbiota in mice treated chronically with Δ9-tetrahydrocannabinol. *PloS one*, 10(12): e0144270.

Costa, J. L. G. P., Maia, L. O., Orlandi-Mattos, P., Villares, J. C., and Esteves, M. a. F. (2011). Neurobiologia da Cannabis: do sistema endocanabinoide aos transtornos por uso de Cannabis. *Jornal Brasileiro De Psiquiatria*, 60(2): 111–122. https://doi.org/10.1590/s0047-20852011000200006.

Dakal, T. C., Xiao, F., Bhusal, C. K., Sabapathy, P. C., Segal, R., Chen, J. et al. (2025). Lipids dysregulation in diseases: core concepts, targets and treatment strategies. *Lipids in Health and Disease*, 24(1): 61.

Dakal, T. C., Xiao, F., Bhusal, C. K., Sabapathy, P. C., Segal, R., Chen, J. et al. (2025). Lipids dysregulation in diseases: core concepts, targets and treatment strategies. *Lipids in Health and Disease*, 24(1): 61.

de Oliveira Carvalho, H., de Melo Santos, A., de Lima Teixeira dos Santos, A. V. T., Gonçalves, D. E. S., Picanço, K. R. T., Souza, B. S. F. E. et al. (2024). *Cannabis sativa* L. fixed oil and its nanoemulsion: Effect on diabetes and dyslipidemia induced in rats. *Pharmacognosy Magazine*, 20(3): 908–920.

Ditchfield, J. (2014). *The medical cannabis guidebook : The definitive guide to using and growing medicinal marijuana.* Green Candy Press.

Duggan, P. J. (2021). The chemistry of cannabis and cannabinoids. *Australian Journal of Chemistry*, 74(6): 369–387. https://doi.org/10.1071/ch21006.

Dziemitko, S., Harasim-Symbor, E., and Chabowski, A. (2023). How do phytocannabinoids affect cardiovascular health? An update on the most common cardiovascular diseases. *Therapeutic Advances in Chronic Disease,* 14. https://doi.org/10.1177/20406223221143239.

Eitan, A., Gover, O., Sulimani, L., Meiri, D., and Schwartz, B. (2023). The effect of orally administered δ9-tetrahydrocannabinol (THC) and cannabidiol (CBD) on obesity parameters in mice. *International Journal of Molecular Sciences*, 24(18): 13797.

El-Mernissi, R., El Menyiy, N., Metouekel, A., Zouhri, A., El-Mernissi, Y., Siddique, F. et al. (2024). Characterization of phenolic compounds and evaluation of anti-diabetic potential in *Cannabis sativa* L. seeds: *In vivo, in vitro*, and *in silico* studies. *Open Life Sciences*, 19(1): 20221024.

Englund, A., Morrison, P. D., Nottage, J., Hague, D., Kane, F., Bonaccorso, S. et al. (2012). Cannabidiol inhibits THC-elicited paranoid symptoms and hippocampal-dependent memory impairment. *Journal of Psychopharmacology*, 27(1): 19–27. https://doi.org/10.1177/0269881112460109.

Filipe Lacerda Leopoldino, Teixeira, L., Maria, A., Alice, A., Karina, Santiago, A. V., Silva, H. R., and Márcia, R. (2025). *Epidemiologia Nutricional Da Hipertensão Arterial Sistêmica*. https://doi.org/10.47094/978-65-6036-811-8/21-39.

Franco-Arroyo, N. N., Viveros-Paredes, J. M., Zepeda-Morales, A. S. M., Roldán, E., Márquez-Aguirre, A. L., Zepeda-Nuño, J. S. et al. (2022). β-Caryophyllene, a dietary cannabinoid, protects against metabolic and immune dysregulation in a diet-induced obesity mouse model. *Journal of Medicinal Food*, 25(10): 993–1002.

García-Gurrola, A., Martínez, A. L., Wall-Medrano, A., Olivas-Aguirre, F. J., Ochoa-Ruiz, E., and Escobar-Puentes, A. A. (2024). Phytochemistry, anti-cancer, and anti-diabetic properties of plant-based foods from mexican agrobiodiversity: A Review. *Foods*, 13(24): 4176.

Grotenhermen, F. (2003). Pharmacokinetics and pharmacodynamics of cannabinoids. *Clinical pharmacokinetics*, 42(4): 327–360. https://doi.org/10.2165/00003088-200342040-00003.

Harasim-Symbor, E., Bielawiec, P., Pedzinska-Betiuk, A., Weresa, J., Malinowska, B., Konstantynowicz-Nowicka, K. et al. (2024). Cannabidiol treatment changes myocardial lipid profile in spontaneously hypertensive rats. *Nutrition, Metabolism, and Cardiovascular Diseases: NMCD*, 34(12): 2817–2833. https://doi.org/10.1016/j.numecd.2023.07.007.

Honório, K. M., Arroio, A., and Da Silva, A. B. F. (2006). Aspectos terapêuticos de compostos da planta *Cannabis sativa. Química Nova*, 29(2): 318–325. https://doi.org/10.1590/s0100-40422006000200024.

Ignatowska-Jankowska, B., Jankowski, M. M., and Swiergiel, A. H. (2011). Cannabidiol decreases body weight gain in rats: involvement of CB2 receptors. *Neuroscience letters*, 490(1): 82-84.

International Diabetes Federation. (2024). *IDF diabetes atlas* (10th ed.). International Diabetes Federation. https://diabetesatlas.org/data-by-location/global/?utm_source=chatgpt.com.

Kaur, S., Garg, A., and Kaushal, N. (2021). Hempseed (*Cannabis sativa*) offers effective alternative over statins in ameliorating hypercholesterolemia associated nephropathy. *Clinical Biochemistry*, 93: 104–111.

Kaushal, N., Dhadwal, S., and Kaur, P. (2020a). Ameliorative effects of hempseed (*Cannabis sativa*) against hypercholesterolemia associated cardiovascular changes. *Nutrition, Metabolism and Cardiovascular Diseases*, 30(2): 330–338.

Kaushal, N., Gupta, M., and Kulshreshtha, E. (2020b). Hempseed (*Cannabis sativa*) lipid fractions alleviate high-fat diet-induced fatty liver disease through regulation of inflammation and oxidative stress. *Heliyon*, 6(7).

Khamseekaew, J., Duangjinda, M., Maneesai, P., Labjit, C., Rattanakanokchai, S., Rongpan, S. et al. (2025). *Cannabis sativa* L. Leaf Oil Displays Cardiovascular Protective Effects in Hypertensive Rats. *Int. J. Mol. Sci.*, 26: 1897. https://doi.org/ 10.3390/ijms26051897.

Krzyżewska, A., Baranowska-Kuczko, M., Kasacka, I., and Kozłowska, H. (2023). Cannabidiol alleviates right ventricular fibrosis by inhibiting the transforming growth factor β pathway in monocrotaline-induced pulmonary hypertension in rats. *Biochimica et Biophysica Acta (BBA) - Molecular Basis of Disease*, 1869(6): 166753–166753. https://doi.org/10.1016/j.bbadis.2023.166753.

Lee, H., Kim, S., Son, Y., Kim, S., Kim, H. J., Jo, H. et al. (2025). National trends in dyslipidemia prevalence, awareness, treatment, and control in South Korea from 2005 to 2022. *Scientific Reports*, 15(1): 1–17.

Levendal, R. A., Schumann, D., Donath, M., and Frost, C. L. (2012). Cannabis exposure associated with weight reduction and β-cell protection in an obese rat model. *Phytomedicine*, 19(7): 575–582.

Liu, T., Zhao, D., and Qi, Y. (2022). Global trends in the epidemiology and management of dyslipidemia. *Journal of Clinical Medicine*, 11(21): 6377.

Lowe, H., Toyang, N., Steele, B., Bryant, J., and Ngwa, W. (2021). The endocannabinoid system: a potential target for the treatment of various diseases. *International Journal Of Molecular Sciences*, 22(17): 9472.

Malachias, M. et al. 7ª Diretriz Brasileira de Hipertensão Arterial: Capítulo 5 - Decisão e Metas Terapêuticas. Arq Bras Cardiol., v. 107, n. 3, p. 25–29, set. 2016.

Martin, S. S., Aday, A. W., Allen, N. B., Almarzooq, Z. I., Anderson, C. A. M., Arora, P. et al. (2025). 2025 heart disease and stroke statistics: A report of US and global data from the American Heart Association. *Circulation,* 151(e41): e41–e660. https://doi.org/10.1161/CIR.0000000000001303.

Mensah, E., Tabrizchi, R., and Daneshtalab, N. (2022). Pharmacognosy and effects of cannabinoids in the vascular system. *ACS Pharmacology & Translational Science,* 5(11): 1034–1049. https://doi.org/10.1021/acsptsci.2c00141.

Moran, B. M., Abdel-Wahab, Y. H., Flatt, P. R., and McKillop, A. M. (2014). Evaluation of the insulin releasing and glucose lowering effects of GPR120 activation in pancreatic β cells. *Diabetes, Obesity and Metabolism*, 16(11): 1128–1139.

Munteanu, C., Mihai, M., Dulf, F., Ona, A., Muntean, L., Ranga, F. et al. (2023). Biochemical changes induced by the administration of *Cannabis sativa* seeds in diabetic wistar rats. *Nutrients*, 15(13): 2944.

Nuutinen, T. (2018). Medicinal properties of terpenes found in *Cannabis sativa* and *Humulus lupulus*. *European Journal of Medicinal Chemistry*, 157: 198–228.

Pagano, C., Savarese, B., Coppola, L., Navarra, G., Avilia, G., Laezza, C. et al. (2023). Cannabinoids in the modulation of oxidative signaling. *International Journal of Molecular Sciences*, 24(3): 2513.

Pattnaik, F., Nanda, S., Mohanty, S., Dalai, A. K., Kumar, V., Ponnusamy, S. K. et al. (2022). Cannabis: Chemistry, extraction and therapeutic applications. *Chemosphere*, 289: 133012.

Pereyra, E. V., Godoy Coto, J., Velez Rueda, J. O., Cavalli, F. A., González Arbelaez, L. F., Fantinelli, J. C. et al. (2025). Beneficial consequences of one-month oral treatment with cannabis oil on cardiac hypertrophy and the mitochondrial pool in spontaneously hypertensive rats. *Cannabis and Cannabinoid Research.* https://doi.org/10.1089/can.2024.0066.

Pirillo, A., Casula, M., Olmastroni, E., Norata, G. D., and Catapano, A. L. (2021). Global epidemiology of dyslipidaemias. *Nature Reviews Cardiology*, 18(10): 689–700.

Poyatos, L., Pérez-Acevedo, A. P., Papaseit, E., Pérez-Mañá, C., Martin, S., Hladun, O. et al. (2020). Oral administration of cannabis and Δ-9-tetrahydrocannabinol (THC) preparations: a systematic review. *Medicina*, 56(6): 309.

Reckelhoff, J. F. (2018). Gender differences in hypertension. *Current Opinion in Nephrology and Hypertension*, 27(3): 176–181. https://doi.org/10.1097/mnh.0000000000000404.

Rhee, M., Lee, J., Lee, E. Y., Yoon, K. H., and Lee, S. H. (2024). Lipid variability induces endothelial dysfunction by increasing inflammation and oxidative stress. *Endocrinology and Metabolism*, 39(3): 511–520.

Rorabaugh, B. R., Guindon, J., and Morgan, D. J. (2023). Role of cannabinoid signaling in cardiovascular function and ischemic injury. *Journal of Pharmacology and Experimental Therapeutics,* 387(3): 265–276. https://doi.org/10.1124/jpet.123.001665

Rubino, F., Cummings, D. E., Eckel, R. H., Cohen, R. V., Wilding, J. P., Brown, W. A. et al. (2025). Definition and diagnostic criteria of clinical obesity. *The Lancet Diabetes & Endocrinology.*

Sánchez, L., Peyraube, R., and Bouso, J. C. (2015). *Marihuana como medicina? Usos médicos y terapéuticos del cannabis y los cannabinoides.* México Unido contra la Delincuencia A.C.

Small, E. (2017). *Cannabis: A Complete Guide.* Boca Raton, FL: CRC Press.

Szlas, A., Kurek, J. M., and Krejpcio, Z. (2022). The potential of L-arginine in prevention and treatment of disturbed carbohydrate and lipid metabolism—a review. *Nutrients*, 14(5): 961.

Viana, T. R. X., Venute, L., Coelho, A., Souza, D. R., Deus, R. X., C, C., Pontes, E. A. S et al. (2024). Cannabis medicinal: O Poder Terapêutico. In *EDITORA CRV eBooks*. https://doi.org/10.24824/978652516100.6

Won, J. C., Kwon, H. S., Moon, S. S., Chun, S. W., Kim, C. H., Park, I. B. et al. (2020). γ-Linolenic acid versus α-lipoic acid for treating painful diabetic neuropathy in adults: a 12-week, double-placebo, randomized, noninferiority trial. *Diabetes Metab. J.*, 44(4): 542–554.

World Health Organization. (2023). *Global report on hypertension: The race against a silent killer*. Geneva: WHO. https://www.who.int/publications/i/item/9789240081062

World Health Organization. (2024). *Obesity and overweight*. https://www.who.int/news-room/fact-sheets/detail/obesity-and-overweight.

World Obesity Federation. (2024). *World Obesity Atlas 2024*. https://www.worldobesity.org/news/world-obesity-atlas-2024

World Obesity Federation. (2024). *World Obesity Atlas 2024.* https://www.worldobesity.org/news/world-obesity-atlas-2024

Yameny, A. A. (2024). Diabetes Mellitus Overview 2024. Journal of Bioscience and Applied Research, 10(3), 641-645.

Zheng, T., BouSaba, J., Taylor, A., Dilmaghani, S., Busciglio, I., Carlson, P. et al. (2023). A randomized, controlled trial of efficacy and safety of cannabidiol in idiopathic and diabetic gastroparesis. *Clinical Gastroenterology and Hepatology*, 21(13): 3405–3414.

Section 3
Toxicity and Risk Assessment

Chapter 12

Risks and Benefits of Cannabis and Cannabinoids in Psychiatry

Paulo Sousa Lima Junior,[1,*] *Melciades Norberto,*[1] *Italo Moita*[2] and *Chistiane M. Feitosa*[1]

1. Introduction

The interest in *Cannabis sativa* and its components, including Δ9-tetrahydrocannabinol (THC) and cannabidiol (CBD) (Figure 1), has grown significantly in the field of psychiatry (Maccarrone et al. 2023). This has been driven both by the increasing legalization and acceptance of cannabis use for medicinal and recreational purposes in various regions of the world and by the identification of potential therapeutic effects of certain cannabinoids in a variety of mental disorders (Bonaccorso et al. 2019).

However, the relationship between cannabis and mental health is complex and varied, with evidence suggesting both significant risks and potential benefits, aspects that require rigorous research to elucidate pharmacological mechanisms, delimit clinical indications, and mitigate possible harm, especially in vulnerable populations, such as adolescents or individuals with a predisposition to psychotic disorders (Hill et al. 2022).

On the one hand, scientific literature has shown an association between cannabis use, particularly in adolescents and young adults, and an increased risk of developing schizophrenia and other psychotic disorders, with studies indicating that factors such as age of onset of use, frequency and duration of consumption can significantly influence this risk, as evidenced by longitudinal research that points to greater vulnerability in users who start before the age of 15 or consume high-potency varieties (e.g., with a high THC content) (Villate et al. 2024). This suggests a complex interaction between genetic predisposition, brain development, and environmental exposure, reinforcing the need for preventive policies aimed at greater clarification of the limits between recreational use and neuropsychiatric damage (Villate et al. 2024).

[1] Laboratory of Research in Medicinal Plants and Experimental Neurochemistry, Federal University of Piauí, 64.049-550, Ininga, Teresina, PI, Brazil.

[2] State University of Maranhao, Central Street, Godofredo Viana, 1300. Medical Course, 65901-050, Imperatriz, Maranhão, Brazil.

* Corresponding author: pjrfarmacia36@ufpi.edu.br

DOI: 10.1201/9781003668190-15

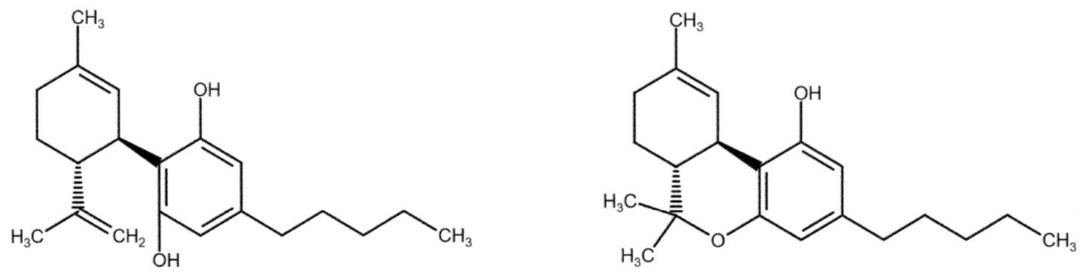

Cannabidiol **Tetrahydrocannabinol**

Figure 1: Chemical structures of cannabidiol (CBD) and tetrahydrocannabinol (THC), the two main active components of the cannabis plant.

Additionally, the ratio between THC and CBD in cannabis products appears to be a crucial factor, with preparations high in THC and low in CBD, such as what is known as "skunk," being considered less safe in terms of the risk of psychotic symptoms (Cavaleri et al. 2024). In fact, THC exposure has been shown to modulate brain function and psychopathology in ways that may contribute to the development of psychotic symptoms in vulnerable individuals, and symptoms similar to acute psychosis have also been observed following oral cannabis administration (Sepehr et al. 2025).

On the other hand, cannabidiol (CBD), another phytocannabinoid abundant in *Cannabis sativa*, has emerged as a substance with therapeutic potential for various psychiatric disorders, and research has explored its efficacy and safety in the treatment of conditions such as: substance use disorders, chronic psychosis and anxiety, both alone and in combination with other treatments, as shown by preclinical studies associating CBD with the modulation of serotoninergic (5-HT1A) and cannabinoid (CB1/CB2) receptors (Rong et al. 2017). Such mechanisms may explain its anxiolytic and antipsychotic effects, in addition to clinical evidence, such as placebo-controlled trials, which indicate symptom reduction in patients with refractory schizophrenia and post-traumatic stress disorder (PTSD) (Bonaccorso et al. 2019).

Although challenges such as variability in bioavailability and lack of dose standardization persist, randomized clinical studies highlight the therapeutic potential of CBD in psychopathological conditions, with pharmacological activities distinct from THC, including anxiolytic, antipsychotic, and neuroprotective properties, as well as modulating the serotonergic system (mechanisms relevant to psychiatric disorders) (McGuire et al. 2018). In addition, evidence suggests that CBD can attenuate psychotomimetic effects and cognitive impairment induced by THC; however, integrating its use into clinical practice requires rigorous protocols and longitudinal studies that validate its safety and efficacy (Chuang et al. 2021; Coles et al. 2023; Wegener 2024).

Therefore, this chapter explores the complex duality of cannabinoids in psychiatry, analyzing both the potential therapeutic benefits of CBD and THC and their neuropsychiatric risks, especially in vulnerable populations, to provide a considered view of the current evidence and discuss its clinical and public health implications, guiding the debate on safe and judicious integration into mental health care.

1.1 Definition and Classification of Cannabinoids and Their Uses in Psychiatry

Cannabinoids are a vast and diverse class of chemical compounds that interact with the endocannabinoid system, a complex cell signaling network present in mammals and other organisms. Their classification is fundamental to understanding their origins, properties, and therapeutic potential. Traditionally, cannabinoids are grouped into three main categories: phytocannabinoids, endocannabinoids, and synthetic cannabinoids (Zou and Kumar 2018). Phytocannabinoids are natural compounds derived from plants, with the species *C sativa* L. being their primary and best-known source. This plant is notable for producing a myriad of chemical substances, including at least 66 compounds identified as cannabinoids (Hanuš et al. 2016). Among these, Δ9-tetrahydrocannabinol (THC) and cannabidiol (CBD) stand out as the most extensively studied and characterized due to their pronounced biological activities and therapeutic relevance (Simiyu et al. 2022).

Endocannabinoids, on the other hand, are cannabinoids produced endogenously by animal organisms, including humans (Pagano et al. 2022). These natural lipid substances function as retrograde neurotransmitters and neuromodulators, playing crucial roles in regulating a wide range of physiological processes (Śmiarowska et al. 2022). The most prominent and well-characterized endocannabinoids are N-arachidonoyl ethanolamine, commonly known as anandamide (AEA), and 2-arachidonoyl glycerol (2-AG) (Mock et al. 2023).

The third category encompasses synthetic cannabinoids, which are compounds designed and produced in laboratories. These compounds are designed to mimic the effects of natural cannabinoids by interacting with cannabinoid receptors in a similar way, although often with different affinity, potency, and selectivity profiles (Roque-Bravo et al. 2022).

The class of synthetic cannabinoids is structurally diverse and includes both substances developed for scientific and therapeutic research purposes, such as Dronabinol (a synthetic form of THC) and nabilone (a semi-synthetic analog of THC), as well as a growing number of illicit compounds (Lurie et al. 2023). The latter, often referred to as "new psychoactive substances" (NSP), can have exacerbated potency and significantly more dangerous adverse effect profiles compared to phytocannabinoids, posing a public health challenge (Ayman Alzu'bi et al. 2024).

The tripartite classification of cannabinoids is not merely taxonomic; it reflects the historical trajectory of scientific research in this area and carries with it distinct pharmacological and therapeutic implications for each group. The discovery and study of phytocannabinoids, driven by interest in the effects of the *Cannabis sativa* plant, was the starting point that subsequently led to the identification of the endocannabinoid system and its endogenous components (Śmiarowska et al. 2022).

This knowledge, for instance, has stimulated the development of synthetic cannabinoids, both as research tools to dissect the mechanisms of the endocannabinoid system and as potential therapeutic agents with optimized pharmacokinetic or pharmacodynamic properties (Roque-Bravo et al. 2022).

1.2 Endocannabinoid System (ECS)

To unlock the therapeutic potential of cannabinoids, it is essential to understand the biology of the Endocannabinoid System (ECS), a true master regulator of our body's balance, whose discovery represented a milestone for neurobiology comparable to the revelation of the endogenous opioid system, all driven by research on the effects of Cannabis sativa.

It is a remarkably complex biological signaling system present throughout the body, composed of three central elements that work in harmony to regulate a wide range of physiological processes, such as mood, memory, appetite, sleep, pain perception, and immune response. The first of these components is endocannabinoids, lipid-based neurotransmitters our bodies produce as needed, the best known of which are anandamide (AEA) and 2-arachidonoylglycerol (2-AG) (Maccarrone et al. 2023).

The second are cannabinoid receptors, mainly CB1 receptors, found predominantly in the central nervous system and responsible for the psychoactive effects of THC, and CB2 receptors,

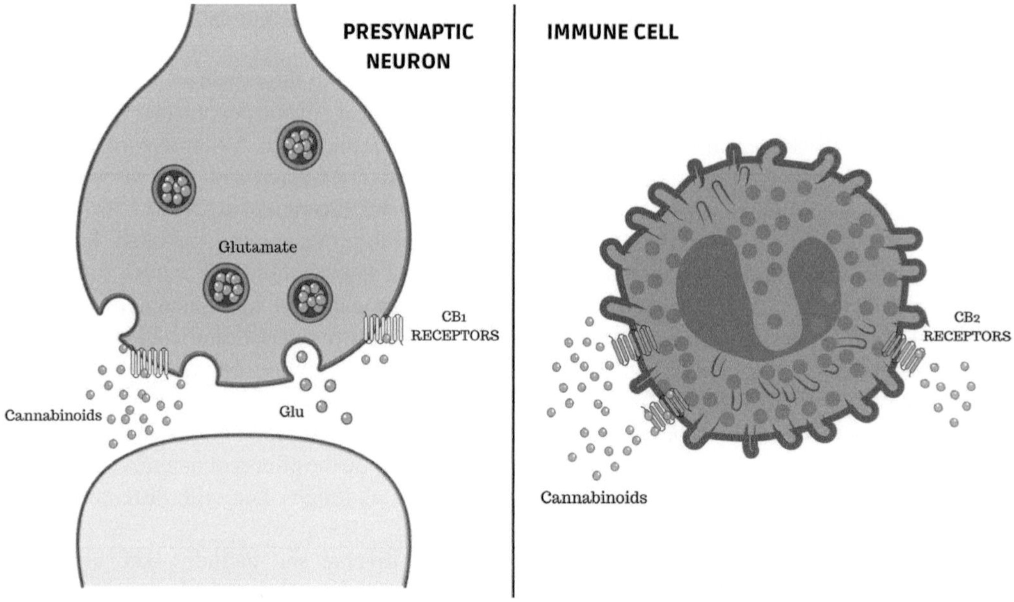

Figure 2: Schematic of cannabinoid-mediated signaling in a presynaptic neuron expressing CB1 receptors and in an immune cell expressing CB2 receptors.

located mainly in immune system cells and associated with the modulation of inflammation and pain (Figure 2). The third pillar is metabolic enzymes, such as FAAH and MAGL, which synthesize and degrade endocannabinoids, ensuring that their signals are localized and temporary. By interacting with this regulatory system, cannabis-derived compounds can modulate dysregulated physiological processes in various pathologies (Miao et al. 2024).

The *Cannabis sativa* plant produces more than a hundred phytocannabinoids, but the fundamental dichotomy between THC and CBD underpins the entire discussion about its medicinal use, determining its applications, safety, and regulatory status. Delta-9-tetrahydrocannabinol (THC) is the main psychoactive component, acting as a partial agonist of CB1 receptors in the brain. By mimicking anandamide, it produces both desired therapeutic effects, such as analgesia, antiemesis, and appetite stimulation, and adverse effects, which include euphoria, anxiety, paranoia, and memory impairment (Li et al. 2024).

In stark contrast, cannabidiol (CBD) is a non-psychoactive compound, making it much more attractive for pharmaceutical development. Its pharmacology is more complex; it has low affinity for CB1 and CB2 receptors and acts as a negative allosteric modulator on the CB1 receptor, which can attenuate the unwanted effects of THC (Black et al. 2019).

The therapeutic benefits of CBD appear to derive from its interactions with multiple targets, including serotonin receptors (5-HT1A) and ion channels (TRPV1), as well as its ability to inhibit FAAH enzyme, increasing endogenous anandamide levels. This varied pharmacology suggests a broad spectrum of activity but also makes it difficult to identify a single mechanism of action. This complex interaction between plant compounds has given rise to the "entourage effect" theory, which posits a therapeutic synergy in whole-plant extracts, a plausible concept that nevertheless challenges the research and regulatory paradigm based on single compounds (Miao et al. 2024).

2. Therapeutic Potential in Psychiatric Disorders

Currently, in neuropsychiatry there is much discussion about the benefits that the use of cannabinoids can bring to the health of human beings, and how research in this area has had significant results for modern medicine; however, there is still an impasse that is very important to take into account because the inappropriate use of cannabinoids can cause severe damage to health (Connor et al. 2021). As a result, there is a major conflict between the benefits and risks of using this chemical compound, which has been the subject of numerous studies on its potential as a pharmacological drug.

As mentioned above, the composition of cannabinoids has been the subject of research due to their benefits, as they contain bioactive principles with therapeutic properties (Leinen et al. 2023). One of the main benefits that has been studied is the reduction of anxiety and stress. According to research carried out by Leinen et al. (2023), cannabinoids have great potential for relieving anxiety and have a good safety profile when it comes to adverse effects, thus showing promising results. Cannabinoids, especially cannabidiol (CBD), interact with the endocannabinoid system, which is a complex network of receptors and molecules that help regulate various functions. 9 assist in the regulation of various physiological functions of the human body, when this interaction occurs (Maccarrone et al. 2023).

Weighing up the aforementioned risks and benefits, research into the therapeutic potential of cannabinoids, particularly cannabidiol (CBD) and, to a lesser extent, synthetic agonists, for psychiatric disorders has generated significant scientific interest, although the field is still developing, with evidence of efficacy and safety varying considerably between conditions (Bonaccorso et al. 2019). The focus is on specific molecules and well-defined conditions, given the pharmacological complexity of the endocannabinoid system and the well-established risks associated with tetrahydrocannabinol (THC), especially in vulnerable psychiatric populations (Bilbao and Spanagel 2022).

2.1 Anxiety Disorders

In the anxiety disorders spectrum, CBD has emerged as the most researched cannabinoid, with a distinct pharmacological profile from THC (Coles et al. 2023). Preclinical and clinical studies suggest that CBD exerts anxiolytic effects through multiple mechanisms, including partial agonism of 5-HT1A receptors, modulation of glutamatergic and GABAergic neurotransmission, and potential influence on hippocampal neurogenesis (Luján and Valverde 2020; Miao et al. 2024). Placebo-controlled trials in humans have demonstrated acute reductions in anxiety induced by simulated stress, particularly in social anxiety disorder (SAD) (Bergamaschi et al. 2011). A seminal study used the public speaking test (SPST) model, showing that single doses of CBD (600 mg) administered before the test significantly reduced subjective anxiety, cognitive discomfort and autonomic symptoms in patients with SAD, compared to placebo, with an effect comparable to that of ipsapirone (a 5-HT1A agonist) and superior to alprazolam in some parameters (Zuardi et al. 1993; Bergamaschi et al. 2011).

For generalized anxiety disorder (GAD), the data are scarcer and less consistent, as observational studies and small open trials suggest potential benefits, but larger, long-term controlled trials are needed to confirm clinical efficacy and establish dosing protocols (Shannon et al. 2019). In panic disorder, research is even more limited, with mainly preclinical evidence or case studies, in need of robust investigation. The central concern remains the potential acute and chronic anxiogenesis associated with THC, contraindicating its unsupervised use in these disorders (Shannon et al. 2019; Narayan et al. 2022).

2.2 Depression and Mood Disorders

In the context of depression and other mood disorders, cannabidiol (CBD) has shown considerable antidepressant potential in animal studies, an effect thought to result not from direct action on cannabinoid receptors, but rather from its ability to enhance the brain's serotonin system by interacting with the 5-HT1A receptor, a mechanism it shares with some conventional antidepressants (Sales et al. 2018). Furthermore, beyond producing rapid and sustained antidepressant-like effects in animal models, laboratory studies suggest that cannabidiol may also promote the growth of new neurons (a process known as neurogenesis) in the hippocampus, a brain region vital for mood regulation that is often impaired by chronic stress and depression (Campos et al. 2013; Rafaela et al. 2024).

However, despite this promising preclinical data, a significant gap in clinical evidence persists, as systematic reviews have consistently concluded that there are no high-quality randomized controlled trials to support the use of CBD specifically for major depressive disorder (Iffland and Grotenhermen 2017). In fact, most of the existing human data on mood comes from studies where depression was a secondary outcome in trials for other conditions, like chronic pain, or from observational studies and case reports (Bonaccorso et al. 2019; Kuhathasan et al. 2019).

The potential use of CBD is further complicated by major safety concerns, as the only FDA-approved product, Epidiolex, not only carries a warning for an increased risk of depression and suicidal thoughts based on clinical trials where four suicides occurred in the CBD group versus none in the placebo group, but it also poses a significant risk of drug-drug interactions (Iffland and Grotenhermen 2017). This is because CBD inhibits the liver enzymes responsible for breaking down many common psychiatric medications, which can lead to toxic effects (Gaston et al. 2017)

Moreover, Δ9-tetrahydrocannabinol (THC), the main psychoactive component in cannabis, presents a paradox regarding depression because while many individuals report using it for a temporary mood lift, this short-term benefit is overshadowed by substantial evidence of long-term harm, with multiple large-scale studies showing that chronic use not only increases the risk of developing depression but also leads to worse clinical outcomes for those already diagnosed (Gripe et al. 2023; Meier et al. 2016).

Regarding depression, a study by Gripe et al. (2023) indicates that an increase in cannabis use, particularly exceeding ten times per year, correlates with specific risks. For males, this heightened consumption was significantly associated with an elevated risk of depressed mood (relative risk [RR]: 1.49; $p < 0.001$), as well as a greater incidence of suicidal ideation (RR: 3.43; $p = 0.012$). For females, the same pattern of use also suggested an increased risk of suicidal ideation (RR: 2.47; $p = 0.002$).

This is believed to be a consequence of the downregulation of the brain's own CB1 cannabinoid receptors from chronic THC exposure, a process that impairs the endocannabinoid system's natural ability to regulate mood and stress, ultimately creating a detrimental cycle where the substance is used to alleviate symptoms that its long-term use helps perpetuate (Neumeister et al. 2013; Hillard and Liu 2014).

Therefore, based on the current evidence, no cannabinoid product can be recommended as a treatment for depression. High-THC cannabis, in particular, should be discouraged, as the evidence strongly indicates it is more likely to worsen the long-term course of the illness (Black et al. 2019). While CBD may hold future promise, its clinical use must await the results of rigorous Randomised controlled trials (RCTs), and any potential application would require extreme caution due to its safety profile (Iffland and Grotenhermen, 2017). The paradoxical relationship between cannabinoids

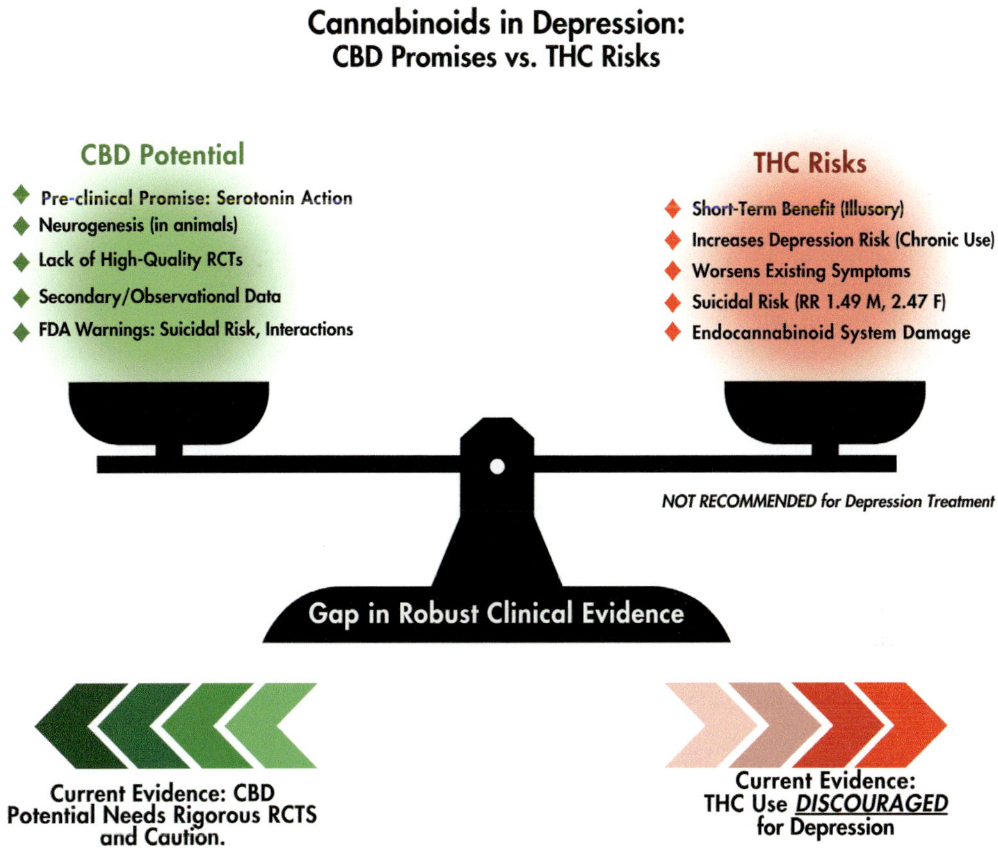

Figure 3: Clinical balance between the potential of cannabidiol (CBD) and the risks of tetrahydrocannabinol (THC) in the treatment of depression.

and depression, highlighting the preclinical promise of CBD against the established risks of THC, is further illustrated in Figure 3.

2.3 Post-Traumatic Stress Disorder (PTSD)

In post-traumatic stress disorder (PTSD), dysfunction of the endocannabinoid system, mainly involving CB1 receptors, has been implicated in the pathophysiology, particularly in the processes of fear extinction and consolidation of aversive memories (Neumeister 2012). While the use of THC-rich cannabis is common among patients, the risks of exacerbation of symptoms, development of dependence, and psychosis are significant; however, clinical trials have focused on synthetic THC agonists or CBD (Hicks et al. 2022; Black et al. 2019).

Studies with nabilone (a synthetic analog of THC) have shown significant efficacy in reducing trauma-related nightmares in military veterans with refractory PTSD, in placebo-controlled trials (Cowling and MacDougall 2019). Furthermore, a retrospective case series on 11 adult PTSD patients showed that oral administration of CBD, in addition to routine psychiatric care, resulted in a 28% reduction in PTSD symptom severity, as measured by the PTSD Checklist for DSM-5 (PCL-5), after eight weeks. The patients received flexible doses of CBD, with an average final dose of 48.64 mg. The mechanisms proposed for CBD's action in PTSD include indirect activation of the endocannabinoid 11 endocannabinoid system, which may facilitate the extinction of aversive memories (Elms et al. 2019).

2.4 Schizophrenia and Psychotic Disorders

Concerning schizophrenia and psychosis, robust epidemiological evidence associates the use of cannabis, particularly high THC potency strains, with an increased risk of developing psychosis, especially in young individuals with genetic vulnerability (Andréasson et al. 1987; Hall and Degenhardt 2008). In addition, THC can precipitate positive (delusions, hallucinations), negative (affective blunting and alogia), and cognitive symptoms in susceptible individuals (Colizzi et al. 2019; Ganesh et al. 2020).

An exploratory, double-blind, randomized, active-controlled clinical trial investigated CBD as monotherapy in patients with acute paranoid schizophrenia. The study showed that both CBD (up to 800 mg/day) and amisulpride (an antipsychotic, also at doses of up to 800 mg/day) improved neurocognitive function with comparable efficacy after four weeks of treatment. Specifically, both groups showed improvements in visual memory and processing speed (Leweke et al. 2021).

Additionally, CBD improved sustained attention and visual-motor coordination, whereas amisulpride improved working memory performance. These cognitive improvements were not systematically associated with increased serum anandamide levels, suggesting that CBD's effects on cognition may be mediated by pathways other than its antipsychotic effects (Leweke et al. 2021).

2.5 Sleep Disorders and Insomnia

The biological basis for the use of cannabis in sleep modulation lies in its interaction with the endocannabinoid system (ECS), as described by Josué Camberos-Barraza et al. (2024), and it is through this pathway that phytocannabinoids such as THC, CBD, and CBN exert their modulatory effects.

THC, the main psychoactive component, exhibits biphasic, dose-dependent effects: it reduces sleep latency at low concentrations, although it consistently suppresses REM sleep (Babson et al. 2017). On the other hand, CBD, which has no intoxicating properties, may have sedative effects when administered in higher doses, probably due to its anxiolytic actions (Shannon et al. 2019).

In addition, CBN, which is a metabolite of THC, has gained prominence as a cannabinoid with sedative potential, with preclinical studies indicating that it may act as a prodrug, i.e., its hypnotic effect would be mainly related to the active metabolite generated after its biotransformation, as evidenced in a study. (Somayaji et al. 2022).

Despite the consistent biological basis and increasingly widespread use, clinical evidence on the efficacy of cannabinoids in the treatment of insomnia is still incipient and marked by low quality, since systematic reviews, such as that conducted by Zhand and Milin (2018), point out that the available studies present a high risk of bias, small samples, and significant methodological heterogeneity, which makes it impossible to conduct robust meta-analyses.

One of the central paradoxes in this field is the discrepancy between patients' positive subjective reports and objective polysomnographic data, which sometimes indicate worsening of sleep architecture, suggesting that cannabinoids may be modifying the perception of sleep rather than promoting it objectively. In addition, the so-called "entourage effect" hypothesis, which proposes a synergy between cannabinoids and terpenes, remains more associated with a marketing narrative than with a clinically validated principle in humans (André et al. 2024; Narayan et al. 2024).

The evaluation of cannabinoids must necessarily include a rigorous analysis of the associated risks, as acute use is generally linked to mild adverse effects such as dizziness and dry mouth, although chronic use presents substantial risks, including the development of tolerance and dependence, with estimated rates reaching up to 50% among daily users (Volkow et al. 2014). Withdrawal syndrome is often marked by severe rebound insomnia, which becomes one of the main factors contributing to relapse among users (Black et al. 2019). In addition, prolonged use has been linked to a decrease in slow-wave sleep (SWS) and to notable cognitive impairments, which tend to intensify the negative effects over time, especially when use becomes habitual or long-standing, and these concerns are further heightened by the fact that the market for cannabinoid-based products remains largely unregulated, leading to the circulation of items with misleading labeling and possible contamination by heavy metals, pesticides, and residual solvents (Bonn-Miller et al. 2017).

Thus, compared to conventional hypnotics, cannabinoids present a distinct risk-benefit profile, as benzodiazepines offer more predictable efficacy but carry a high risk of dependence and a potentially dangerous withdrawal syndrome, whereas cannabinoids demonstrate less consistent efficacy alongside a lower, yet still significant, risk of dependence and a distressing but nonfatal withdrawal; moreover, the growing preference among many patients to use cannabis instead of prescribed medications signals a deep dissatisfaction with the current standard of care (Corroon et al. 2017).

2.6 Substance Use Disorders (SUD)

In the field of substance use disorders (SUD), CBD has been explored as a potential tool due to its anxiolytic and antipsychotic effects and, crucially, its influence on memory and reactivity to drug-related cues (Karimi-Haghighi et al. 2022). Preclinical studies consistently demonstrate that CBD reduces environmental cue-induced drug seeking, self-medication to relieve negative withdrawal symptoms, and vulnerability to relapse in animal models of opioid, cocaine, alcohol, and tobacco dependence (Turna et al. 2019).

Moreover, in a clinical trial with humans to treat heroin use disorder, oral administration of cannabidiol (CBD) at doses of 400 mg and 800 mg significantly reduced both craving and anxiety induced by triggers in abstinent individuals. Notably, the study demonstrated that these beneficial effects persisted for up to 7 days after the last dose, suggesting a strong impact of CBD on the brain's reactivity to these stimuli (Hurd et al. 2019).

Therefore, the central hypothesis is that CBD attenuates the salience of drug-associated cues and interferes with the consolidation and reactivation of reward memories, thus reducing the impulse to use. CBD's apparent lack of intrinsic rewarding properties and low abuse potential increase its appeal for this application, although larger and longer trials, especially for opioids and stimulants, are urgently needed.

Table 1 below summarizes the main benefits and risks that the use of cannabinoids (CBC and THC) presents when treated for each psychiatric disorder that was addressed in topic 2 (therapeutic potential in psychiatric disorders).

Table 1: Main potential benefits and risks of using CBD and THC for psychiatric disorders.

Psychiatric Disorders	Potential Benefits of Using CBD and THC for Psychiatric Disorders	Risk of Using CBD and THC for Psychiatric Disorders	References
Anxiety disorders	Cannabidiol (CBD) has demonstrated anxiolytic effects through multiple mechanisms, acutely reducing anxiety in conditions such as Social Anxiety Disorder.	Some data on Generalized Anxiety Disorder and Panic Disorder are scarce, and Tetrahydrocannabinol (THC) is associated with acute and chronic anxiety.	Bergamaschi et al. 2011; Narayan et al. 2022; Shannon et al. 2019; Zuardi et al. 1993
Depression and mood disorders	In animal studies, CBD shows antidepressant potential by increasing the serotonergic system and promoting neurogenesis.	Clinical evidence is lacking, and products like Epidiolex (CBD) carry warnings about an increased risk of depression. CBD can also cause significant drug interactions. While some use THC to improve mood, chronic use is associated with an increased risk of depression and worse outcomes, with no cannabinoid product currently recommended for depression.	Iffland and Grotenhermen 2017; Sales et al. 2018
Post-Traumatic Stress Disorder (PTSD)	Synthetic THC analogues, such as nabilone, have been shown to reduce trauma-related nightmares, and oral CBD has been shown to decrease the severity of PTSD symptoms. CBD may also help extinguish aversive memories.	The use of THC-rich cannabis by patients with PTSD carries risks such as exacerbation of symptoms, dependence, and psychosis.	Black et al. 2019; Cowling and MacDougall 2019; Hicks et al. 2022
Schizophrenia and Psychotic Disorders	Studies show that CBD improves neurocognitive function in acute paranoid schizophrenia.	Strong evidence links cannabis use, especially high-THC strains, to an increased risk of developing psychosis.	Andréasson et al. 1987; Hall and Degenhardt 2008; Leweke et al. 2021
Sleep Disorders and Insomnia	THC may reduce the time to fall asleep (sleep latency), and CBD, like CBN (a metabolite of THC), may have sedative effects.	Clinical evidence is limited and of low quality, and objective data sometimes indicate worsening sleep architecture.	Babson et al. 2017; Black et al. 2019; Somayaji et al. 2022
Substance Use Disorders (SUD)	CBD is being investigated for its anxiolytic and antipsychotic properties, and its ability to influence memory and drug cue reactivity.	Preclinical studies suggest that CBD reduces drug-seeking behaviors and vulnerability to relapse in several animal models of addiction.	Karimi-Haghighi et al. 2022; Turna et al. 2019

3. Clinical Practice and Future Perspectives

The clinical practice, regulatory landscape and prospects for the use of medical cannabis constitute a rapidly evolving field, centered predominantly on its two main constituents: cannabidiol and Δ9-tetrahydrocannabinol, and while there is robust, high-quality scientific evidence supporting the use of purified CBD for rare and refractory forms of pediatric epilepsy, the evidence base for other conditions, such as chronic pain and 13 anxiety, remains contested and is still crawling towards more effective evidence, as seen in the previous section (Black et al. 2019).

This disparity fuels a notable divergence between regulatory models, contrasting the strictly pharmaceutical approach of the US Food and Drug Administration (FDA) with Brazil's hybrid and judicialized system, where patient activism and court decisions play a central role in defining access (Greenwich Biosciences 2014).

The clinical evaluation of cannabinoids is marked by a significant "gap between evidence and expectation." Public perception often positions cannabis as a panacea, while scientific reality is much more nuanced and hierarchical. At the top of this hierarchy is epilepsy, the vanguard of cannabinoid medicine and the application best validated scientifically (Devinsky et al. 2017).

The development of Epidiolex, an oral solution of highly purified CBD, has set the gold standard. Multiple randomized, double-blind, placebo-controlled clinical trials published in high-impact journals have unequivocally demonstrated its efficacy for seizures associated with devastating syndromes such as Lennox-Gastaut, Dravet, and Tuberous Sclerosis Complex (TSC) (Devinsky et al. 2017; Greenwich Biosciences 2014).

In a study of patients with TSC, for example, a percentage reduction in seizure frequency of 49% was observed in the group receiving cannabidiol (CBD) at a dose of 25 mg/kg/day and 48% in the group with a dose of 50 mg/kg/day, compared to a reduction of 27% in the placebo group. It was this high-quality body of evidence that contributed to the FDA's approval of Epidiolex in 2018, 14 the first plant-derived drug to receive such approval for this and other conditions (Thiele et al. 2021).

However, its effectiveness is accompanied by adverse effects that require monitoring. The most common were diarrhea (occurring in 31% and 56% of patients in the CBD groups, respectively, versus 25% in the placebo group) and drowsiness (13% and 26% in the CBD groups, respectively, versus 9% in the placebo group). Notably, elevated liver transaminases occurred in 18.9% of patients receiving cannabidiol, in contrast to no cases in the placebo group, in addition to significant drug interactions (Thiele et al. 2021).

In stark contrast to the clarity for epilepsy, the use of cannabinoids for chronic neuropathic pain is a complex and controversial field. Although systematic reviews of randomized clinical trials demonstrate statistically significant reductions in pain in many studies, the overall quality of evidence is consistently rated as low to very low (Black et al. 2019).

This uncertainty stems from methodological challenges such as small sample sizes, short study durations, and, crucially, the difficulty of blinding in THC trials, whose psychoactive effects often reveal the active treatment to participants. Most of the evidence involves THC or combinations of THC/CBD, making it difficult to isolate the contribution of each molecule (Straud et al. 2024; Bonn-Miller et al. 2021).

Additionally, the application of cannabinoids in anxiety disorders, although promising in preclinical studies, faces significant clinical obstacles. A key meta-analysis on the subject revealed a critical finding: although the initial analysis showed a large reduction in anxiety symptoms, the effect disappeared after applying statistical corrections for publication bias. This phenomenon, where studies with positive results are more likely to be published, suggests that the current evidence base may be inflated (Bahji et al. 2020).

The stark conclusion is that while CBD may have potential value, its routine use for anxiety is not supported by the available evidence and should be confined to well-designed clinical trials. Meanwhile, research is expanding into other frontiers, with investigations into neuroprotective potential in diseases such as Alzheimer's and Parkinson's, pain studies in conditions such as fibromyalgia, and feasibility assessments for treating symptoms of COVID Longa (Thurgur et al. 2023; Marques and Campos 2024; Strand et al. 2023).

In line with this, the future of cannabinoid medicine is being shaped by an inexorable transition from an herbal approach to a pharmacological paradigm (Pietrafusa et al. 2019). Current clinical research asks drug development questions: What is the pharmacokinetic profile of a specific formulation? How does an isolated molecule affect brain networks? An analysis of clinical trials reveals sophisticated investigations, such as functional magnetic resonance imaging to examine the effects of CBD on brain connectivity (NCT04831294) and detailed pharmacokinetic studies (NCT04280289). Research is expanding into new indications, such as fibromyalgia (NCT04729179) and COVID Longa (NCT04997395), and exploring CBD as a harm reduction agent in Cannabis Use Disorder (NCT06569394) (US National Library of Medicine 2025).

The road ahead is full of challenges and opportunities, as the main challenges are to bridge the evidence gap through high-quality trials, standardize products to ensure consistency and safety, harmonize disparate regulatory frameworks, and fight stigma by educating healthcare professionals and the public. The opportunities, however, are transformative, with research into "minor" cannabinoids (such as CBG and CBN) and terpenes representing a vast frontier for new drug discovery (Li et al. 2024; Arnold et al. 2024).

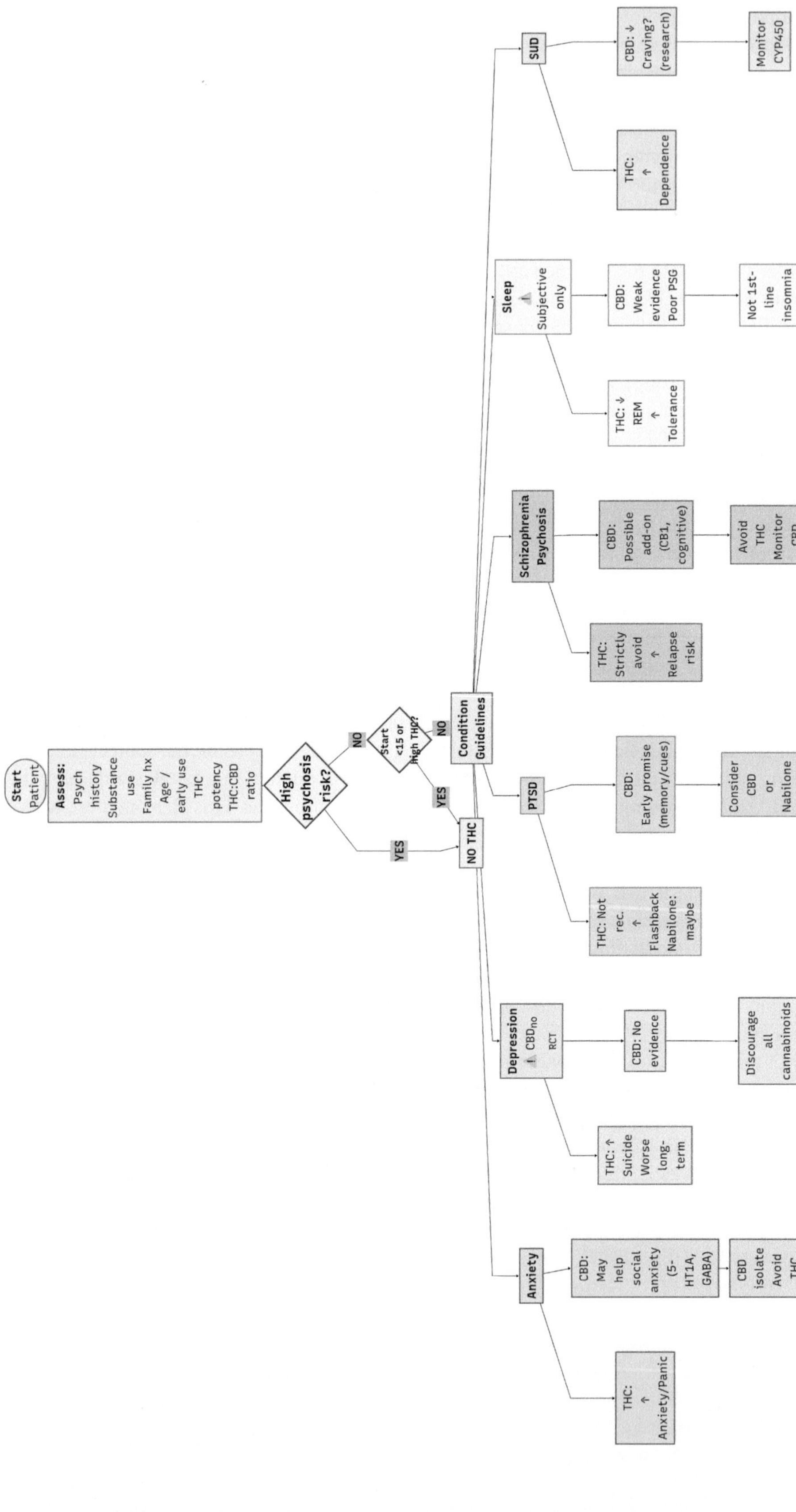

Figure 4: Simplified clinical guidelines for the use of cannabinoids in psychiatry.

Thus, the development of synthetic molecules that target SEC more precisely, such as FAAH (Fatty Acid Amide Hydrolase) inhibitors or selective CB2 agonists, could offer therapeutic benefits with fewer adverse effects. Ultimately, future research could enable personalized medicine by identifying biomarkers to predict patient response and meet unmet patient needs (Tian et al. 2025).

Below you can see a flowchart with simplified clinical guidelines for the use of cannabinoids in psychiatry (Figure 4).

4. Conclusion

In conclusion, the field of cannabinoid therapeutics is defined by a central paradox: as the efficacy of purified CBD for specific epilepsies is well established, setting a gold standard for pharmaceutical evidence, yet for most other popular applications, clinical evidence remains insufficient, fueling a global tension reflected in drastically different regulatory models. Given this, the future points unequivocally towards greater "pharmaceuticalization," in which scientific rigour, from dissecting molecular mechanisms to developing standardized formulations, will be the key to realizing the full therapeutic potential of this class of compounds. So while cannabis' journey from ancient herbal remedy to modern drug class is well underway, its success depends on a continued commitment to science to navigate its complex and promising future.

References

Abernethy, A. (2019, July 25). *Hemp Production and the 2018 Farm Bill*. U.S. Food and Drug Administration. https://www.fda.gov/news-events/congressional-testimony/hemp-production-and-2018-farm-bill-07252019

André, R., Gomes, A. P., Pereira-Leite, C., António Marques-da-Costa, Rodrigues, L. M., Sassano, M. et al. (2024). The Entourage Effect in Cannabis Medicinal Products: A Comprehensive Review. *Pharmaceuticals*, 17(11): 1543–1543. https://doi.org/10.3390/ph17111543

Andréasson, S., Engström, A., Allebeck, P., and Rydberg, U. (1987). Cannabis and Schizophrenia: A longitudinal study of Swedish Conscripts. *The Lancet*, 330(8574): 1483–1486. https://doi.org/10.1016/s0140-6736(87)92620-1

Arnold, J. C., Occelli Hanbury-Brown, C. V., Anderson, L. L., Bedoya-Pérez, M. A., Udoh, M., Sharman, L. A. et al. (2024). A sleepy cannabis constituent: cannabinol and its active metabolite influence sleep architecture in rats. *Neuropsychopharmacology*. https://doi.org/10.1038/s41386-024-02018-7

Ayman Alzu'bi, Almahasneh, F., Ramada Khasawneh, Ejlal Abu-El-Rub, Worood Bani Baker, and Al-Zoubi, R. M. (2024). The synthetic cannabinoids menace: a review of health risks and toxicity. *European Journal of Medical Research*, 29(1). https://doi.org/10.1186/s40001-023-01443-6

Babson, K. A., Sottile, J., and Morabito, D. (2017). Cannabis, Cannabinoids, and Sleep: a Review of the Literature. *Current Psychiatry Reports*, 19(4). https://doi.org/10.1007/s11920-017-0775-9

Bahji, A., Meyyappan, A. C., and Hawken, E. R. (2020). Efficacy and acceptability of cannabinoids for anxiety disorders in adults: A systematic review & meta-analysis. *Journal of Psychiatric Research*, 129: 257–264. https://doi.org/10.1016/j.jpsychires.2020.07.030

Bergamaschi, M. M., Queiroz, R. H. C., Chagas, M. H. N., de Oliveira, D. C. G., De Martinis, B. S., Kapczinski, F. et al. (2011). Cannabidiol Reduces the Anxiety Induced by Simulated Public Speaking in Treatment-Naïve Social Phobia Patients. *Neuropsychopharmacology*, 36(6): 1219–1226. https://doi.org/10.1038/npp.2011.6

Black, N., Stockings, E., Campbell, G., Tran, L. T., Zagic, D., Hall, W. D. et al. (2019). Cannabinoids for the treatment of mental disorders and symptoms of mental disorders: a systematic review and meta-analysis. *The Lancet Psychiatry*, 6(12). https://doi.org/10.1016/s2215-0366(19)30401-8

Bonaccorso, S., Ricciardi, A., Zangani, C., Chiappini, S., and Schifano, F. (2019). Cannabidiol (CBD) use in psychiatric disorders: A systematic review. *NeuroToxicology*, 74: 282–298. https://doi.org/10.1016/j.neuro.2019.08.002

Bonn-Miller, M. O., Loflin, M. J. E., Thomas, B. F., Marcu, J. P., Hyke, T., and Vandrey, R. (2017). Labeling accuracy of cannabidiol extracts sold online. *JAMA*, 318(17): 1708–1709. https://doi.org/10.1001/jama.2017.11909

Bonn-Miller, M. O., Sisley, S., Riggs, P., Yazar-Klosinski, B., Wang, J. B., Loflin, M. J. E. et al. (2021). The short-term impact of 3 smoked cannabis preparations versus placebo on PTSD symptoms: A randomized cross-over clinical trial. *PLOS ONE*, 16(3): e0246990. https://doi.org/10.1371/journal.pone.0246990

Campos, A. C., Ortega, Z., Palazuelos, J., Fogaça, M. V., Aguiar, D. C., Díaz-Alonso, J. et al. (2013). The anxiolytic effect of cannabidiol on chronically stressed mice depends on hippocampal neurogenesis: involvement of the endocannabinoid system. *International Journal of Neuropsychopharmacology*, 16(6): 1407–1419. https://doi.org/10.1017/s1461145712001502

Cavaleri, D., Bartoli, F., Crocamo, C., and Carrà, G. (2024). Acute cognitive and psychiatric effects of cannabinoids. *Italian Journal of Psychiatry*, 1. https://doi.org/10.36180/2421-4469-2024-6

Chuang, S. H., Westenbroek, R. E., Stella, N., and Catterall, W. A. (2021). Combined antiseizure efficacy of cannabidiol and clonazepam in a conditional mouse model of dravet syndrome. *Journal of Experimental Neurology*, 2(2). https://doi.org/10.33696/neurol.2.040

Coles, M., Porto, R. R., Chesworth, R., Steiner-Lim, G., and Karl, T. (2023). therapeutic potential of a combined cannabidiol (cbd) - delta-9-tetrahydrocannabinol (thc) treatment strategy for appswe/ps1δe9 transgenic mice. *IBRO Neuroscience Reports*, 15(388): S388. https://doi.org/10.1016/j.ibneur.2023.08.736

Colizzi, M., Weltens, N., McGuire, P., Lythgoe, D., Williams, S., Van Oudenhove, L. et al. (2019). Delta-9-tetrahydrocannabinol increases striatal glutamate levels in healthy individuals: implications for psychosis. *Molecular Psychiatry*, 25(12): 3231–3240. https://doi.org/10.1038/s41380-019-0374-8

Connor, J. P., Stjepanović, D., Le Foll, B., Hoch, E., Budney, A. J., and Hall, W. D. (2021). Cannabis use and cannabis use disorder. *Nature Reviews Disease Primers*, 7(1): 16. https://doi.org/10.1038/s41572-021-00247-4

Corroon, J., Mischley, L., and Sexton, M. (2017). Cannabis as a substitute for prescription drugs – a cross-sectional study. *Journal of Pain Research*, 10: 989–998. https://doi.org/10.2147/jpr.s134330

Cowling, T., and MacDougall, D. (2019, February 20). *Nabilone for the Treatment of Post-Traumatic Stress Disorder: A Review of Clinical Effectiveness and Guidelines*. Nih.gov; Canadian Agency for Drugs and Technologies in Health. https://www.ncbi.nlm.nih.gov/books/NBK546995/

Devinsky, O., Cross, J. H., Laux, L., Marsh, E., Miller, I., Nabbout, R. et al. (2017). Trial of Cannabidiol for Drug-Resistant Seizures in the Dravet Syndrome. *The New England Journal of Medicine*, 376(21): 2011–2020. https://doi.org/10.1056/NEJMoa1611618

Elms, L., Shannon, S., Hughes, S., and Lewis, N. (2019). Cannabidiol in the Treatment of Post-Traumatic Stress Disorder: A Case Series. *The Journal of Alternative and Complementary Medicine*, 25(4): 392–397. https://doi.org/10.1089/acm.2018.0437

Ganesh, S., Cortes-Briones, J., Ranganathan, M., Radhakrishnan, R., Skosnik, P. D., and D'Souza, D. C. (2020). Psychosis-Relevant Effects of Intravenous Delta-9-Tetrahydrocannabinol: A Mega Analysis of Individual Participant-Data from Human Laboratory Studies. *The International Journal of Neuropsychopharmacology*, 23(9): 559–570. https://doi.org/10.1093/ijnp/pyaa031

Gaston, T. E., Bebin, E. M., Cutter, G. R., Liu, Y., and Szaflarski, J. P. (2017). Interactions between cannabidiol and commonly used antiepileptic drugs. *Epilepsia*, 58(9): 1586–1592. https://doi.org/10.1111/epi.13852

Greenwich Biosciences. (2014). *Epidiolex (cannabidiol) oral solution: Full prescribing information*. Fda.gov. https://www.fda.gov/drugsatfda

Gripe, I., Pape, H., and Thor Norström. (2023). Associations between Cannabis Use and Mental Distress in Young People: a Longitudinal Study. *Journal of Adolescent Health*, 74(3). https://doi.org/10.1016/j.jadohealth.2023.10.003

Hall, W., and Degenhardt, L. (2008). Cannabis use and the risk of developing a psychotic disorder. *World Psychiatry*, 7(2): 68–71. https://doi.org/10.1002/j.2051-5545.2008.tb00158.x

Hanuš, L. O., Meyer, S. M., Muñoz, E., Taglialatela-Scafati, O., and Appendino, G. (2016). Phytocannabinoids: a unified critical inventory. *Natural Product Reports*, 33(12): 1357–1392. https://doi.org/10.1039/c6np00074f

Hicks, T. A., Zaur, A. J., Keeley, J. W., and Amstadter, A. B. (2022). The association between recreational cannabis use and posttraumatic stress disorder: A systematic review and methodological critique of the literature. *Drug and Alcohol Dependence*, 240: 109623. https://doi.org/10.1016/j.drugalcdep.2022.109623

Hill, K. P., Gold, M. S., Nemeroff, C. B., McDonald, W., Grzenda, A., Widge, A. S. et al. (2022). Risks and Benefits of Cannabis and Cannabinoids in Psychiatry. *American Journal of Psychiatry*, 179(2): 98–109. https://doi.org/10.1176/appi.ajp.2021.21030320

Hillard, C., and Liu, Q. (2014). Endocannabinoid Signaling in the Etiology and Treatment of Major Depressive Illness. *Current Pharmaceutical Design*, 20(23): 3795–3811. https://doi.org/10.2174/13816128113196660735

Hurd, Y. L., Spriggs, S., Alishayev, J., Winkel, G., Gurgov, K., Kudrich, C. et al. (2019). Cannabidiol for the Reduction of Cue-Induced Craving and Anxiety in Drug-Abstinent Individuals With Heroin Use Disorder: A Double-Blind Randomized Placebo-Controlled Trial. *American Journal of Psychiatry*, 176(11): 911–922. https://doi.org/10.1176/appi.ajp.2019.18101191

Iffland, K., and Grotenhermen, F. (2017). An update on safety and side effects of cannabidiol: A review of clinical data and relevant animal studies. *Cannabis and Cannabinoid Research*, 2(1): 139–154. https://doi.org/10.1089/can.2016.0034

Josué Camberos-Barraza, Camacho-Zamora, A., Bátiz-Beltrán, J. C., Osuna-Ramos, J. F., Rábago-Monzón, Á. R., Valdez-Flores, M. A. et al. (2024). Sleep, Glial function, and the endocannabinoid system: implications for neuroinflammation and sleep disorders. *International Journal of Molecular Sciences (Online)*, 25(6): 3160–3160. https://doi.org/10.3390/ijms25063160

Karimi-Haghighi, S., Razavi, Y., Iezzi, D., Scheyer, A. F., Manzoni, O., and Haghparast, A. (2022). Cannabidiol and substance use disorder: Dream or reality. *Neuropharmacology*, 207: 108948. https://doi.org/10.1016/j.neuropharm.2022.108948

Kuhathasan, N., Dufort, A., MacKillop, J., Gottschalk, R., Minuzzi, L., and Frey, B. N. (2019). The use of cannabinoids for sleep: A critical review on clinical trials. *Experimental and Clinical Psychopharmacology*, 27(4): 383–401. https://doi.org/10.1037/pha0000285

Leinen, Z. J., Mohan, R., Premadasa, L. S., Acharya, A., Mohan, M., and Byrareddy, S. N. (2023). Therapeutic Potential of Cannabis: A Comprehensive Review of Current and Future Applications. *Biomedicines*, 11(10): 2630. https://doi.org/10.3390/biomedicines11102630

Leweke, F. M., Rohleder, C., Gerth, C. W., Hellmich, M., Pukrop, R., and Koethe, D. (2021). Cannabidiol and amisulpride improve cognition in acute schizophrenia in an explorative, double-blind, active-controlled, randomized clinical trial. *Frontiers in Pharmacology*, 12: 614811. https://doi.org/10.3389/fphar.2021.614811

Li, S., Li, W., Malhi, N. K., Huang, J., Li, Q., Zhou, Z. et al. (2024). Cannabigerol (CBG): A comprehensive review of its molecular mechanisms and therapeutic potential. *Molecules (Basel, Switzerland)*, 29(22): 5471. https://doi.org/10.3390/molecules29225471

Luján, M. Á., and Valverde, O. (2020). The Pro-neurogenic effects of cannabidiol and its potential therapeutic implications in psychiatric disorders. *Frontiers in Behavioral Neuroscience*, 14. https://doi.org/10.3389/fnbeh.2020.00109

Lurie, Y., Nadir, Y., Hoffman, R., Miller, A., Efrati, E., Ring, G. et al. (2023). An outbreak of severe coagulopathy in northern Israel among users of illicit synthetic cannabinoids adulterated with brodifacoum. *Clinical Toxicology*, 61(6): 429–435. https://doi.org/10.1080/15563650.2023.2215402

Maccarrone, M., Vincenzo Di Marzo, Gertsch, J., Grether, U., Howlett, A. C., Hua, T. et al. (2023). Goods and bads of endocannabinoid system as a therapeutic target: Lessons learned after 30 years. *Pharmacological Reviews*, PHARMREV-000600. https://doi.org/10.1124/pharmrev.122.000600

Marques, B. L., and Campos, A. C. (2024). Cannabidiol and Alzheimer's disease. *International Review of Neurobiology*, 121–134. https://doi.org/10.1016/bs.irn.2024.04.014

McGuire, P., Robson, P., Cubala, W. J., Vasile, D., Morrison, P. D., Barron, R. et al. (2018). Cannabidiol (CBD) as an Adjunctive Therapy in Schizophrenia: A Multicenter Randomized Controlled Trial. *American Journal of Psychiatry*, 175(3): 225–231. https://doi.org/10.1176/appi.ajp.2017.17030325

Meier, M. H., Caspi, A., Cerdá, M., Hancox, R. J., Harrington, H., Houts, R. et al. (2016). Associations Between Cannabis Use and Physical Health Problems in Early Midlife. *JAMA Psychiatry*, 73(7): 731. https://doi.org/10.1001/jamapsychiatry.2016.0637

Miao, Y., Zhao, F., and Guan, W. (2024). A novel insight into the antidepressant effect of cannabidiol: possible involvement of the 5-HT1A, CB1, GPR55, and PPARγ receptors. *The International Journal of Neuropsychopharmacology*, 1. https://doi.org/10.1093/ijnp/pyae064

Mock, E. D., Berend Gagestein, and Mario. (2023). Anandamide and other N-acylethanolamines: A class of signaling lipids with therapeutic opportunities. *Progress in Lipid Research*, 89: 101194–101194. https://doi.org/10.1016/j.plipres.2022.101194

Narayan, A. J., Downey, L. A., Manning, B., and Hayley, A. C. (2022). Cannabinoid treatments for anxiety: A systematic review and consideration of the impact of sleep disturbance. *Neuroscience & Biobehavioral Reviews*, 143: 104941. https://doi.org/10.1016/j.neubiorev.2022.104941

Narayan, A. J., Downey, L. A., Rose, S., Lauren Di Natale, and Hayley, A. C. (2024). Cannabidiol for moderate-severe insomnia: a randomized controlled pilot trial of 150 mg of nightly dosing. *Journal of Clinical Sleep Medicine*. https://doi.org/10.5664/jcsm.10998

Neumeister, A. (2012). The endocannabinoid system provides an avenue for evidence-based treatment development for ptsd. *Depression and Anxiety*, 30(2): 93–96. https://doi.org/10.1002/da.22031

Neumeister, A., Normandin, M. D., Pietrzak, R. H., Piomelli, D., Zheng, M. Q., Gujarro-Anton, A. et al. (2013). Elevated brain cannabinoid CB1 receptor availability in post-traumatic stress disorder: a positron emission tomography study. *Molecular Psychiatry*, 18(9): 1034–1040. https://doi.org/10.1038/mp.2013.61

Pagano, C., Navarra, G., Coppola, L., Avilia, G., Bifulco, M., and Laezza, C. (2022). Cannabinoids: Therapeutic Use in Clinical Practice. *International Journal of Molecular Sciences*, 23(6): 3344. https://doi.org/10.3390/ijms23063344

Pietrafusa, N., Ferretti, A., Trivisano, M., de Palma, L., Calabrese, C., Carfì Pavia, G. et al. (2019). Purified cannabidiol for treatment of refractory epilepsies in pediatric patients with developmental and epileptic encephalopathy. *Paediatric Drugs*, 10.1007/s40272-01900341-x. https://doi.org/10.1007/s40272-019-00341-x

Rafaela Oliveira Cochito, Antônio Palma Miracco, Bruna Zorzo Marques, Luiz, J., Matheus, Roberto Fontanella Dinatt, Sousa, P. et al. (2024). Integrative review on the role of BDNF and cannabidiol in neuroplasticity. *Brazilian Journal of Development*, 10(2): e67068–e67068. https://doi.org/10.34117/bjdv10n2-013

Rong, C., Lee, Y., Carmona, N. E., Cha, D. S., Ragguett, R.-M., Rosenblat, J. D. et al. (2017). Cannabidiol in medical marijuana: Research vistas and potential opportunities. *Pharmacological Research*, 121: 213–218. https://doi.org/10.1016/j.phrs.2017.05.005

Roque-Bravo, R., Silva, R. S., Malheiro, R. F., Carmo, H., Carvalho, F., da Silva, D. D. et al. (2022). Synthetic Cannabinoids: A Pharmacological and Toxicological Overview. *Annual Review of Pharmacology and Toxicology*, 63(1). https://doi.org/10.1146/annurev-pharmtox-031122-113758

Sales, A. J., Fogaça, M. V., Sartim, A. G., Pereira, V. S., Wegener, G., Guimarães, F. S. et al. (2018). Cannabidiol induces rapid and sustained antidepressant-like effects through increased bdnf signaling and synaptogenesis in the prefrontal cortex. *Molecular Neurobiology*, 56(2): 1070–1081. https://doi.org/10.1007/s12035-018-1143-4

Sepehr Pourebrahim, Ahmad, T., Rottmann, E., Schulze, J., and Scheller, B. (2025). Does Cannabis Use Contribute to Schizophrenia? A Causation Analysis Based on Epidemiological Evidence. *Biomolecules*, 15(3): 368–368. https://doi.org/10.3390/biom15030368

Shannon, S., Lewis, N., Lee, H., and Hughes, S. (2019). Cannabidiol in Anxiety and Sleep: A Large Case Series. *The Permanente Journal*, 23(1). https://doi.org/10.7812/tpp/18-041

Simiyu, D. C., Jang, J. H., and Lee, O. R. (2022). Understanding Cannabis sativa L.: Current Status of Propagation, Use, Legalization, and Haploid-Inducer-Mediated Genetic Engineering. *Plants*, 11(9): 1236. https://doi.org/10.3390/plants11091236

Śmiarowska, M., Białecka, M., and Machoy-Mokrzyńska, A. (2022). Cannabis and cannabinoids: pharmacology and therapeutic potential. *Neurologia I Neurochirurgia Polska*, 56(1): 4–13. https://doi.org/10.5603/PJNNS.a2022.0015

Strand, N. H., Maloney, J., Kraus, M., Wie, C., Turkiewicz, M., Gomez, D. A. et al. (2023). Cannabis for the treatment of fibromyalgia: A systematic review. *Biomedicines*, 11(6): 1621. https://doi.org/10.3390/biomedicines11061621

Straud, C. L., Roache, J. D., Ginsburg, B. C., Baig, R. M., King, V. L., Barron, S. et al. (2024). Enhancing massed prolonged exposure with cannabidiol to improve posttraumatic stress disorder: Design and methodology of a pilot randomized clinical trial. *Contemporary Clinical Trials Communications*, 38: 101270. https://doi.org/10.1016/j.conctc.2024.101270

Thiele, E. A., Bebin, E. M., Bhathal, H., Jansen, F. E., Kotulska, K., Lawson, J. A. et al. (2021). Add-on Cannabidiol Treatment for Drug-Resistant Seizures in Tuberous Sclerosis Complex. *JAMA Neurology*, 78(3): 285. https://doi.org/10.1001/jamaneurol.2020.4607

Thurgur, H., Schlag, A. K., Iveson, E., Hosseini, A., Lynskey, M., and Nutt, D. J. (2023). Cannabis-based medicinal products (CBMPs) for the treatment of Long COVID symptoms: current and potential applications. *Exploration of Medicine*, 487–503. https://doi.org/10.37349/emed.2023.00158

Tian, N., Yang, C., Du, Y., Chen, M., Li, B., Li, D. et al. (2025). Cannabinoid receptor 2 selective agonist ameliorates adjuvant-induced arthritis by modulating the balance between Treg and Th17 cells. *Frontiers in Pharmacology*, 16. https://doi.org/10.3389/fphar.2025.1532518

Turna, J., Syan, S. K., Frey, B. N., Rush, B., Costello, M. J., Weiss, M. et al. (2019). Cannabidiol as a novel candidate alcohol use disorder pharmacotherapy: A systematic review. *Alcoholism: Clinical and Experimental Research*, 43(4): 550–563. https://doi.org/10.1111/acer.13964

US National Library of Medicine. (2025). *Clinicaltrials.gov*. Clinicaltrials.gov. https://clinicaltrials.gov/

Villate, A., Olivares, M., Aresatz Usobiaga, Unzueta-Larrinaga, P., Rocío Barrena-Barbadillo, Callado, L. F. et al. (2024). Uncovering metabolic dysregulation in schizophrenia and cannabis use disorder through untargeted plasma lipidomics. *Scientific Reports*, 14(1). https://doi.org/10.1038/s41598-024-83288-5

Volkow, N. D., Baler, R. D., Compton, W. M., and Weiss, S. R. B. (2014). Adverse health effects of marijuana use. *New England Journal of Medicine*, 370(23): 2219–2227. https://doi.org/10.1056/nejmra1402309

Wegener, G. (2024). Advancing the understanding of cannabinoids in psychiatry. *Acta Neuropsychiatrica*, 36(5): 251–252. https://doi.org/10.1017/neu.2024.47

Zanelati, T., Biojone, C., Moreira, F., Guimarães, F., and Joca, S. (2009). Antidepressant-like effects of cannabidiol in mice: possible involvement of 5-HT1A receptors. *British Journal of Pharmacology*, 159(1): 122–128. https://doi.org/10.1111/j.1476-5381.2009.00521.x

Zhand, N., and Milin, R. (2018). What do we know about the pharmacotheraputic management of insomnia in cannabis withdrawal: A systematic review. *The American Journal on Addictions*, 27(6): 453–464. https://doi.org/10.1111/ajad.12783

Zou, S., and Kumar, U. (2018). Cannabinoid receptors and the endocannabinoid system: Signaling and function in the central nervous system. *International Journal of Molecular Sciences*, 19(3): 833. https://doi.org/10.3390/ijms19030833

Zuardi, A. W., Cosme, R. A., Graeff, F. G., and Guimarães, F. S. (1993). Effects of ipsapirone and cannabidiol on human experimental anxiety. *Journal of Psychopharmacology*, 7(1_suppl): 82–88. https://doi.org/10.1177/026988119300700112

CHAPTER 13

Cannabis Use and the Risk of Psychosis or Schizophrenia

Shweta Jaiswal, Divya Zambre, Pavan Ugalmugale, Rishabh Agade, Bhagyashree Kokate and *Veena S. Belgamwar**

1. Introduction

Cannabis use has risen sharply worldwide. By 2021, an estimated 219 million people reported using cannabis, about a 21% increase over 2011 levels. Use rates vary widely (past-year prevalence from < 1% to > 40%) and have climbed with legalization in many regions. Simultaneously, product potency has surged: high-tetrahydrocannabinol preparations (e.g., "skunk" strains and concentrates) are far more common than a decade ago. These trends (increased use and potency) could raise the population risk of cannabis-related psychosis (Wang et al. 2024). A large and growing epidemiological literature links cannabis exposure to later psychotic disorders. Longitudinal and case-control studies consistently find that regular or heavy cannabis users have roughly 2–399× higher odds of developing schizophrenia or related psychoses than never-users (Hall and Degenhardt 2008; Marconi et al. 2016). For instance, Hall and Degenhardt (2008) observed that "regular cannabis use predicts an increased risk of schizophrenia and of reporting psychotic symptoms" even after adjusting for confounders. Meta-analyses confirm this dose-response relationship. Marconi et al. (2016) reported that the heaviest cannabis users had an odds ratio ≈ of 3.90 for schizophrenia versus non-users. First-episode psychosis case–control studies mirror these findings: in the large EU-GEI sample, daily cannabis users had ≈ 3.2× higher odds of psychosis (≈ 4.8× for daily use of high-THC cannabis) compared to never-users (Di Forti et al. 2019). Likewise, national registry studies find elevated risk: for example, individuals with a cannabis use disorder had about 4× the incidence of schizophrenia relative to those without. These consistent associations—typically robust to statistical control of other factors—suggest that cannabis use likely plays a causal role in precipitating psychosis in vulnerable people. Cannabis's biological effects provide plausible mechanisms for the link to psychosis. Δ^9-tetrahydrocannabinol (THC), the main psychoactive cannabinoid, is a partial agonist at CB1 cannabinoid receptors and powerfully increases dopamine release in mesolimbic pathways (Bossong and Niesink 2010; Pertwee 2006). This mirrors a core neurochemical feature of schizophrenia. In healthy volunteers, acute THC can transiently induce positive psychotic-like symptoms (e.g., paranoia and perceptual distortions) and impair cognition (D'Souza et al. 2004). Repeated exposure to high-THC, low-CBD cannabis has been epidemiologically linked to higher schizophrenia risk (Volkow et al. 2017). Crucially, the endocannabinoid system is highly active

Department of Pharmaceutical Sciences, Rashtrasant Tukadoji Maharaj Nagpur University.
* Corresponding author: vbelgamwar@gmail.com

DOI: 10.1201/9781003668190-16

during brain development: CB1 receptor expression peaks in adolescence, coinciding with synaptic pruning and cortical maturation (Rubino and Parolaro 2016). Exogenous cannabinoids during this sensitive window may disrupt neural development, such as by altering glutamate/GABA balance or pruning dynamics, thereby increasing long-term liability to psychotic disorders. Not everyone who uses cannabis develops psychosis. Instead, risk depends on individual vulnerability. Under a diathesis–stress model, cannabis acts as a trigger mainly in those with preexisting risk factors. Genetic predisposition is one key factor: for instance, the COMT *Val^158Met* polymorphism modulates cannabis response (Caspi et al. 2005). *Val/Val* individuals (who catabolize dopamine more rapidly) exhibit more pronounced THC-induced psychotic symptoms than *Met* carriers. Other dopamine-related gene variants (e.g., *AKT1*) have been similarly implicated, though the evidence is mixed.

Three notable moderating factors are:

- Genetic/Familial Risk: A personal or family history of schizophrenia greatly amplifies cannabis's impact. For instance, individuals with a familial schizophrenia background who use cannabis are ~2.5–10× more likely to develop psychosis than comparable non-users (Moore et al. 2007).
- Early Cannabis Exposure: Adolescence is uniquely vulnerable. Each year, younger at first cannabis use is linked to substantially higher later psychotic symptoms (e.g., one study found each additional year of adolescent use nearly doubled the odds of adult hallucinations). The developing brain, rich in CB_1 receptors and undergoing extensive pruning, is especially sensitive to cannabinoid disruption (Fergusson and Boden 2008; Mustonen et al. 2018).
- Social/Environmental Stress: Chronic adversity and social context amplify risk. For example, one longitudinal study found cannabis raised psychosis risk only among urban-raised youths (with negligible effect in rural users). Ongoing stressors such as childhood trauma or social isolation chronically upregulate dopamine and immune pathways; cannabis exposure may then unmask these dysregulated circuits (Harley et al. 2010; Kuepper et al. 2011). In practice, these factors combine additively. An adolescent with multiple vulnerabilities—e.g., high-risk genetics, family schizophrenia history, early trauma, and daily high-THC use—would lie at the end of risk, whereas an adult without such predispositions might escape any lasting psychosis (Johnson et al. 2023).

Investigating cannabis-induced psychosis (CIP) is important for both science and policy. Public health significance: The explosive growth in cannabis use and potency means exposure is widespread, especially among youths. Even a partial causal role implies many cases at the population level—cohort data suggest roughly 5–10% of schizophrenia cases in high-use regions may be attributable to cannabis (Hjorthøj et al. 2021). CIP provides a "natural experiment" into schizophrenia onset (D'Souza et al. 2004). Patients whose psychotic episodes closely follow cannabis use offer a window into early disease mechanisms. Studying these cases can reveal how exogenous cannabinoids, acting in concert with genetic and developmental vulnerabilities, precipitate persistent psychotic disorders. Identifying modifiable risk factors guides intervention. For instance, education campaigns can warn adolescents and high-risk individuals about cannabis harms, while regulations (such as capping THC potency or raising the legal age of use) could help reduce the incidence of cannabis-related psychosis. Figure 1 summarizes the pathways through which cannabis use contributes to psychotic symptoms, relapse, and transition to schizophrenia across different risk populations.

2. Neurobiology of Psychosis and Schizophrenia

2.1 Neurodevelopmental Basis and Pathophysiology of Psychotic Disorders

Psychotic disorders, including schizophrenia, are widely recognized as neurodevelopmental conditions resulting from complex interactions between genetic predispositions and environmental

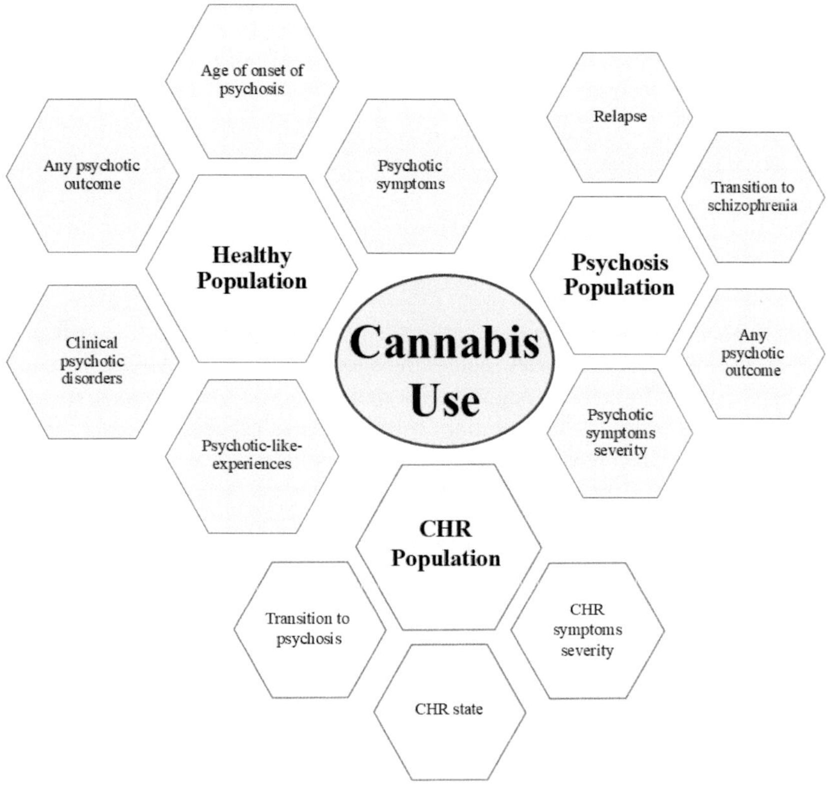

Figure 1: This figure represents the effect of cannabis consumption on the healthy population, CHR (Clinical high risk) population, and psychotic disorders.

insults that affect brain development during critical periods such as prenatal stages, childhood, and adolescence (Fatemi and Folsom 2009). Neurodevelopmental models posit that aberrations in neural circuit formation, synaptic pruning, and myelination underlie the cognitive and perceptual disturbances characteristic of psychosis (Rapoport et al. 2012; Weinberger 1987). Structural neuroimaging studies consistently demonstrate abnormalities in brain regions involved in higher-order cognition and sensory processing, including reduced gray matter volume in the prefrontal cortex, hippocampus, and temporal lobes, as well as altered white matter integrity (Fatemi and Folsom 2009; Thompson et al. 2001; Vita et al. 2012). These structural changes are thought to reflect disrupted neurodevelopmental processes and synaptic dysfunction. The positive, negative and cognitive symptoms in terms of schizophrenia are influenced by the dysregulation of neurotransmitter systems, particularly dopamine, glutamate and gamma-aminobutyric acid (GABA), which is linked to psychosis at the cellular and molecular level (Howes and Kapur 2009; Lisman et al. 2008). Aberrant synaptic pruning during adolescence is a fundamental neurodevelopmental mechanism linked to schizophrenia. By clearing surplus synapses, this process, which is carried out by microglia, the immune cells that live in the brain, is crucial for improving neural circuits (Sekar et al. 2016). Over-pruning has been correlated with patients' decreased synaptic density, which may be the cause of cognitive impairments and changed neural connectivity linked to psychosis (Paolicelli et al. 2011). These alterations may be exacerbated by neuroinflammation, which involves activated microglia, elevated pro-inflammatory cytokines, and impaired neuronal function (Müller 2014). Importantly, early-life environmental factors such as prenatal infections, obstetric complications, childhood trauma, and cannabis exposure can influence neurodevelopmental trajectories, potentially triggering the onset of psychotic disorders in genetically susceptible individuals.

2.2 Neurotransmitter Systems in Psychosis

While the dopaminergic system has long been central to models of psychosis, emerging evidence supports a multifaceted neurotransmitter dysfunction:

- Dopamine System: The classical dopamine hypothesis posits that hyperactivity of dopaminergic transmission in mesolimbic pathways contributes to positive symptoms such as hallucinations and delusions, while hypodopaminergia in the prefrontal cortex is associated with negative symptoms and cognitive impairments (Howes and Kapur 2009; Müller 2014). Dopamine dysregulation is modulated by interactions with other neurotransmitter systems and influenced by developmental trajectories.
- Glutamate System: Glutamate, the primary excitatory neurotransmitter, is critically involved in synaptic plasticity and neural communication. The N-methyl-D-aspartate (NMDA) receptor hypofunction hypothesis suggests that reduced NMDA receptor activity on inhibitory interneurons leads to cortical disinhibition, contributing to psychosis (Coyle 2012; Javitt and Zukin 1991). NMDA receptor antagonists like ketamine produce psychosis-like symptoms, supporting glutamatergic involvement.
- GABAergic System: Gamma-aminobutyric acid (GABA), the major inhibitory neurotransmitter, is essential for maintaining excitatory-inhibitory balance. Dysfunction in GABAergic interneurons, particularly parvalbumin-positive interneurons, impairs cortical oscillations and synchrony, disrupting cognition and sensory processing in schizophrenia (Lewis et al. 2012).
- Serotonin System: Serotonergic pathways modulate dopamine activity and have been implicated in schizophrenia pathophysiology. Serotonin 2A receptor antagonism forms the basis of atypical antipsychotic drugs, highlighting its role in symptom modulation.

2.3 Dopaminergic and Endocannabinoid System Interactions

Modulating neurotransmitter release and neural circuitry linked to psychosis depends critically on the endocannabinoid system (ECS). The ECS comprises endogenous ligands, including anandamide and 2- 2-arachidonoylglycerol (2-AG), their receptors (CB1 and CB2), and enzymes that control synthesis and degradation (Pertwee 2006). The ECS interacts closely with the dopaminergic system. CB1 receptors are extensively expressed in brain areas rich in dopaminergic neurons and linked to psychosis, including the prefrontal cortex, hippocampal area, and the basal ganglia at synapses. At synapses, endocannabinoids control dopaminergic activity by adjusting neurotransmitter release. Activation of CB1 receptors, for instance, can indirectly increase dopamine release in the mesolimbic pathway, producing possibly psychotic-like effects(Bossong and Niesink 2010; Pertwee 2006). Exogenous cannabinoids found in cannabis, including Δ9-tetrahydrocannabinol (THC), function as partial agonists at CB1 receptors, stimulating endogenous cannabinoids but with more potential and longer duration. The psychotomimetic effects of THC could result from dysregulation of this system, producing aberrant dopaminergic signalling and changed glutamate release (Volkow et al. 2016). On the other hand, cannabidiol (CBD) might have antipsychotic and neuroprotective actions through integrated processes, including indirect modulation of ECS and other neurotransmitter systems (Leweke et al. 2012). Furthermore, ECS dysregulation itself has been linked to schizophrenia pathophysiology; changed endocannabinoid levels and receptor expression seen in patients suggest this. About cannabis use, the dynamic interaction between the dopamine and ECS systems, together with glutamatergic and GABAergic modulation, creates a neurochemical substrate that supports the onset and development of psychosis and schizophrenia.

2.4 Relevance to Cannabis-Induced Mental Health Effects

Understanding cannabis associated psychosis implies a neurobiological basis derived from the interactions between the dopaminergic and endocannabinoid systems. In healthy people, acute THC exposure causes brief psychotomimetic reactions, including paranoia and perceptual abnormalities that mimic positive symptoms of schizophrenia (D'Souza et al. 2004). These effects are hypothesised to result from disturbance of normal ECS functioning and THC-induced dysregulation of dopamine signalling (Howes et al. 2012). Chronic and heavy cannabis use, particularly with high-THC, low-CBD strains, is associated with an increased risk of developing persistent psychotic disorders (Di Forti et al. 2015; D'Souza et al. 2004; Howes and Kapur 2009). CBD, another major cannabinoid, exhibits antipsychotic and anxiolytic properties and may mitigate some adverse effects of THC through antagonistic or modulatory effects at CB1 receptors and other targets (Leweke et al. 2012). The THC/CBD ratio, therefore, critically influences the neuropsychiatric outcome of cannabis use. Adolescence is a sensitive period during which the brain undergoes significant neurodevelopmental changes, including synapse pruning and maturation of dopaminergic pathways (Gogtay et al. 2004). Cannabis use during this window may interfere with these processes, increasing vulnerability to psychosis later in life (Rubino and Parolaro 2016). In summary, the neurobiology of psychosis and schizophrenia involves complex disruptions in dopaminergic and endocannabinoid signaling, which cannabis use can exacerbate or trigger in susceptible individuals. Understanding these mechanisms is essential for developing targeted prevention and intervention strategies.

3. Psychoactive Components of Cannabis and Their Effects

The use of extracts from the cannabis plant for medicinal purposes dates back to ancient China around 2900 BC (Russo 2007). At that time, cannabis was employed in various forms to address several health issues, including joint pain, muscle spasms, gout, and malaria. By approximately 1000 BC, in India, cannabis was utilized for its therapeutic effects as a pain reliever, sedative, tranquilizer, and anti-inflammatory (Touw 1981). In the early 1800s, Western medicine began investigating the medical potential of cannabis. Its psychoactive effects are primarily attributed to delta-9-tetrahydrocannabinol (delta-9-THC), a specific compound found in the plant. Another major component, cannabidiol (CBD), extracted from *Cannabis sativa*, is known for its diverse biological effects and health benefits, notably without inducing psychoactive effects (Mouslech and Valla 2009). Research indicates that CBD's activity is closely associated with the human endocannabinoid system, which was identified following the discovery of cannabinoid receptor 1 (CB1). This system comprises two primary receptors, CB1 and CB2, and naturally occurring ligands known as endocannabinoids (Pertwee 2008). The two key endocannabinoids—anandamide (AEA) and 2-arachidonoylglycerol (2-AG)—originate from arachidonic acid. These compounds influence the function of both CB1 and CB2 receptors (Rathod and Agrawal, 2024). The major phytocannabinoids differ structurally, which contributes to their distinct pharmacological effects (Figure 2). Enzymes such as fatty acid amide hydrolase (FAAH) and monoacylglycerol lipase (MAGL) regulate their concentrations by degrading AEA and 2-AG, respectively. CB1 receptors are primarily located in the central nervous system, particularly in brain regions linked to motor function, emotions, motivation, and energy regulation. They are also present in organs such as the heart, liver, pancreas, muscles, fat tissues, and reproductive system. On the other hand, CB2 receptors are mostly found in immune-related cells, including leukocytes, and in organs involved in immune responses, such as the spleen, thymus, and bone marrow (Nguyen et al. 2017). The therapeutic effects of cannabidiol (CBD) are primarily attributed to its interaction with the endocannabinoid system (ECS). Interestingly, CBD does not attach directly to the primary (orthosteric) binding sites of the CB1 and CB2 receptors. Instead, studies have shown that it acts through allosteric modulation of these receptors. For instance, CBD functions as an inverse agonist or antagonist at CB1 receptors with an affinity (Ki) of 3.3–4.8 nM, and as an antagonist at CB2 receptors with a Ki of approximately 4.3 nM (as shown in Table 1). Within the ECS, CBD also modulates endocannabinoid levels by interacting with fatty acid-binding proteins, with an EC50 of 27.5 μM (Tham et al. 2019).

Beyond the ECS, CBD has demonstrated significant activity on transient receptor potential vanilloid channels (TRPVs). It activates TRPV1 with an EC50 of 1 μM, TRPV2 at 1.25 μM, TRPV3

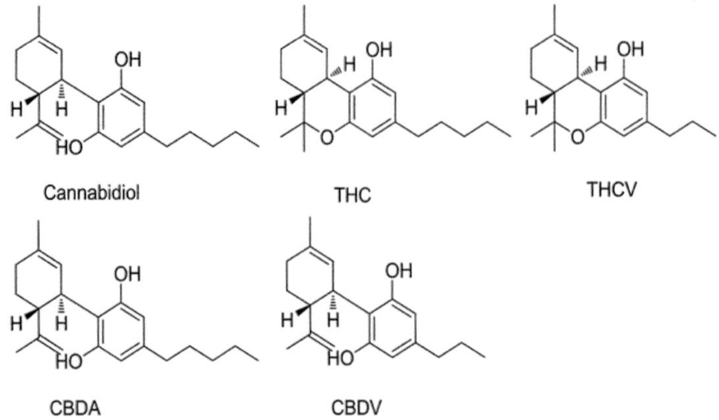

Figure 2: Chemical structures of CBD, THC, THCV, CBDA, and CBDV.

Table 1: Pharmacodynamic properties of CBD at related receptors.

Receptor	Affinity (nM)	Function	References
CB1	Ki = 3.3 ~ 4.9 nM	Inverse agonist/antagonist	(Tham et al. 2019; Thomas et al. 2007)
	IC_{50} = 0.27–0.96 mM	Negative allosteric modulators	(Laprairie et al. 2015)
CB2	Ki = 4.3 μM	Antagonist	(Martínez-Pinilla et al. 2017)
	EC_{50} = 503 nM	Inverse agonist	(Thomas et al. 2007)
	IC_{50} = 3 nM	Negative allosteric modulators	(Martínez-Pinilla et al. 2017)
GPR55	IC_{50} = 445 nM	Antagonist	(Ryberg et al. 2007)
TPPA1	EC_{50} = 110 nM	Agonist	(De Petrocellis et al. 2011)
TRPV1	EC_{50} = 1000 nM	Agonist	(Bisogno et al. 2001; De Petrocellis et al. 2011)
TRPV2	EC_{50} = 1250 nM	Agonist	(De Petrocellis et al. 2011)
TRPV3	EC_{50} = 3700 nM	Agonist	(De Petrocellis et al. 2012)
TRPV4	EC_{50} = 800 nM	Agonist	(De Petrocellis et al. 2012)
TRPM8	IC_{50} = 160 nM	Antagonist	(De Petrocellis et al. 2008)
$5\text{-}HT_{1}A$	N.D.	Indirect agonist	(Russo et al. 2005)
PPARγ	EC_{50} = 2010 nM	Agonist	(Granja et al. 2012)
FAAH	27.5 μM	Inhibitor	(Bisogno et al. 2001)
D2	Ki = 11 nM at $D2_{high}$	Partial agonist	(Ryberg et al. 2007)
	Ki = 2800 nM at $D2_{low}$		

at 3.7 μM, and TRPV4 at 0.8 μM. Additionally, CBD interacts with the peroxisome proliferator-activated receptor gamma (PPARγ), with an EC50 of 2 μM (see Table 2). Other notable molecular targets under investigation include the G-protein-coupled receptor GPR55 (EC50 of 445 nM), various serotonin (5-HT) receptors, GABA_A receptors, and the TRPM8 receptor. Table 1 summarizes the receptor affinities and functional roles related to CBD. Despite these findings, the exact biological mechanisms behind CBD's broad effects remain not fully understood.

Among the various receptors influenced by cannabidiol (CBD), FAAH, 5-HT1A, and TRPV1 have been identified as key players in its antipsychotic effects. Its antidepressant and anti-anxiety actions are thought to stem from CBD's ability to prevent the breakdown of anandamide (AEA) and its interaction with the 5-HT1A serotonin receptor. CBD also shows strong affinity for several targets associated with epilepsy, such as TRPV channels, T-type calcium channels, serotonin

Table 2: Key epidemiological studies of cannabis use and psychotic disorders.

Design/ Population	Cannabis Exposure	Outcome (DSM/ ICD)	Effect Size (OR/HR) (95% CI)	Study (Year)
Prospective cohorts and cross-sectional (66,816 individuals)	Heaviest use vs nonuse	Psychotic disorders (ICD/DSM)	OR = 3.90 (2.84–5.34)	(Marconi et al. 2016) (meta-analysis)
Case-control (901 FEP patients vs 1,237 controls, Europe)	Daily use; high-potency daily use	First-episode psychosis (ICD-10)	OR ≈3.2 (2.2–4.1) for daily use; 4.8 (2.5–6.3) for daily high-potency	(Di Forti et al. 2019) (EU-GEI)
Denmark national registry cohort (N≈7.2M, 1972–2016)	Cannabis use disorder (ICD)	Schizophrenia (ICD-10 F20)	Adjusted HR ≈4.0 (approx. 3–6 range)	(Hjorthøj et al. 2021)
Ontario population cohort (N=13.6M, 2006–2022)	Cannabis use disorder (ICD-10 F12x/T40.7)	Schizophrenia (ICD-10 F20x/ F25x)	8.9% incidence in CUD vs 0.6% without (annualized; PARF↑ 3.7→10.3%)	(Myran et al. 2025)
Review of 83 studies comparing substance users vs non-users	Any cannabis use (vs. none)	Age at psychosis onset (mixed)	Cannabis users had psychosis onset 2.70 years earlier (SD diff –0.414)	(Large et al. 2011) meta-analysis

receptors, and GPR55. Additionally, CBD interacts with calcium channels, which are implicated in the development of epilepsy. When it comes to sleep regulation, CBD is known to inhibit FAAH, thereby increasing AEA levels, and also suppress GABA receptors—both mechanisms that may influence sleep patterns. Research has also linked CBD to cardiovascular regulation through its interactions with CB1, TRPV1, PPARs, and 5-HT1A receptors. Its potential in managing diabetes may be due to its ability to reduce the production of inflammatory cytokines such as IFN-γ and TNF-α, and to limit T-cell proliferation. For pain management, CB1, CB2, and GPR2 are suggested as key targets. Meanwhile, the antitumor activity of CBD is believed to be largely mediated through its effects on TRPV channels.

3.1 The Effects of Cannabis on Mental Health

Recreational cannabis use has been linked to lasting negative effects on mental well-being, particularly among younger individuals, who may be more vulnerable (Niesink and van Laar 2013). Although the age at which people begin using cannabis is decreasing, societal concern is growing about its long-term impact on adolescent mental and social development. Research highlights a strong association between cannabis use and a heightened risk of cognitive decline, depression, anxiety, paranoia, psychosis, and schizophrenia (Schoeler and Bhattacharyya 2013). Early cannabis exposure has also been tied to the emergence of symptoms within the schizophrenia spectrum (Atakan 2012). The connection between cannabis and psychotic disorders such as schizophrenia has been consistently observed. Cannabis use is notably higher in individuals with schizophrenia compared to the general population, and prolonged use may induce psychotic episodes. This risk appears to be influenced by multiple factors, including the potency and amount of cannabis consumed. Higher doses and more potent strains are particularly associated with increased risk for chronic psychosis, although the biological mechanisms that explain individual susceptibility remain unclear. While most recreational users do not develop severe or permanent psychological problems, cannabis use can negatively impact mental functioning (Campos et al. 2012). Adverse effects depend on various factors, including age of first use, dosage, frequency, and the user's genetic and psychological profile. Between 15% and 50% of users may experience short-term psychotic episodes, typically resolving without medical intervention. Evidence suggests individuals predisposed to psychosis—such as those with low cerebrospinal anandamide levels or a family history of psychotic disorders—are susceptible to the effects of cannabis. In particular, those with high schizotypy traits or in ultra-high-risk categories experience more intense psychosis-like symptoms (Leweke et al. 2012).

High THC doses can trigger temporary psychotic responses even in those without a history of mental illness, with more severe effects in new or occasional users. Strains with higher THC content, like "skunk" or sinsemilla, are more frequently associated with first-time psychotic episodes and relapse in schizophrenia. THC affects brain regions responsible for memory, attention, motor skills, and perception, with peak impairment occurring within one to two hours of use (Hallak et al. 2010). There is growing evidence of dysfunction in the endocannabinoid system among schizophrenia patients, which might be linked to their characteristic cognitive deficits. THC mimics these deficits by impairing attention and memory. This similarity is fueling research into cannabinoid-based pharmacological treatments. Cannabis-based medications were once commonly prescribed but fell out of favor in the mid-20th century due to inconsistent potency, unpredictable responses, side effects like anxiety and confusion, and the introduction of more stable alternatives like aspirin and barbiturates (Hunault et al. 2009). Today, cannabis extracts and synthetic cannabinoids are largely prohibited in many regions.

3.2 CBD-THC Ratio and Its Effects

Although CBD has not consistently shown symptom-relieving properties, it may protect against the negative effects of THC. Some studies suggest CBD reduces THC-induced psychotic symptoms when administered either before or alongside THC. However, CBD is usually found in cannabis resin and is rarely present in herbal cannabis (Zuardi et al. 1982). In early research, Rottanburg and colleagues observed a connection between CBD absence in certain cannabis strains and a higher incidence of psychosis. Additionally, it appears that higher CBD levels might reduce the rewarding ("wanting") sensation of THC, potentially lowering addiction risk. Still, there's insufficient evidence to confirm that hashish, which contains more CBD, is less addictive than more potent herbal cannabis (Rottanburg et al. 1982). Brain imaging studies suggest CBD and THC influence different brain areas. For instance, during tasks involving memory, emotion, and speech processing, CBD and THC exhibit opposing effects in regions such as the hippocampus, amygdala, and prefrontal cortex. These findings may explain their contrasting behavioral and psychological impacts. THC is known to trigger transient hallucinations and disrupt sensory processing, particularly in users predisposed to psychosis. CBD has also been linked to reduced brain activation in addiction-related circuits, supporting its potential protective role. Still, not all studies support these findings, and variability in cannabis strain and usage patterns continues to complicate research outcomes (Dalton et al. 1976).

3.3 CBD's Antipsychotic Potential

Evidence suggests that CBD could be beneficial in treating several psychiatric and neurological disorders, including anxiety, depression, and psychosis. Notably, CBD seems to mitigate THC-induced anxiety and psychosis-like symptoms. While its binding to cannabinoid receptors is weak, CBD may counteract THC by preventing the breakdown of anandamide, thereby indirectly reducing THC activity at these receptors. Higher levels of anandamide have been linked to fewer psychotic symptoms, and boosting its concentration through CBD has shown promise in slowing the progression of early psychosis. Clinical trials have demonstrated that CBD is as effective as certain antipsychotic medications like amisulpride, with fewer side effects such as weight gain, hormonal disruption, or motor impairments. CBD has also been shown to reduce drug-induced motor abnormalities and does not cause catalepsy, unlike some traditional antipsychotics. These findings align CBD with atypical antipsychotic profiles, suggesting it could be a safer alternative (Hallak et al. 2010). Furthermore, in preclinical models, CBD reduced hyperactivity caused by stimulants without inducing harmful side effects. Although CBD does not significantly alter the activity of dopamine or serotonin systems, it exerts a wide range of pharmacological effects across multiple brain pathways. Its antipsychotic benefits may arise from modulating neurotransmitters indirectly, including promoting neurogenesis in the hippocampus, which could be beneficial for cognitive dysfunction in schizophrenia (Campos et al. 2012). In behavioral studies, CBD reversed symptoms related to psychosis without causing sedation or movement disorders commonly associated with antipsychotics like haloperidol. In fact, it produced effects similar to those of clozapine, another atypical antipsychotic, increasing activity in cognitive brain regions without overstimulating motor areas. CBD may also help regulate brain activity disrupted by other psychosis models, including those involving glutamate receptor antagonists (Leweke et al. 2012). However, it does not affect dopamine reuptake or directly alter dopaminergic activity, suggesting a unique mechanism of action compared to traditional treatments. In non-clinical studies, higher CBD content in cannabis was linked to fewer self-reported psychotic symptoms, but not other mental health issues.

3.4 Neuroprotective Effects of CBD

CBD has demonstrated neuroprotective, anticonvulsant, and anxiolytic properties in various studies. While it has minimal impact on normal brain function, its therapeutic effects emerge when the endocannabinoid system is disrupted, such as by THC or external stressors. CBD also acts as an antioxidant and anti-inflammatory agent, mechanisms that may be relevant for treating neurological conditions such as Alzheimer's, Huntington's, and Parkinson's disease. It appears capable of producing these effects independently of CB1 and CB2 receptors, possibly providing broader neuroprotection. However, current research offers limited support for CBD's cognitive benefits. Although some studies suggest it may improve attention or memory in certain populations, others report mixed results. For example, one study found that a 600 mg dose of CBD impaired selective attention in schizophrenia patients, likely due to its sedative properties (Alger and Kim 2011).

4. Epidemiological Evidence Linking Cannabis to Psychosis

Cannabis is one of the most widely used psychoactive substances globally, with recent estimates of 228 million users in 2022. Over the past two decades, many countries have liberalized medical or recreational cannabis laws, leading to a higher prevalence of use (Wang et al. 2024). These trends have raised concerns about potential harms. A large body of evidence now links cannabis use to later development of psychotic disorders. In particular, longitudinal and case-control studies consistently find that regular or heavy cannabis use in adolescence or young adulthood is associated with an elevated risk of schizophrenia or other psychoses. For instance, Hall and Degenhardt (2008) concluded that "regular cannabis use predicts an increased risk of schizophrenia and of reporting psychotic symptoms" even after adjusting for confounders. Systematic meta-analyses report roughly 2–3× higher odds of psychosis in cannabis users versus nonusers. Importantly, most studies use standardized diagnostic criteria (DSM or ICD) and prospective designs, strengthening the validity of the association (Hall and Degenhardt 2008); (Marconi et al. 2016). Given the high societal burden of psychotic disorders, understanding the epidemiological link between cannabis and psychosis is of major public health interest.

4.1 Global Epidemiological Trends

Cannabis is now the most commonly used illicit drug worldwide. By 2021, an estimated 219 million people reported cannabis use, up 21% from 2011. Use rates vary widely by region, with past-year prevalence ranging from < 1% to over 40% in some countries. As of early 2024, 40+ countries had introduced new medical or recreational cannabis laws, and studies show legalization is associated with substantially higher use. For example, pooled data indicate past-year cannabis prevalence ~ 12.0% in legalized countries versus ~5.4% in non-legalized countries. In the United States, adolescent cannabis use rose 4% from 2008–2019 following state legalization. Alongside rising use, potency has increased. High-THC cannabis products (e.g., "skunk," concentrates) are more prevalent now than a decade ago. Higher THC concentration is biologically plausible to enhance psychotogenic effects. These trends (greater use and potency) could increase the population risk for cannabis-related psychosis. Global schizophrenia incidence remains roughly 0.5–0.7 per 1,000 person-years (lifetime risk ~ 0.7–1%), with little evidence of sharp recent changes. However, registry-based studies show that the population-attributable fraction (PAF) of schizophrenia linked to cannabis use has been rising. For example, a Danish national cohort (1972–2016) found the PAF for cannabis use disorder (CUD) in schizophrenia increased from ~ 2% in 1995 to ~ 6–8% by 2010 (Hjorthøj et al. 2021). Similarly, a large Canadian cohort (Ontario 2006–2022; N=13.6 million) found the PAF of schizophrenia attributable to CUD nearly tripled, from 3.7% pre-legalization to 10.3% post-legalization (Myran et al. 2025). In that study, 8.9% of individuals diagnosed with CUD later developed schizophrenia, compared to 0.6% without CUD. These figures suggest that a growing minority of schizophrenia cases (on the order of 5–10%) may be linked to cannabis in populations with high use.

4.2 Findings From Cohort, Case-Control, and Population-Based Studies

A wealth of epidemiological studies of various designs have examined the cannabis–psychosis link. Longitudinal cohorts (prospective birth cohorts, national registries, military conscripts) generally find that earlier cannabis use predicts later psychotic outcomes, even after adjusting for confounders. For instance, the landmark Dunedin birth cohort (New Zealand) showed that adolescent cannabis use was associated with a higher risk of schizophreniform disorder in young adulthood. A recent meta-analysis integrating these data reported that chronic or heavy cannabis users have markedly elevated risk: pooled odds ratios (ORs) are on the order of ~ 3–4 for "hard" outcomes. Specifically, Marconi et al. found a logistic model OR of 3.90 (95% CI 2.84–5.34) for schizophrenia or related psychoses among the heaviest cannabis users versus nonusers. Similarly, a pooled analysis of cohort and cross-sectional studies found a summary OR of 2.88 (95% CI 2.24–3.70) for psychosis (schizophrenia or psychotic experiences) in cannabis users. These analyses confirm a consistent association: one meta-analysis reported a roughly 4-fold increase in risk among the most frequent users, compared with ~2-fold for average users. In nearly all studies, the direction of effect was positive, and most individual estimates were statistically significant. Importantly, these associations are not confined to cross-sectional designs: even in cohort studies that excluded baseline cases of psychosis, cannabis use remained a robust risk marker. Case-control studies of first-episode psychosis (FEP) further illustrate the association. The EU-GEI multicenter study (Lancet Psychiatry 2019) compared 901 FEP patients to 1,237 population controls across 11 sites. It found that daily cannabis use carried significantly increased odds of psychotic disorder: adjusted OR ≈ 3.2 (95% CI 2.2–4.1) vs never-users (Di Forti et al. 2019). The risk was even higher for daily use of high-potency cannabis (THC ≥ 10%): OR ≈ 4.8 (95% CI 2.5–6.3) (Di Forti et al. 2019). Remarkably, the fraction of psychosis cases attributable to high-potency cannabis ranged from 12.2% overall up to 50.3% in Amsterdam (Di Forti et al. 2019). A London case-control study similarly estimated that 1 in 3 first-episode psychosis cases was linked to high-potency cannabis use in that setting. These controlled studies, which collected detailed usage history and applied DSM/ICD diagnoses, consistently support a dose-dependent risk gradient. Population-based registry studies have also documented the link. In Denmark, Hjorthøj et al. (2021) used nationwide registers (N≈7.2 million) to compare individuals with and without cannabis use disorder (CUD). Those with CUD had an adjusted hazard ratio of ≈4 for incident schizophrenia throughout 1972–2016 (Hjorthøj et al. 2021). Notably, the proportion of schizophrenia cases with prior CUD rose from ~ 2% in 1995 to ~ 6–8% by 2010 (Hjorthøj et al. 2021), tracking the increase in cannabis availability and potency. In Ontario, the population-based cohort described above found 8.9% of persons with CUD later diagnosed with schizophrenia, versus only 0.6% of those without CUD (Myran et al. 2025). The corresponding relative risk is roughly 14-fold higher in CUD patients, although demographic and clinical confounding may inflate this estimate. Collectively, these large-scale studies underscore that the association emerges in naturalistic settings rather than in specialized samples.

4.3 Association With Early-Onset and Dose-Dependent Risk

Several findings highlight that younger age at first use and greater intensity of use amplify psychosis risk. The onset of cannabis use during adolescence appears particularly hazardous. The pooled analysis by Pourebrahim et al. (2025) noted a "twofold-higher risk" of schizophrenia for cannabis exposure during adolescence compared to use in adulthood. Consistent with this, meta-analytic data show that individuals who use cannabis tend to manifest psychotic illnesses 2–3 years earlier than non-users. These observations suggest that cannabis may accelerate the emergence of psychosis. Dose-response relationships are also evident. Epidemiologic reviews consistently report that heavier, more frequent, or more potent cannabis use confers a higher risk. For example, Marconi et al. observed progressively higher ORs with increasing use: the heaviest users had an OR $\approx$ 3.9 compared with nonusers, while the average risk across all users was about 2-fold. In a similar analysis, the strongest associations were observed in cohorts with severe use categories: nearly a 4-fold risk in cohort designs and 5-fold in case-control designs for the highest exposure groups. Case-control studies reinforce this pattern: in EU-GEI, daily high-potency users had ~ 5× odds of psychosis (Di Forti et al. 2019), compared to ~ 3× for daily use of typical cannabis. In sum, there is a clear dose-dependent gradient, with heavier use (frequency, duration, and THC potency) linked to progressively greater psychosis odds (Marconi et al. 2016). This meets a key epidemiologic criterion for causality. Notably, high-THC strains ("skunk") have expanded in markets, and these potent products are likely driving the observed dose effect. Pourebrahim et al. (2025) explicitly highlight that risk "increases with a high cannabis THC concentration and increased frequency of use," possibly reflecting disruption of synaptic plasticity during neurodevelopment.

4.4 Temporal Sequence: Cannabis Use Preceding Psychotic Symptoms

Establishing that cannabis use precedes psychotic illness is crucial to causal inference. Many prospective studies have demonstrated that cannabis exposure typically occurs years before psychosis onset. Hall and Degenhardt (2008) reviewed longitudinal evidence and concluded that regular cannabis use precedes and predicts psychosis, and that the relationship is not explained by self-medication of prodromal symptoms. Likewise, meta-analyses of first-episode cases find that cannabis use was reported before any psychotic diagnosis in almost all study designs. Marconi et al. specifically excluded subjects who had psychotic symptoms at baseline, ensuring that cannabis use was antecedent; their pooled analysis still found a strong association. In fact, sensitivity analyses in these studies (limited to first-onset cases) show virtually identical effect sizes to those in full samples, suggesting reverse causation is unlikely. Moreover, as noted, cannabis-using patients have an earlier age at onset of illness. On average, schizophrenia begins about 2.7 years sooner in those with a history of cannabis use. This temporal shift implies that cannabis is a risk factor accelerating illness emergence, rather than a consequence. In summary, the temporal relationship is consistently observed: cannabis use in adolescence/young adulthood typically antedates psychotic symptoms by several years, reinforcing a likely contributory role in pathogenesis.

4.5 Neurobiological Plausibility and Mechanistic Evidence

The cannabis–psychosis link is supported by coherent neurobiological pathways. Δ9-tetrahydrocannabinol (THC), the primary psychoactive compound in cannabis, is a partial agonist at brain cannabinoid type 1 (CB1) receptors, which modulate key neurotransmitter systems. CB1 receptors are abundant in areas involved in psychosis, including the prefrontal cortex, hippocampus, and basal ganglia. THC's action disrupts endocannabinoid signaling by altering glutamate and GABA release via retrograde inhibition, thereby affecting downstream dopamine circuits (Bloomfield et al. 2016). Acute THC administration has been shown to increase dopaminergic activity transiently—for instance, animal studies and one human neuroimaging provocation study demonstrated THC-induced dopamine release and neuronal firing. Dysregulated dopamine is a core feature of psychosis, so this provides a mechanistic bridge. Over chronic use, adaptive changes occur: imaging studies suggest reduced dopamine synthesis and blunted dopaminergic responses in regular cannabis users, which may predispose to psychotic symptomatology. Experimental evidence in humans underscores plausibility. Intravenous THC challenge in healthy volunteers reliably induces short-lived psychotic-like symptoms (e.g., paranoia and hallucinations). Importantly, cannabis contains both THC and cannabidiol (CBD), but higher-THC/low-CBD strains are most strongly implicated in risk. Genetic factors also intertwine: some studies suggest that genetic variants (e.g., in COMT or AKT1) moderate an individual's sensitivity to cannabis-induced psychosis, indicating an interaction between genetic vulnerability and cannabis exposure. Finally, neurodevelopment may amplify risk. The adolescent brain is undergoing maturation of synaptic pruning and endocannabinoid regulation. Pourebrahim et al. point to a "selective cannabis toxicity on synaptic plasticity in adolescence". In animal models, adolescent THC exposure produces enduring changes in cortical circuitry and behavior. While exact pathways remain under investigation, the convergence of human and animal data, from molecular to behavioral levels, makes a causal link biologically plausible (Pourebrahim et al. 2025).

4.6 Challenges in Establishing Causality

Despite robust associations, proving causality is challenging. Observational studies are subject to confounding and bias. Cannabis users often differ from non-users in many ways (genetics, environment, other substance use) that may also influence psychosis risk. Although most studies adjust for covariates (age, sex, socioeconomic status, other drug use, and family history), residual confounding is always possible. For example, unmeasured factors like childhood trauma or urbanicity might correlate with both cannabis use and psychosis onset. Pooled estimates from raw data (as in the meta-analyses above) are typically unadjusted, and these effect sizes may be inflated by such confounding. Indeed, one meta-analysis noted that fully adjusted ORs were ~ 45% lower than unadjusted ones (Marconi et al. 2016). Reverse causation is another concern: prodromal psychotic symptoms might lead to self-medication with cannabis. However, the prospective design of many key studies (excluding subjects with baseline symptoms) argues against this. Moreover, consistent temporal lag (cannabis use preceding symptoms by years) and the observed dose-response pattern are hard to attribute to reverse causation. Cannabis exposure is often based on self-report (with variable accuracy), and "use" can range from occasional to daily. Standardized diagnostic criteria are used for outcomes, but psychosis itself exists on a spectrum (from subclinical psychotic experiences to full-blown schizophrenia). Studies vary in outcome definitions (schizophrenia diagnosis vs psychotic-like symptoms), which can introduce heterogeneity. Finally, ethical constraints preclude randomized trials of cannabis use over many years to the onset of psychosis, so evidence must come from observational designs or quasi-experiments. Genetic approaches (Mendelian randomization) provide some support for a causal effect of cannabis on schizophrenia risk, but results suggest only a modest causal estimate. In sum, while the Bradford Hill criteria (temporality, dose-response, and coherence with biology) lean toward causality, the evidence cannot prove causation beyond doubt. The residual possibility of confounding, selection bias, or shared liability cannot be fully eliminated.

5. Clinical Features of Cannabis-Associated Psychosis

Cannabis, an internationally used psychotropic drug, has come under increasing scrutiny owing to its potential to induce psychosis in vulnerable subjects. Cannabis-induced psychosis (CIP) is a clinical syndrome characterised by the development of psychotic symptoms in response to cannabis use. Different psychiatric nomenclatures have developed diagnostic criteria for CIP, such as the Diagnostic and Statistical Manual of Mental Disorders, Fifth Edition (DSM-5) (American Psychiatric Association 2021) and the International Classification of Diseases, Tenth Edition (ICD-10) (World Health Organisation 1992).

5.1 Diagnostic Criteria of CIP

DSM-5 diagnoses CIP when a person is affected by psychotic symptoms, i.e., hallucinations, delusions, disorganized thinking, and negative symptoms, within a brief time of cannabis consumption (American Psychiatric Association 2021).

Diagnostic criteria of CIP include:

Presence of Psychotic Symptoms: The patient must display one or more of the following psychotic symptoms: hallucinations, delusions, disorganised thinking, and negative symptoms.

Temporal Association: Appearance of psychotic symptoms ought to be within a short time frame after the use of cannabis, typically between 30 minutes and 1 hour (Large et al. 2011).

Cannabis Use: The patient should have used cannabis before the onset of symptoms of psychosis.

As Large et al. (2011) said, "the temporal association between cannabis use and development of psychotic symptoms is an essential component in the diagnosis of CIP." Freeman et al. (2007) also refer to excluding other possible causes of psychotic symptoms, and in their view, "a complete medical and psychiatric assessment is needed to rule out other possible causes of the psychotic symptoms." Individuals with a history of CIP can still experience chronic psychosis symptoms even when isolated from cannabis (Larkin and Read 2008). Cognitive deficit and adverse social function have also been associated with CIP (Kessler et al. 2005). As Moore et al. (2007) note, "the risk of schizophrenia is greatly elevated in people who have CIP, especially if there is a family risk of psychotic disorder." Again, Larkin and Read (2008) note that long-term psychotic symptoms can be experienced by individuals with CIP even when cannabis use has ceased, which underlines the value of continuing monitoring and intervention over time.

5.2 Acute vs. Persistent Symptoms in Cannabis-Induced Psychosis

Cannabis that was once relegated to the fringes of decent society now experiences a global explosion of decriminalization and legalization. Where advocates highlight its potential curative utility, concerns remain, particularly regarding the potential for CIP. Understanding the nuances of CIP appropriately facilitates appropriate diagnosis, effective management, and policy. The current chapter examines a critically significant distinction between persistent and acute symptoms of CIP, presents their diagnostic criteria, clinical presentations, and potential long-term impact, and concludes by advocating a more sophisticated, evidence-based approach to this nuanced disorder. CIP involves the development of psychotic symptoms, such as hallucinations, delusions, disorganized thinking, and negative symptoms, with cannabis use. The definitional point of difference remains symptom duration. Acute psychosis in this category means fleeting psychotic symptoms that arise in close temporal relation to cannabis use and resolve with a definable time interval following abstinence. Persistent psychosis involves a more prolonged illness course duration in that psychosis symptoms are ongoing and continue to persist in an elongated time interval following intoxication and abstinence, which can mature into a chronic psychotic disorder in the form of schizophrenia. The Diagnostic and Statistical Manual of Mental Disorders, Fifth Edition (DSM-5) outlines "Cannabis-Induced Psychotic Disorder" criteria in detail (American Psychiatric Association 2021). According to the DSM-5 definition, psychotic symptoms shall arise during/shortly after cannabis intoxication/withdrawal. Notably, to differentiate this disorder from an independent primary psychotic disorder, DSM-5 stipulates that an independent primary psychotic disorder cannot better explain symptoms, and symptoms cannot persist for a long duration (i.e., for over one month) post-cessation of cannabis use.

The "one-month rule" forms an essential criterion in differentiating an acute, transient CIP from a longer-duration psychotic illness. However, even this "one-month rule" has its caveats. Its opponents argue that it is an arbitrary time-point and can in no way do justice to the subtle clinical reality wherein the psychosis continuum from an acute to chronic condition can be gradual and less sharply definable (Large et al. 2011). Once again, vulnerabilities of a genetic nature for psychosis or of a subclinical nature for psychotic experiences can have a significant impact on the duration and shape of symptoms.

5.3 Clinical Presentation of CIP

The clinical presentation of CIP can vary considerably, influenced by factors such as the potency of the cannabis consumed, the individual's pre-existing vulnerabilities, and the route of administration.

Acute CIP often manifests with florid psychotic symptoms, including:

- Hallucinations: These can be auditory (hearing voices), visual (seeing things that are not there), or tactile (feeling sensations on the skin).
- Delusions: Fixed, false beliefs that are resistant to reason. Common delusions in CIP include paranoia (belief that one is being persecuted), grandiosity (belief in having special powers or abilities), and ideas of reference (belief that unrelated events have special significance for oneself).
- Disorganized Thought: Difficulty organizing thoughts, resulting in incoherent speech, illogical reasoning, and tangential thinking.
- Disorganized Behavior: Erratic or unpredictable behavior, ranging from agitation and hyperactivity to catatonia.

These acute symptoms are typically observed during or immediately after cannabis intoxication, often accompanied by anxiety, panic, and derealization (feeling detached from reality). Cannabis withdrawal may also cause psychotic symptoms in certain people, though less frequently. Notably, in acute CIP, these symptoms should resolve and ultimately return to baseline completely within days to weeks of cannabis abstinence. Chronic CIP has a more complex and concerning picture. Initially, it might appear similar to acute CIP, but the key point is that the psychotic symptoms persist beyond the expected duration. These symptoms can linger for months or even years, and they can evolve into a chronic psychotic disorder such as schizophrenia or schizoaffective disorder.

Individuals with chronic CIP most commonly experience:

- Persistent Hallucinations and Delusions: While the intensity of these symptoms may fluctuate, they do not completely resolve.
- Negative Symptoms: These include affective flattening (reduced emotional expression), alogia (poverty of speech), avolition (lack of motivation), and anhedonia (inability to experience pleasure).
- Cognitive Impairment: Difficulties with attention, memory, and executive function.
- Social and Occupational Dysfunction: Impaired ability to maintain relationships, attend school, or hold a job.

Acute and chronic CIP may not be distinguishable absolutely. A gradual development of a chronic psychosis from an acute psychosis will be seen in some patients, while others will have remission followed by a relapse. Also, chronic CIP cannot be distinguished from a primary psychotic disorder superimposed on it.

5.4 Etiology: Risk Factors and Mechanisms

The actual processes underlying CIP remain to be studied, but several factors are thought to be responsible for its cause.

- Cannabis Potency: High-potency cannabis products, particularly those with high levels of THC (tetrahydrocannabinol), are associated with an increased risk of CIP (Di Forti et al. 2015).
- Frequency and Duration of Use: Frequent and prolonged cannabis use is another significant risk factor.
- Genetic Vulnerability: Individuals with a family history of psychosis or schizotypal personality traits are more susceptible to developing CIP.
- Age of Onset: Early-onset cannabis use (i.e., before the age of 18) is associated with a greater risk of developing chronic psychotic disorders (Fergusson and Boden 2008).
- Pre-existing Mental Health Conditions: Individuals with pre-existing anxiety, depression, or other mental health conditions may be more vulnerable to developing CIP.

Neurobiological evidence suggests that delta-9-tetrahydrocannabinol (THC), the primary psychoactive constituent of cannabis, disrupts dopaminergic signaling within the brain, particularly in the mesolimbic pathway—a neural circuit integral to reward processing, motivation, and the pathogenesis of psychotic disorders. Moreover, cannabis use modulates the endocannabinoid system, which is critically involved in the regulation of mood, cognitive function, and the stress response. The progression from acute to persistent cannabis-induced psychosis (CIP) is hypothesised to involve a multifaceted interaction among genetic predisposition, environmental influences, and neurobiological mechanisms. Chronic exposure to cannabis may induce neuroplastic alterations that facilitate the transition to a sustained psychotic disorder. In individuals with underlying genetic vulnerabilities, cannabis may function as a precipitating factor that accelerates the onset of psychosis.

5.5 Treatment Strategies

The treatment of CIP depends on the severity and duration of symptoms.

Acute CIP typically requires symptomatic management, including:

- Cessation of Cannabis Use: This is the first and most crucial step in treatment.
- Supportive Care: Providing a safe and supportive environment, reassurance, and crisis intervention.
- Pharmacological Intervention: In some cases, antipsychotic medications may be necessary to manage severe psychotic symptoms. Benzodiazepines may be used to manage anxiety and agitation.

Persistent CIP requires a more comprehensive and long-term treatment approach, similar to that used for primary psychotic disorders.

- Antipsychotic Medications: These are the cornerstone of treatment for persistent psychosis.
- Psychosocial Interventions: Cognitive behavioral therapy (CBT), family therapy, and social skills training can help individuals manage symptoms, improve coping skills, and enhance social functioning.
- Rehabilitation Services: Vocational rehabilitation, supported employment, and educational support can help individuals regain their independence and reintegrate into society.

It is crucial to emphasize the importance of early intervention in both acute and persistent CIP. Early diagnosis and treatment can improve outcomes and reduce the risk of long-term disability.

5.6 Transition From Cannabis-Induced Psychosis to Schizophrenia

"The association of cannabis use with psychosis, particularly schizophrenia, remains a matter of controversy. Whereas cannabis use has been associated with a higher risk of psychotic disorders, the shape of this association, particularly in terms of conversion from cannabis-induced psychosis (CIP) to schizophrenia, remains to be clarified. The current paper tries to present what has so far come out about this conversion in terms of evidence for causality, predictors of chronic psychosis symptoms, and problems in the differentiation of CIP from early onset/comorbid schizophrenia. The association of psychosis with cannabis has been established well enough, with numerous studies demonstrating a higher prevalence of cannabis use among schizophrenia patients (Semple et al. 2005). Establishing a causal relationship is much more difficult. The vulnerability-stress theory posits that cannabis is a "stressor" that can reveal hidden vulnerability to psychosis in susceptible individuals (Caspi et al. 2005). It would mean that cannabis actually does not cause schizophrenia directly, but it accelerates or precipitates the onset among already susceptible individuals. The evidence for this vulnerability-stress model is robust. Genetic studies have identified individual genes for schizophrenia and for being more vulnerable to cannabis's effects (Zheng et al. 2022). Besides this, a history of psychosis in one's family, trauma in childhood, and pre-existing subclinical psychosis symptoms (e.g., odd perceptual experiences, magical thinking) have all been shown to have a high risk for developing psychosis among cannabis-using individuals (van Os et al. 2002). These predictors suggest that individuals with pre-existing vulnerabilities are at higher risk for chronic psychosis when they consume cannabis. However, the question of whether cannabis can directly induce a schizophrenic disorder in individuals without pre-existing vulnerabilities remains a point of contention. While some argue that cannabis can act as a primary causal agent for psychosis, particularly with high-potency products and early onset of use, the current evidence leans more towards the acceleration/precipitation model. Distinguishing between these two scenarios is crucial for both clinical management and public health interventions. Cannabis-induced psychosis is typically characterized by the onset of psychotic symptoms (e.g., hallucinations, delusions, and disorganized thinking) in close temporal proximity to cannabis use, with resolution of symptoms within a relatively short period (days to weeks) after cessation of use (American Psychiatric Association 2021). However, a significant proportion of individuals diagnosed with CIP go on to develop schizophrenia or another persistent psychotic disorder (Carvalho and Vieira-Coelho 2022). Identifying factors that predict this transition is critical for early intervention and improved outcomes.

Several factors have been identified as potential predictors of psychosis persistence following CIP:

- Severity and Nature of Initial Psychotic Symptoms: More severe psychotic symptoms at the initial presentation, particularly those aligning with the diagnostic criteria for schizophrenia (e.g., bizarre delusions and negative symptoms), are associated with a higher risk of transitioning to schizophrenia (Arendt et al. 2005). The presence of negative symptoms like blunted affect, avolition, and alogia during the acute CIP episode is particularly concerning.
- Duration of Cannabis Use and Age of Onset: Longer duration of cannabis use, particularly regular and heavy use, and younger age at the onset of cannabis use are associated with a greater risk of persistent psychosis. Younger brains are still developing and may be more vulnerable to the potentially neurotoxic effects of cannabis.ha
- Family History of Psychosis: As mentioned earlier, a family history of psychosis significantly increases the risk of developing schizophrenia after CIP. This highlights the importance of considering genetic vulnerability in the diagnostic and prognostic assessment.
- Co-occurring Substance Use Disorders: The presence of other substance use disorders, particularly stimulant use, can complicate the clinical picture and increase the likelihood of persistent psychosis (Henquet et al. 2005). Polysubstance use can exacerbate psychotic symptoms and interfere with treatment adherence.

- Neurocognitive Deficits: Studies have shown that individuals who transition from CIP to schizophrenia often exhibit neurocognitive deficits, particularly in attention, working memory, and executive function, even after the acute psychotic symptoms have subsided. These deficits may reflect underlying neurobiological vulnerabilities.

Identifying these predictors allows clinicians to stratify patients based on their risk of developing schizophrenia after CIP and tailor interventions accordingly. High-risk individuals may benefit from more intensive monitoring, early antipsychotic treatment, and comprehensive psychosocial support.

5.7 The Diagnostic Dilemma: Differentiating CIP From Early or Comorbid Schizophrenia

One of the major challenges in clinical practice is differentiating between true CIP, which resolves completely after cessation of cannabis use, and early-stage schizophrenia that is triggered or exacerbated by cannabis. The diagnostic criteria for CIP require that the psychotic symptoms resolve completely after a period of abstinence from cannabis. However, in many cases, it can be difficult to determine whether residual symptoms are due to the lingering effects of cannabis or represent the beginning of a chronic psychotic disorder.

Several factors can complicate the diagnostic process:

- Retrospective Reporting Bias: Individuals may under-report their cannabis use or have difficulty accurately recalling the temporal relationship between cannabis use and the onset of psychotic symptoms.
- Comorbid Substance Use Disorders: As mentioned earlier, the presence of other substance use disorders can confound the clinical picture and make it difficult to isolate the specific effects of cannabis.
- Subclinical Psychotic Symptoms: Individuals may have pre-existing subclinical psychotic symptoms that are exacerbated by cannabis, making it difficult to determine whether the psychosis is truly cannabis-induced or merely unmasked.
- Lack of Standardized Diagnostic Criteria: There is a lack of standardized diagnostic criteria for CIP, resulting in inconsistent diagnoses and treatment.

To improve diagnostic accuracy, clinicians should:

- Obtain a Detailed History of Substance Use: A thorough history of cannabis and other substance use, including the frequency, duration, and potency of substances used, is crucial.
- Conduct Serial Assessments: Repeated assessments of psychotic symptoms over time, both during and after periods of abstinence from cannabis, are necessary to determine whether symptoms are resolving or persisting.
- Consider Neurocognitive Testing: Neurocognitive testing can help identify underlying neurocognitive deficits that may suggest a vulnerability to schizophrenia.
- Obtain Collateral Information: Gathering information from family members or other close contacts can provide valuable insights into the individual's premorbid functioning and substance use history.

5.8 Diagnostic and Clinical Management Challenges

Diagnosis of CIP has been challenging as the symptoms overlap with other psychiatric disorders, for example, schizophrenia (SZ) and bipolar disorder (BD) (Cosgrove and McTavish 2018). Diagnostic and Statistical Manual of Mental Disorders, 5th Edition (DSM-5) has a precise diagnosis of cannabis-induced psychotic disorder, where there must be psychotic symptoms within 1 hour of cannabis consumption (American Psychiatric Association 2013). Diagnosis of CIP has been challenging as most of the CIP patients are capable of fulfilling SZ or BD, thereby making it challenging to ascertain if cannabis consumption is causative of psychosis (Myles et al. 2012). The Journal of Clinical

Psychopharmacology study confirmed that 25% of CIP patients also met diagnostic criteria for SZ, demonstrating the complexity of the diagnosis (Koskinen et al. 2010). In addition, an incorrect time frame between cannabis initiation and the onset of psychotic symptoms can complicate the confirmation of a causal relationship (D'Souza et al. 2009). As D'Souza et al. (2016) explained, "the relationship between cannabis consumption and psychosis is complex, and the diagnosis of CIP requires a careful assessment of the patient's history, symptoms, and substance use patterns." There are many issues concerning the clinical treatment of CIP, particularly the treatment. There has been a trend of using antipsychotic medications, e.g., risperidone and olanzapine, in managing psychosis symptoms, but their efficacy in the treatment of CIP has been poor (Hall and Degenhardt 2008). In a Journal of Clinical Psychopharmacology study, antipsychotic medications decreased psychosis symptoms in CIP patients. Nevertheless, the response rate was less than in SZ (Koskinen et al. 2010).

6. Individual Susceptibility to Cannabis-Induced Psychosis

6.1 Genetic Vulnerability

The risk of psychotic reactions to cannabis is heavily modulated by individual vulnerability. Genetic predisposition plays a central role: almost all repeatedly identified risk loci affect dopamine signaling or its regulation. For instance, the COMT Val158Met polymorphism is the most-studied gene: carriers of the Val (high-enzyme activity) allele tend to catabolize prefrontal dopamine more rapidly, leaving lower extracellular dopamine levels. Multiple studies report that Val-allele carriers are particularly sensitive to cannabis. A cohort of adolescent cannabis users with the COMT Val/Val genotype was far more likely to develop psychotic symptoms or schizophreniform disorders than Met/Met homozygotes (Vaessen et al. 2018). Subsequent experiments and patient samples confirmed that the Val variant is associated with more frequent THC-induced psychotic experiences, earlier onset of symptoms, and higher THC sensitivity. By contrast, Met carriers show a relative resilience to cannabis's psychotic effects. This gene's impact is often contingent on other risk factors, but overall, the systematic review by Carvalho and Vieira-Coelho (2022) notes that the COMT rs4680 Val allele "has been associated with cannabis use–induced psychotic experiences, with earlier age at onset of these experiences, and with more responsive THC-induced psychosis." In short, COMT Val/Val appears to be a liability genotype for cannabis-triggered psychosis (Carvalho and Vieira-Coelho 2022). Beyond COMT, several other polymorphisms in dopaminergic genes modulate cannabis psychosis risk. AKT1 (a kinase involved in dopamine signaling) has one of the strongest replications. The rs2494732 C allele (especially CC homozygotes) doubles the odds of psychotic disorder among heavy cannabis users. For instance, Di Forti et al. (2012) showed that first-episode patients carrying AKT1 C/C who had used cannabis were about twice as likely to develop psychosis as T/T users. It was found that healthy volunteers with AKT1 risk genotypes experienced more acute psychotic-like effects of THC (Di Forti et al. 2012). Although some recent studies failed to replicate AKT1's effect, the preponderance of evidence still implicates this gene (Morgan et al. 2016). Similarly, DRD2 variants appear relevant. A particular intronic SNP (rs1076560) in the dopamine D2 receptor gene was associated with a striking 3-fold higher rate of cannabis-related psychosis in one Dutch study. Likewise, the dopamine transporter gene DAT1 (SLC6A3) 3′-UTR VNTR polymorphism has been linked to THC sensitivity: carriers of the "9-repeat" allele (which increases synaptic dopamine) showed significantly greater midbrain and striatal responses to THC and more psychotic symptoms in placebo-controlled testing. These genes fit the broader pattern: Carvalho and Vieira-Coelho emphasize that "the majority of identified risk polymorphisms are related directly (COMT, DRD2, and DAT) or indirectly (AKT1) to the dopaminergic system" (Carvalho and Vieira-Coelho 2022). This converges on the classic dopamine-salience hypothesis of psychosis, in which aberrant dopamine signaling (now unmasked by cannabis) triggers psychotic experiences. Other susceptibility loci fall outside the core dopamine pathway but still affect related neural circuits. A genome-wide association study of cannabis-induced hallucinations found significant SNPs near

CHRM3 (the cholinergic muscarinic-3 receptor) in European Americans. Blockade of muscarinic receptors is known to induce psychotic symptoms, so a CHRM3 link makes biological sense. Similarly, one genome-wide interaction study (GWEIS) by Boks et al. identified a SNP (rs7958311) in P2RX7 (the purinergic P2X7 receptor) that was associated with high levels of cannabis-related psychotic experiences in regular users. This suggests immune-related pathways may also contribute (Boks et al. 2020). By contrast, studies of other candidates (e.g., BDNF and FAAH) have yielded null or inconsistent results. For example, polymorphisms in FAAH (an endocannabinoid-degrading enzyme) have not been reliably linked to cannabis-induced psychosis in recent large samples (Cheng et al. 2019). Altogether, the genetic picture is complex and polygenic, but dopaminergic genes (COMT, AKT1, DRD2, and DAT) stand out as the most robust modulators of cannabis psychosis risk.

6.2 Environmental Risk Factors

Environmental factors likewise play a key role in modulating individual susceptibility. A strong body of epidemiological evidence has long shown that childhood adversity dramatically raises psychosis risk. Meta-analyses indicate that physical abuse, sexual abuse, emotional abuse, neglect, or early parental loss each roughly doubles or triples the likelihood of later psychotic disorder. For instance, a recent review found that most forms of childhood maltreatment confer around a 2–3× increase in schizophrenia or related psychosis risk. Importantly, early trauma appears to "create an enduring vulnerability" to psychosis that may not manifest until further stressors occur (Harley et al. 2010). For example, a study showed that individuals with childhood abuse combined with subsequent life stressors had synergistically higher odds of subclinical psychotic experiences—far beyond the individual effects of abuse or later stress alone. In that study, the addition of cannabis use also increased psychosis likelihood, albeit with a somewhat smaller effect (Begemann et al. 2017). Nonetheless, the implication is clear: a history of trauma primes the brain to respond abnormally to later insults—including cannabis exposure. Urbanity and social stress are additional environmental contributors. Growing up in a city (as opposed to the countryside) is well-established as a schizophrenia risk factor. One landmark longitudinal study found that adolescent cannabis users from urban environments had a much higher incidence of psychotic symptoms over 10 years than similar users from rural areas. In statistical terms, cannabis use raised psychosis risk significantly only for those raised in urban settings; among rural youths, the effect was negligible. As Kuepper et al. conclude, "Environmental influences associated with urban upbringing may increase vulnerability to the psychotomimetic effects of cannabis use" (Kuepper et al. 2011). Mechanistically, urban stressors (overcrowding, noise, and social fragmentation) are thought to chronically activate the stress-response and dopaminergic systems. Chronic social stress (e.g., peer victimization, discrimination, or social isolation) similarly sensitizes dopaminergic and immune pathways. For example, rodent models show that prolonged social defeat or stress increases dopamine release and behavioral sensitivity to psychotomimetic (Fett et al. 2019). Clinically, having a chronically stressful life or belonging to a marginalized minority group is known to elevate psychosis incidence. Although cannabis use prevalence may vary across these groups, the heightened baseline risk suggests an interaction: social adversity and cannabis together can overload already vulnerable systems. Indeed, one large study noted that the effect of genetics (PRS) and cannabis differed between African- versus European-ancestry subgroups, hypothesizing that unequal exposure to racism or urban stress may modulate cannabis's impact (van Os et al. 2005). Critically, genes and environment do not operate in isolation but interact. The classic example is again COMT Val^158^Met. It was reported that adolescent cannabis users carrying the COMT Val allele were far more likely to develop schizophreniform symptoms than Met carriers. Vinkers et al. observed that heavy cannabis-using youth showed a marked rise in subclinical psychosis only if they were Val/Val homozygotes with histories of maltreatment (Vinkers et al. 2013).

6.3 High-Risk Populations

Adolescents stand out as high-risk. The developing brain is uniquely sensitive to exogenous cannabinoids, and epidemiological data confirm that early-onset use is particularly pernicious (Kalayasiri et al. 2010). For example, Canadian public health reviewers note that initiating cannabis use before age 16 substantially increases the likelihood of psychosis. Consistent with this, population studies find that each year of regular cannabis use in adolescence nearly doubles the odds of hallucinations (OR 1.92) and more than doubles the odds of paranoid ideation (OR 2.33) later in life (Mustonen et al. 2018). Large cohorts also show that adolescent cannabis users manifest psychotic symptoms at younger ages: UK Biobank analyses indicate cannabis use is linked to earlier onset of unusual psychotic experiences. In practical terms, a teenager using cannabis daily is not only adding the direct effects of THC but also perturbing a brain still undergoing synaptic pruning and myelination—potentially derailing normal neural development in ways that increase psychosis risk (Mackie et al. 2021). Likewise, individuals with a family history of psychosis or schizophrenia are at much higher risk when they use cannabis. This is a classic diathesis–stress scenario: a genetic predisposition already exists, so cannabis acts as a trigger. Public health data emphasize this danger: for example, Health Canada notes that people with a familial psychosis history who use cannabis are "2.5 to 10 times more likely to develop psychosis" than non-users with the same family history. In other words, among genetically vulnerable lineages, cannabis substantially amplifies risk. Patients with comorbid mental health disorders may also represent a high-risk subgroup, although the literature here is less clear-cut. Cannabis use is notably common in people with mood, anxiety, or personality disorders, and these conditions share some neurobiological pathways with psychosis. For instance, an anxious or depressed individual may use cannabis to self-medicate, inadvertently precipitating psychotic symptoms. At the very least, the presence of any psychiatric illness signals a lower threshold for dysregulation. Although systematic reviews have not quantified this risk as precisely as family history or age, it is widely accepted that patients in a prodromal ("ultra-high-risk") phase for psychosis who also use cannabis tend to convert more rapidly to full psychosis. In sum, populations characterized by preexisting vulnerability—young age, genetic/familial predisposition, or concurrent psychiatric illness—exhibit markedly higher cannabis-psychosis rates in practice (Pelayo-Terán et al. 2012).

6.4 Cumulative Risk Model

All of these findings underscore a cumulative risk model of cannabis-induced psychosis. Rather than any single factor, it is the synergy of predispositions and exposures that determines outcome. Conceptually, one can imagine plotting risk as the sum of weighted contributions: polygenic risk score, presence of high-risk alleles (e.g., COMT Val and AKT1 CC), severity of childhood trauma, degree of urban/social stress, age at onset of use, and dose/frequency/potency of cannabis. Each factor pushes an individual further along a vulnerability continuum (Wainberg et al. 2021). For example, a teenager with COMT Val/Val, a parental history of schizophrenia, who grew up in a high-stress neighborhood and uses high-THC cannabis daily would sit at the extreme end of that continuum—effectively guaranteed to experience some psychotic manifestations eventually. Conversely, an adult without family history, without traumatic stress, using cannabis infrequently and only in low doses, might never encounter anything beyond mild transient effects (Mustonen et al. 2018). This multifactorial perspective is reflected in recent research and theory. Johnson et al. explicitly describe cannabis psychosis risk as additive: schizophrenia PRS and cannabis exposure (especially early/heavy use) "combine to increase an individual's vulnerability" in a linear way. Their data showed that genetic liability and cannabis dependence each independently predicted unusual cannabis-related experiences, suggesting that one does not simply "substitute" for the other but rather piles risk upon risk (Johnson et al. 2023). Carvalho and Vieira-Coelho similarly advocate a broad approach, calling for polygenic and epigenetic profiling to eventually enable "pharmacogenetic-guided cannabis use"—essentially tailoring risk assessments and even therapeutic recommendations to the person's genomics. They note that personalized models that account for multiple genes, environmental exposures, and development stages are needed. In their words, integrated risk stratification might "allow a better and more rational use of cannabis" by matching "appropriate therapy based on the genetic/epigenetic background"(Carvalho and Vieira-Coelho 2022).

In summary, individual susceptibility to cannabis-induced psychosis emerges from a complex interplay of many factors. Genetic polymorphisms in dopamine-related and other signaling pathways set a baseline sensitivity: variants like COMT Val, AKT1 rs2494732 C, DRD2 rs1076560 T, DAT1 9-repeat, and others each tilt the balance toward psychosis when challenged by THC. Environmental adversities (childhood trauma, urban stress, social defeat) lower that threshold further. These forces interact (e.g., COMT×trauma×cannabis, or polygenic risk×early use) to amplify risk, often in roughly additive ways. Certain groups exemplify the highest risk—notably adolescents, people with a family history of psychosis, and those with other psychiatric comorbidities—because they typically carry more of these vulnerabilities at once. The overall model is one of cumulative liability: no single gene or exposure is deterministic, but the sum of one's genetic load and life history determines how dangerous cannabis use will be. This integrated view has important practical implications. It suggests that risk assessment for cannabis-induced psychosis must be personalized. A thorough evaluation would consider the user's genotype profile (or PRS), psychiatric and family history, trauma history, and social context. Ultimately, tools such as polygenic risk scores combined with environmental risk algorithms could quantify an individual's susceptibility. Such models are still in development, but early evidence (e.g., UK Biobank analyses) indicates they can stratify risk meaningfully. Clinically, this could guide counseling: for example, warning a young person with multiple risk factors that their chances of cannabis-triggered psychosis are very high, or considering alternative therapies to cannabinoid products for high-genetic-risk patients. Carvalho and Vieira-Coelho even envision "pharmacogenetic-guided cannabis use," analogous to how genetics now guide medication choice in oncology or pain management.

Susceptibility to cannabis-induced psychosis reflects the aggregate of genetic, developmental, and environmental risks. A highly academic consensus has emerged that, while THC can produce transient psychotic-like effects in anyone, only those with sufficient predisposing "hits" will develop enduring or severe symptoms. This means that research and public health must focus not just on cannabis exposure itself, but on the context of individual vulnerability. Ongoing genetic studies (including broad genome-wide scans and PRS work) and longitudinal cohorts are beginning to map out this landscape with greater precision. The hope is that with these insights—e.g., identifying a dangerous COMT/AKT1 genotype combination or quantifying an exposome score—we can predict who is most at risk and intervene early, perhaps before psychosis fully manifests. Thus, a multifactorial, personalized risk model is emerging as the paradigm for understanding, predicting, and ultimately preventing cannabis-related psychosis.

7. Structural and Functional Alterations in Cannabis-Induced Psychosis

Cannabis-induced psychosis (CIP) is characterized by acute psychotic episodes precipitated by cannabis use, which typically remit upon cessation of use. It offers a unique model for exploring the neural mechanisms underlying psychosis and the neurobiological impact of cannabis on brain structure and function.

7.1 Structural Gray Matter Abnormalities

Advancements in structural brain imaging—particularly magnetic resonance imaging (MRI)—have enabled detailed exploration of gray matter volume (GMV) in individuals with CIP. Comparative studies between CIP patients, healthy controls, and individuals with chronic schizophrenia (SZ) have sought to delineate both shared and distinct neural alterations. These investigations aim to identify whether the neuroanatomical profile of CIP aligns more closely with normative brain structure or with the structural abnormalities characteristic of SZ. A consistent finding across multiple studies is a reduction in GMV within the prefrontal cortex (PFC) among individuals with CIP. The PFC plays a central role in executive function, working memory, and cognitive control—domains frequently impaired in psychosis. A meta-analysis by Lorenzetti et al. (2019) reported that chronic cannabis use is associated with diminished PFC volume, suggesting that repeated exposure—particularly among individuals with pre-existing vulnerabilities—may interfere with PFC maturation and functionality, potentially increasing susceptibility to psychotic episodes. The temporal lobe, especially the hippocampus and amygdala, has also garnered interest. These regions are critical for memory consolidation, emotional regulation, and contextual processing—functions often disrupted in psychotic states. Some studies have noted hippocampal volume reductions in individuals with CIP, which may underlie cognitive deficits frequently observed in these patients (Radhakrishnan et al. 2014). However, findings have not always been consistent, emphasizing the need for larger, rigorously controlled studies to clarify the relationships among cannabis use, structural brain changes, and psychosis. Importantly, comparative analyses of CIP and SZ suggest nuanced differences in GMV alterations. Schizophrenia is typically associated with widespread gray matter reductions across multiple brain regions, whereas CIP appears to involve more localized changes, particularly within the PFC and temporal lobe (Bloomfield et al. 2016). These distinctions imply that, while CIP shares certain clinical features with SZ, it may arise from partially distinct neurobiological processes.

7.2 Functional Dysconnectivity: Insights From fMRI and EEG/ERP

Functional imaging modalities, such as functional MRI (fMRI) and electroencephalography (EEG), including event-related potentials (ERPs), provide insights into brain activity and connectivity patterns. These tools have been instrumental in highlighting how brain regions coordinate—or fail to coordinate—their activity in individuals with psychosis, including those with CIP. Resting-state functional connectivity (rs-FC) studies have revealed disruptions in core neural networks in CIP. Altered activity within the default mode network (DMN), a system engaged during internally focused thought and self-referential processing, has been observed in CIP populations (Bossong et al. 2013). Reductions in functional connectivity within the DMN may reflect impaired self-monitoring and difficulties distinguishing internal thoughts from external stimuli—hallmarks of psychotic symptoms. Disruptions in connectivity between the PFC and subcortical regions, such as the thalamus and striatum, have also been documented. The thalamus serves as a critical sensory relay, while the striatum is involved in motivation and reward processing. Altered interactions between these regions and the PFC could contribute to the cognitive and sensory disturbances frequently observed in CIP (Curran et al. 2016), including impaired sensory gating, attention deficits, and the emergence of hallucinations or delusional beliefs. ERP studies provide further evidence of functional abnormalities. Reduced amplitude of the P300 component—a waveform associated with attentional allocation and the processing of novel stimuli—has been reported in individuals with CIP (D'Souza et al. 2012). This suggests that individuals experiencing cannabis-induced psychosis may struggle to appropriately direct cognitive resources to relevant environmental cues, leading to disorganized thought processes and impaired reality testing.

7.3 Cognitive Impairments in CIP: Memory, Attention, and Executive Dysfunction

Understanding cognitive dysfunction in CIP requires a broader consideration of how cannabis affects cognition in general. While acute or recreational use can cause transient cognitive slowing, chronic heavy cannabis use, particularly when initiated during adolescence, is linked to persistent deficits in attention, memory, and executive functioning (Volkow et al. 2014; Meier et al. 2012). These impairments are largely attributed to cannabis's influence on the endocannabinoid system—a critical modulator of synaptic plasticity and neuronal signaling, especially in regions such as the PFC and hippocampus. CIP represents a more severe form of cannabis-related cognitive disruption. Triggered by the psychoactive component of cannabis, Δ9-tetrahydrocannabinol (THC),

CIP involves acute psychotic episodes that can leave lasting cognitive sequelae even after the resolution of psychotic symptoms. Memory impairments are among the most frequently reported cognitive deficits in CIP. Both short- and long-term memory may be compromised, affecting the ability to learn, recall, and organize personal experiences. Working memory deficits are particularly problematic, often manifesting as difficulty retaining and manipulating information needed for daily tasks (Jager et al. 2006). Verbal learning and episodic memory impairments can affect the retention of names, conversations, or factual information (Joyce and Roiser 2007), while deficits in visual-spatial memory may lead to disorientation and trouble recalling visual details (Nuechterlein et al. 2008). Attention is similarly affected. Individuals with CIP often exhibit impairments across various domains of attention—sustained, selective, and divided—which can severely limit academic and occupational performance (Solowij et al. 2002). Executive functions, which govern planning, decision-making, impulse control, and goal-oriented behavior, are also vulnerable. CIP has been associated with poor cognitive flexibility, reduced inhibitory control, and diminished problem-solving abilities (Grant et al. 2003). These deficits reflect broader disruptions in the neural circuitry supporting complex cognitive operations and are critical targets for intervention and rehabilitation.

7.4 Persistent Deficits Following Early-Onset Cannabis Use

Historically, CIP was considered a short-lived condition resolving with the cessation of cannabis use. However, emerging data indicate that when cannabis use begins in adolescence, CIP can produce long-term neurocognitive impairment. Adolescence is a critical window of brain maturation (involving synaptic pruning and myelination), and exogenous cannabinoids can derail this process. Longitudinal cohort studies provide stark evidence; for instance, follow-up of the Dunedin cohort found that individuals who used cannabis heavily from a young age showed significant cognitive decline by mid-adulthood across multiple domains (processing speed, verbal memory, executive function) (Wilkinson et al. 2014). On average, early-onset heavy users lost about 8 IQ points, and these deficits did not fully recover with abstinence. Similarly, chronic users who started before age 15 perform worse on sustained attention, impulse control, and executive tasks than later-onset users or nonusers. These findings suggest that CIP precipitated during the vulnerable adolescent brain can leave enduring scars. Moreover, epidemiological data indicate CIP is relatively common among first-episode psychosis cases in areas of heavy cannabis use: some studies estimate that up to 25–50% of young psychotic patients have a history of cannabis-triggered psychosis. The trend toward higher-potency cannabis (with more THC) may be driving an increase in CIP cases over the past decade. In sum, early-onset cannabis exposure not only precipitates acute psychosis but also heightens the risk of persistent cognitive and functional deficits (Wilkinson et al. 2014).

7.5 Neurobiological Mechanisms

Several mechanisms likely underlie these structural and cognitive abnormalities.

THC Neurotoxicity: Δ^9-THC exerts direct effects on brain cells. Animal and human studies suggest that heavy or prolonged THC exposure can damage developing neurons and disrupt neurotransmitter systems (notably dopamine and glutamate pathways critical for cognition). Regions rich in CB1 receptors (e.g., hippocampus, PFC) are especially vulnerable, as evidenced by volume loss and synaptic changes in these areas (Burggren et al. 2019).

Developmental Disruption: Cannabis may interfere with normal neurodevelopment. The endocannabinoid system plays a regulatory role in neurogenesis and synaptic pruning during adolescence. Exogenous cannabinoids (THC) introduced during this period can perturb neural connectivity and circuit refinement, leading to aberrant brain maturation. This is supported by findings that prenatal or adolescent cannabinoid exposure alters cortical development and later cognitive function.

Gene-Environment Interactions: Genetic vulnerability modulates CIP risk. Certain alleles (e.g., the COMT Val158Met variant or AKT1 polymorphisms) interact with cannabis exposure to increase psychosis risk. For instance, individuals with the COMT Val/Val genotype who use cannabis (especially if abused or in the context of childhood stress) show a markedly higher likelihood of psychotic outcomes compared to Met carriers (Wilkinson et al. 2014). These findings imply that inherited differences in dopamine metabolism or intracellular signaling can amplify the effect of THC.

Neuroinflammation: Chronic cannabis use can activate immune pathways in the brain. Microglial cells express cannabinoid receptors, and dysregulated activation may release pro-inflammatory cytokines, leading to neural injury. Although direct human evidence is still emerging, preclinical models show that prolonged THC exposure can induce neuroinflammatory states that impair cognition. In sum, CIP likely arises from a toxic synergy: THC intoxication triggers psychosis on a background of neurodevelopmental disruption, amplified by genetic predisposition and inflammatory processes.

7.6 Clinical Implications: Prevention and Intervention

Screening and Early Intervention: Clinicians treating young people should routinely assess cannabis use, especially in adolescents or those with a family history of psychosis. Early-onset cannabis use is a red flag: because adolescent brains are particularly susceptible, early use significantly raises the risk of CIP and lasting deficits. Clinicians must be vigilant to psychosocial stressors (e.g., childhood trauma) that compound cannabis risk. For individuals who develop CIP, prompt treatment of the psychotic episode is essential (typically antipsychotic medication and supportive care), but equally important is addressing the cannabis use itself.

Psychosocial Treatments: Motivational interviewing and cognitive-behavioral interventions have demonstrated efficacy in reducing cannabis use and improving outcomes. For example, many early-psychosis programs now incorporate psychoeducation and motivational enhancement to curb use (Aydin et al. 2016). Formal programs (group therapy and cognitive-behavioral therapy targeting substance use) should be offered whenever possible; in practice, however, few early-intervention services have dedicated cannabis-targeted treatments (Burggren et al. 2019), highlighting a gap in care. Cognitive remediation therapy may also be beneficial for recovering lost skills.

Harm Reduction: Public health efforts should emphasize the risks of heavy cannabis use, particularly high-THC products, for youth. Educational campaigns in schools and communities can inform adolescents that early and frequent use can alter brain development and precipitate psychosis. Harm-reduction strategies (promoting lower-potency preparations and discouraging daily use, especially among teens) are prudent. Clinicians should counsel young patients and families that abstinence or delayed initiation is the safest course. Policymakers might consider regulating cannabis potency and implementing age restrictions to protect developing brains.

Together, a proactive strategy of screening, education, and targeted intervention can mitigate the neuropsychiatric harm of cannabis. By identifying high-risk individuals (based on age, use patterns, and genetics) and intervening early, it may be possible to prevent CIP onset or reduce its long-term impact on cognition and functional outcome.

8. Conclusion

Existing research indicates that cannabis use is a significant contributor to the development of schizophrenia. Findings from meta-analyses and long-term studies consistently demonstrate that frequent consumption of cannabis, particularly high-potency strains, is linked to a heightened risk of psychotic disorders. In fact, heavy cannabis users face a three- to fourfold increase in the likelihood of developing schizophrenia compared to those who abstain. Additionally, there is strong evidence of a dose-dependent effect: earlier initiation, more frequent usage, and higher levels of THC all amplify the risk. However, cannabis use alone does not lead to psychosis in all individuals.

Current theoretical models suggest a complex interplay of factors, where cannabis interacts with genetic predispositions (such as schizophrenia-related genes or COMT variants), developmental timing, and psychosocial challenges. This supports the "multiple-hit" or "ecological" framework of schizophrenia, in which substance use acts as a trigger or accelerator in genetically or biologically vulnerable individuals.

Neurobiologically, Δ^9-THC's affinity for CB1 receptors provides a direct link to psychosis-related circuitry. THC's ability to acutely induce schizophrenia-like symptoms in healthy subjects underscores the plausibility of causality. Its interaction with the dopamine system (stimulating mesolimbic release) aligns with the dopamine hypothesis of psychosis. Simultaneously, cannabis impacts glutamatergic and GABAergic transmission and alters the regulation of neurotrophic factors during development. In particular, adolescent cannabis exposure may disrupt synaptic pruning and cortical maturation, creating enduring abnormalities in brain networks. Animal models of prenatal or adolescent cannabinoid exposure exhibit long-lasting dopamine dysregulation and behavior resembling psychosis, lending mechanistic support. These insights have practical consequences. In clinical settings, psychiatrists and pediatricians should routinely inquire about cannabis use, particularly in youths with prodromal symptoms or a family history of psychosis—patients who report heavy use of high-THC cannabis warrant close monitoring and early intervention. Cognitive-behavioral and motivational interventions can be offered to reduce cannabis intake among at-risk individuals. From a public health standpoint, policymakers should consider measures to limit youth access to high-potency cannabis and to inform the public about psychosis risks. Indeed, mathematical models estimate that curtailing adolescent cannabis use could substantially reduce the population burden of schizophrenia.

Causal links can only be established with more sophisticated designs (e.g., prospective cohorts with genetic data, natural experiments around legalization, and ethically permissible human pharmacological studies). Better quantification of individual THC and CBD exposure is needed in epidemiological work. Genetic and biomarker studies (e.g., imaging of ECS function) may clarify why some users develop psychosis while others do not. Additionally, the roles of cannabidiol (CBD), which may have antipsychotic or neuroprotective effects, and of newer synthetic cannabinoids in modulating risk merit investigation. Ultimately, a comprehensive understanding will emerge from integrating population data with cellular and circuit-level studies of how cannabinoids interact with brain development and neurotransmission. In closing, the current evidence supports a nuanced conclusion: cannabis use contributes to schizophrenia risk through biological and environmental interactions, but it is one factor in a complex etiology. A balanced risk model recognizes that while most users do not become psychotic, a nontrivial subset does, and often those cases involve heavy, high-THC use in a vulnerable context. Awareness of these links should inform clinical assessment (including substance use histories in psychiatric care) and guide public health strategies aimed at mitigating this preventable pathway to serious mental illness.

References

Acting on persecutory delusions: The importance of safety seeking. (2007). *Behaviour Research and Therapy*, 45(1): 89–99.

Alger, B. E., and Kim, J. (2011). Supply and demand for endocannabinoids. *Trends in Neurosciences*, 34(6): 304–315.

American Psychiatric Association. (2021). *Diagnostic and Statistical Manual of Mental Disorders (DSM-5)*. American Psychiatric Publishing.

Arendt, M., Rosenberg, R., Foldager, L., Perto, G., and Munk-Jørgensen, P. (2005). Cannabis-induced psychosis and subsequent schizophrenia-spectrum disorders: follow-up study of 535 incident cases. *The British Journal of Psychiatry : The Journal of Mental Science*, 187: 510–515.

Atakan, Z. (2012). Cannabis, a complex plant: different compounds and different effects on individuals. *Therapeutic Advances in Psychopharmacology*, 2(6): 241–254.

Aydin, C., Tibbo, P. G., and Ursuliak, Z. (2016). Psychosocial Interventions in Reducing Cannabis Use in Early Phase Psychosis. *The Canadian Journal of Psychiatry*. https://doi.org/10.1177/0706743716639931

Begemann, M. J. H., Stotijn, E., Schutte, M. J. L., Heringa, S. M., and Sommer, I. E. C. (2017). Letter to the Editor: Beyond childhood trauma - stressful events early and later in life in relation to psychotic experiences. *Psychological Medicine*, 47(15): 2731–2736.

Bisogno, T., Hanus, L., De Petrocellis, L., Tchilibon, S., Ponde, D. E., Brandi, I. et al. (2001). Molecular targets for cannabidiol and its synthetic analogues: effect on vanilloid VR1 receptors and on the cellular uptake and enzymatic hydrolysis of anandamide. *British Journal of Pharmacology*, 134(4): 845–852.

Bloomfield, M. A. P., Ashok, A. H., Volkow, N. D., and Howes, O. D. (2016). The effects of Δ9-tetrahydrocannabinol on the dopamine system. *Nature*, 539(7629): 369.

Boks, M. P., He, Y., Schubart, C. D., van Gastel, W., Elkrief, L., Huguet, G. et al. (2020). Cannabinoids and psychotic symptoms: A potential role for a genetic variant in the P2X purinoceptor 7 (P2RX7) gene. *Brain, Behavior, and Immunity*, 88: 573–581.

Bossong, M. G., Martijn Jansma, J., van Hell, H. H., Jager, G., Kahn, R. S., and Ramsey, N. F. (2013). Default Mode Network in the Effects of Δ9-Tetrahydrocannabinol (THC) on Human Executive Function. *PLOS ONE*, 8(7): e70074.

Bossong, M. G., and Niesink, R. J. M. (2010). Adolescent brain maturation, the endogenous cannabinoid system and the neurobiology of cannabis-induced schizophrenia. *Progress in Neurobiology*, 92(3): 370–385.

Burggren, A. C., Shirazi, A., Ginder, N., and London, E. D. (2019). Cannabis effects on brain structure, function, and cognition: considerations for medical uses of cannabis and its derivatives. *The American Journal of Drug and Alcohol Abuse*, 45(6). https://doi.org/10.1080/00952990.2019.1634086

Campos, A. C., Moreira, F. A., Gomes, F. V., Del Bel, E. A., and Guimarães, F. S. (2012). Multiple mechanisms involved in the large-spectrum therapeutic potential of cannabidiol in psychiatric disorders. *Philosophical Transactions of the Royal Society of London. Series B, Biological Sciences*, 367(1607): 3364–3378.

Carvalho, C., and Vieira-Coelho, M. A. (2022). Cannabis induced psychosis: A systematic review on the role of genetic polymorphisms. *Pharmacological Research*, 181: 106258.

Caspi, A., Moffitt, T. E., Cannon, M., McClay, J., Murray, R., Harrington, H. et al. (2005). Moderation of the effect of adolescent-onset cannabis use on adult psychosis by a functional polymorphism in the catechol-O-methyltransferase gene: longitudinal evidence of a gene X environment interaction. *Biological Psychiatry*, 57(10): 1117–1127.

Cheng, Z., Phokaew, C., Chou, Y.-L., Lai, D., Meyers, J. L., Agrawal, A. et al. (2019). A regulatory variant of CHRM3 is associated with cannabis-induced hallucinations in European Americans. *Translational Psychiatry*, 9(1): 309.

Coyle, J. T. (2012). NMDA receptor and schizophrenia: a brief history. *Schizophrenia Bulletin*, 38(5): 920–926.

Curran, H. V., Freeman, T. P., Mokrysz, C., Lewis, D. A., Morgan, C. J. A., and Parsons, L. H. (2016). Keep off the grass? Cannabis, cognition and addiction. *Nature Reviews Neuroscience*, 17(5): 293–306.

Dalton, W. S., Martz, R., Lemberger, L., Rodda, B. E., and Forney, R. B. (1976). Influence of cannabidiol on delta-9-tetrahydrocannabinol effects. *Clinical Pharmacology and Therapeutics*, 19(3): 300–309.

De Petrocellis, L., Ligresti, A., Moriello, A. S., Allarà, M., Bisogno, T., Petrosino, S. et al. (2011). Effects of cannabinoids and cannabinoid-enriched Cannabis extracts on TRP channels and endocannabinoid metabolic enzymes. *British Journal of Pharmacology*, 163(7): 1479–1494.

De Petrocellis, L., Orlando, P., Moriello, A. S., Aviello, G., Stott, C., Izzo, A. A. et al. (2012). Cannabinoid actions at TRPV channels: effects on TRPV3 and TRPV4 and their potential relevance to gastrointestinal inflammation. *Acta Physiologica (Oxford, England)*, 204(2): 255–266.

De Petrocellis, L., Vellani, V., Schiano-Moriello, A., Marini, P., Magherini, P. C., Orlando, P. et al. (2008). Plant-derived cannabinoids modulate the activity of transient receptor potential channels of ankyrin type-1 and melastatin type-8. *The Journal of Pharmacology and Experimental Therapeutics*, 325(3): 1007–1015.

Di Forti, M., Iyegbe, C., Sallis, H., Kolliakou, A., Falcone, M. A., Paparelli, A. et al. (2012). Confirmation that the AKT1 (rs2494732) genotype influences the risk of psychosis in cannabis users. *Biological Psychiatry*, 72(10): 811–816.

Di Forti, M., Marconi, A., Carra, E., Fraietta, S., Trotta, A., Bonomo, M. et al. (2015). Proportion of patients in south London with first-episode psychosis attributable to use of high potency cannabis: a case-control study. *The Lancet. Psychiatry*, 2(3): 233–238.

Di Forti, M., Quattrone, D., Freeman, T. P., Tripoli, G., Gayer-Anderson, C., Quigley, H. et al. (2019). The contribution of cannabis use to variation in the incidence of psychotic disorder across Europe (EU-GEI): a multicentre case-control study. *The Lancet. Psychiatry*, 6(5). https://doi.org/10.1016/S2215-0366(19)30048-3

D'Souza, D. C., Fridberg, D. J., Skosnik, P. D., Williams, A., Roach, B., Singh, N. et al. (2012). Dose-Related Modulation of Event-Related Potentials to Novel and Target Stimuli by Intravenous Δ9-THC in Humans. *Neuropsychopharmacology*, 37(7): 1632–1646.

D'Souza, D. C., Perry, E., MacDougall, L., Ammerman, Y., Cooper, T., Wu, Y.-T. et al. (2004). The psychotomimetic effects of intravenous delta-9-tetrahydrocannabinol in healthy individuals: implications for psychosis.

Neuropsychopharmacology : Official Publication of the American College of Neuropsychopharmacology, 29(8): 1558–1572.

D'Souza, D. C., Sewell, R. A., and Ranganathan, M. (2009). Cannabis and psychosis/schizophrenia: human studies. *European Archives of Psychiatry and Clinical Neuroscience*, 259(7). https://doi.org/10.1007/s00406-009-0024-2

Fatemi, S. H., and Folsom, T. D. (2009). The neurodevelopmental hypothesis of schizophrenia, revisited. *Schizophrenia Bulletin*, 35(3): 528–548.

Fergusson, D. M., and Boden, J. M. (2008). Cannabis use and later life outcomes. *Addiction*, 103(6): 969–976.

Fett, A.-K. J., Lemmers-Jansen, I. L. J., and Krabbendam, L. (2019). Psychosis and urbanicity: a review of the recent literature from epidemiology to neurourbanism. *Current Opinion in Psychiatry*, 32(3): 232–241.

Gogtay, N., Giedd, J. N., Lusk, L., Hayashi, K. M., Greenstein, D., Vaituzis, A. C. et al. (2004). Dynamic mapping of human cortical development during childhood through early adulthood. *Proceedings of the National Academy of Sciences of the United States of America*, 101(21): 8174–8179.

Granja, A. G., Carrillo-Salinas, F., Pagani, A., Gómez-Cañas, M., Negri, R., Navarrete, C. et al. (2012). A cannabigerol quinone alleviates neuroinflammation in a chronic model of multiple sclerosis. *Journal of Neuroimmune Pharmacology : The Official Journal of the Society on NeuroImmune Pharmacology*, 7(4): 1002–1016.

Grant, I., Gonzalez, R., Carey, C. L., Natarajan, L., and Wolfson, T. (2003). Non-acute (residual) neurocognitive effects of cannabis use: a meta-analytic study. *Journal of the International Neuropsychological Society : JINS*, 9(5): 679–689.

Hallak, J. E. C., Machado-de-Sousa, J. P., Crippa, J. A. S., Sanches, R. F., Trzesniak, C., Chaves, C. et al. (2010). Performance of schizophrenic patients in the Stroop Color Word Test and electrodermal responsiveness after acute administration of cannabidiol (CBD). *Revista Brasileira de Psiquiatria (Sao Paulo, Brazil : 1999)*, 32(1): 56–61.

Hall, W., and Degenhardt, L. (2008). Cannabis use and the risk of developing a psychotic disorder. *World Psychiatry: Official Journal of the World Psychiatric Association (WPA)*, 7(2). https://doi.org/10.1002/j.2051-5545.2008.tb00158.x

Harley, M., Kelleher, I., Clarke, M., Lynch, F., Arseneault, L., Connor, D. et al. (2010). Cannabis use and childhood trauma interact additively to increase the risk of psychotic symptoms in adolescence. *Psychological Medicine*, 40(10): 1627–1634.

Henquet, C., Murray, R., Linszen, D., and van Os, J. (2005). The environment and schizophrenia: the role of cannabis use. *Schizophrenia Bulletin*, 31(3): 608–612.

Hjorthøj, C., Posselt, C. M., and Nordentoft, M. (2021). Development Over Time of the Population-Attributable Risk Fraction for Cannabis Use Disorder in Schizophrenia in Denmark. *JAMA Psychiatry*, 78(9). https://doi.org/10.1001/jamapsychiatry.2021.1471

Howes, O. D., Kambeitz, J., Kim, E., Stahl, D., Slifstein, M., Abi-Dargham, A. et al. (2012). The nature of dopamine dysfunction in schizophrenia and what this means for treatment. *Archives of General Psychiatry*, 69(8): 776–786.

Howes, O. D., and Kapur, S. (2009). The dopamine hypothesis of schizophrenia: version III--the final common pathway. *Schizophrenia Bulletin*, 35(3): 549–562.

Hunault, C. C., Mensinga, T. T., Böcker, K. B. E., Schipper, C. M. A., Kruidenier, M., Leenders, M. E. C. et al. (2009). Cognitive and psychomotor effects in males after smoking a combination of tobacco and cannabis containing up to 69 mg delta-9-tetrahydrocannabinol (THC). *Psychopharmacology*, 204(1): 85–94.

Jager, G., Kahn, R. S., Van Den Brink, W., Van Ree, J. M., and Ramsey, N. F. (2006). Long-term effects of frequent cannabis use on working memory and attention: an fMRI study. *Psychopharmacology*, 185(3): 358–368.

Javitt, D. C., and Zukin, S. R. (1991). Recent advances in the phencyclidine model of schizophrenia. *The American Journal of Psychiatry*, 148(10): 1301–1308.

Johnson, E. C., Colbert, S. M. C., Jeffries, P. W., Tillman, R., Bigdeli, T. B., Karcher, N. R. et al. (2023). Associations Between Cannabis Use, Polygenic Liability for Schizophrenia, and Cannabis-related Experiences in a Sample of Cannabis Users. *Schizophrenia Bulletin*, 49(3): 778–787.

Joyce, E. M., and Roiser, J. P. (2007). Cognitive heterogeneity in schizophrenia. *Current Opinion in Psychiatry*, 20(3): 268.

Kalayasiri, R., Gelernter, J., Farrer, L., Weiss, R., Brady, K., Gueorguieva, R. et al. (2010). Adolescent cannabis use increases risk for cocaine-induced paranoia. *Drug and Alcohol Dependence*, 107(2-3): 196–201.

Kessler, R. C., Berglund, P., Demler, O., Jin, R., Merikangas, K. R., and Walters, E. E. (2005). Lifetime Prevalence and Age-of-Onset Distributions of DSM-IV Disorders in the National Comorbidity Survey Replication. *Archives of General Psychiatry*, 62(6): 593–602.

Koskinen, J., Löhönen, J., Koponen, H., Isohanni, M., and Miettunen, J. (2010). Rate of cannabis use disorders in clinical samples of patients with schizophrenia: a meta-analysis. *Schizophrenia Bulletin*, 36(6): 1115–1130.

Kuepper, R., van Os, J., Lieb, R., Wittchen, H.-U., and Henquet, C. (2011). Do cannabis and urbanicity co-participate in causing psychosis? Evidence from a 10-year follow-up cohort study. *Psychological Medicine*, 41(10): 2121–2129.

Kuepper, R., van Os, J., Lieb, R., Wittchen, H.-U., Höfler, M., and Henquet, C. (2011). Continued cannabis use and risk of incidence and persistence of psychotic symptoms: 10 year follow-up cohort study. *BMJ (Clinical Research Ed.)*, 342: d738.

Laprairie, R. B., Bagher, A. M., Kelly, M. E. M., and Denovan-Wright, E. M. (2015). Cannabidiol is a negative allosteric modulator of the cannabinoid CB1 receptor. *British Journal of Pharmacology*, 172(20): 4790–4805.

Large, M., Sharma, S., Compton, M. T., Slade, T., and Nielssen, O. (2011). Cannabis use and earlier onset of psychosis: a systematic meta-analysis. *Archives of General Psychiatry*, 68(6). https://doi.org/10.1001/archgenpsychiatry.2011.5

Larkin, W., and Read, J. (2008). Childhood trauma and psychosis: evidence, pathways, and implications. *Journal of Postgraduate Medicine*, 54(4): 287–293.

Leweke, F. M., Piomelli, D., Pahlisch, F., Muhl, D., Gerth, C. W., Hoyer, C. et al. (2012). Cannabidiol enhances anandamide signaling and alleviates psychotic symptoms of schizophrenia. *Translational Psychiatry*, 2(3): e94.

Lewis, D. A., Curley, A. A., Glausier, J. R., and Volk, D. W. (2012). Cortical parvalbumin interneurons and cognitive dysfunction in schizophrenia. *Trends in Neurosciences*, 35(1): 57–67.

Lisman, J. E., Coyle, J. T., Green, R. W., Javitt, D. C., Benes, F. M., Heckers, S., and Grace, A. A. (2008). Circuit-based framework for understanding neurotransmitter and risk gene interactions in schizophrenia. *Trends in Neurosciences*, 31(5): 234–242.

Lorenzetti, V., Chye, Y., Silva, P., Solowij, N., and Roberts, C. A. (2019). Does regular cannabis use affect neuroanatomy? An updated systematic review and meta-analysis of structural neuroimaging studies. *European Archives of Psychiatry and Clinical Neuroscience*, 269(1): 59–71.

Mackie, C. J., Wilson, J., Freeman, T. P., Craft, S., Escamilla De La Torre, T., and Lynskey, M. T. (2021). A latent class analysis of cannabis use products in a general population sample of adolescents and their association with paranoia, hallucinations, cognitive disorganisation and grandiosity. *Addictive Behaviors*, 117: 106837.

Marconi, A., Di Forti, M., Lewis, C. M., Murray, R. M., and Vassos, E. (2016). Meta-analysis of the Association Between the Level of Cannabis Use and Risk of Psychosis. *Schizophrenia Bulletin*, 42(5): 1262.

Martínez-Pinilla, E., Varani, K., Reyes-Resina, I., Angelats, E., Vincenzi, F., Ferreiro-Vera, C. et al. (2017). Binding and Signaling Studies Disclose a Potential Allosteric Site for Cannabidiol in Cannabinoid CB Receptors. *Frontiers in Pharmacology*, 8: 744.

Meier, M. H., Caspi, A., Ambler, A., Harrington, H., Houts, R., Keefe, R. S. E. et al. (2012). Persistent cannabis users show neuropsychological decline from childhood to midlife. *Proceedings of the National Academy of Sciences*, 109(40): E2657–E2664.

Moore, T. H. M., Zammit, S., Lingford-Hughes, A., Barnes, T. R. E., Jones, P. B., Burke, M. et al. (2007). Cannabis use and risk of psychotic or affective mental health outcomes: a systematic review. *Lancet (London, England)*, 370(9584): 319–328.

Morgan, C. J. A., Freeman, T. P., Powell, J., and Curran, H. V. (2016). AKT1 genotype moderates the acute psychotomimetic effects of naturalistically smoked cannabis in young cannabis smokers. *Translational Psychiatry*, 6(2): e738.

Mouslech, Z., and Valla, V. (2009). Endocannabinoid system: An overview of its potential in current medical practice. *Neuro Endocrinology Letters*, 30(2): 153–179.

Müller, N. (2014). Immunology of Schizophrenia. *Neuroimmunomodulation*, 21(2-3): 109–116.

Mustonen, A., Niemelä, S., Nordström, T., Murray, G. K., Mäki, P., Jääskeläinen, E., and Miettunen, J. (2018). Adolescent cannabis use, baseline prodromal symptoms and the risk of psychosis. *The British Journal of Psychiatry : The Journal of Mental Science*, 212(4): 227–233.

Myles, N., Newall, H., Nielssen, O., and Large, M. (2012). The association between cannabis use and earlier age at onset of schizophrenia and other psychoses: meta-analysis of possible confounding factors. *Current Pharmaceutical Design*, 18(32): 5055–5069.

Myran, D. T., Pugliese, M., Harrison, L. D., Solmi, M., Anderson, K. K., Fiedorowicz, J. G. et al. (2025). Changes in Incident Schizophrenia Diagnoses Associated With Cannabis Use Disorder After Cannabis Legalization. *JAMA Network Open*, 8(2): e2457868.

Nguyen, T., Li, J.-X., Thomas, B. F., Wiley, J. L., Kenakin, T. P., and Zhang, Y. (2017). Allosteric Modulation: An Alternate Approach Targeting the Cannabinoid CB1 Receptor. *Medicinal Research Reviews*, 37(3): 441–474.

Niesink, R. J. M., and van Laar, M. W. (2013). Does Cannabidiol Protect Against Adverse Psychological Effects of THC? *Frontiers in Psychiatry*, 4: 130.

Nuechterlein, K. H., Green, M. F., Kern, R. S., Baade, L. E., Barch, D. M., Cohen, J. D. et al. (2008). The MATRICS Consensus Cognitive Battery, Part 1: Test Selection, Reliability, and Validity. *American Journal of Psychiatry*. https://doi.org/10.1176/appi.ajp.2007.07010042

Paolicelli, R. C., Bolasco, G., Pagani, F., Maggi, L., Scianni, M., Panzanelli, P. et al. (2011). Synaptic pruning by microglia is necessary for normal brain development. *Science (New York, N.Y.)*, 333(6048): 1456–1458.

Pelayo-Terán, J. M., Suárez-Pinilla, P., Chadi, N., and Crespo-Facorro, B. (2012). Gene-environment interactions underlying the effect of cannabis in first episode psychosis. *Current Pharmaceutical Design*, 18(32): 5024–5035.

Pertwee, R. G. (2006). The pharmacology of cannabinoid receptors and their ligands: an overview. *International Journal of Obesity (2005)*, 30 Suppl 1: S13–S18.

Pertwee, R. G. (2008). The diverse CB1 and CB2 receptor pharmacology of three plant cannabinoids: delta9-tetrahydrocannabinol, cannabidiol and delta9-tetrahydrocannabivarin. *British Journal of Pharmacology*, 153(2): 199–215.

Pourebrahim, S., Ahmad, T., Rottmann, E., Schulze, J., and Scheller, B. (2025). Does Cannabis Use Contribute to Schizophrenia? A Causation Analysis Based on Epidemiological Evidence. *Biomolecules*, 15(3): 368.

Radhakrishnan, R., Wilkinson, S. T., and D'Souza, D. C. (2014). Gone to Pot – A Review of the Association between Cannabis and Psychosis. *Frontiers in Psychiatry*, 5: 72718.

Rapoport, J. L., Giedd, J. N., and Gogtay, N. (2012). Neurodevelopmental model of schizophrenia: update 2012. *Molecular Psychiatry*, 17(12): 1228–1238.

Rathod, S. S., and Agrawal, Y. O. (2024). Phytocannabinoids as Potential Multitargeting Neuroprotectants in Alzheimer's Disease. *Current Drug Research Reviews*, 16(2): 94–110.

Rottanburg, D., Robins, A. H., Ben-Arie, O., Teggin, A., and Elk, R. (1982). Cannabis-associated psychosis with hypomanic features. *Lancet (London, England)*, 2(8312): 1364–1366.

Rubino, T., and Parolaro, D. (2016). The Impact of Exposure to Cannabinoids in Adolescence: Insights From Animal Models. *Biological Psychiatry*, 79(7): 578–585.

Russo, E. B. (2007). History of cannabis and its preparations in saga, science, and sobriquet. *Chemistry and Biodiversity*, 4(8): 1614–1648.

Russo, E. B., Burnett, A., Hall, B., and Parker, K. K. (2005). Agonistic properties of cannabidiol at 5-HT1a receptors. *Neurochemical Research*, 30(8): 1037–1043.

Ryberg, E., Larsson, N., Sjögren, S., Hjorth, S., Hermansson, N.-O., Leonova, J. et al. (2007). The orphan receptor GPR55 is a novel cannabinoid receptor. *British Journal of Pharmacology*, 152(7): 1092–1101.

Schoeler, T., and Bhattacharyya, S. (2013). The effect of cannabis use on memory function: an update. *Substance Abuse and Rehabilitation*, 4: 11–27.

Sekar, A., Bialas, A. R., de Rivera, H., Davis, A., Hammond, T. R., Kamitaki, N. et al. (2016). Schizophrenia risk from complex variation of complement component 4. *Nature*, 530(7589): 177–183.

Semple, D. M., McIntosh, A. M., and Lawrie, S. M. (2005). Cannabis as a risk factor for psychosis: systematic review. *Journal of Psychopharmacology (Oxford, England)*, 19(2): 187–194.

Solowij, N., Stephens, R. S., Roffman, R. A., Babor, T., Kadden, R., Miller, M. et al. (2002). Cognitive functioning of long-term heavy cannabis users seeking treatment. *JAMA*, 287(9): 1123–1131.

Tham, M., Yilmaz, O., Alaverdashvili, M., Kelly, M. E. M., Denovan-Wright, E. M., and Laprairie, R. B. (2019). Allosteric and orthosteric pharmacology of cannabidiol and cannabidiol-dimethylheptyl at the type 1 and type 2 cannabinoid receptors. *British Journal of Pharmacology*, 176(10): 1455–1469.

Thomas, A., Baillie, G. L., Phillips, A. M., Razdan, R. K., Ross, R. A., and Pertwee, R. G. (2007). Cannabidiol displays unexpectedly high potency as an antagonist of CB1 and CB2 receptor agonists *in vitro*. *British Journal of Pharmacology*, 150(5): 613–623.

Thompson, P. M., Vidal, C., Giedd, J. N., Gochman, P., Blumenthal, J., Nicolson, R. et al. (2001). Mapping adolescent brain change reveals dynamic wave of accelerated gray matter loss in very early-onset schizophrenia. *Proceedings of the National Academy of Sciences of the United States of America*, 98(20): 11650–11655.

Touw, M. (1981). The religious and medicinal uses of Cannabis in China, India and Tibet. *Journal of Psychoactive Drugs*, 13(1): 23–34.

Vaessen, T. S. J., de Jong, L., Schäfer, A. T., Damen, T., Uittenboogaard, A., Krolinski, P. et al. (2018). The interaction between cannabis use and the Val158Met polymorphism of the COMT gene in psychosis: A transdiagnostic meta - analysis. *PloS One*, 13(2): e0192658.

van Os, J., Bak, M., Hanssen, M., Bijl, R. V., de Graaf, R., and Verdoux, H. (2002). Cannabis use and psychosis: a longitudinal population-based study. *American Journal of Epidemiology*, 156(4): 319–327.

van Os, J., Krabbendam, L., Myin-Germeys, I., and Delespaul, P. (2005). The schizophrenia envirome. *Current Opinion in Psychiatry*, 18(2): 141–145.

Vinkers, C. H., Van Gastel, W. A., Schubart, C. D., Van Eijk, K. R., Luykx, J. J., Van Winkel, R. et al. (2013). The effect of childhood maltreatment and cannabis use on adult psychotic symptoms is modified by the COMT Val^{158}Met polymorphism. *Schizophrenia Research*, 150(1): 303–311.

Vita, A., De Peri, L., Deste, G., and Sacchetti, E. (2012). Progressive loss of cortical gray matter in schizophrenia: a meta-analysis and meta-regression of longitudinal MRI studies. *Translational Psychiatry*, 2(11): e190.

Volkow, N. D., Baler, R. D., Compton, W. M., and Weiss, S. R. B. (2014). Adverse health effects of marijuana use. *The New England Journal of Medicine*, 370(23): 2219–2227.

Volkow, N. D., Hampson, A. J., and Baler, R. D. (2017). Don't Worry, Be Happy: Endocannabinoids and Cannabis at the Intersection of Stress and Reward. *Annual Review of Pharmacology and Toxicology*, 57: 285–308.

Volkow, N. D., Swanson, J. M., Evins, A. E., DeLisi, L. E., Meier, M. H., Gonzalez, R. et al. (2016). Effects of Cannabis Use on Human Behavior, Including Cognition, Motivation, and Psychosis: A Review. *JAMA Psychiatry*, 73(3): 292–297.

Wainberg, M., Jacobs, G. R., di Forti, M., and Tripathy, S. J. (2021). Cannabis, schizophrenia genetic risk, and psychotic experiences: a cross-sectional study of 109,308 participants from the UK Biobank. *Translational Psychiatry*, 11(1): 211.

Wang, Q., Qin, Z., Xing, X., Zhu, H., and Jia, Z. (2024). Prevalence of Cannabis Use around the World: A Systematic Review and Meta-Analysis, 2000-2024. *China CDC Weekly*, 6(25): 597–604.

Weinberger, D. R. (1987). Implications of normal brain development for the pathogenesis of schizophrenia. *Archives of General Psychiatry*, 44(7): 660–669.

Wilkinson, S. T., Radhakrishnan, R., and D'Souza, D. C. (2014). Impact of Cannabis Use on the Development of Psychotic Disorders. *Current Addiction Reports*, 1(2): 115–128.

World Health Organization. (1992). International classification of diseases (10th ed.). Geneva: World Health Organization.

Zheng, S., Chan, S. K. W., and Lee, J. (2022). Managing treatment resistance in schizophrenia: A joint study in Hong Kong and Singapore. *Frontiers in Psychiatry*, 13. https://doi.org/10.3389/fpsyt.2022.1005373

Zuardi, A. W., Shirakawa, I., Finkelfarb, E., and Karniol, I. G. (1982). Action of cannabidiol on the anxiety and other effects produced by delta 9-THC in normal subjects. *Psychopharmacology*, 76(3): 245–250.

Chapter 14

Cannabis and Pregnancy

Implications for Maternal and Child Health

Bhagyashree Kokate, Swati Bodhankar, Deepali Chaudhary and *Veena S. Belgamwar**

1. Introduction

Marijuana, which comes from the plants *Cannabis sativa* and *C indica*, has more than 100 pharmacologically active ingredients, classified as cannabinoids. THC and CBD are the most well-known and widely researched. THC is accountable for the drug's psychotropic effects, which make it euphoric and intoxicating, whereas CBD is not intoxicating and has drawn interest due to its potential use as a medicine. For thousands of years, cannabis has been used in various cultures for therapeutic, spiritual, and leisure purposes. In modern society, it has become the world's most widely consumed illegal psychoactive drug, second only to alcohol, tobacco, and caffeine in total use. About 219 million individuals, or about 4.3% of the world's population aged 15 to 64, reported cannabis use in the last year, based on the 2023 United Nations Office on Drugs and Crime (UNODC 2023). A complex interaction between socioeconomic factors, legal restrictions, cultural norms, and public health concerns shapes the global cannabis use landscape (Gabarin et al. 2023; Doyle 2025).

Cannabis, illegal in most places for decades, has been radically revalued in the last 20 years. In North America, Europe, and some Latin American and Asian countries, where drug policy reform has resulted in the decriminalization or legalization of cannabis for both medical and recreational purposes, this paradigm shift has been especially pronounced (Fischer et al. 2017; Hall and Lynskey 2020; Mollner 2022). These policy reforms have created new opportunities for medicinal research, economic investment, and social justice reform. They have also created legitimate concerns, however, about the risks to public health, including elevated rates of cannabis use disorder, increasing mental illness such as anxiety and psychosis, impaired cognitive function, and elevated rates of impaired driving (Meier et al. 2012; Volkow et al. 2014; Di Forti et al. 2019).

The rising prevalence of cannabis use among expectant mothers is quite concerning, particularly in areas where legalization has increased accessibility and decreased perceived risks. Most pregnant individuals self-medicate with cannabis for frequent gestational symptoms like nausea, vomiting (*hyperemesis gravidarum*), insomnia, anxiety, and pain. This is encouraged by the absence of regulatory control, deceptive marketing labels, and sparse guidance from healthcare providers.

Department of Pharmaceutical Sciences, Rashtrasant Tukadoji Maharaj Nagpur University, Nagpur, Maharashtra, India.
* Corresponding author: vbelgamwar@gmail.com

DOI: 10.1201/9781003668190-17

Although growing anecdotal experience and observational studies increasingly suggest cannabis use during pregnancy is not a major safety concern, the empirical literature on the topic remains sparse, variable, and replete with methodological difficulties.

Researchers have identified relationships between prenatal cannabis use and several perinatal adverse outcomes, such as low birth weight, preterm delivery, small-for-gestational-age infants, and offspring developmental impairment in cognition, behaviour, and executive function (Micalizzi et al. 2024; Lo et al. 2025; Tadesse et al. 2024). These associations, however, are often confounded by variables like the use of tobacco, alcohol, or other drugs concurrently; variation in cannabis potency and method of use; socioeconomic and psychosocial stressors; and study design and outcome variable variability.

Furthermore, the endocannabinoid system, which plays a crucial role in functions like neurodevelopment, placentation, and immune modulation, may be particularly susceptible to perturbation by exogenous cannabinoids like THC during pregnancy (Mahintamani et al. 2025). These speculative biological mechanisms highlight the possibility of harm but remain inadequately explained. Additionally, metabolic disruptions such as increased risk of childhood obesity and diabetes have been linked to prenatal cannabis exposure (Vanin et al. 2023; Moore 2024).

A lack of uniform clinical guidelines, combined with inconsistent risk communication by clinicians, also complicates clinical decision-making and hinders public understanding. Most clinicians express discomfort or uncertainty in counselling pregnant women regarding the use of cannabis because they receive inadequate training and evidence-based information. As stronger cannabis products become more accessible, the risks to maternal and child health increase in proportion (Antonia Biggs et al. 2025; Krishnan and Yen 2025). In light of these nuances, it has become important to have rigorous longitudinal and multidisciplinary research that investigates the short- and long-term consequences of prenatal cannabis exposure. These studies would aim to control for confounding variables, use objective biomarkers of exposure, and measure outcomes across developmental stages. It is intended to generate solid evidence that can guide regulatory policy, impact public health communications, and inform clinical practice. Finally, an active, evidence-based, and morally sound research agenda is necessary to safeguard maternal and child health in the age of cannabis normalization.

Cannabis use during pregnancy messes up the mother's metabolism, the placenta's function, and the baby's development, which can have harmful effects in the short and long term. New research shows that even early or short-term exposure to cannabis during pregnancy can slow foetal growth, change the way the brain develops, and raise the risk of obesity, diabetes, and heart disease later in life. There is a greater need for future preclinical and clinical studies to look into how different ways of exposing people to cannabinoids and different mixtures of cannabinoid components may work together to harm reproductive health. This literature review's goal is to stress the need for more targeted research, better public health education, and better healthcare support to deal with the use of edible cannabis during pregnancy in this high-risk group.

2. Composition of Cannabis

Cannabis is known to have a very complex chemical profile. Various studies have reported more than 550 different compounds in cannabis. These include > 140 cannabinoids, 120 terpenes, 50 hydrocarbons, 46 phenolic or polyphenolic compounds, 34 sugars, 25 ketones and aldehydes, along with many kinds of organic acids, fatty acids, amino acids, esters, lactones, phytosterols, alkaloids, vitamins, and biogenic amines (Aizpurua-Olaizola et al. 2016; ElSohly and Slad 2006).

Tetrahydrocannabinol (THC) is the primary psychoactive ingredient in cannabis. The well-known psychoactive and physiological effects of cannabis are attributed to a number of additional cannabinoids, including cannabidiol (CBD). Several methods, including smoking, vaping, and consuming cannabis edibles, can release, consume, or inhale these chemicals. Numerous mental and physical side effects, such as euphoria, altered perception of time, increased appetite, difficulty concentrating, short-term memory impairment, and clumsiness, can result from cannabis use or inhalation. Cannabis has emerged with promising potential in medical use for the treatment of numerous conditions, such as chronic pain, nausea, anxiety, and inflammation (Whiting et al. 2015; Berman et al. 2018). In order to alleviate symptoms like anxiety, insomnia, pain, and nausea, cannabis use during pregnancy is now more widely accepted as safe or better than other treatments like prescription drugs (Chang et al. 2019; Jarlenski et al. 2017). Health professionals who treat pregnant patients should have this conversation with them about the available evidence and make sure that they are all in agreement when weighing the risks of cannabis use against alternative treatments. For various reasons, including a lack of expertise in this area, healthcare providers have stated that they might not have this conversation with their pregnant patients (Holland et al. 2016).

The public is increasingly coming to believe that cannabis is safe, even during pregnancy. From 2005 to 2015, pregnant women who reported using cannabis within the previous 30 days were almost three times more likely to believe that frequent use of cannabis is not harmful (Jarlenski et al., 2017; Tadesse et al. 2025). Interestingly, even though the perception that regular cannabis use has no risk was significantly lower among pregnant people who reported no recent cannabis use, it still increased dramatically in the same period (Jarlenski et al. 2017). While it is rare for people to begin using cannabis in pregnancy, more than half of those who report frequent use pre-pregnancy continue use in pregnancy, with about one-third reporting daily use in pregnancy (Satti et al. 2022).

Cannabinoids primarily interact with cannabinoid receptor types 1 and 2 (CB1 and CB2, respectively), but they can also interact with other receptors such as serotonin receptors and vanilloid-type transient receptor potential (TRPV) channels, which result in the physiological effects of cannabis, including psychoactivity or euphoria, motor impairment, analgesia, and immunomodulation (Newmeyer et al. 2017; Herreros et al. 2019; Howlett and Abood 2017). The onset of effects is typically felt within a few minutes when smoked and within about 30–60 minutes when eaten. These effects last for 2–6 hours, depending on the amount used and the cultivar's concentration of THC or CBD. Each cannabis compound, on its own, may have a well-defined physiological effect, but certain combinations of chemicals (as found in plant extracts) can have a synergistic physiological effect or a so-called "entourage effect" (Anand et al. 2021; Russo, 2019). In addition to these hard-to-define entourage effects, the chemical profiles and concentrations of each compound can vary dramatically among cannabis cultivars, even differ depending on the plant age, harvest conditions, storage conditions, and growth conditions (Russo 2011; Zager et al. 2019).

2.1 Major Cannabinoids and Their Potential

2.1.1 Tetrahydrocannabinol (THC)

Cannabis-derived Δ9-tetrahydrocannabivarin (THCV) differs from more widely used cannabinoids like Δ9-tetrahydrocannabinol (THC) due to its distinct characteristics. The absence of psychotropic effects is THCV's primary advantage over THC. According to research on rodents, THCV reduces hunger, promotes fullness, and boosts energy metabolism, which makes it a potentially effective treatment for type 2 diabetes and obesity. Previous research has shown the differences between THCV and THC in terms of energy regulation, glucose metabolism, and glycaemic control. Additionally, THCV's effects on dyslipidemia and glycaemic control in people with type 2 diabetes demonstrated lower fasting plasma glucose concentrations when compared to a placebo group. THC, on the other hand, is indicated in individuals with cachexia; however, THCV's uniquely diverse properties provide neuroprotection, appetite suppression, glycaemic control, and reduced side effects, among other things, making it a potential priority candidate for the development of clinically useful therapies in the future. Hopefully, THCV could offer an optional platform for the treatment of critical illnesses (Abioye et al. 2020; Khalsa et al. 2022).

The cannabis plant contains tetrahydrocannabivarin, which is not psychotropic. THCV has been proposed as a potential treatment for a variety of clinical diseases, including schizophrenia, epilepsy, nausea, obesity, and some skin conditions, due to its many pharmacologic effects, which include anti-psychotic, anti-inflammatory, and immunomodulatory qualities. Diabetes and its complications, diabetic cardiovascular dysfunction, cancer, pain, neurodegeneration, cardiovascular disease, obesity and metabolic syndrome, nephropathy, retinopathy, and neuropathy are among the disorders that THCV may be able to cure due to oxidative stress and inflammation (Mendoza 2025; Abioye et al. 2020).

2.1.2 Cannabidiol (CBD)

Cannabidiol, or CBD, is a component of the *Cannabis sativa* plant that does not have psychotropic activity (Boggs et al. 2018; Figure 1). Its therapeutic potential, with anxiolytic, anti-inflammatory, and antiemetic effects, has led to increased use in the United States (Iffland and Grotenhermen 2017). There is limited data regarding the use of cannabidiol while pregnant, despite the rising use of the drug to treat symptoms like nausea and chronic pain among pregnant women (Dickson et al. 2018). Cannabidiol disrupted trophoblast turnover and placental remodelling, as revealed by an *in vitro* investigation into the drug's action upon trophoblast cells as well as placental activity (Brown et al. 2017). As shown in a study in mice, the drug transfer from the mother's blood to the foetus's blood was quick, and the drug became concentrated in the foetus's liver, brain, and gastrointestinal system.

Cannabinoids connect with the body via the endocannabinoid system, which serves as a critical balancing system in almost all living organisms. The endocannabinoid system is an endogenous system composed of substances, metabolic enzymes, and cannabinoid receptors CB1 and CB2, which aid the body in achieving homeostasis by modulating pain and inflammation. Phyto-cannabinoids are the plant counter parts of human endocannabinoids, for instance, 2-arachidonoylglycerol and anandamide, and mimic these two CB1 and CB2 receptors.

They have been shown to have antibacterial activity, especially against Staphylococcus species, which are often involved in skin infections, and *Cutibacterium acnes* (*C. acnes*), a causative bacterium of acne. Cannabinoids also have antioxidant activity, which can help minimize free-radical-induced skin damage and photoaging. The effects of cannabinoids on the skin's immune system may result from modulation of cytokine secretion and the suppression of immune cell functions. In autoimmune dermatological disorders such as psoriasis or atopic dermatitis, the immune system's suppression, often associated with these conditions, may paradoxically reduce inflammation and symptom severity. The action mechanisms of cannabinoids in skin diseases are multifaceted and warrant further investigation. Still, preliminary findings indicate that cannabinoids have therapeutic potential for skin disease, with effective and safe outcomes (Kwiecień and Kowalczuk 2023).

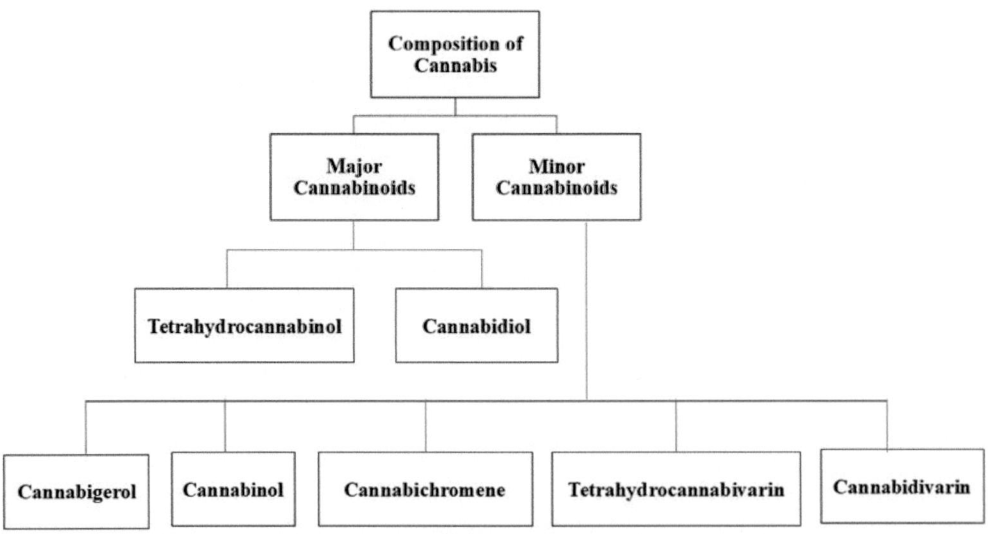

Figure 1: Composition of cannabis showing all major and minor cannabinoids.

2.2 Minor Cannabinoids and Their Potential

2.1.1 Cannabigerol (CBG)

Like other cannabinoids, CBG has demonstrated potential neuroprotective effects, mainly as a result of its interactions with the ECS. The ECS is essential for controlling a number of physiological functions, including those of the nervous system, as was previously mentioned. Alzheimer's disease, Parkinson's disease, multiple sclerosis (MS), and other neurodegenerative diseases are linked to neuroinflammation, which CBG may help lower. The possible neuroprotective effects of CBG were investigated in two mouse models of Huntington's disease in an initial study. In this study, CBG therapy partially restored gene expression associated with Huntington's disease in mice and enhanced motor function in mice with the disease. A major contributing factor to neurodegenerative diseases is oxidative stress, and antioxidants can shield neurons from the damage caused by free radicals. In 2020, a study investigated the neuroprotective properties of CBG, as well as CBD, in rat hypothalamus cells (Hypo-E22 cells) and tissue (Li et al. 2024; Jastrząb et al. 2022).

2.1.2 Cannabinol (CBN)

Similar to other cannabinoids, CBG has demonstrated possible neuroprotective qualities, mostly as a result of its interactions with the ECS. Multiple sclerosis (MS), Parkinson's disease, Alzheimer's disease, and other neurodegenerative diseases are linked to neuroinflammation, which CBG may help lower. In two mouse models of Huntington's disease, a preliminary investigation examined the possible neuroprotective effects of CBG. In this study, CBG treatment partially normalized gene expression associated with Huntington's disease in mice and enhanced motor function in mice with the disease. Neurodegenerative diseases are mainly caused by oxidative stress, and antioxidants can help shield neurons from the damage caused by free radicals. A 2020 study examined the neuroprotective effects of CBD and CBG in rat hypothalamic cells (Hypo-E22 cells) and tissue (Singh et al. 2023).

2.1.3 Cannabichromene (CBC)

Arguments have been made that cannabichromene is useful for various treatments, including anti-inflammatory, anticonvulsant, antimicrobial, and antinociceptive functions. The attention on medical attributes of cannabinoids has mainly been focused on Δ9-tetrahydrocannabinol and cannabidiol. The above studies on CBC suggest that this phytocannabinoid has potential medicinal value that needs further study. With increased availability of hemp, CBC products are sold over-the-counter and frequently used, with little to no investigation of their safety or efficacy (Turner et al. 1981).

2.1.4 Tetrahydrocannabivarin (THCV)

A lesser-known cannabinoid that comes from Cannabis sativa, tetrahydrocannabivarin (THCV), has become a promising new therapeutic option (Wargent et al. 2013). Cannabis-derived Δ9-tetrahydrocannabivarin (THCV) differs from more widely used cannabinoids like Δ9-tetrahydrocannabinol (THC) due to its distinct characteristics. The absence of psychotropic effects is THCV's primary advantage over THC. According to research on rodents, THCV reduces hunger, promotes fullness, and boosts energy metabolism, which makes it a potentially effective treatment for type 2 diabetes and obesity. Previous research has shown the differences between THCV and THC in terms of energy regulation, glucose metabolism, and glycaemic control. Additionally, THCV's effects on dyslipidemia and glycaemic control in people with type 2 diabetes demonstrated lower fasting plasma glucose concentrations when compared to a placebo group. THC, on the other hand, is indicated in individuals with cachexia; however, THCV's uniquely diverse properties provide neuroprotection, appetite suppression, glycaemic control, and reduced side effects, among other things, making it a potential priority candidate for the development of clinically useful therapies in the future. Hopefully, THCV could offer an optional platform for the treatment of critical illnesses (Abioye et al. 2020; Khalsa et al. 2022).

The cannabis plant contains tetrahydrocannabivarin, which is not psychotropic. THCV has been proposed as a potential treatment for a variety of clinical diseases, including schizophrenia, epilepsy, nausea, obesity, and some skin conditions, due to its many pharmacologic effects, which include anti-psychotic, anti-inflammatory, and immunomodulatory qualities. Diabetes and its complications, diabetic cardiovascular dysfunction, cancer, pain, neurodegeneration, cardiovascular disease, obesity and metabolic syndrome, nephropathy, retinopathy, and neuropathy are among the disorders that THCV may be able to cure due to oxidative stress and inflammation (Mendoza 2025; Abioye et al. 2020).

2.2.5 Cannabidivarin (CBDV)

Cannabidivarin (CBDV) is a minor cannabinoid in cannabis that's structurally similar to cannabidiol (CBD), but not the same. Like many cannabinoids, CBDV has possible health benefits. Researchers first discovered CBDV in cannabis in 1969 (Tomagra et al. 2025). It is believed that CBDV shares many of the same benefits as CBD because the two compounds are so structurally similar. CBDV is almost molecularly identical to CBD, except it has fewer carbons on its side chain. In 2019, researchers found that CBDV may treat symptoms of ulcerative colitis. The study found that CBDV's anti-inflammatory effects lower intestinal inflammation while balancing gut microbiota. It may also reduce nausea, according to animal studies. Cannabidivarin (CBDV) is a safe, non-psychoactive phytocannabinoid isolated from *Cannabis sativa*. Although CBDV is usually a minor constituent of naturally occurring cannabinoids found in cannabis, CBDV has been attracting great interest owing to its potential benefits to clinical conditions that cannabidiol (CBD) cannot effectively treat. Owing to its lipophilicity and blood-brain barrier (BBB) permeability, CBDV has attracted significant attention for its potential to modulate the course of neurological diseases. Moreover, CBDV enhanced morphine-induced analgesia by specifically inhibiting chronic morphine-induced glial activation and pro-inflammatory factor expression in the nucleus accumbens (Wang et al. 2022; Hurley et al. 2022).

3. Cannabis Use in Pregnancy and Its Implications for Foetal and Neonatal Development

One of the most prevalent pregnancy symptoms, especially during the first trimester, is nausea. More and more pregnant women are using cannabis to ease their discomfort (Baja and Domingues 2024). Cannabis use has changed dramatically over the past few decades, going from being primarily illegal to becoming more widely accepted and legal.

One of the many cannabinoids that readily cross the placenta and enter the foetal bloodstream is tetrahydrocannabinol. Cannabis exposure during pregnancy can interfere with the foetal endogenous cannabinoid signaling system, which has several roles in embryo development. Disruption of endocannabinoid signaling has been shown to impact foetal neurodevelopment and cause abnormalities in neural wiring in both humans and animals. Previous studies have shown that children of cannabis users during pregnancy were less focused and attentive than children of non-users. It is necessary to conduct larger studies that can adequately account for confounding in cannabis-outcome correlations. Children exposed to cannabis during pregnancy had a 50% increased risk of being diagnosed with autism during the trial; these associations persisted even after controlling for confounders.

Additionally, children exposed to cannabis during pregnancy appeared to be slightly more likely to develop learning difficulties, attention-deficit hyperactivity disorder, and intellectual disabilities than children who were not exposed. However, after matching and covariate adjustment, these correlations shrank in size (increasing by 11–22%) and failed to reach statistical significance at conventional levels. The primary association between maternal cannabis use and autism spectrum disorder (ASD) persisted in sensitivity analysis by other substance use, income, and preterm birth. The development of the foetal central nervous system may be impacted by drug exposure during pregnancy. Animal research indicates that prenatal harm to the growing central nervous system continues to affect foetal, neonatal, infant, and childhood development. Neuroimaging studies have linked cannabis exposure during pregnancy to changes in the brain that are specific to certain regions and genes. The foetal brain develops during pregnancy, especially during the first trimester. Prenatal injuries are now associated with neurodevelopmental issues and central nervous system abnormalities. The foetal endocannabinoid type 1 receptor, the main mechanism through which cannabis acts on the brain, is expressed at the human equivalent of 5–6 weeks of gestation, according to research conducted on animals. Pregnancy-related cannabis use may have complex relationships with potential neurological effects on the foetus that may be mediated or confused. Prematurity, the foetal and postnatal environments, the kind and amount of substances a person was exposed to, their genetic profile, and environmental factors could all be factors. Cannabis has both therapeutic and recreational uses. Further research is needed to determine the effects of legalizing cannabis in many jurisdictions, as well as the timing and quantity of cannabis use in relation to pregnancy and childhood health outcomes. To further remove any potential residual confounding bias in this field, new analytical methods are required (Corsi et al. 2020). But even with its increasing acceptance, medical professionals and expectant mothers continue to have serious concerns about the safety of cannabis use during pregnancy.

4. Pharmacokinetics of Cannabis in Pregnancy

It is reasonable to speculate that exposure to THC during pregnancy may result in long-term alterations in neuronal development. The possibility that THC exposure during pregnancy could cause long-term changes in neuronal development is plausible. However, understanding the potential effects of cannabis use during pregnancy requires knowledge of the duration, total amount, and degree of THC exposure to the foetus and foetal brain after maternal cannabis use. While the pharmacokinetics (PK) of THC and its metabolites in adult humans have been studied following intravenous (IV), oral, and inhalation administration, little is known about how cannabis PK varies during pregnancy, as well as the transfer of THC from mother to foetus and foetal PK. Moreover, the overall foetal toxicity may be affected by the method of cannabis ingestion (oral, inhalation, and different smoking techniques) (Grant et al. 2018).

The primary psychoactive component of cannabis is (-)-Δ-tetrahydrocannabinol (THC), and there is proof that THC and its metabolites can easily cross the placenta. Human THC is primarily broken down into the active form 11-hydroxy-THC (11-OH-THC) and the inactive form 11-nor-9-carboxy-THC (THC-COOH) by the cytochrome P450 (CYP) enzyme cytochrome P450. Despite our increasing knowledge of cannabinoid metabolism by cytochrome P450 enzymes, little is known about the roles of transporters in cannabis disposition, including exposure of the mother and foetus during pregnancy (Chen et al. 2021). The area under the concentration-time curve (AUC) of THC in foetal plasma is roughly 30% of the maternal plasma AUC of THC, according to a previous study that used a catheterized pregnant macaque model.

4.1 Mechanisms of Potential Harm

The highest prevalence was observed among women aged 15 to 24 years, whose use increased from 4.9% in 2012 to 6.5% in 2017. The Screening for Pregnancy Endpoints (SCOPE) study, which includes nulliparous women from Australia, New Zealand, Ireland, and the UK who gave birth to a singleton between 2004 and 2011, found that approximately 4% of pregnant women self-reported using cannabis. These studies show that cannabis use during pregnancy has generally increased in developed countries. Furthermore, since most studies only use self-reports, the actual prevalence of cannabis use among expectant mothers may be underreported. Furthermore, even though there is evidence to support the physiological benefits of cannabis-derived products during pregnancy, particularly in the treatment of chronic pain, spasticity, sleep disorders, nausea, and vomiting, very little research has been done on these benefits or the potential effects of non-psychoactive components when consumed alone. The mechanism of action of Δ 9-THC led to the discovery of the endocannabinoid system (ECS), which is composed of endocannabinoids, their metabolic enzymes, and cannabinoid receptors. In addition to its role in modulating the neurological, immunological, and endocrine systems, there is mounting evidence that the ECS plays a role in reproductive processes such as fertilization, implantation, embryonic development, and placental expansion. Therefore, exposure to insults that can interfere with ECS signaling may lead to unfavorable reproductive and pregnancy outcomes. Reports on the consequences of cannabis use in pregnant women are often conflicting. Although many studies have connected prenatal cannabis use to stillbirth, preterm birth, small for gestational age, low birth weight, and increased admission to neonatal critical care units, some researchers have found no connection between it and poor pregnancy or neonatal outcomes (Martínez-Peña et al. 2021).

The primary psychoactive ingredient in marijuana and other cannabis-based preparations, Δ9-tetrahydrocannabinol (THC), can cross the placental barrier and expose the foetus. Because the foetus's brain is particularly susceptible to the mother's drug use, prenatal cannabis exposure (PCE) has been demonstrated to change the child's behaviour and cognitive abilities. The cannabinoid receptor type 1 (CB1R) is expressed and functionally associated with signaling pathways early in the embryonic brain's development. Given that CB1R is crucial for CNS development, affecting synaptogenesis, neuronal cell migration, and proliferation, as well as functional synaptic architecture and signal transduction, persistent cognitive deficits after PCE are not surprising. Compared to other drugs of abuse, less is known about the mechanisms underlying the cognitive deficits brought on by PCE, despite recent studies demonstrating the long-term effects of prenatal and perinatal cannabis exposure (Pinky et al. 2023).

4.2 Foetal and Neonatal Development: Observed Implications

About half of pregnant women who use cannabis continue to use it during pregnancy, particularly during the first trimester's organogenesis, when the foetus is at its most vulnerable. The rapid passage of delta-9-tetrahydrocannabinol, the primary active component in cannabis, crosses the placenta, raising concerns about potential harm to the foetus and the unborn child. The limited information currently available suggests that cannabis use during pregnancy may be associated with poor foetal neurodevelopment, stillbirth, and intrauterine growth restriction. A prior meta-analysis found that when prenatal tobacco use was included, significant associations between prenatal cannabis use and higher rates of low birthweight (LBW) and preterm delivery disappeared. In actuality, cannabis potency has increased recently, and usage habits have changed as well (Lo et al. 2024; Figure 2).

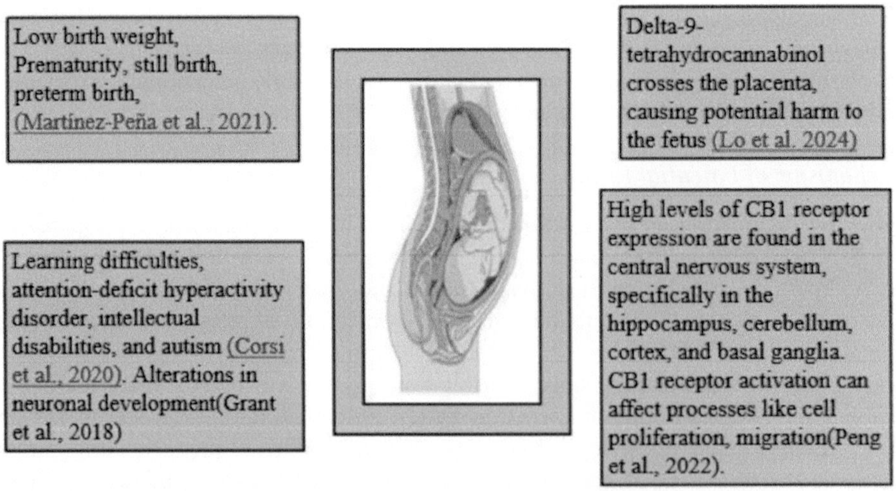

Figure 2: Effects of cannabis use during pregnancy on foetal development.

4.3 Birth Growth and Outcomes

Numerous studies and meta-analyses have found an independent association between cannabis use during pregnancy and an increased risk of PTB, SGA, and perinatal death. The dosage, frequency, timing, and potency of cannabis use should be the focus of future research in this area (Lo et al. 2024).

4.4 Neurodevelopmental, Behavioural and Mental Health Outcomes

The main cause for worry is the possible effects of cannabis use on foetal neurodevelopment (Figure 3). Research has repeatedly demonstrated links between cannabis use by mothers and minor but noteworthy deficiencies in children's executive functioning, attention, impulse control, and memory. We need to improve our scientific knowledge and train medical professionals in this field (Roncero et al. 2020). Out of 250 children, 80 (32%) were exposed to cannabis, per research by Keim et al. (2024). Pregnant women who reported using alcohol, tobacco, or other drugs ranged from 22% to 39%. Most families were below the poverty line. Of the children, 155 were Black/ African American and non-Hispanic (62%), 34 were multiracial and non-Hispanic (14%), 50 were White and non-Hispanic (20%), and 11 were Hispanic (4%). Children exposed to cannabis had age-corrected standard scores for attention and inhibitory control (National Institutes of Health Toolbox) that were roughly 0.4 SDs lower than those who were not ($\beta = -6.1$ points; 95% CI, −10.8 to −1.4) after controlling for confounders and propensity score weighting. Children who were exposed also displayed worse task-organizational skills and increased hostility. We need to improve our scientific knowledge and train medical professionals in this field (Roncero et al. 2020).

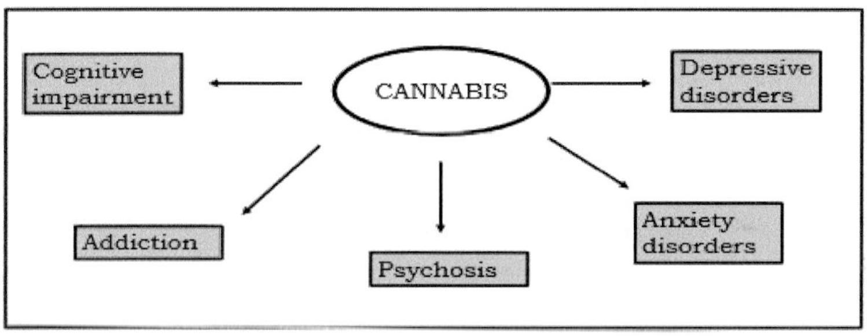

Figure 3: Effect of cannabis on mental health.

5. Challenges in Research and Clinical Practice

Self-reporting Bias: Much of the data relies on maternal self-reporting of cannabis use, which can be subject to recall bias and social desirability bias (Sainz et al. 2025).

Confounding Factors: It is hard to control for the myriad of confounding variables that can influence pregnancy outcomes, including the use of other substances (tobacco and alcohol), socioeconomic status, nutrition, and stress levels (Sainz et al. 2025).

Variability in Cannabis Products: Because the potency and content of cannabis products vary widely, it is difficult to generalize results. The evaluation of dosage and exposure is made more difficult by the growing availability of edible cannabis products, oils, and concentrates (Wohrer et al. 2024).

Ethical Considerations: Randomized controlled trials on pregnant individuals cannot be conducted because it is ethically prohibited. Therefore, research is largely observational, limiting causal inferences (Wohrer et al. 2024).

Lack of Clear Guidelines: Pregnant patients and healthcare professionals are left in the dark by the absence of clear, evidence-based guidelines regarding cannabis use during pregnancy from major medical organizations. Although many have cautioned, it remains difficult to obtain definitive medical advice (Wohrer et al. 2024).

6. Cannabis Use in Pregnancy: Implications for Child Health and Neurodevelopment

In recent decades, there has been a change in the legality and acceptance of cannabis use in society, especially in its different forms like marijuana. Pregnancy-related cannabis exposure is associated with an increased risk of specific adverse neuropsychiatric effects in the developing foetus. Poor executive function, attention problems, thought-related problems, social problems, attentional problems, violence, psychosis proneness, psychotic-like experiences, and ASD are some of these effects (Andrade et al. 2025).

Unfortunately, the use of this substance by women of reproductive age, particularly during pregnancy, has evolved along with this environment. Cannabis is frequently thought of as a harmless chemical when contrasted with other illegal drugs or even some prescription drugs. However, the scientific understanding of cannabis's effects on a developing foetus and child is complicated, so its potential effects on health and neurodevelopment should be carefully considered. With the help of scientific literature, this chapter will examine the current understanding of cannabis use during pregnancy, its physiological mechanisms of action, and its known and suspected effects on foetal development, infant health, and long-term neurodevelopmental outcomes. Several studies have demonstrated that cannabis exposure during pregnancy has a range of often contradictory effects on the foetus's health. The primary psychoactive component of cannabis, delta-9-tetrahydrocannabinol (THC), readily crosses the placenta and exposes the developing foetus to its effects. There are many cannabinoid receptors (CB1 and CB2) in the foetal brain and throughout the body. These receptors are critical for immunological response, synaptic plasticity, and neurodevelopment, according to Costa et al. (2020) and Song et al. (2020). Because THC can bind to these receptors, it may interfere with these complex processes if it is present during important foetal developmental stages. Since other cannabinoids interact with the endocannabinoid system even though they are not psychoactive, research on their effects on development is still ongoing. While other factors, such as maternal nutrition, socioeconomic status, and polysubstance use, often complicate these correlations, some research suggests that maternal cannabis use may be linked to poorer birth outcomes, such as stillbirth, preterm birth, and lower birth weight. A meta-analysis, for instance, suggested a higher risk of low birth weight but cautioned that confounding variables were probably important. Neonatal abstinence syndrome (NAS), a condition marked by withdrawal symptoms, appears to be less common and less severe in children born to pregnant women who used cannabis than in children exposed to opioids (Andrade et al. 2025).

Given the potential for increased use among pregnant women and the fact that cannabis is being thoroughly studied as a novel treatment for a number of illnesses, such as cancer, multiple sclerosis, and epilepsy, significant efforts must be made immediately to evaluate the potential effects of exposure on the foetus. For instance, oromucosal spray (Sativex) has been approved by the European Union for the treatment of spasticity associated with multiple sclerosis. Several problems hamper research on cannabis use during pregnancy. First, underreporting and social shame may cause self-reported cannabis use to be erroneous. Second, it may be challenging to pinpoint the precise effects of cannabis because many pregnant women who use it also use other drugs, like alcohol and tobacco. Thirdly, THC content in modern products has risen dramatically, and cannabis consumption patterns and potencies have changed over time (Grant et al. 2018).

6.1 Methodological Hurdles in Prenatal Cannabis Research

Despite significant advancements, there are still many obstacles to fully understanding the effects of cannabis use during pregnancy in both clinical and experimental settings. The THC concentrations used in *in vitro* and animal studies differ significantly. THC is frequently given in mouse experiments at doses ranging from 2 to 10 mg/kg, resulting in plasma concentrations that are comparable to those attained through cannabis smoking. Considering the growing potency of commercially available cannabis products, these amounts are especially important. The THC content of the majority of commercially available products was less than 2% at the beginning of the 20th century. Nevertheless, these products have grown in popularity recently and now frequently have THC concentrations higher than 20–30%. This notable increase in potency prompts worries that the studies' conclusions might understate the possible dangers of contemporary cannabis products (Krishnan and Yen 2025).

Future research should prioritize large-scale prospective longitudinal cohort studies that closely monitor expecting moms from conception to infancy. To thoroughly account for a wide range of confounders, including lifestyle choices, socioeconomic characteristics, and co-exposures, these studies require advanced statistical modelling tools. To accurately measure substance use, this will require the use of comprehensive questionnaires, linking medical data, and collecting biological samples (such as urine, hair, and saliva) at different intervals. For instance, a hypothetical large-scale project known as the Cannabis and Pregnancy Study (CaPS) might recruit expectant mothers early in pregnancy, collect detailed information on all facets of substance use and lifestyle, and track the children into early adolescence to assess behavioural patterns and developmental outcomes (Gao et al. 2025).

6.2 Biomarkers of Exposure and Effect

The current methods of measuring cannabis exposure are susceptible to recollection bias and underreporting. Future research should focus on developing and validating more objective biomarkers of cannabis exposure and its metabolites. Measuring active metabolites of THC (like 11-hydroxy-THC and THC-OOH) in maternal blood, urine, meconium, and neonatal hair can provide a more accurate and temporally defined picture of exposure. The underlying causes of harm may also be revealed by research on biomarkers of developmental damage downstream of cannabis exposure, such as epigenetic changes or levels of particular protein expression in foetal tissues or newborn samples. The creation and validation of reliable hair cannabis analysis is necessary to comprehend dosage and usage duration (Chaput et al. 2024).

6.3 Impact of Different Cannabinoids and Product Types

THC and CBD are the most common of the more than 100 cannabinoids found in the cannabis plant. However, the neurodevelopmental effects of CBD, which is generally considered non-intoxicating, may differ significantly from those of THC. Furthermore, the increasing availability of diverse cannabis products, including edibles, tinctures, concentrates, and vaporized forms, each with varying cannabinoid profiles and potential delivery systems, complicates generalization. Future research must differentiate the effects of THC, CBD, and their ratios within these diverse product types. Studies employing controlled administration of specific cannabinoid formulations in animal models, followed by carefully designed human studies comparing exposure to specific product types, are essential. For instance, research investigating the impact of high-CBD, low-THC formulations on maternal anxiety and subsequent foetal development, compared to high-THC products, is warranted (Simei et al. 2024).

7. Investigating Mechanisms of Action and Developmental Pathways

Determining particular risks and vulnerabilities requires an understanding of how cannabis compounds interact with the growing foetal brain and body. Foetal development is closely linked to the endocannabinoid system (ECS), a sophisticated signalling network involved in neurodevelopment, mood regulation, and appetite. Exogenous cannabinoids can interact with this system, potentially disrupting critical developmental processes (Martínez-Peña et al. 2021).

7.1 Preclinical In Vitro and In Vivo Models

Robust preclinical research remains crucial for elucidating the biological mechanisms of prenatal cannabis exposure. Studies utilizing cell cultures (e.g., neural progenitor cells, placental cells) exposed to specific cannabinoids at physiologically relevant concentrations can provide insights into cellular toxicity, signal transduction pathways, and gene expression changes. Animal models, particularly rodents, enable control for genetic background and environmental factors, allowing for the investigation of dose-dependent effects on neurodevelopment, behaviour, and reproductive outcomes across generations. Research by Krishnan and Yen (2025) highlights the potential of animal models to explore the impact of prenatal cannabis on ECS development.

7.2 Neurodevelopmental Trajectories and Long-Term Outcomes

The most significant concern surrounding prenatal cannabis exposure relates to potential long-term neurodevelopmental and behavioural consequences in offspring. Future research must move beyond immediate birth outcomes to investigate the impact on cognitive function (e.g., memory, attention, and executive function), emotional regulation, social behaviours, and the risk of specific psychiatric disorders (e.g., ADHD, anxiety, depression, and psychosis) in childhood and adolescence. Longitudinal studies will be critical for tracking these developmental trajectories. For instance, studies examining the impact on executive function development, as explored by Gunn et al. (2021), are essential for understanding potential long-term cognitive deficits.

7.3 Placental Function and Foetal Growth

The placenta plays a critical role in nutrient and oxygen transfer to the foetus. Cannabis compounds can cross the placental barrier, and their effects on placental vascularization, nutrient transport, and hormonal signalling need further investigation. Research exploring alterations in placental gene expression, protein synthesis, and microvascular function following maternal cannabis exposure could reveal mechanisms underlying potential issues like intrauterine growth restriction (IUGR) or preterm birth. Studies investigating the impact of cannabinoids on placental gene expression are crucial for this understanding (Brett et al. 2014).

8. Addressing Clinical Questions and Guiding Public Health Recommendations

As cannabis use in pregnancy continues, there is an urgent need for clinical guidance and evidence-based recommendations for healthcare providers and expectant parents.

8.1 Clinical Trials and Intervention Studies

To conclusively establish causality and dose-response relationships, carefully planned, placebo-controlled clinical trials are required, despite the ethical challenges they present. These studies may concentrate on particular demographics or results, like how cannabis (more especially, THC vs. CBD) affects pregnant women's anxiety or nausea (Panday et al. 2022). Additionally, it could be highly beneficial to investigate possible ways to lessen any negative effects of cannabis exposure during pregnancy, such as behavioural therapies or nutritional supplements.

8.2 Developing Evidence-Based Clinical Guidelines

There is currently uncertainty regarding the safe use of cannabis during pregnancy, which makes the creation of evidence-based treatment guidelines necessary. This calls for combining the available data, recognizing its shortcomings, and offering precise, helpful advice to medical professionals regarding the diagnosis, counselling, and care of pregnant cannabis users (Towobola et al. 2023).

8.3 Public Health Messaging and Education

Accurate and detailed public health messages are essential, so that parents-to-be are informed about the possible dangers and unknowns related to cannabis use during pregnancy. This calls for honest communication of scientific facts, steering clear of both panic and oversimplification. The educational campaigns are to stress the point of cannabis abstinence during pregnancy and lactation; however, they are also to provide the non-confrontational side as well as the means of assistance for those who find it difficult to give up (Gerede et al. 2024).

9. Future Research Directions in Cannabis Use During Pregnancy

The legal and social landscape surrounding cannabis has undergone a dramatic transformation in recent decades, with widespread decriminalization and legalization leading to increased accessibility and, consequently, a rise in reported cannabis use across various demographics, including pregnant individuals. This shift, however, has outpaced our scientific understanding of the potential impacts of cannabis and its compounds, particularly cannabidiol (CBD) and delta-9-tetrahydrocannabinol (THC), on foetal development and long-term child health. While anecdotal evidence and observational studies suggest potential risks, definitive conclusions remain elusive due to a confluence of methodological challenges, ethical considerations, and the complex nature of cannabis products themselves. Therefore, future research endeavours must adopt a rigorous, multidisciplinary, and ethically sound approach to illuminate this critical area of public health (Farrelly et al. 2023).

To better understand the effects of prenatal cannabis exposure, integrative research approaches that link biological pathways with clinical outcomes are required. The expanding and shifting patterns in cannabis use must be considered in future studies.

Future research should aim to comprehensively document maternal cannabis exposure by detailing its duration, frequency, and intensity. Incorporating objective biomarkers—such as THC and its metabolites in maternal blood, urine, cord blood, and breast milk—will enhance the accuracy and reliability of exposure assessment. Determining how PCE modifies metabolic, cardiovascular, and neurodevelopmental pathways over the course of a person's life requires research that combines imaging, epigenetic, and immunologic profiling with clinical data. A comprehensive understanding of other effects of early cannabis exposure on long-term health and disease risk will be made possible by longitudinal birth cohorts that incorporate neuroimaging, cognitive tests, cardiometabolic phenotyping, and other indicators. Furthermore, epigenetic analysis may identify susceptibility biomarkers and guide personalized risk assessment, given the growing evidence of sex-specific vulnerabilities and the wide range of individual responses to PCE. Lastly, specific methods to enhance anticipatory counselling are still needed to integrate research findings into clinical practice. (Krishnan and Yen 2025).

9.1 Ethical Considerations

Ethical considerations are paramount in all research involving pregnant individuals and their offspring (Simei et al. 2024).

9.1.1 Informed Consent and Vulnerable Populations

Rigorous informed consent processes that clearly articulate the potential risks and the exploratory nature of research are essential. Special attention must be paid to ensuring that pregnant individuals from vulnerable populations are not disproportionately burdened by research participation and that their autonomy is respected (Simei et al. 2024).

9.1.2 Minimizing Risk and Maximizing Benefit

Research designs must prioritize the safety and well-being of both the pregnant individual and the foetus. This may involve focusing on observational studies, using less invasive data-collection methods, and ensuring immediate clinical follow-up for participants (Arellano et al. 2023).

9.1.3 Interdisciplinary Collaboration

Addressing the complexities of prenatal cannabis exposure demands a collaborative approach involving obstetricians, paediatricians, neonatologists, pharmacologists, toxicologists, neuroscientists, geneticists, statisticians, and public health experts. Such collaboration will foster a holistic understanding and lead to more comprehensive and impactful research (Arellano et al. 2023).

10. Growing Legalization and Perceived Safety of Cannabis

Cannabis and cannabinoid-infused products are gaining general acceptance as mainstream consumer products and traditional medical drugs. Many states have established their own regimes of laws to control the manufacturing, processing, safety testing, and sale of a vast range of cannabis-based products, but these products remain scheduled as Schedule I drugs, the most restrictive federal drug classification in the United States, because of the disparity between state and federal law, federal agencies have limited regulatory control over the cannabis industry and its consumer protection. By way of example, federal regulations against heavy metals or the use of pesticides cannot be applied to or enforced against a Schedule I drug, federally illegal by definition. Therefore, the future of the United States' legalization of cannabis seems to have great potential as well as great risk (Bahji and Stephenson 2019). Proponents of legalization have emphasized the potential to eradicate the marijuana black market, improve quality and safety control, increase tax revenues, improve the availability of medical cannabis, and lower gang-related drug violence. As legalization regimes are established in multiple countries, public health professionals are increasingly synthesizing decades of knowledge from other policy areas to inform effective cannabis policy (Chiu et al. 2022). Conversely, opponents of legalization have stressed concerns about cannabis's addictive potential, second-hand cannabis exposure, potential exacerbation of underlying and established mental illnesses, as well as alterations in perception and attitudes towards cannabis, particularly those that affect safety and driving. Cannabis is used to treat a wide range of symptoms and medical ailments; however, because of limitations in technique, sample size, and research time, there is insufficient scientific evidence to support its claimed therapeutic benefit in some conditions and its safety for long-term usage. Personal beliefs and cannabis-related experiences would significantly influence individual preferences about the legalization of cannabis. Over time, support for legalizing cannabis has grown in the United States. Over the past 50 years, there has been a significant shift in the legal regulation of cannabis use in the US for both medical and non-medical purposes (Farrelly et al. 2023). The federal government of the United States enacted criminal laws that forbade the use of cannabis in any form in 1970.

Although cannabis was illegal on a federal level, Oregon was the first state to solely impose a fine for possession of the drug in 1973. Several other states followed suit, but over the following 20 years, US state and federal cannabis laws largely remained the same. Because cannabis policy is changing quickly and support for legalizing marijuana is growing, it is critical to understand how the public views cannabis and the harms it poses. Although the federal Controlled Substances Act prohibits marijuana use in the United States and the Drug Enforcement Agency lists it as a Schedule I substance, some states have enacted laws allowing its sale and possession for both medical and recreational use. As of September 2020, medical marijuana is allowed in 33 states and the District of Columbia (Murray and Di Forti 2016). As more states and municipalities enact laws allowing access to marijuana, it is critical to comprehend how the general population views the drug and the risks it poses. The way that the general public views substance use can influence what is viewed as a problem and the guidance that is given to those who are struggling. Public attitudes can also affect patterns of substance use (Blest-Hopley et al. 2020)

Public opinions may also have an impact on marijuana consumption patterns. Concerns regarding legalization have been raised about marijuana's growing potency. The primary psychoactive component of marijuana, Δ9-tetrahydrocannabinol (THC), has typically been the centre of discussions about potency. Cannabis legalization's effect on road safety is a significant public issue (Resko et al. 2020), and it may be a determining factor in people's voting decisions. For instance, Looby et al. (2007) discovered that if accurate and trustworthy roadside sobriety tests were available, adults were more likely to change their minds and support legalization. The precise effect of legalizing marijuana on traffic safety is yet unknown, despite worries. Due to state-level differences in traffic fatality reporting and the difficulties of connecting detected marijuana use with intoxication, it is difficult to determine the causal impact of legalization on road safety (Chen and French 2023). Because of the way THC is metabolized, roadside testing for impairment while under the influence of marijuana is more difficult than it is for alcohol; evidence of marijuana usage does not always imply current impairment (González-Sala et al. 2023). There is disagreement over what constitutes impairment, even though new forensic techniques are being developed to detect recent marijuana use (Stanton et al. 2022). Legalization for both medical and recreational purposes has sparked worries about how marijuana use may affect workplace safety and performance. While there is a dearth of research on marijuana use and employment outcomes, some data suggest that drug use is linked to lower levels of work dedication and increased employee turnover. However, there is conflicting research regarding marijuana's potential impact on worker safety. Compared with random drug testing, one study revealed no changes in the number of positive tests performed after an accident. Another small study found that habitual marijuana users' night shift interruptions were lessened by marijuana usage (Resko et al. 2020). Employers who have procedures for drug testing employees and the use or possession of narcotics in the workplace may have difficulties if recreational marijuana is legalized. However, workplace safety and work performance remain major considerations in the debate over legalization. Because cannabis policy is changing quickly and support for legalizing marijuana is growing, it is critical for preventive efforts to understand how the public views cannabis and the harms it poses (Farrelly et al. 2023).

The public's perception of marijuana's potency and the possible health effects of legalization are important to discuss. Finding elements linked to attitudes and beliefs can help focus preventative and educational initiatives by improving our understanding of risk perception and health behaviours. We specifically concentrate on underlying assumptions, such as whether people acknowledge that marijuana is more potent than it was in the past and if they anticipate that legalization will have a detrimental impact on employee safety and traffic safety, expanding on studies on opinions regarding the legalization of marijuana (Farmer et al. 2022). We take into account political orientation, marijuana use (within the last year or more than a year ago), sentiments toward legalization, and demographics (age, gender, race, and education). Drawing from previous research, we postulated that younger age, male gender, white or African American race, higher educational attainment, marijuana use, support for legalization, and left-leaning political beliefs would all be linked to higher likelihoods of acknowledging marijuana's greater potency and lower likelihoods of anticipating detrimental public health effects from legalization (Murray et al. 2017).

According to the latest estimates from the United Nations Office on Drugs and Crime (UNODC), there were over 188 million cannabis users in 2017, making it one of the most widely used psychoactive drugs in the world. International drug control conventions, such as the 1961 UN Single Convention on Narcotic Drugs, have maintained that cannabis is still illegal, but since at least the 1960s, opponents have argued against its criminalization for a variety of reasons (Ransing et al. 2022). For instance, although cannabis usage is common among young adults, it is thought to be less harmful than illegal substances like alcohol and tobacco (Midgette and Reuter 2019). By subjecting users to the criminal justice system, which has disproportionately impacted underprivileged minority populations, particularly Black and Hispanic communities, the criminalization of cannabis use and possession has probably caused more harm than benefit. Legalization might assist in rebuilding these communities by expunging arrests and utilizing the money raised by the retail cannabis industry to restore justice. Reducing the illegal cannabis market would significantly lower the expenses of enforcing cannabis prohibition. Lastly, improved management and regulation of cannabis products would be possible with a legal retail market. For instance, adults would be shielded from contaminants like heavy metals and fungi, as well as from dangerously high doses of THC. Colorado and Washington passed referendums to legalize the possession and retail sale of non-medical cannabis in 2012, making it possible for retail sales to begin in 2014. Legalizing cannabis usage for non-medical purposes may have a net positive impact, but there are worries about growing risks to public health. The adverse physical health effects of cannabis remain largely unclear, as epidemiological studies are challenging to conduct partly due to its legal status and the high prevalence of concurrent tobacco use among cannabis users worldwide (Matheson and Le Foll 2020). One recurring finding is that long-term, strong cannabis use is linked to respiratory issues such as chronic bronchitis. There is little evidence to support the idea that cannabis usage may increase the risk of testicular cancer and cardiovascular disease. Recently, cannabis hyperemesis syndrome (CHS) has been identified as a serious risk factor for long-term cannabis use. Since cannabis has antiemetic properties, CHS is a paradoxical side effect of using the drug. It is characterized by nausea, vomiting, and abdominal pain that has no known cause, but is believed to be caused by alterations in the endocannabinoid system and the ensuing dysregulation of stress and anxiety responses. Regular cannabis usage has been shown to have far more detrimental long-term psychological impacts, while causality is still up for debate. Cross-sectional studies have shown a substantial decline in cognitive function brought on by frequent, heavy cannabis use, raising concerns about potential impairments in psychosocial functioning and educational/vocational success (Xing and Shi 2024). At least a dozen prospective longitudinal studies have shown a link between cannabis usage and a higher chance of developing psychotic symptoms or illness in the future since the late 1980s. Strong evidence from laboratory, clinical, and animal research has linked cannabis use to an increased risk of psychosis. There are significant regional and national differences in the legal status of cannabis.

Despite cannabis's widespread prohibition on a global scale, laws on its usage are gradually being relaxed. More countries around the world, including the Netherlands, Portugal, and some regions of Australia, have decriminalized. In addition, some US states, Peru, Germany, New Zealand, and the Netherlands have legalized medical marijuana. As of right now, the only three nations that have national legalization of cannabis use for recreational purposes are Canada, Uruguay, and Malta. Additionally, in 2012, some US states started legalizing cannabis for recreational use (Aditya and Al Fatih 2022). By 2023, almost half of these states had done so. Anti-legalization arguments, on the other hand, include the potential for legalization to result in a rise in teenage use and a rise in cannabis-impaired driving. The potential negative effects of these legislative changes on driving-related outcomes are another crucial topic, given the detrimental effects of cannabis on driving abilities and its association with motor vehicle accidents (Bowler et al. 1998; Marcu 2020; Summers 2018).

The German government has the intention of legalizing the use of cannabis for recreational purposes. The move is to control the quality of the drug, stop the flow of counterfeit products, and protect children. The most important elements of the move were formulated in October 2022 and forwarded to the European Commission for assessment. The launch of a controlled system of supply of cannabis to adults will improve the protection of children, enhance consumer health, and address the problems associated with the black market. To assess the viability of these goals, a study was conducted to describe the current status of research on the impact of controlled cannabis sales using an international literature review and input from field professionals. To achieve this purpose, it is necessary to examine the scientific research and field experience in countries that have not only legalized and decriminalized the cultivation and possession of cannabis for personal use but have also granted legality to the commercial cultivation and trade of recreational cannabis. This review must be conducted in countries that have followed alternative forms of legalization, i.e., decriminalization of cultivation and possession for private use. A few countries that have followed such alternative forms are Canada, Uruguay, the different states of the United States, Switzerland, and the Netherlands (Cabral Barata et al. 2022; Xing and Shi 2024).

10.1 Legalization Trends

In the 1990s and early 2000s, movements supporting medical use of cannabis sparked the trend toward its legalization (National Academies of Sciences, Engineering, and Medicine, 2017). Germany, Australia, the UK, Israel, and Thailand are among the more than 50 nations that have authorized or partially legalized cannabis for medical use (Fischer et al. 2017). Additionally, more jurisdictions are moving toward complete legalization for recreational use. The first nation to legalize cannabis for recreational use was Uruguay (2013), followed by Canada (2018) (Hall and Lynskey 2020). While cannabis is still illegal at the federal level in the United States, more than 20 states and the District of Columbia have legalized its recreational use, and many more have allowed its medical use (Volkow et al. 2014). Several European nations, including Malta, Switzerland, and the Netherlands, are investigating or establishing regulated cannabis markets (EMCDDA 2023).

10.2 Perceived Safety and Social Acceptance

The public's perception of cannabis has likewise drastically changed as legalization has expanded (Young-Wolff et al. 2017). Risk perception is declining, especially among adolescents and young people, according to surveys conducted in North America and some parts of Europe (Miech et al. 2021). Cannabis is being promoted as a wellness product in certain places and is increasingly seen as a "safe" or "natural" substitute for drugs like alcohol or tobacco (Zuckerman et al. 2021). Cannabis use has become more accepted as a result of the growth of CBD (cannabidiol) products, which are frequently promoted as calming, pain-relieving, or anxiety-reducing (Fischer et al. 2017). The portrayal of cannabis as a comparatively safe or even advantageous drug has also been influenced by social media, popular culture, and aggressive marketing from the growing cannabis sector (Zuckerman et al. 2021).

10.3 Concerns and Misconceptions

The growing consensus that cannabis is harmless, however, does not entirely match the state of science about its effects (Volkow et al. 2014). Cannabis use carries some risks, even while it may provide therapeutic advantages for illnesses like multiple sclerosis, epilepsy, and chronic pain (National Academies of Sciences, Engineering, and Medicine 2017). Now widely available in legal markets, high-THC cannabis strains have been linked to deleterious effects on teenage brain development, addiction, psychosis risk, and cognitive impairment (Meier et al. 2012; Di Forti et al. 2019).

Furthermore, especially among young people, the notion that legalization removes danger may result in earlier initiation, increased usage, and a lack of prudence (Santaella-Tenorio et al. 2017). Increases in traffic accidents, ER visits, and unintentional child consumption have been observed by public health officials in several legalized areas (Volkow et al. 2014).

10.4 Balancing Legalization With Public Health

As legalization increases, striking a balance between corporate interests, public health safeguards, and individual liberty becomes increasingly difficult (Haden and Emerson 2014). Lawmakers are increasingly focusing on effective cannabis regulation, including measures such as quality control, age restrictions, harm-reduction strategies, advertising bans, and public education (Fischer et al. 2017).

Additionally, long-term studies on cannabis use are becoming increasingly important, especially given its impact on society, mental health, and cognitive function (National Academies of Sciences, Engineering, and Medicine 2017).

10.5 Maternal Health Implications

Cannabis use may decrease adherence to prenatal treatment because it can affect cognition, attention, and decision-making (Narayanan et al. 2025). Co-using cannabis with alcohol or tobacco increases the hazards to the health of both the mother and the foetus (Ko et al. 2015). New information points to links with anaemia, high blood pressure, and a higher requirement for caesarean sections (Corsi et al. 2019). Particularly at crucial stages of neurodevelopment, THC readily crosses the placenta and attaches itself to foetal cannabinoid receptors (El Marroun et al. 2009). Cannabis use during pregnancy has been connected to: reduced executive function, deficits in language and memory, behavioural issues, increased impulsivity, low weight at birth, premature birth, and small for gestational age (SGA) (Gunn et al. 2016; Bertrand et al. 2018).

Breast milk contains THC, which can linger for days or weeks. Babies exposed through breastfeeding may show signs of poor eating, sedation, and altered motor development (Bertrand et al. 2018). Marijuana exposure in newborns is not associated with any dysmorphic traits. Infants exposed to marijuana during pregnancy are more likely to be underweight at birth. A smaller head circumference could be observed, particularly if tobacco use is concurrent. Neonates exposed to marijuana do not exhibit any withdrawal symptoms. However, the results of the clinical examination may be consistent with withdrawal from other substances, such as nicotine or opioids, because these newborns are at a very high risk of being exposed to several drugs. Marijuana use during pregnancy can cause increased trembling, a high-pitched cry, and changed reactions to visual cues. Between 2% and 5% of expectant mothers self-report using marijuana during their pregnancy (Corsi et al. 2025).

These rates among low-income urban women range from 14 to 28%. Cannabis usage during pregnancy is becoming more common, most likely as a result of its easy accessibility after legalization, perceived safety, and its anti-nausea effects. A high incidence of other substance use disorders is also linked to marijuana usage. This increases the danger of multiple exposures for both the mother and the foetus. Marijuana usage during pregnancy has been linked in several studies to an increased risk of spontaneous preterm birth. Some research has linked marijuana consumption during pregnancy to a considerable drop in birth weight, while other studies show no difference when controlling for other maternal drug use (Shukla and Doshi 2023).

During pregnancy, women may use cannabis for pleasure, to treat pregnancy-related issues, including nausea and vomiting, and to manage stress; many of these women seem to be ignorant of the hazards associated with pregnancy. Women who are of reproductive age are increasingly using cannabis, both before and during pregnancy. For example, 9.9% of 16,556 women of reproductive age who participated in a study using data from the 2016 Behavioural Risk Factor Surveillance System from 12 US states reported using marijuana at the time of the survey. Before getting pregnant, cannabis use is also common (Gerede et al. 2024).

For instance, 5% of 1,228 women in a secondary review of data from the Effects of Aspirin in Gestation and Reproduction experiment, which was carried out at four clinical locations in the US, reported using cannabis during their infertility attempts. Additionally, cannabis use is common during pregnancy. For instance, in the 2016–2017 Pregnancy Risk Assessment Monitoring System, a survey of 1,147 women in New Hampshire, 5.5% reported using cannabis during pregnancy, most often as an antiemetic (Andrade 2024).

Cannabis users may also participate in behaviours affecting maternal and child health, such as poor nutrition, inconsistent prenatal care, and increased risk of interpersonal violence (Richardson et al. 2016). It is challenging to distinguish cannabis's isolated effects on health outcomes due to these confounding factors (Van Boekel et al. 2013).

10.6 Implications and Public Health Needs

Accurate identification of predictors and risk factors of cannabis use can assist in designing screening tools and targeted interventions (Mark et al. 2016). Validated, nonjudgmental questions about cannabis and other substances should be part of routine pregnancy screenings (Sugarman and Califf 2014). Public health strategies must address interconnected lifestyle, sociodemographic, and psychological issues beyond individual drug use (Beauchamp and Childress 2019).

10.7 Policy, Legal, and Considerations for Cannabis

The evolving landscape of cannabis legislation worldwide has created a complex matrix of policy, legal, and ethical challenges for researchers, policymakers, and healthcare providers. Although public attitudes toward cannabis have grown more favourable, the divergence between state and federal laws, especially in countries like the United States, has generated significant barriers to scientific investigation and evidence-based policymaking (Hall and Weier 2015; National Academies of Sciences, Engineering, and Medicine 2017).

10.8 Legal Heterogeneity and Its Impact on Research

The patchwork of cannabis regulations across jurisdictions—ranging from full legalization to complete prohibition—poses a major obstacle to conducting rigorous research. In the US, while many states have legalized medical and/or recreational cannabis, federal classification of cannabis as a Schedule I drug under the Controlled Substances Act restricts funding, access to quality-controlled samples, and approval for clinical trials (Pacula and Smart 2017). This inconsistency hampers efforts to standardize studies and undermines the generalizability of findings across regions.

10.9 Informed Consent and Stigma in Study Recruitment

There are numerous reasons why patients use cannabis, many of which may be poorly understood or mostly unknown to medical professionals. Among the many alleged advantages of cannabis are its analgesic and anxiolytic qualities as well as its proven efficacy as a neuroleptic drug in the treatment of ailments, including seizure disorders and muscle stiffness. Cannabis' immunosuppressive and antineoplastic qualities have been empirically confirmed, making it useful for cancer patients in the prevention and treatment of chemotherapy-induced nausea, vomiting, and appetite regulation (Greene et al. 2023).

Chronic pain and multiple sclerosis are the two most prevalent conditions for medical cannabis prescriptions, both of which have strong proof of effectiveness. Other illnesses that are frequently mentioned include post-traumatic stress disorder, HIV/AIDS, and glaucoma. However, cannabis is not typically regarded as a drug by the majority of Western medical professionals, nor does it have any bearing on standard prescribing procedures for such diseases. Subjective norms or perceived or recognized risks could be the cause. In these situations, individuals may use cannabis to treat their ailments in place of traditional medications. The pooled prevalence of replacing medicinal cannabis pharmaceuticals is 60%, according to a recent comprehensive review and meta-analysis. The most often substituted medications are narcotics/opioids, anxiolytics, and antidepressants (Pratt et al. 2019).

Cannabis users have consistently shown reluctance to discuss their associated use behaviours and patterns with healthcare providers, even in the face of successful legislative initiatives to promote social acceptance. Bias, stigma, fear of the repercussions, and the unclear importance of disclosure are all mentioned in the suggested justification. Additionally, carers are not well-versed in the human endocannabinoid system and its pertinent therapeutic consequences, nor are they readily equipped with formal education to have productive interactions with patients about cannabis usage (King et al. 2024).

Among other issues, cannabis is frequently left out of medication reconciliation records due to a lack of regulatory standards, which further reduces routine awareness. Since the provider's decisions are not supported by thorough data or the patient's holistic perspective, these shortcomings eventually hinder their ability to make decisions. Cannabis users are therefore more likely to experience negative outcomes such as drug interactions, poor anaesthesia response, increased surgical pain medication dosages, or exacerbated illness states, as observed in other stigmatized situations(Borojevic and Söhner 2025).

10.10 Risk Communication in Research Settings

Implementing cannabis communication strategies should include a number of essential components. First and foremost, as public health professionals, we must employ clear, focused language to fairly and appropriately notify people of the dangers to themselves and others that are currently understood. Secondly, our messaging should be organized to minimize the negative effects on individuals who decide to consume cannabis. Third, we should be careful not to use stigma, fear, and stereotypes while educating the public about cannabis. The principles of risk communication, which frequently take the shape of "be first, be right, and be credible," are addressed by these components (Steiner et al. 2019).

10.11 Implications for Funding, Regulatory Approval, and Publication

Over the past twenty years, federal funding for cannabis research has grown tenfold as government agencies at all levels have had to make tough choices about public health, product safety, and criminal law. But since cannabis laws and policies change quickly, researchers' capacity to produce timely, thorough data that informs policy changes has not kept up. This emphasizes the need for state governments to play a larger role in addressing the financial shortfall. Although federal funding for cannabis is well-established, little is known about how states finance cannabis research or the scope of state and university-level collaborations to enhance funding prospects for scientific study on cannabis. This study examines the present state government funding levels for cannabis research, as well as the financial distribution processes (Balla et al. 2025).

11. Conclusion

Cannabis usage during pregnancy has become a growing source of concern because of the possible negative effects it may have on the woman and her unborn child. Cannabis usage has been linked to a higher risk of pregnancy-related issues, including an early birth and a low birth weight. It has also been linked to possible detrimental impacts on emotional and mental health. According to studies, cannabis exposure during pregnancy can have a detrimental effect on the placenta's function and the foetus's growth. Placental insufficiency and limited foetal growth may result from this. According to longitudinal research, children exposed to cannabis during pregnancy face additional long-term developmental difficulties, including behavioural problems, poor academic performance, and diminished cognitive ability. A thorough and well-coordinated approach is necessary to address the issue of cannabis use during pregnancy. Initiatives in research, education, and public health policy should all be coordinated and integrated using this approach. Marijuana users who are pregnant are more likely to use other substances, such as alcohol, be underweight, and have worse social and educational standing. According to several findings, marijuana consumption is linked to anxiety and sadness. Pregnant women who use marijuana are more likely to experience anaemia and spontaneous preterm birth. Marijuana smoke contains carcinogenic and respiratory pollutants, similar to tobacco smoke. When marijuana and tobacco are used together, the risk of maternal asthma and preeclampsia is higher than when tobacco is used alone. To improve results and patient safety, primary care doctors, obstetricians, social workers, pharmacists, and psychologists who work with women who use pharmaceuticals must collaborate as a cohesive team. Comprehensive counselling should ideally be provided before conception and at every patient interaction. Women should also undergo drug usage screening and, if required, be referred to rehabilitation facilities.

References

Abioye, A., Ayodele, O., Marinkovic, A., Patidar, R., Akinwekomi, A., and Sanyaolu, A. (2020). Δ9-Tetrahydrocannabivarin (THCV): a commentary on potential therapeutic benefit for the management of obesity and diabetes. *Journal of Cannabis Research*, 2(1): 6.

Abrams, S. S., El-Ch Contact, P., and LaMarca, P. P. (2020). Amniotic fluid is a potential source for assessing fetal cannabis exposure. *Journal of Perinatology*, 40(10): 1479–1485.

Aizpurua-Olaizola, O., Soydaner, U., Öztürk, E., Schibano, D., Simsir, Y., Navarro, P. et al. (2016). Evolution of the cannabinoid and terpene content during the growth of Cannabis sativa plants. *Journal of Natural Products*, 79(2): 324–331. https://doi.org/10.1021/acs.jnatprod.5b00949

Anand, U., Scalabrini, A., Gonzalez, M. I., Altemimi, A. B., and Prasad, M. N. V. (2021). Cannabis and cannabinoid pharmacology: Potential anti-inflammatory and anti-cancer properties. *Frontiers in Pharmacology*, 12: 653481. https://doi.org/10.3389/fphar.2021.653481

Andrade C. (2025). Maternal Cannabis Use During Pregnancy and Neuropsychiatric Adverse Outcomes During Childhood and Early Adult Life. *The Journal of Clinical Psychiatry*, 86(1): 24f15753. https://doi.org/10.4088/JCP.24f15753

Andrade, C. (2024). Maternal Cannabis Use During Pregnancy and Maternal and Neonatal Adverse Outcomes. *The Journal of Clinical Psychiatry*, 85(4). https://doi.org/10.4088/JCP.24f15611

Antonia Biggs, M., Raifman, S., Zaugg, C., and Roberts, S. C. M. (2025). Pregnant and Recently Pregnant People's Views on Policies That Punish Pregnant People Who Use Cannabis. *Substance Use and Misuse*, 845–853.

Arellano, L., Alcubilla, P., and Leguízamo, L. (2023). Ethical considerations in informed consent. In *Ethics - Scientific Research, Ethical Issues, Artificial Intelligence and Education [Working Title]*. IntechOpen.

Astley, S. J., Milburn, L. G., Walters, D. G., and Grella, C. E. (2011). Association of prenatal cannabis exposure with the development of childhood attention problems. *Child Abuse and Neglect*, 35(4): 233–248.

Bahji, A., and Stephenson, C. (2019). International Perspectives on the Implications of Cannabis Legalization: A Systematic Review and Thematic Analysis. *International Journal of Environmental Research and Public Health*, 16(17): 3095.

Baja, I. and Domingues, R.M.S. (2024). The Effects of Cannabis Use during Pregnanacy on Low Birth Weight and Preterm Birth: A Systematic Review and Meta-analysis. *American Journal of Perinatology*, 41(01): 017:030.

Balla, A., Boyle, R. G., and Dempsey, C. (2025). State funding for cannabis research: an analysis of funding mechanisms and levels. *Journal of Cannabis Research*, 7(1): 1–9.

Bannigan, P., Evans, J. C., and Allen, C. (2022). Shifting the Paradigm on Cannabis Safety. *Cannabis and Cannabinoid Research*, 7(1): 3–10.

Berman, P., Sulimani, L., Golan-Gueta, I., and Meiri, D. (2018). Medicinal cannabis: Historical perspectives and current usage in Israel. *Israel Medical Association Journal*, 20(3): 141–146.

Blest-Hopley, G., Giampietro, V., and Bhattacharyya, S. (2020). A systematic review of human neuroimaging evidence of memory-related functional alterations associated with cannabis use complemented with preclinical and human evidence of memory performance alterations. *Brain Sciences*, 10(2): 102.

Boggs, D. L., Nguyen, J. D., Morgenson, D., Taffe, M. A., and Ranganathan, M. (2018). Clinical and preclinical evidence for functional interactions of cannabidiol and Δ^9-tetrahydrocannabinol. *Neuropsychopharmacology*, 43(1): 142–154. https://doi.org/10.1038/npp.2017.209

Borojevic, V., and Söhner, F. (2025). Detecting and understanding potential stigma among medical cannabis users in Germany. *BMC Public Health*, 25(1): 1–14.

Borrelli, F., Fasolino, I., Romano, B., Capasso, R., Maiello, F., Coppola, D. et al. (2013). Beneficial effect of the non-psychotropic plant cannabinoid cannabigerol on experimental inflammatory bowel disease. *Biochemical Pharmacology*, 85(9): 1306–1316. https://doi.org/10.1016/j.bcp.2013.01.017

Bowler, S., Donovan, T., Tolbert, C., and Tolbert, C. J. (1998). *Citizens as Legislators: Direct Democracy in the United States*.

Brents, L. K., Reichard, E. E., Zimmerman, S. M., Moran, J. H., and Fantegrossi, W. E. (2015). Prenatal cannabinoid exposure: Animal models and potential developmental outcomes. *Birth Defects Research Part C: Embryo Today: Reviews*, 105(1): 53–69. https://doi.org/10.1002/bdrc.21091

Brett, K. E., Ferraro, Z. M., Yockell-Lelievre, J., Gruslin, A., and Adamo, K. B. (2014). Maternal-fetal nutrient transport in pregnancy pathologies: the role of the placenta. *International Journal of Molecular Sciences*, 15(9): 16153–16185.

Brown, Q. L., Sarvet, A. L., Shmulewitz, D., Martins, S. S., Wall, M. M., and Hasin, D. S. (2017). Trends in marijuana use among pregnant and nonpregnant reproductive-aged women, 2002–2014. *Obstetrics and Gynecology,* 129(4): 653–660. https://doi.org/10.1097/AOG.0000000000001945

Cabral Barata, P., Ferreira, F., and Oliveira, C. (2022). Non-medical cannabis use: international policies and outcomes overview. An outline for Portugal. *Trends in Psychiatry and Psychotherapy*, 44: e20200239.

Cameron, R. S., Perono, G. A., Natale, C. D., Petrik, J. J., Holloway, A. C., and Hardy, D. B. (2025). The impact of cannabinoids on reproductive function. *Reproduction (Cambridge, England)*, 169(5). https://doi.org/10.1530/REP-24-0369

Cannabidiol Safety: A Review. *Current Drug Safety*, 18(4): 465–473.

Cascio, M. G., Gauson, L. A., Stevenson, L. A., Ross, R. A., and Pertwee, R. G. (2010). Evidence that the plant cannabinoid cannabigerol is a highly potent α2-adrenoceptor agonist and moderately potent 5HT1A receptor antagonist. *British Journal of Pharmacology*, 159(1): 129–141. https://doi.org/10.1111/j.1476-5381.2009.00515.x

Chandra, S., Avula, B., and Duke, R. C. (2019). The association between maternal marijuana use during pregnancy and adverse perinatal outcomes. *Cannabis and Cannabinoid Research*, 4(1): 1–7.

Chang, C. J., Lee, F. K., Chen, J. K., Huang, Y. C., Chen, P. J., Chen, C. H. et al. (2020). Association between prenatal cannabis exposure and behavioural problems in children: A systematic review and meta-analysis. *Journal of the American Medical Directors Association* 21(9): 1225–1232.e4.

Chang, J. C., Tarr, J. A., Holland, C. L., Rubio, D., Rodriguez, K. L., Kraemer, K. L. et al. (2019). Self-reported prenatal cannabis use and perceptions of risk. *Obstetrics and Gynecology*, 133(1): 98–103. https://doi.org/10.1097/AOG.0000000000003011

Chaput, K. H., McMorris, C. A., Metcalfe, A., Ringham, C., McNeil, D., Konschuh, S. et al. (2024). Development and validation of the Cannabis Exposure in Pregnancy Tool (CEPT): a mixed methods study. *BMC Pregnancy and Childbirth*, 24(1): 1–12.

Chen, W., and French, M. T. (2023). Marijuana legalization and traffic fatalities revisited. *Southern Economic Journal*, 90(2): 259–276.

Chen, X., Unadkat, J. D., and Mao, Q. (2023). Maternal and Fetal Exposure to (-)-Δ-tetrahydrocannabinol and Its Major Metabolites in Pregnant Mice Is Differentially Impacted by P-glycoprotein and Breast Cancer Resistance Protein. *Drug Metabolism and Disposition: The Biological Fate of Chemicals*, 51(3): 269–275.

Chiu, V., Hall, W., Chan, G., Hides, L., and Leung, J. (2022). A Systematic Review of Trends in US Attitudes toward Cannabis Legalization. *Substance Use and Misuse*, 57(7): 1052–1061.

Clinical Epigenetics. (2023). Prenatal delta-9-tetrahydrocannabinol exposure is associated with changes in rhesus macaque DNA methylation enriched for autism genes. *Clinical Epigenetics,* 15: 104. https://doi.org/10.1186/s13148-023-01519-4

Conner, M., Littenberg, M. E., Drake, R. L., Levitt, P. S., Ghandi, P. A., Levitt, L. N. et al. (2014). Prenatal exposure to cannabis: effects on fetal development and offspring behaviour." *Journal of the American Osteopathic Association*, 114(10): 731–739.

Coppola, M., and Mondola, R. (2022). Delta-8-THC: A legal high? *Toxicology Letters*, 359: 20–25. https://doi.org/10.1016/j.toxlet.2021.12.001

Corsi, D. J., Donelle, J., Sucha, E., Hawken, S., Hsu, H., El-Chaâr, D. et al. (2020). Maternal cannabis use in pregnancy and child neurodevelopmental outcomes. *Nature Medicine*, 26(10): 1536–1540.

Corsi, D. J., Morris, T. T., Reed, Z. E., and Davey Smith, G. (2025). Maternal cannabis use in pregnancy, perinatal outcomes, and cognitive development in offspring: a longitudinal analysis of the ALSPAC cohort using paternal cannabis use as a negative control exposure. *European Journal of Epidemiology*, 40(5): 549–562.

Costa, R., Giuffrida, S., and Giordano, G. (2020). The endocannabinoid system in brain development: a critical review. *Current Opinion in Pharmacology*, 53: 86–93.

DeLong, G. T., Wolf, C. E., Poklis, J. L., Lichtman, A. H., and Wiley, J. L. (2010). Pharmacological evaluation of the natural constituent of Cannabis sativa, cannabichromene and its modulation by cannabidiol. *Pharmacology Biochemistry and Behavior,* 96(4): 584–588. https://doi.org/10.1016/j.pbb.2010.07.026

Di Forti, M., Quattrone, D., Freeman, T. P., Tripoli, G., Gayer-Anderson, C., Quigley, H. et al. (2019). The contribution of cannabis use to variation in the incidence of psychotic disorder across Europe (EU-GEI): A multicentre case-control study. *The Lancet Psychiatry,* 6(5): 427–436. https://doi.org/10.1016/S2215-0366(19)30048-3

Dickson, B., Mansfield, C., Guiahi, M., and Little, T. (2018). Recommendations for pregnancy and cannabis use. *Canadian Family Physician,* 64(6): 408–409.

Doyle, R. (2025). *The Impact of Marijuana Edibles on Fetal Development in Pregnant Adolescents and Young Mothers* [Western Michigan University]. https://scholarworks.wmich.edu/honors_theses/3932

ElSohly, M. A., and Slade, D. (2006). Chemical constituents of marijuana: The complex mixture of natural cannabinoids. *Life Sciences*, 78(5): 539–548. https://doi.org/10.1016/j.lfs.2005.09.011

Farmer, C. M., Monfort, S. S., and Woods, A. N. (2022). Changes in Traffic Crash Rates After Legalization of Marijuana: Results by Crash Severity. *Journal of Studies on Alcohol and Drugs*, 83(4): 494–501.

Farrelly, K. N., Wardell, J. D., Marsden, E., Scarfe, M. L., Najdzionek, P., Turna, J. et al. (2023). The impact of recreational cannabis legalization on cannabis use and associated outcomes: A systematic review. *Substance Abuse: Research and Treatment*. https://doi.org/10.1177/11782218231172054

Fischer, B., Russell, C., Sabioni, P., van den Brink, W., Le Foll, B., Hall, W. et al. (2017). Lower-risk cannabis use guidelines: A comprehensive update of evidence and recommendations. *American Journal of Public Health*, 107(8): e1–e12. https://doi.org/10.2105/AJPH.2017.303818

Gabarin, A., Yarmolinsky, L., Budovsky, A., Khalfin, B., and Ben-Shabat, S. (2023). Cannabis as a Source of Approved Drugs: A New Look at an Old Problem. *Molecules*, 28(23): 7686.

Gao, Y., Xiang, L., Yi, H., Song, J., Sun, D., Xu, B., Zhang, G., and Wu, I. X. (2025). Confounder adjustment in observational studies investigating multiple risk factors: a methodological study. *BMC Medicine*, 23(1): 132.

Gerede, A., Stavros, S., Chatzakis, C., Vavoulidis, E., Papasozomenou, P., Domali, E., Nikolettos, K., Oikonomou, E., Potiris, A., Tsikouras, P., and Nikolettos, N. (2024). Cannabis Use during Pregnancy: An Update. *Medicina*, 60(10): 1691.

Gerede, A., Stavros, S., Chatzakis, C., Vavoulidis, E., Papasozomenou, P., Domali, E. et al. (2024). Cannabis Use during Pregnancy: An Update. *Medicina*, 60(10): 1691s.

Goldschmidt, L., Richardson, G. A., and Astley, S. J. (2019). Prenatal cannabis use and child development: a longitudinal study. *Child Development*, 90(3): e291-e305.

González-Sala, F., Tortosa-Pérez, M., Peñaranda-Ortega, M., and Tortosa, F. (2023). Effects of Cannabis Legalization on Road Safety. A Literature Review. *International Journal of Environmental Research and Public Health*, 20(5): 4655.

Grant, K. S., Petroff, R., Isoherranen, N., Stella, N., and Burbacher, T. M. (2018). Cannabis use during pregnancy: Pharmacokinetics and effects on child development. *Pharmacology and Therapeutics*, 182: 133–151.

Grant, Kimberly S., Rebekah Petroff, Nina Isoherranen, Nephi Stella, and Thomas M. Burbacher. (2018). Cannabis Use during Pregnancy: Pharmacokinetics and Effects on Child Development. *Pharmacology and Therapeutics*, 182 (February): 133–51.

Gunn, C. P., Skelly, L. A., Smith, L. M., Leppert, J. K., Pester, J. N., and Leppert, J. (2021). Prenatal cannabis exposure and executive function in children. *Addictive Behaviors*, 113: 106702.

Hadzigeorgiou, G. V., C. K. Tsilimigaki, D. K. Dimopoulos, E. L. Giannakopoulou, F. G. Kalfane, and D. G. Kalfane. 2019. Cannabis Use in pregnancy: a review of the current evidence. *Current Pharmaceutical Biotechnology*, 20(11): 915–922.

Hall, W., and Lynskey, M. (2020). Assessing the public health impacts of legalizing recreational cannabis use: The US experience. *World Psychiatry*, 19(2): 179–186. https://doi.org/10.1002/wps.20735

Herreros, I., Monleón, D., and de la Torre, R. (2019). Cannabinoid receptor signaling in neurodevelopment. *Brain Plasticity*, 5(1): 37–53. https://doi.org/10.3233/BPL-190081

Hilderbrand, R. L. (2020). Delta-8-THC and delta-10-THC: Emerging cannabinoids. *Cannabis Science and Technology*, 3(5): 32–39.

Hill, A. J., Weston, S. E., Jones, N. A., Smith, I., and Whalley, B. J. (2013). Cannabidivarin is anticonvulsant in mouse and rat models of epilepsy. *Epilepsia*, 54(4): 747–758. https://doi.org/10.1111/epi.12079

Holland, C. L., Rubio, D., Rodriguez, K. L., Kraemer, K. L., Day, N., Arnold, R. M. et al. (2016). Self-reported use of marijuana during pregnancy: Correlation between use, perception, and perinatal outcomes. *Obstetrics and Gynecology*, 127(4): 681–687. https://doi.org/10.1097/AOG.0000000000001352

Howlett, A. C., and Abood, M. E. (2017). CB1 and CB2 receptor pharmacology. *Neuropharmacology*, 124: 5–17. https://doi.org/10.1016/j.neuropharm.2017.03.002. http://www.librar.ca.gov/crb

Huestis, M. A., Mitchell, S. M., and Jordan, G. D. (2019). Hair cannabinoid analysis of chronic cannabis use. *Journal of Chromatography B: Analytical Technologies in the Biomedical and Life Sciences*, 1129: 121830.

Hurley, E. N., Ellaway, C. J., Johnson, A. M., Truong, L., Gordon, R., Galettis, P. et al. (2022). Efficacy and safety of cannabidivarin treatment of epilepsy in girls with Rett syndrome: A phase 1 clinical trial. *Epilepsia*, 63(7): 1736–1747.

Iannotti, F. A., Hill, C. L., Leo, A., Alhusaini, A., Soubrane, C., Mazzarella, E. et al. (2014). Non-psychotropic plant cannabinoids, cannabidivarin (CBDV) and cannabigerol (CBG), activate and desensitize TRPV1 channels in vitro: Potential for the treatment of neuronal hyperexcitability. *Neurochemistry International*, 75: 59–70. https://doi.org/10.1016/j.neuint.2014.06.006

Iffland, K., and Grotenhermen, F. (2017). An update on safety and side effects of cannabidiol: A review of clinical data and relevant animal studies. *Cannabis and Cannabinoid Research*, 2(1): 139–154. https://doi.org/10.1089/can.2016.0034

Jarlenski, M., Koma, J. W., Zank, J., Bodnar, L. M., Bogen, D. L., and Chang, J. C. (2017). Trends in perception of risk of regular marijuana use among US pregnant and nonpregnant reproductive-aged women. *American Journal of Obstetrics and Gynecology*, 217(6): 705–707. https://doi.org/10.1016/j.ajog.2017.07.016

Jastrząb, A., Jarocka-Karpowicz, I., and Skrzydlewska, E. (2022). The Origin and Biomedical Relevance of Cannabigerol. *International Journal of Molecular Sciences*, 23(14): 7929.

Keim, S. A., Fried, P., Yeates, K. O., Boone, K. M., Vrantsidis, D. M., Dean, A. et al. (2024). Prenatal Cannabis Exposure and Executive Function and Aggressive Behavior at Age 5 Years. *JAMA pediatrics*, 178(12): 1316–1325. https://doi.org/10.1001/jamapediatrics.2024.4352

Khalsa, J. H., Bunt, G., Blum, K., Maggirwar, S. B., Galanter, M., and Potenza, M. N. (2022). Review: Cannabinoids as Medicinals. *Current Addiction Reports*, 9(4): 630–646.

King, D. D., Gill, C. J., Cadieux, C. S., and Singh, N. (2024). The role of stigma in cannabis use disclosure: an exploratory study. *Harm Reduction Journal*, 21(1): 1–13.

Krishnan, P., and Yen, E. (2025). The changing landscape of cannabis use: impact on maternal health and neonatal outcomes. *Pediatric Research*, 1–11.

Kruger, J. S., and Kruger, D. J. (2022). Delta-8-THC use and perceived effects: Results from a national study. *Journal of Cannabis Research,* 4(1): 5. https://doi.org/10.1186/s42238-022-00091-5

Kwiecień, E., and Kowalczuk, D. (2023). Therapeutic Potential of Minor Cannabinoids in Dermatological Diseases-A Synthetic Review. *Molecules (Basel, Switzerland)*, 28(16). https://doi.org/10.3390/molecules28166149

Lindelöf, H., Hammarsjö, A., Voss, U., Gaetana Piticchio, S., Conner, P., Papadogiannakis, N. et al. (2025). Genome sequencing in a cohort of 32 fetuses with genetic skeletal disorders. *European Journal of Human Genetics : EJHG*. https://doi.org/10.1038/s41431-025-01886-x

Lo, J. O., Ayers, C. K., Yeddala, S., Shaw, B., Robalino, S., Ward, R. et al. (2025). Prenatal cannabis use and neonatal outcomes: A systematic review and meta-analysis. *JAMA Pediatrics*. Advance online publication. https://doi.org/10.1001/jamapediatrics.2025.0689

Lo, J. O., Shaw, B., Robalino, S., Ayers, C. K., Durbin, S., Rushkin, M. C. et al. (2024). Cannabis Use in Pregnancy and Neonatal Outcomes: A Systematic Review and Meta-Analysis. *Cannabis and Cannabinoid Research*, 9(2): 470–485.https://doi.org/10.1089/can.2022.0262

Mahintamani, T., Mukherjee, D., and Basu, D. (2025). Cannabis and psychopathology: 2024 Snapshot of a meandering journey. *Indian Journal of Psychiatry*, 67(3): 283–302.

Marcu, J. (2020). The legalization of cannabinoid products and standardizing cannabis-drug development in the United States: a brief report. *Dialogues in Clinical Neuroscience*, 22(3): 289–293.

Martínez-Peña, A. A., Perono, G. A., Gritis, S. A., Sharma, R., Selvakumar, S., Walker, O. S. et al. (2021). The Impact of Early Life Exposure to Cannabis: The Role of the Endocannabinoid System. *International Journal of Molecular Sciences*, 22(16): 8576.

Martínez-Peña, A. A., Perono, G. A., Gritis, S. A., Sharma, R., Selvakumar, S., Walker, O. S. et al. (2021). The Impact of Early Life Exposure to Cannabis: The Role of the Endocannabinoid System. *International Journal of Molecular Sciences*, 22(16): 8576.

Matheson, J., and Le Foll, B. (2020). Cannabis Legalization and Acute Harm From High Potency Cannabis Products: A Narrative Review and Recommendations for Public Health. *Frontiers in Psychiatry*, 11: 591979.

Meier, M. H., Caspi, A., Ambler, A., Harrington, H., Houts, R., Keefe, R. S. et al. (2012). Persistent cannabis users show neuropsychological decline from childhood to midlife. *Proceedings of the National Academy of Sciences*, 109(40): E2657–E2664. https://doi.org/10.1073/pnas.1206820109

Mendoza, S. (2025). The role of tetrahydrocannabivarin (THCV) in metabolic disorders: A promising cannabinoid for diabetes and weight management. *AIMS Neuroscience*, *12*(neurosci-12-01-003), 32–43.

Metz, T. D., and Borgelt, L. M. (2018). Marijuana Use in Pregnancy and While Breastfeeding. *Obstetrics and Gynecology*, 132(5): 1198–1210.

Micalizzi, L., Aston, E. R., Nesi, J., Price, D., and Gunn, R. L. (2024). A Descriptive Analysis of a Popular Pregnancy Forum: Comments on the Developmental Consequences of Cannabis Use on Offspring. *Journal of Studies on Alcohol and Drugs*. https://doi.org/10.15288/jsad.23-00019

Midgette, G., and Reuter, P. (2019). Has Cannabis Use Among Youth Increased After Changes in Its Legal Status? A Commentary on Use of Monitoring the Future for Analyses of Changes in State Cannabis Laws. *Prevention Science*, 21(1): 137–145.

Mollner, K. (2022). Global Impacts of Legalization and Decriminalization of Marijuana and Cannabis. *Journal of Toxicology and Risk Assessment*, 8(1): 046.

Moore, B. F. (2024). Prenatal exposure to cannabis: Effects on childhood obesity and cardiometabolic health. *Current Obesity Reports*, 13(1): 154–166. https://doi.org/10.1007/s13679-023-00544-x

Murray, R. M., and Di Forti, M. (2016). Cannabis and Psychosis: What Degree of Proof Do We Require? *Biological Psychiatry*, 79(7): 514–515.

Murray, R. M., Englund, A., Abi-Dargham, A., Lewis, D. A., Di Forti, M., Davies, C. et al. (2017). Cannabis-associated psychosis: Neural substrate and clinical impact. *Neuropharmacology*, 124: 89–104.

Nachnani, R., Raup-Konsavage, W. M., and Vrana, K. E. (2021). The pharmacological case for cannabigerol. *The Journal of Pharmacology and Experimental Therapeutics*, 376(2): 204–212. https://doi.org/10.1124/jpet.120.000280

Narayanan, P., Bertrand, K., Waalen, J., Chambers, C., Ferran, K., and Bandoli, G. (2025). The Effect of Cannabis Consumption During Lactation on the Macronutrient Concentrations in Breast Milk. *Breastfeeding Medicine*. https://doi.org/10.1089/bfm.2024.0083

National Academies of Sciences, Engineering, and Medicine. (2017). *The health effects of cannabis and cannabinoids: The current state of evidence and recommendations for research*. The National Academies Press. https://doi.org/10.17226/24625

Newmeyer, M. N., Swortwood, M. J., Abulseoud, O. A., and Huestis, M. A. (2017). Subjective and physiological effects after controlled Sativex and oral THC administration. pp. 235–254. *In*: Pacher, P., Mechoulam, R., and Huestis, M. A. (Eds.). *Handbook of Cannabis*. Oxford University Press.

Panday, J., Taneja, S., Popoola, A., Pack, R., Greyson, D., McDonald, S. D., Black, M., Murray-Davis, B., Darling, E., and Vanstone, M. (2022). Clinician responses to cannabis use during pregnancy and lactation: a systematic review and integrative mixed-methods research synthesis. *Family Practice*, 39(3): 504–514.

Peng, H., Li, H., Wei, Y., Zhang, R., Chang, X., Meng, L., Wang, K. et al. (2023). Effects of prenatal exposure to THC on hippocampal neural development in offspring. *Toxicology Letters*, 374: 48–56. https://doi.org/10.1016/j.toxlet.2022.12.007

Pertwee, R. G. (2008). The diverse CB1 and CB2 receptor pharmacology of three plant cannabinoids: Δ9-tetrahydrocannabinol, cannabidiol and Δ9-tetrahydrocannabivarin. *British Journal of Pharmacology*, 153(2): 199–215. https://doi.org/10.1038/sj.bjp.0707442

Pinky, P. D., Bloemer, J., Smith, W. D., Du, Y., Heslin, R. T., Setti, S. E. et al. (2023). Prenatal cannabinoid exposure elicits memory deficits associated with reduced psa-ncam expression, altered glutamatergic signaling, and adaptations in hippocampal synaptic plasticity. *Cells*, 12(21): 2525. https://doi.org/10.3390/cells12212525

Poudel, A., Pradhananga, D., and Shrestha, A. (2023). Emerging cannabinoids: Pharmacology and toxicology of delta-10-THC. *Frontiers in Pharmacology*, 14: 1020157. https://doi.org/10.3389/fphar.2023.1020157

Pratt, M., Stevens, A., Thuku, M., Butler, C., Skidmore, B., Wieland, L. S. et al. (2019). Benefits and harms of medical cannabis: a scoping review of systematic reviews. *Systematic Reviews*, 8(1): 320.

Rae-Grant, A., Day, G. S., Marrie, R. A., Rabinstein, A., Cree, B. A. C., Gronseth, G. S. et al. (2018). Practice guideline recommendations summary: Disease-modifying therapies for adults with multiple sclerosis: Report of the Guideline Development, Dissemination, and Implementation Subcommittee of the American Academy of Neurology. *Neurology*, 90(17): 777–788. https://doi.org/10.1212/WNL.0000000000005347

Ransing, R., de la Rosa, P. A., Pereira-Sanchez, V., Handuleh, J. I. M., Jerotic, S., Gupta, A. K. et al. (2022). Current state of cannabis use, policies, and research across sixteen countries: cross-country comparisons and international perspectives. *Trends in psychiatry and psychotherapy*, 44(Suppl 1). e20210263. https://doi.org/10.47626/2237-6089-2021-0263

Resko, S. M., Szechy, K. A., Early, T. J., Ellis, J. D., Hicks, D., and Agius, E. (2020). Perceptions of public health consequences of marijuana legalization. *Addiction Research and Theory*, 29(3): 255–262. https://doi.org/10.1080/16066359.2020.1823971

Rideout, N. (2023, July 6). THC use during pregnancy linked to changes in fetal development. *OHSU News*. https://news.ohsu.edu/2023/07/06/thc-use-during-pregnancy-linked-to-changes-in-fetal-development

Roncero, C., Valriberas-Herrero, I., Mezzatesta-Gava, M., Villegas, J. L., Aguilar, L., and Grau-López, L. (2020). Cannabis use during pregnancy and its relationship with fetal developmental outcomes and psychiatric disorders. A systematic review. *Reproductive Health*, 17(1): 25.

Russo, E. B. (2011). Taming THC: Potential cannabis synergy and phytocannabinoid-terpenoid entourage effects. *British Journal of Pharmacology,* 163(7): 1344–1364. https://doi.org/10.1111/j.1476-5381.2011.01238.x

Russo, E. B. (2019). The case for the entourage effect and conventional breeding of clinical cannabis: No "strain," no gain. *Frontiers in Plant Science,* 9: 1969. https://doi.org/10.3389/fpls.2018.01969

Russo, E. B., and Marcu, J. P. (2017). Cannabis pharmacology: The usual suspects and a few promising leads. *Cannabis and Cannabinoid Research*, 2(1): 61–67. https://doi.org/10.1089/can.2017.0012

Sainz, K., Ulibarri, H., Arroyo, A., Herrera, D. G., Hamilton, B., Ruffley, K., Robinson, M., and Marchand, G. J. (2025). Meta-analysis of maternal and neonatal outcomes of cannabis use in pregnancy current to March 2024. *Maternal Health, Neonatology and Perinatology*, 11(1): 1–22.

Satti, D., Frank, C., and Jones, A. (2022). Cannabis use in pregnancy: Changing trends and implications. *Journal of Maternal-Fetal and Neonatal Medicine*, 35(20): 3907–3914. https://doi.org/10.1080/14767058.2021.1911511

Shukla, S., and Doshi, H. (2023). Marijuana and Maternal, Perinatal, and Neonatal Outcomes. In *StatPearls*. StatPearls Publishing.

Simei, J. L. Q., Souza, J. D. R., Pedrazzi, J. F., Guimarães, F. S., Campos, A. C., Zuardi, A. et al. (2024). Research and Clinical Practice Involving the Use of Cannabis Products, with Emphasis on Cannabidiol: A Narrative Review. *Pharmaceuticals*, 17(12): 1644.

Singh, C., Rao, K., Yadav, N., Vashist, Y., Chugh, P., Bansal, N., and Minocha, N. (2023). Current Cannabidiol Safety: A Review. *Current Drug Safety*, 18(4): 465–473.

Solmi, M., De Toffol, M., Kim, J. Y., Choi, M. J., Stubbs, B., Thompson, T. et al. (2023). Balancing risks and benefits of cannabis use: umbrella review of meta-analyses of randomised controlled trials and observational studies. *BMJ*, 382. https://doi.org/10.1136/bmj-2022-072348

Song, L., Zhang, Y., Zhang, C., and Li, T. (2020). The endocannabinoid system and its role in brain development and neurodevelopmental disorders. *Frontiers in Pharmacology*, 11: 568212.

Stanton, D. L., Sr, Makin, D., Stohr, M., Lovrich, N. P., Willits, D., Hemmens, C. et al. (2022). Law enforcement perceptions of cannabis legalization effects on policing: challenges of major policy change implementation at the street level. *Contemporary Drug Problems*. https://doi.org/10.1177/00914509211053660

Steiner, L., Nicol, A.-M., and Eykelbosh, A. (2019). How we talk about "Pot" matters: strategies for improved cannabis risk communication. *Environmental Health Review*, 62(1): 8–13.

Summers, D. J. (2018). *The Business of Cannabis: New Policies for the New Marijuana Industry*. Bloomsbury Publishing USA.

Tadesse, A. W., Ayano, G., Dachew, B. A., Tusa, B. S., Damtie, Y., Betts, K. et al. (2024). The association between prenatal cannabis use and congenital birth defects in offspring: A cumulative meta-analysis. *Neurotoxicology and Teratology*, 102: 107340. https://doi.org/10.1016/j.ntt.2024.107340

Tomagra, G., Gandlevskiy, N., Rosso, E., Bonardi, M., Binello, A., Carabelli, V. et al. (2025). THC, CBD and minor cannabinoid CBDV differently modulate hippocampal neurons firing. *Neurotoxicology*, 108: 180–190.

Tortoriello, G., Morris, C. V., Alpar, A., Fuzik, J., Shirran, S. L., Calvigioni, D. et al. (2014). Miswiring the brain: Δ9-tetrahydrocannabinol disrupts cortical development by inducing an SCG10 degradation pathway. *The EMBO Journal*, 33(7): 668–685. https://doi.org/10.1002/embj.201385978

Towobola, A., Towobola, B., Nair, B., and Makwana, A. (2023). The ethics and management of cannabis use in pregnancy following decriminalisation and licensing for medical use: narrative review. *BJPsych Bulletin*, 47(1): 28–37.

Turner, C. E., Elsohly, M. A., and Boeren, E. G. (1981). Constituents of Cannabis sativa L. XVII. A review of the natural constituents. *Journal of Natural Products*, 43(2): 169–234.

U.S. Food and Drug Administration. (2022). *5 Things to Know About Delta-8 THC*. https://www.fda.gov/consumers/consumer-updates/5-things-know-about-delta-8-thc

United Nations Office on Drugs and Crime (UNODC). (2023). *World Drug Report 2023*. https://www.unodc.org/unodc/en/data-and-analysis/world-drug-report-2023.html

Vandermeer, J. W., Patel, S. N., and Lassi, M. M. (2019). Neonatal abstinence syndrome: A review of management and outcomes. *The Journal of Maternal-Fetal and Neonatal Medicine*, 32(18): 3200–3207.

Vanin, S. R., Hardy, D. B., and Schulich School of Medicine and Dentistry. (2023, November 9). Prenatal exposure to cannabis may increase diabetes risk in offspring. *Schulich*

Vázquez, C. M., and Vazquez, F. (2019). Prenatal cannabis exposure affects maternal care and adult offspring behaviour in mice. *Neuroscience Letters*, 704: 147–153.

Volkow, N. D., Baler, R. D., Compton, W. M., and Weiss, S. R. (2014). Adverse health effects of marijuana use. *New England Journal of Medicine*, 370(23): 2219–2227. https://doi.org/10.1056/NEJMra1402309

Volkow, N. D., Espinosa, P. S., and Mercado, A. (2016). Effects of cannabis on the developing brain. *The American Journal on Addictions*, 25(5): 379:381.

Waller, S. S., Randall, S. A., O'Donnell, K., Eiden, R. D., and Short, G. (2019). Maternal cannabis use before and during pregnancy: Associations with birth outcomes. *Journal of Perinatology*, 39(1): 50–58.

Wang, X., Lin, C., Wu, S., Zhang, T., Wang, Y., Jiang, Y., and Wang, X. (2022). Cannabidivarin alleviates neuroinflammation by targeting TLR4 co-receptor MD2 and improves morphine-mediated analgesia. *Frontiers in Immunology*, 13: 929222.

Wargent, E. T., Zaibi, M. S., Silvestri, C., Hislop, D. C., Stocker, C. J., Stott, C. G. et al. (2013). The cannabinoid Δ9-tetrahydrocannabivarin (Δ9-THCV) ameliorates insulin sensitivity in two mouse models of obesity. *Nutrition and Diabetes*, 3(5): e68. https://doi.org/10.1038/nutd.2013.9

Whiting, P. F., Wolff, R. F., Deshpande, S., Di Nisio, M., Duffy, S., Hernandez, A. V. et al. (2015). Cannabinoids for medical use: A systematic review and meta-analysis. *JAMA*, 313(24): 2456–2473. https://doi.org/10.1001/jama.2015.6358

Wohrer, F., Ngo, H., DiDomenico, J., Ma, X., Roberts, M. H., and Bakhireva, L. N. (2024). Potentially modifiable risk and protective factors affecting mental and emotional wellness in pregnancy. *Frontiers in Human Neuroscience*, 18: 1323297.

Xing, J., and Shi, Y. (2024). Cannabis consumers' preferences for legal and illegal cannabis: evidence from a discrete choice experiment. *BMC Public Health*, 24(1): 2397.

Zager, J. J., Barhum, Y., and Shohami, E. (2019). The role of cannabis cultivar variability in neurodevelopmental outcomes. *Journal of Cannabis Research*, 1(1): 2. https://doi.org/10.1186/s42238-019-0002-0

Zamberletti, E., Boggs, J., and Petrella, C. (2020). Emerging therapeutic applications of cannabidiol in the context of neurological disorders: A review. *Frontiers in Neurology*, 11: 546752.

Zamberletti, E., Marengo, L., Gabaglio, M., Piscitelli, F., Castiglioni, C., Ligresti, A. et al. (2012). Cannabinol and neuroprotection in a murine model of neurodegeneration. *Psychopharmacology*, 224(4): 537–546. https://doi.org/10.1007/s00213-012-2785-0

Section 4
Regulations and Socio-Economic Perspectives

Chapter 15

Regulations, Legalization, and Social Impact

Marcília Pinheiro da Costa, Marcia dos Santos Rizzo, Valéria Carlos de Sousa, Igor Frederico da Silveira Ramos* and *Talissa Brenda de Castro Lopes*

1. Introduction

The Cannabis genus (Cannabaceae) has been cultivated for centuries for various uses, including food, medicine, recreation, and religious rituals (De Souza et al. 2022). The term cannabis includes the species *Cannabis sativa*, *Cannabis indica*, and *Cannabis ruderalis*, as well as additional species and subspecies of *Cannabis sativa* (Hong et al. 2024). Cannabis is the most commonly used recreational drug worldwide. As discussions on decriminalization and legalization of its use advance, the topic has gained significant attention in social and scientific circles in many countries (Chandy et al. 2024). Supporters of cannabis legalization have advanced the following advantages: enhanced quality control and increased availability for medicinal use, augmented tax revenue, and a reduction in the illegal market and gang violence. Conversely, opponents emphasize the potential risks associated with cannabis use, including the possibility of addiction, mental health concerns, and behavioural changes (Bahji and Stephenson 2019).

Over time, several nations have independently implemented regulatory measures allowing access to various cannabis-containing products. The legalization of medicinal cannabis use in some U.S. states and Canada in the 1990s inspired countries in Europe, Oceania, Africa, and Asia to adopt similar policies (Hall et al. 2019). Notably, most countries with regulatory guidelines for medical cannabis access are concentrated in the Americas and Europe (De Souza et al. 2022). The result of these advances is access to cannabis-based medicinal products (CBMPs), which is a collective term to describe a formulation or other product containing cannabis or its derivatives for medicinal use in humans (Banerjee et al. 2022). These products used in medical cannabis treatment include: (a) raw herbal cannabis; (b) cannabis extract; and (c) cannabinoid compounds, including natural cannabinoids [delta-9-tetrahydrocannabinol (THC); cannabidiol (CBD)] and synthetic cannabinoids (Abuhasira et al. 2018).

Considering this global scenario, it is crucial to understand and assess the effects of these regulations on the medicinal use of cannabis and their impact on public health. To ensure ongoing monitoring of access and aid in the development of effective health policies and regulations, numerous challenges must be addressed (Ransing et al. 2022; Mekonen et al. 2025). Figure 1 illustrates a sequence of steps from the use and legalization of cannabis to its acceptance as a medicinal product.

Graduate Program of Pharmaceutical Science, Federal University of Piauí, Teresina, PI, 64049-550, Brazil.
* Corresponding author: marciliapc@ufpi.edu.br

DOI: 10.1201/9781003668190-19

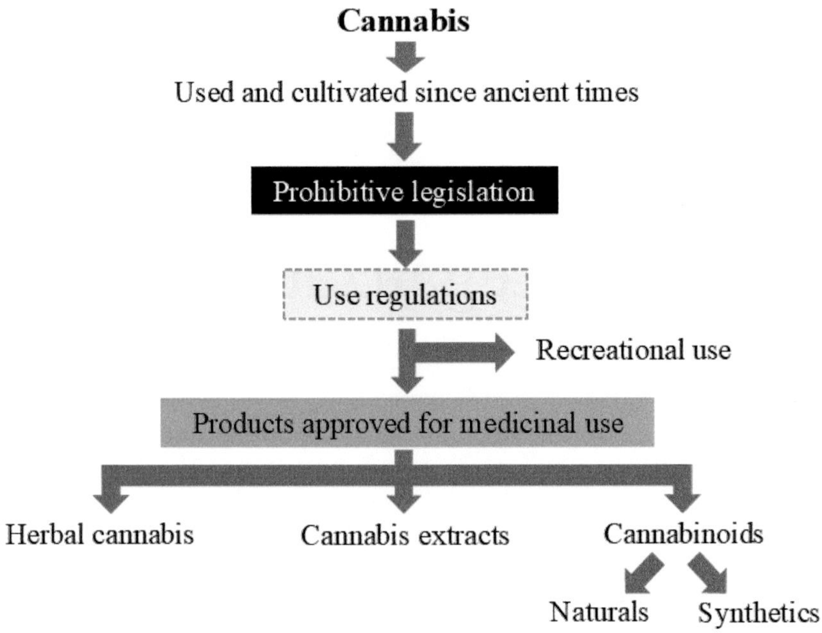

Figure 1: Illustration of how cannabis use has evolved, leading to cannabis-based medicinal products (CBMPs).

In this regard, this chapter focuses on the various authorization models for the use of medicinal cannabis in practice around the world. This analysis will help us better understand the evolution, challenges, and effects of such regulations.

2. International Organizations in Global Cannabis Legislation

Cannabis regulation is heavily influenced by international organizations that establish guidelines, conventions, and recommendations shaping national policies. The United Nations (UN) plays a vital role in setting global standards for drugs, including cannabis (Bewley-Taylor 2013).

In the U.S. in 1937, the Marihuana Tax Act 15 criminalized cannabis use, causing its consumption to decline rapidly. This Tax Act was comparable to the one imposed on other narcotics by the Harrison Act (Abuhasira et al. 2018; Hong et al. 2024).

In 1961, cannabis, cannabis resins, and extracts were classified under Schedule I and Schedule IV. Schedule I covers substances that, among other things, can be converted into substances with a potential for abuse similar to cannabis, cannabis resin, or cocaine. Schedule IV includes substances that are particularly susceptible to abuse and can cause harmful effects. This risk is not offset by significant therapeutic benefits that are not found in substances outside of Schedule IV (Abuhasira et al. 2018). According to the 1961 Single Convention on Narcotic Drugs, cannabis was listed among the most controlled substances for many years, restricting its use and trade (Bewley-Taylor 2013).

In 1970, the U.S. passed the Controlled Substances Act (CSA), which classified cannabis as a Schedule I drug. The CSA reaffirmed the strictest possible federal control of cannabis, and it continues to be the foundation for federal regulation of cannabis today. In 1972, the National Commission on Marihuana and Drug Abuse (The Shafer Commission) considered that cannabis was not a serious health threat and favored social measures for regulation rather than criminalization, similar to controls used for alcohol. Despite the recommendations of the Shafer Commission, cannabis has remained classified in Schedule I (Hong et al. 2024).

In 2019, the World Health Organization (WHO) Expert Committee on Drug Dependence (ECDD) recommended removing cannabis and cannabis resin from Schedule IV of the 1961 UN convention, while retaining them in Schedule I (ECDD2019) (De Souza et al. 2022). In December 2020, the United Nations Commission on Narcotic Drugs (CND) followed the ECDD's recommendation (United Nations Commission on Narcotic Drugs 2020) (De Souza et al. 2022). The WHO played a crucial role in scientifically reviewing cannabis to support evidence-based policies. The WHO'S ECDD conducted reviews that led to the reclassification of cannabis based on its medicinal properties and features, influencing the decisions of the Commission on Narcotic Drugs (WHO 2019). This historic decision moved cannabis out of the strictest category, recognizing its medicinal benefits and removing barriers to clinical and research use, encouraging countries to revisit their domestic laws (UNODC 2020; Banerjee et al. 2022). Figure 2 illustrates a timeline of key milestones in cannabis legislation.

Another concern with the increasing legalization for medicinal use was the quality of the inputs. It is known that cultivation and primary processing of cannabis affect the quality of the active pharmaceutical ingredients, so these steps should comply with the provisions of the UN Conventions and the WHO guidelines on good agricultural and collection practices for medicinal plants. These guidelines have been recommended to other countries, including a quality control system for plant inputs, from cultivation to distribution (Lipnik-Štangelj and Razinger 2020).

The Organization of American States (OAS) operates regionally, promoting cooperation among countries in the Americas on cannabis and drug policies overall, with support from the Inter-American Drug Abuse Control Commission (CICAD). The OAS has backed various policy approaches, including harm reduction, decriminalization, and regulation (CICAD 2022).

Therefore, the UN, WHO, and OAS are essential to the worldwide effort to decriminalize and legalize cannabis for both medicinal and recreational purposes. These organizations also observe the global shift in policies related to cannabis use and trade, facilitate international discussion, and fully support the development of legal frameworks.

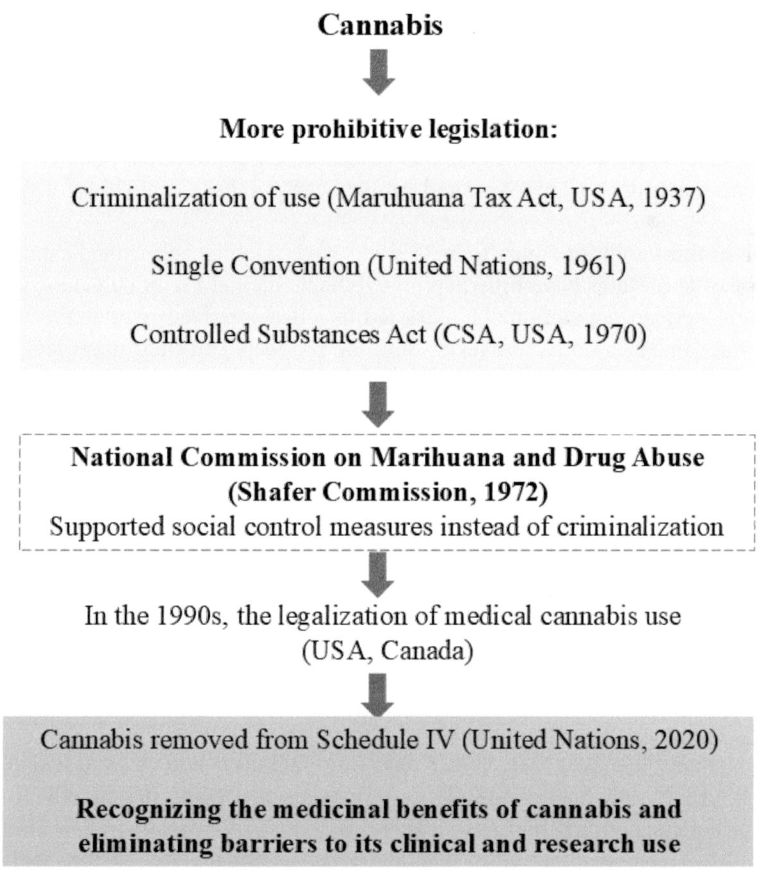

Figure 2: Legislative milestones on cannabis and its legalization for medicinal use.

3. Regulations and Legalization on the Continents

Given that the legality and use of cannabis vary considerably from country to country and region to region, this topic will focus on the prohibition or controlled use of medical cannabis in countries where these legal aspects are well established.

3.1 North America

The legalization of cannabis for medicinal use is being led by three different regulatory systems in North America: the U.S., Canada, and Mexico.

3.1.1 U.S.

After nearly a century of prohibiting the use, possession, and sale of *Cannabis sativa* for medicinal and recreational purposes, the U.S. has begun initiating movements and legal reforms at the state level. These efforts have led to the establishment of regulated markets to accommodate the ongoing changes in cannabis legalization (Firth et al. 2020; Lee 2023).

However, the legalization process in the U.S. occurred in a decentralized manner because, under federal law, cannabis is classified as a Schedule I drug, meaning it is not accepted for medical use and has a high potential for abuse (2025). Conversely, some states have passed their laws governing the medical and recreational use of cannabis. These regulations include requirements for consumption, as well as regulations related to cultivation, distribution, sale, and taxation. These regulations differ considerably among U.S. states (Cerdá et al. 2020; Pacula et al. 2023).

In 1996, Californians approved the use of cannabis for the treatment of nausea, weight loss, pain, muscle spasms, and other severe medical conditions. Since then, more than 30 jurisdictions in the U.S. have legalized the medical use of cannabis in various forms. The regulations differ from state to state regarding the medical conditions recognized, the types of products permitted, and the methods of obtaining them, whether through home cultivation or purchasing from dispensaries. Some states limit the use of cannabis to products with high cannabidiol (CBD) content and low tetrahydrocannabinol (THC) content. In contrast, more liberal states allow patients to use cannabis for any condition that a doctor approves, and patients can purchase cannabis at dispensaries (Hall et al. 2019).

As a result of this evolution, more than 35 states have established medical cannabis programs. Thus, over 50% of U.S. states have fully authorized the medicinal use of cannabis, which accounts for 72% of the American population. This has led to a decentralized regulatory model, in which each state operates independently. However, both the products and their users technically remain in violation of U.S. federal law (Hall and Lynskey 2020; Fortin et al. 2022; Hameed et al. 2023; Farrelly et al. 2023).

3.1.2 Canada

Canada was one of the first countries to approve a medical cannabis access program in 1999. The regulations governing patient eligibility and legal sources of supply have changed over time. With this evolution, Canada has created a regulated national cannabis industry that offers products in different dosage forms (Shim et al. 2023).

Medical cannabis was legalized in Canada in 2001, and over the next two decades, regulations were put in place to improve access for patients (Hall et al. 2023). In 2001, Health Canada established the Medical Marijuana Access Regulations, which required patients to apply for authorization to possess cannabis. This regulation stipulated that patients must provide written documentation from their physician, stating that they were either receiving palliative care or experiencing debilitating symptoms from specific medical conditions or treatments that could not be effectively managed with conventional medications (Shim et al. 2023).

In 2013, Health Canada replaced the Medical Access to Cannabis Regulations with the Cannabis for Medical Purposes Regulations, which came into effect on April 1, 2014. These new regulations eliminated Health Canada's role in authorizing patient access to medical cannabis, shifting that responsibility to physicians (Shim et al. 2023).

3.1.3 Mexico

In 2021, Mexico enacted regulations for the medicinal use of cannabis aimed at managing, controlling, promoting, and overseeing the health aspects of raw materials, pharmacological derivatives, and cannabis-based medications. The approval of the General Health Law on Health Control for the Production, Research, and Medicinal Use of Cannabis and its Pharmacological Derivatives facilitated controlled and safe access to cannabis-based treatments for patients with specific illnesses. This represented a significant milestone in the journey toward comprehensive regulation of medicinal cannabis in Mexico (Ruiz and Garcia 2025).

3.2 South America

South America presents a diverse landscape of cannabis regulation, with countries at varying stages of legalization and distinct control models (Alvarez et al. 2023). A significant advancement in the region has been the establishment of legal frameworks for medical cannabis in several countries, including Brazil, Argentina, Uruguay, Bolivia, Chile, Colombia, Costa Rica, Ecuador, Panama, Paraguay, and Peru (Durán-Martínez and Pennell, 2024). However, Venezuela, Guyana, and French Guiana have not yet legalized the medicinal use of cannabis (De Souza et al. 2022).

3.2.1 Brazil

In Brazil, the use of medicinal cannabis requires a medical prescription and authorization from the National Health Surveillance Agency – ANVISA (De Souza et al. 2022). In 2015, ANVISA issued a regulatory decision that removed cannabidiol from the list of prohibited substances and repositioned it on the list of controlled drugs in class C1, which means that it requires a medical prescription (Brasil 2015a).

In the same year, RDC No. 17 established standards and procedures for the importation of cannabidiol-based products for non-commercial use, marking a significant milestone in the regulation of licensed medicines in Brazil (Brasil 2015b). The most recent rules for importing cannabis-derived products in Brazil are outlined in RDC No. 660/2022. This regulation specifies the criteria and procedures for individuals to import cannabis derivatives for personal use, provided they have a prescription from a qualified healthcare professional to treat various medical conditions (Brasil 2022).

3.2.2 Argentina

In Argentina, cannabis regulation began with Law No. 27,350, enacted in March 2017. This law established the first legal framework for cannabis in a non-punitive sense, focusing specifically on its medicinal use (Aguilar et al. 2022). Law No. 27,350 addresses "Medical and Scientific Research on the Medicinal Use of the Cannabis Plant and its Derivatives" and aims to create a regulatory framework for research into the medicinal, therapeutic, and analgesic applications of cannabis and its derivatives.

Additionally, this law established the National Program for the Study and Research of the Medicinal Use of the Cannabis Plant, its Derivatives, and Unconventional Treatments, which operates under the supervision of the Argentine Ministry of Health (De Vito 2017). Known as the "Medicinal Cannabis Law," it established mechanisms to ensure free access to treatment for individuals enrolled in the Cannabis Program (Fraga and Prado 2025).

In 2020, Decree 883 (DCTO-2020-883-APN-PTE-Law, No. 27,350 Regulation) was approved, establishing medical and scientific research into the medicinal use of the cannabis plant and its derivatives. This regulation was a step forward, as it ended the ban imposed over the last 60 years on the cultivation of cannabis in the country. The decree allows restricted access to cannabis derivatives for medicinal, therapeutic, and palliative use by individuals and communities, allowing for authorized individual and community production of cannabis (Sedan et al. 2023).

Another significant advancement was the regulation of Argentina's cannabis production chain through the passage of Law No. 27,669 in 2022. The law establishes a regulatory framework to promote the development of the medical cannabis and industrial hemp industry, aiming to regulate the national production, commercialization, and export of cannabis and its derivatives for medicinal, scientific research, and industrial purposes (Argentina 2022).

3.2.3 Uruguay

In 2013, Uruguay became the first country in the world to legalize the cultivation and sale of cannabis under Law No. 19,172 on "Marijuana and its derivatives." According to Guido et al. (2020) and Alvarez et al. (2023), this law covers the "state control and regulation of importation, production, acquisition, storage, marketing, and distribution."

3.2.4 Colombia

Colombia is another pioneering model in Latin America, focusing on the medicinal and economic use of cannabis (Cubillos Sanchez 2021). Due to its geographical location, which provides suitable climatic conditions for cannabis production practically all year round, Colombia has positioned itself as one of the leading exporters of cannabis (Rosero-Ceballos et al. 2025). Since 2015, Colombia has made significant progress in regulating the medicinal and scientific use of cannabis, allowing its cultivation for therapeutic, industrial, and research purposes.

3.2.5 Paraguay, Bolivia, Chile, and Peru

In Paraguay, Congress passed Law No. 6,007/2017, creating a national scientific and medical research program on cannabis, as well as a national registry that gives patients free access to these products. However, the law did not remove medical cannabis from the list of illegal drugs, nor did it legalize home cultivation (Durán-Martínez and Pennell 2024).

Bolivia allows the medicinal use of cannabis, but not its production. Access requires import licenses (Durán-Martínez and Pennell 2024).

Chile became the first Latin American country to legalize the cultivation of cannabis for medicinal use. In 2013, cannabis cultivation was authorized in La Florida, a municipality in the Santiago metropolitan area, to produce oils for two hundred patients in a clinical study. Then, in 2015, the Secretariat of Public Health issued Resolution 432, which allowed the use of cannabis oil in medical treatments. They also issued Decree 84, which authorized the sale of the oil in pharmacies with a prescription (Duran-Martinez and Pennell 2024).

In 2019, Peru passed Law No. 30,681, which regulates the medicinal and therapeutic use of cannabis and its derivatives (Guido et al. 2020). The law states that the Peruvian General Directorate of Medicines, Supplies, and Drugs is responsible for issuing licenses for production, importation, commercialization, and inspection (Lima 2019).

3.3 Europe

Cannabis and cannabinoids play a role in pharmacotherapy across European Union member states (Lipnik-Štangelj and Razinger 2020). However, cannabis regulatory models differ across countries based on their legal traditions and public health policies. In Europe, the most commonly authorized medicinal cannabis products are standardized cannabinoid-based medicines. Only six European countries—the Netherlands, Italy, Germany, Portugal, the Czech Republic, and Denmark—have programs that permit patients to access cannabis, such as herbal preparations (Fortin et al. 2022).

Medicinal cannabis cultivation in the European Union is currently allowed in Austria, the Czech Republic, Italy, Germany, Greece, Malta, the Netherlands, and Portugal. All of these member states have established a cannabis cultivation authority and outlined its responsibilities (Lipnik-Štangelj and Razinger 2020).

The Netherlands was the first European Union (EU) member state to develop a strategy to give patients access to medical cannabis in 1998. At that time, the goal of this initiative was to grow cannabis that met pharmaceutical standards and to make it available for research and development of approved medical products. In 2001, the Netherlands revised its medical cannabis policy to allow patients with a prescription to access it. Since then, more EU member states have made cannabis accessible for medical purposes (Knöss et al. 2019).

Italy has regulations governing the use of medicinal cannabis. Cannabis for this purpose is produced by the Pharmaceutical Chemical Military Facility in Florence (Baratta et al. 2021). In Italy, cannabis has been a prescription drug since 1998 (Cortellini et al. 2019), and in 2015, the prescription of cannabis for medical use and its pharmaceutical preparations were regulated (Russo et al. 2021).

In 2017, Germany legalized prescribing cannabis flowers for medical use, removing the previous requirement that patients go through a one-year legal process to get permission for its use (Manthey et al. 2024). In 2018, the United Kingdom regulated the medicinal use of cannabis, mainly due to pressure from patients and media coverage caused by reports of improvements in intractable epilepsy in children (Schlag et al. 2020).

In Portugal, Law No. 33/2018 legalized the use of medicines, preparations, and substances derived from the cannabis plant for medicinal purposes. The law was supported by Decree-Law No. 8/2019, which regulated the cultivation, extraction, and commercial activities related to these formulations. In 2019, the National Institute of Pharmacy and Medicines issued a list of conditions for which the use of cannabinoids for medicinal purposes was approved, with the caveat that they should only be prescribed when conventional treatments with authorized medications did not work or caused significant adverse effects (Silva et al. 2021).

In France, medical cannabis remains illegal. The country has one of the strictest illicit drug laws in Europe (Wallez et al. 2024). However, in 2021, a nationwide experimental medicinal cannabis program was launched to feasibly provide medicinal cannabis to people with serious chronic illnesses that are not adequately relieved by other treatments (Barré et al. 2024; Wallez et al. 2024).

In Spain, the medical use of cannabis is not yet regulated. However, in 2022, the Spanish Congress approved a report examining experiences regulating cannabis for medical purposes and has already established the Spanish Medical Cannabis Association (AECAME) (CMS, 2024). As shown in this topic, the legalization of cannabis for medicinal use in the European Union varies widely, and there is a trend toward regulation in some countries that have not yet implemented it.

3.4 Asia-Pacific and Africa

Cannabis policies in Asia and Africa are generally much more restrictive. Several countries have strict laws on the use, cultivation, and sale of the plant, along with penalties (Areesantichai et al. 2020; Thippaiah et al. 2025).

Recently, many countries in the Asia-Pacific region, including East and South Asia, Southeast Asia, and Oceania, have legalized medical cannabis. In Australia, New Zealand, and Thailand, medicinal use has been legalized, while in South Korea and Singapore, it is limited. It remains illegal in China, Japan, Cambodia, Indonesia, Laos, Malaysia, Myanmar, the Philippines, and Vietnam (Areesantichai et al. 2020).

In 2016, Australia became the first country in the Asia-Pacific region to legalize medical cannabis. Laws for personal use and cultivation were enacted by the Australian Capital Territory Legislative Assembly in 2019 and took effect in 2020 (Areesantichai et al. 2020).

Thailand became the first country in Asia to permit the use and possession of cannabis leaves in February 2021, and the entire plant in June 2022, following approval for medicinal use in 2019 (Kalayasiri and Boonthae 2023).

Africa has the fewest countries with authorization for medical cannabis use. Although cannabis is widely used across the continent as an illegal recreational drug in many countries, its medical potential is often overlooked (Adebisi and Olaoye 2022). In Africa, only South Africa, Kenya, and Ethiopia have legalized cannabis for medical purposes (Ransing et al. 2022).

4. Cannabis-Derived Medicines Approved for Medicinal Use

Of the hundreds of different molecules found in cannabis, the most abundant, most studied, and most pharmacologically interesting phytocannabinoids are delta-9-tetrahydrocannabinol (THC) and cannabidiol (CBD) (Fortin et al. 2022; Chandy et al. 2024).

To date, the U.S. Food and Drug Administration (FDA) has approved four drugs: the synthetic cannabinoid, Epidiolex®; and three synthetic THC drugs: Marinol® (dronabinol), Syndros® (dronabinol), and Cesamet® (nabilone) (Chandy et al. 2024; Hong et al. 2024). Epidiolex® has been approved by the FDA for treating chemotherapy-induced nausea and vomiting and epilepsy (Chandy et al. 2024). The medication has also received approval for the treatment of seizures in patients diagnosed with Lennox-Gastaut syndrome, Dravet syndrome, or tuberous sclerosis complex, provided that the patient is at least two years of age. Marinol® and Syndros® are approved for managing HIV/AIDS-induced anorexia and chemotherapy-induced nausea and vomiting (CINV) in patients who do not respond well to standard antiemetics (Hong et al. 2024).

The majority of European countries have outlawed the use of herbal cannabis, while cannabinoid-based medicines are legal in many of them. Cannabinoid-based medicines, particularly nabiximols, have achieved widespread acceptance and are authorized for use in most European Union countries (Abuhasira et al. 2018).

In 2016, China showed promising results from research on Cannabidiol (CBD) for epilepsy, gout, Parkinson's disease, autism, depression, and Alzheimer's disease. In 2019, Japan authorized trials with Epidiolex (Areesantichai et al. 2020).

5. Social Impact

The potential risks associated with cannabis use have raised concerns among government authorities in several countries, leading to the development of legislation regarding its consumption, cultivation, and sale (De Souza et al. 2022). These laws initially caused nearly all countries to implement prohibitions as a primary strategy to reduce cannabis use, mainly influenced by political and religious reasons (Ransing et al. 2022).

Laws and regulations are evolving worldwide. Since the late 1980s, many countries have gradually shifted away from strict prohibition policies and adopted alternative approaches (Decorte 2020). Awareness of the therapeutic benefits and potential of cannabis-based medical products has increased, leading to the legalization of medicinal cannabis in many nations (De Souza et al. 2022).

Clinical trials with cannabis products have been employed for various medical conditions, including chronic pain, some treatment-resistant epilepsies, amyotrophic lateral sclerosis, psychological and psychiatric disorders, Parkinson's disease, Alzheimer's disease, and nausea and vomiting caused by chemotherapy (Fortin et al. 2022; De Souza et al. 2022; Banerjee et al. 2022). Despite the benefits of cannabis-based products in relieving suffering for many patients unresponsive to traditional treatments, issues related to cannabis use disorders, adverse effects, and drug interactions must also be addressed (Kocis et al. 2023; Hall et al. 2025). Therefore, further research is needed to support these therapeutic indications and to understand the risks associated with long-term use of these products (De Souza et al. 2022).

Sociopolitical factors, religion, culture, clinical practice, and policies and programs across countries often influence cannabis dependence or abuse. This use can also cause behavioral changes that lead to aggression, school dropout, and disability, as well as high socioeconomic costs (Ransing et al. 2022). Bahji and Stephenson (2019) posit that cannabis use can induce short-term effects, including impairment of short-term memory, motor coordination, and judgment. In the long term, disorders are worsened by dependence, impaired brain development, decreased educational and cognitive performance, and a higher risk of chronic psychotic disorders, among other factors. Furthermore, fatal harm is also a concern for people who regularly use cannabinoids or are dependent, including the risks of injury, car accidents, and suicide.

To prevent patients from turning to the illegal cannabis market or self-cultivation, implementing price control policies for cannabis-based medicines is essential to stop abusive practices. Globally, cannabis is the most widely used illegal drug, and government authorities have acknowledged the failures of repressive policies in controlling its abuse, along with the negative consequences, such as increasing social injustices and inefficient use of public resources (De Souza et al. 2022).

Therefore, understanding all these factors related to beneficial use and its risks is important to guide public health policies on cannabis use more broadly (Ransing et al. 2022). However, the consequences of widespread legalization and liberalization of cannabis growing worldwide are unpredictable, and the results will only be known in the future (Bahji and Stephenson 2019).

6. Conclusion and Perspectives

Growing international recognition of the medicinal properties of cannabis and its derivatives has increased interest among researchers and the pharmaceutical industry. This has caused some countries to enact state laws that conflict with federal laws. The breadth of these laws has been crucial for regulating all stakeholders, including producers and traders of inputs and products, healthcare professionals, and patients.

Currently, beyond medicinal use, cannabis has gained popularity in many countries that have decriminalized access, personal possession, and recreational use. Additionally, non-medicinal and cannabis-based medicinal products are expanding in the market. The widespread availability of these products sparks much public health debate and calls for educational policies to inform society about abuse, addiction, and other adverse events. Failing to follow legal requirements related to the production, access, and use of cannabis and its derivatives can result in serious social and public health issues.

Therefore, laws governing medicinal cannabis must be strictly enforced to ensure product quality, the credibility of clinical research, control over access to products, patient safety, and the success of treatments.

References

Abuhasira, R., Shbiro, L., and Landschaft, Y. (2018). Medical use of cannabis and cannabinoids containing products-Regulations in Europe and North America. *European Journal of Internal Medicine*, 49: 2–6.

Adebisi, Y., and Olaoye, D. (2022). Medical Use of Cannabis in Africa: The Pharmacists' Perspective. *Innovations in Pharmacy*, 13(1): 8.

Aguilar, Ó., Díaz, M. C., and Romero, L. (2022). Citizen science towards the regulation of medical cannabis in Argentina. *Tapuya: Latin American Science, Technology and Society*, 5: 2100037.

Alvarez, E., Queirolo, R., and Sotto, B. (2023). Conflicting forces in the implementation of medicinal cannabis regulation in Uruguay. *Journal of Cannabis Research*, 5(1): 26.

Areesantichai, C., Perngparn, U., and Pilley, C. (2020). Current cannabis-related situation in the Asia-Pacific region. *Current Opinion in Psychiatry*, 33(4): 352–359.

ARGENTINA. Ley n.º 27669, de 26 de maio de 2022. Marco regulatorio para el desarrollo de la industria del cannabis medicinal y el cáñamo industrial. Available at: <https://www.argentina.gob.ar/normativa/nacional/ley-27669-365303/texto>. Accessed:14/06/25.

Baratta, F., Simiele, M., Pignata, I., Ravetto Enri, L., Torta, R., De Luca, A. et al. (2021). Cannabis-based oral formulations for medical purposes: preparation, quality and stability. *Pharmaceuticals*, 14(2): 171.

Barré, T., Cazorla, G., Di Beo, V., Lopez, F., Radoszycki, L., Maradan, G. et al. (2024). Acceptability of and attitudes to the therapeutic use of cannabis and cannabidiol in people with Parkinson's disease: A French survey. *Clinical Parkinsonism & Related Disorders*, 11: 100286.

Bahji, A., and Stephenson, C. (2019). International Perspectives on the Implications of Cannabis Legalization: A Systematic Review & Thematic Analysis. *International Journal of Environmental Research and Public Health*, 16(17): 3095.

Banerjee, R., Erridge, S., Salazar, O., Mangal, N., Couch, D., Pacchetti, B. et al. (2022). Real World Evidence in Medical Cannabis Research. *Therapeutic Innovation & Regulatory Science*, 56: 8–14.

Bewley-Taylor, D. R. (2013). Towards revision of the UN drug control conventions: Harnessing like-mindedness. *International Journal of Drug Policy*, 24(1): 60–68.

BRASIL. Agência Nacional de Vigilância Sanitária - ANVISA (2015a) Resolução da Diretoria Colegiada – RDC n. 3, de 26 de janeiro de 2015. Diário Oficial da União 1(19): 37.

BRASIL. Agência Nacional de Vigilância Sanitária - ANVISA (2015b) Resolução da Diretoria Colegiada – RDC n. 17, de 6 de maio de 2015. Diário Oficial da União 1(86): 43.

BRASIL. Agência Nacional de Vigilância Sanitária – ANVISA (2022) Resolução da Diretoria Colegiada – RDC n. 660, de 30 de março de 2022. Diário Oficial da União 1: 199.

Cáceres Guido, P., Riva, N., Calle, G., Dell'Orso, M., Gatto, M., Sberna, N. et al. (2020). Medicinal cannabis in Latin America: History, current state of regulation, and the role of the pharmacist in a new clinical experience with cannabidiol oil. *Journal of the American Pharmacists Association*, 60: 212–215.

Cerdá, M., Mauro, C., Hamilton, A., Levy, N. S., Santaella-Tenorio, J., Hasin, D. et al. (2020). Association Between Recreational Marijuana Legalization in the United States and Changes in Marijuana Use and Cannabis Use Disorder From 2008 to 2016. *JAMA Psychiatry*, 77(2): 165–171.

Chandy, M., Nishiga, M., Wei, T. T., Hamburg, N. M., Nadeau, K., and Wu, J. C. (2024). Adverse Impact of Cannabis on Human Health. *Annual Review of Medicine*, 75: 353–367.

CMS (2024). Cannabis law and legislation in Spain. Available at: <https://cms.law/en/int/expert-guides/cms-expert-guide-to-a-legal-roadmap-to-cannabis/spain#:~:text=United%20Arab%20Emirates-,Medical%20 use,medicinal%20cannabis%20is%20not%20regulated> Accessed:14/06/25.

COMISIÓN INTERAMERICANA PARA EL CONTROL DEL ABUSO DE DROGAS - CICAD (2022) Informe sobre políticas de drogas en las Américas. Washington, D.C.: OEA. Available at: <https://www.oas.org/es/cicad/>. Accessed:15/06/25.

Cortellini, A., Porzio, G., Cofini, V., Necozione, S., Giusti, R., Marchetti, P. et al. (2019). What cancer patients actually know regarding medical cannabis? A cross-sectional survey with a critical analysis of the current attitudes. *Journal of Oncology Pharmacy Practice*, 25(6): 1439–1444.

Cubillos Sánchez, P. A. (2020). Cannabis for medical and scientific purposes: the Colombian landscape. *Colombian Journal of Anesthesiology*, 49: e954. https://www.revcolanest.com.co/index.php/rca/article/view/954.

DEA – Drug Enforcement Administration. Schedules of Controlled Substances: Rescheduling of Marijuana. Washington DC (2024). Available at: <https://www.dea.gov/sites/default/files/2024-05/Scheduling%20 NPRM%20508.pdf > Accessed:15/06/25.

Decorte, T., Lenton, S., and Wilkins, C. (2020). Legalizing Cannabis: Experiences, Lessons and Scenarios. New York: Routledge.

De Souza, M. R., Henriques, A. T., and Limberger, R. P. (2022). Medical cannabis regulation: an overview of models around the world with emphasis on the Brazilian scenario. *Journal of Cannabis Research*, 4: 33.

De Vito, E. L. (2017). Argentina tiene su primera ley sobre el uso medicinal de la planta de cannabis. Historia y perspectivas. *Medicina*, 77(5): 388–393.

Durán-Martínez, A., and Pennell, C. (2024). Change from Above or Pressure from Below? The Diffusion of Cannabis Reform in Latin America. *Bulletin of Latin American Research*, 43: 347–361.

Farrelly, K. N., Wardell, J. D., Marsden, E., Scarfe, M. L., Najdzionek, P., Turna, J. et al. (2023). The Impact of Recreational Cannabis Legalization on Cannabis Use and Associated Outcomes: A Systematic Review. *Substance Abuse: Research and Treatment*, 17: 117822182311720.

Firth, C. L., Hajat, A., Dilley, J. A., Braun, M., and Maher, J. E. (2020). Implications of Cannabis Legalization on Juvenile Justice Outcomes and Racial Disparities. *American Journal of Preventive Medicine*, 58(4): 562–569.

Fortin, D., Marcellin, F., Carrieri, P., Mancini, J., and Barré, T. (2022). Medical Cannabis: Toward a New Policy and Health Model for an Ancient Medicine. *Frontiers in Public Health*, 10: 904291.

Fraga, P., and Prado, M. (2025). A construção de um direito: A regulamentação da Cannabis medicinal na Argentina e no Brasil. *Saúde e Sociedade*, 34(1): 1–12.

Hall, W., and Lynskey, M. (2020). Assessing the public health impacts of legalizing recreational cannabis use: the US experience. *World Psychiatry*, 19(2): 179–186.

Hall, W., Manthey, J., and Stjepanović, D (2025). Cannabis use and cannabis use disorders and their treatment in Europe. *European Archives of Psychiatry and Clinical Neuroscience*, 275: 307–313.

Hall, W., Stjepanović, D., Caulkins, J., Lynskey, M., Leung, J., Campbell, G. et al. (2019). Public health implications of legalising the production and sale of cannabis for medicinal and recreational use. *Lancet* (London, England), 394(10208): 1580–1590.

Hall, W., Stjepanović, D., Dawson, D., and Leung, J. (2023). The implementation and public health impacts of cannabis legalization in Canada: a systematic review. *Addiction*, 118: 2062–2072.

Hameed, M., Prasad, S., Jain, E., Dogrul, B. N., Al-Oleimat, A., Pokhrel, B. et al. (2023). Medical Cannabis for Chronic Nonmalignant Pain Management. *Current Pain and Headache Reports*, 27(4): 57–63.

Hong, G., Sideris, A., Waldman, S., Stauffer, J., and Wu, C. L. (2024). Legal and Regulatory Aspects of Medical Cannabis in the United States. *Anesthesia and Analgesia*, 138: 31–41.

Kalayasiri, R., and Boonthae, S. (2023). Trends of cannabis use and related harms before and after legalization for recreational purpose in a developing country in Asia. *BMC Public Health*, 23(1): 911.

Knöss, W., Van de Velde, M., Sandvos, C., and Cremer-Schaeffer, P. (2019). Key elements of legal environments for medical use of cannabis in different countries. Schlüsselelemente der rechtlichen Rahmenbedingungen für die medizinische Nutzung von Cannabis in verschiedenen Ländern. Bundesgesundheitsblatt, Gesundheitsforschung, Gesundheitsschutz, 62(7): 855–860.

Kocis, P. T., Mallinson, D. J., and Servinsky, Jr. T. J. (2024). Cannabinoid Awareness, Reporting Use to Health Care Providers, and Perceptions Regarding Safety - Pennsylvania, March 2023-April 2023. *Medical Cannabis and Cannabinoids*, 7(1): 119–124.

Lee, C. K. (2023). Medicinal cannabis law in the USA: history, movements, trends, and countertrends. *Brazilian Journal of Pain*, 6(1): 7–11.

Levinsohn, E. A., and Hill, K. P. (2020). Clinical uses of cannabis and cannabinoids in the United States. *Journal of The Neurological Sciences*, 411: 116717.

LIMA, Congreso de la República (2019). Decreto Supremo que aprueba el Reglamento de la Ley N° 30681, de 23 de Febrero de 2019. Ley que regula el uso medicinal y terapéutico del Cannabis y sus derivados - DECRETO SUPREMO - N° 005-2019-SA - SALUD. Available at: <https://busquedas.elperuano.pe/dispositivo/NL/1744045-2>. Accessed:15/06/25.

Lipnik-Štangelj, M, and Razinger, B. (2020). A regulatory take on cannabis and cannabinoids for medicinal use in the European Union. *Archives of Industrial Hygiene and Toxicology*, 71(1): 12–18.

Manthey, J., Rehm, J., and Verthein, U. (2024). Germany's cannabis act: a catalyst for European drug policy reform? The Lancet Regional Health. *Europe*, 42: 100929.

Mekonen Yimer, T., Hoch, E., Fischer, B., Dawson, D., and Hall, W. (2025). The adverse public health effects of non-medical cannabis legalisation in Canada and the USA. *The Lancet Public Health*, 10(2): e148–e159.

Mendoza-Chuctaya, G. (2022). Legalisation of medicinal marijuana in Perú. *Revista Colombiana de Psiquiatría*, 51(1): 4–5.

Pacula, R. (2022). Relationships of Cannabis Policy Liberalization with Alcohol Use and Co-Use with Cannabis: A Narrative Review. *Alcohol Research: Current Reviews*, 42(1): 6.

Ransing, R., De La Rosa, P. A., Pereira-Sanchez, V., Handuleh, J. I. M., Jerotic, S., Gupta, A. K. et al. (2022). Current state of cannabis use, policies, and research across sixteen countries: cross-country comparisons and international perspectives. *Trends in Psychiatry and Psychotherapy*, 44(1): e20210263.

Rosero-Ceballos, E. L., and Meneses-Medina, P. A. (2025). Factores socioeconómicos que contribuyen al debate sobre la regulación del consumo de cannabis en Colombia. *Equidad Y Desarrollo*, 4: 1–23.

Ruiz, E. A., and García, J. L. M. (2025). Cannabis medicinal no México: uma análise do projeto de lei para sua regulamentação. *Saúde e Sociedade*, 34(1): 1–14.

Russo, E., Cannas, C., Rivetti, M. S., Villa, C., and Rebesco, B. (2021). Innovative Clinical-Organizational Model to Ensure Appropriateness and Quality in the Management of Medical Cannabis: An Italian Regional Case. *Healthcare*, 9(11): 1425.

Schlag, A. K., Baldwin, D. S., Barnes, M., Bazire, S., Coathup, R., Curran, H. V. et al. (2020). Medical cannabis in the UK: From principle to practice. *Journal of Psychopharmacology*, 34(9): 931–937.

Sedan, D., Vaccarini, C., Demetrio, P., Morante, M., Montiel, R., Saurí, A. et al. (2023). Cannabinoid Content in Cannabis Flowers and Homemade Cannabis-Based Products Used for Therapeutic Purposes in Argentina. *Cannabis and Cannabinoid Research*, 8: 197–206.

Shim, M., Nguyen, H., and Grootendorst, P. (2023). Lessons from 20 years of medical cannabis use in Canada. *PLOS One*, 18: e0271079.

Silva, R. G., Remtula, S. P., and Gonçalves, T. C. (2021). Canabinoides na dor crónica: uma revisão baseada na evidência. *Revista Portuguesa de Clínica Geral*, 37: 133–144.

Thippaiah, S. M., and Gude, J. G. (2025). Recreational Use of Cannabis: Insights from India and Other Asian Countries. *Journal of Psychiatry Spectrum*, 4(3): 211–217.

UNITED NATIONS OFFICE ON DRUGS AND CRIME - UNODC (2020). World drug report 2020. Viena: UNODC. Available at: <https://www.unodc.org/doc/wdr2016/WDR_2016_Chapter_1_Cannabis.pdf >. Accessed: 10/06/25

Wallez, S., Kousignian, I., Hecker, I., Rezag Bara, S. F., Andersen, A. J., Melchior, M. et al. (2024). Factors associated with the use of cannabis for self-medication by adults: data from the French TEMPO cohort study. *Journal of Cannabis Research*, 6(1): 19.

WORLD HEALTH ORGANIZATION (WHO). Critical review report: Cannabidiol - CBD (2018) 40th Expert Committee on Drug Dependence Meeting. Geneva: WHO. Available at: <https://www.who.int/publications/m/item/cannabidiol>. Accessed:10/06/25

Chapter 16

Global Cannabis Policies and Regulatory Frameworks

A Comparative Overview

Pedro Vitor Oliveira Silva Furtado,[1,*] *João Paulo da Silva Gomes,*[1]
Juliana de Sousa Figuerêdo,[1] *Patrícia e Silva Alves,*[1] *Maria Gabryella Castro Moita,*[2]
Maria das Dores Alves de Oliveira[1] and *Chistiane Mendes Feitosa*[1]

1. Introduction

Although widely outlawed in several countries, *Cannabis sativa* has a history of millennia of use by the human species, with records of cultivation dating back some 12,000 years in the Central Asian region. The plant has traditionally been used as food, as a raw material for textiles, and especially for medicinal and pharmacological purposes. With its global spread between the 19th and 20th centuries, cannabis became part of the formulation of various products in countries such as Brazil, which, paradoxically, was one of the first in Latin America to institute a ban on its use, through the so-called "Pito do Pango Law" in 1830. At the time, this legislation reflected a movement of social and moral control, consolidating the criminalization of the plant even in therapeutic contexts (Pierro Neto et al. 2023; Carvalho 2014; Zuardi 2006).

Belonging to the *Cannabaceae* family and the cannabis genus, *Cannabis sativa L.* is a species with a wide phytochemical diversity, containing hundreds of active compounds, among which the cannabinoids stand out. The complexity of its chemical composition and the interaction between its constituents make scientific studies more challenging. Although there has been substantial progress in proving its therapeutic properties, the incorporation of cannabis derivatives into the pharmaceutical market requires proof of quality, efficacy, and safety, as well as compliance with strict regulatory standards to avoid risks to public health, such as intoxication and adverse effects. Despite its potential, the inclusion of cannabis in the clinical context requires a therapeutic model that considers both scientific criteria and the subjective aspects of health care, such as patient autonomy and building effective therapeutic bonds (De Faria and Winkler 2021; ElSohly and Slade 2005; Russo 2016).

[1] Centro de Ciências da Natureza, Universidade Federal do Piauí, 64049-550, Teresina, Brazil.
[2] Instituto Federal do Piauí - Campus Teresina Central, 64000-040, Teresina, Brazil.
* Corresponding author: pedrovitor_furtado@hotmail.com

DOI: 10.1201/9781003668190-20

The contemporary regulatory models applied to cannabis range from total prohibition to full legalization, including decriminalization and exclusively medicinal legalization. Each of these models reflects different political, health, and socio-cultural configurations. During the 20th century, the hegemony of the prohibitionist paradigm, anchored in moral, health, and public safety discourses, led to the criminalization of the cultivation, possession, and use of the plant—even in therapeutic contexts. This paradigm was consolidated by international regulations, such as the 1961 Single Convention on Narcotic Drugs, which imposed severe restrictions on research and the medical application of cannabis, reinforcing the social stigma associated with its use. However, since the 21st century, there has been a regulatory shift driven by scientific evidence about cannabinoids, especially Δ9-tetrahydrocannabinol (THC) and cannabidiol (CBD), as well as social pressure for access to alternative treatments. In this context, different countries have adopted more flexible regulatory frameworks aimed at reducing harm, expanding access to treatments, and increasing the economic value of the plant (Fraga and Brandão 2025; Martins and Posso 2023; Fischer et al. 2022).

Although cannabis regulatory models have different impacts, recent analysis indicates that simple legislative change does not ensure uniform social and health outcomes. Studies highlight that decriminalization, while reducing the criminal burden on users, does not eliminate the illicit market or necessarily promote safe and equitable access, as legal frameworks often remain fragmented and unclear. Medical legalization, while expanding therapeutic possibilities and encouraging scientific research, still faces regulatory challenges related to product standardization and integration into public health systems. Full legalization, on the other hand, in addition to broadly regulating the production chain, requires robust control mechanisms and preventive policies to mitigate the potential increase in problematic consumption, which requires a delicate balance between individual freedom, collective health, and social justice. In addition, the global context shows that reforms must be accompanied by rigorous epidemiological monitoring and continuous legislative adjustments, taking into account the cultural, economic, and political specificities of each country, so that regulatory progress effectively contributes to harm reduction (Svrakic et al. 2012; Hussain et al. 2021; Hall 2020).

2. Theoretical and Methodological Foundations

The heterogeneity of cannabis regulatory models worldwide, driven by distinct historical, cultural, and political realities, underscores the need for a comparative study to identify the patterns, advances, and limitations intrinsic to each regulatory approach. This comparative analysis, based on a qualitative methodology involving documentary review, legislative analysis, and study of specialized literature, selects representative countries across both geopolitics and regulatory diversity, ranging from total prohibition to full legalization. The choice of cases also took into account socio-cultural relevance and the availability of consistent data to ensure the validity of the analysis. This procedure aims to foster an understanding of the legal, social, and health implications of drug policies, thereby improving public health strategies and the formulation of evidence-based policies (Hussain et al. 2021; Hall 2020).

3. North America and Latin America

3.1 Canada

Canada became the second country globally, after only Uruguay, to legalize, produce, sell, and regulate the use of cannabis for recreational or non-medical purposes, which occurred through the Cannabis Act in October 2018, and the first in the G7. Therapeutic use was legalized in 2001 (Hall et al. 2023).

In which a system of state control over the possession, cultivation, production, distribution, and sale of the species was established, to protect young people from access to products derived from the plant, ensure that adults can obtain controlled-quality cannabis products, and consequently prevent criminal organizations from profiting from the trade of the substance, rigorously throughout the country's territory. Therefore, the Canadian model chose to prioritize consumer health protection, reducing the illegal market, and public safety (Ng et al. 2022; Rubin-kahana et al. 2022).

The Cannabis Law established a minimum age of 18 for consuming the substance, with possession restricted to 30 grams in public spaces and permission for home cultivation of up to 4 plants per residence, as well as the sharing of cannabis with other adults. However, some cities like Quebec and Manitoba have decided to prohibit home cultivation (Hall et al. 2023; Rubin-kahana et al. 2022).

The impacts of cannabis consumption, along with cannabis legislation and regulation in Canada, have indicated an increase among adults; however, there has been no significant increase or decrease among adolescents/students. A reduction in prison populations and cannabis prices has also been observed. Consequently, there was a considerable decrease in crime among young people aged 12 to 17, among both boys and girls. However, consumer demand and access to safe products still require regulatory adjustments (Hall et al. 2020).

In short, the legalization of cannabis in Canada has proven to be an innovative policy that balances freedom and state control. However, despite bringing economic and social benefits, the system still faces adjustments that require constant adaptations, so that, in the future, Canadian legislation can serve as a model for other nations regarding cannabis regulation, documenting and demonstrating advances and complexities from implementation, transition, and consolidation (Mekonen et al. 2025).

3.2 United States

The cannabis landscape in the United States is complex, with a duality between federal and state laws that creates both challenges and opportunities (Ortega-Bolaños et al. 2024). At the federal level, cannabis is classified as a Schedule I drug, indicating a high potential for abuse and a lack of acceptable medical use (Meneze et al. 2024; Shankar and Gupta 2024). However, many states have legalized cannabis for medicinal or recreational purposes, creating a conflict with federal law (Kamyab et al. 2023). This divergence between federal and state laws has created a series of challenges and tensions for patients, providers, and companies in the medicinal product sector, with an emphasis on cannabis (Perlman et al. 2021).

State legalization has generated debates about the impact on public health (Auguskani 2025). It is noteworthy that proponents highlight the therapeutic potential of medicinal cannabis, while critics express concerns about increased consumption and adverse effects on mental health (Kamyab et al. 2023; Nargis 2025). Furthermore, some studies suggest that legalizing medical cannabis may be associated with lower rates of opioid concentrations, substances derived from opium that function by acting on opioid receptors in the brain, producing pain relief and sedation effects, and overdose deaths (Hasin et al. 2017).

Economically, state legalization has created new industries and tax revenues (Berk 2025). However, cannabis companies face obstacles due to discrepancies between federal laws, including difficulties accessing banking services and tax deductions (Kamyab et al. 2023). The lack of clarity in federal-level regulation also creates uncertainty for investors and businesses (Coggon and Kamunge-Kpodo 2022). Furthermore, the lack of understanding regarding federal-level regulation creates uncertainty for investors and hinders interstate expansion (Brill et al. 2024). As a result, the lack of clarity regarding federal legalization creates an atmosphere of insecurity for companies and individuals operating in the cannabis industry, as well as for states that have legalized cannabis (Mallinson et al. 2020).

Rights advocates argue that states should have autonomy to determine their own policies without federal interference (Mallinson et al. 2020). They are more aware of responding to the needs and concerns of their citizens through a unique and appropriate approach (Coggon and Kamunge-Kpodo 2022). On the other hand, proponents of federal law argue that the federal government has the right to continue to classify it as a dangerous substance and that state legalization undermines efforts to prevent drug use and protect public health (Miller and Saad 2017).

The coexistence of federal and state laws presents challenges for marginalized groups that can lead to cannabis-related offenses (Tobey et al. 2019), such as detention and deportation, even if these actions are legal under state law (Bruzelius and Martins 2024). As of 2023, many states have legalized cannabis for medicinal or recreational purposes, and more states are expected to follow suit in the coming years (Hong et al. 2023). The future of cannabis policy in the United States remains uncertain, but the coexistence of federal and state laws will continue to shape the legal, economic, and social landscape in the coming years (Sandler et al. 2019).

Therefore, the duality between federal and state legislation regarding cannabis consumption in the United States is an issue with significant implications for public health, the economy, and social justice. As the landscape evolves, it is important to ensure consistent, jurisprudentially supported legalization to mitigate future impacts on different political and social approaches (Schauer 2021; Nargis 2025).

3.3 Uruguay

In 2013, Uruguay became the first country in the world to regulate the cannabis market, marking changes in global drug policies (Boidi et al. 2016; Tesalonika and Kusumawardani 2019). This pioneering decision, led by then-President José Mujica, addressed public health and safety issues by removing the cannabis market from the control of criminal groups and placing it under state control (Alvarez et al. 2023). Uruguayan law allows access to this substance through three means: home cultivation, cannabis clubs, and pharmacies (Queirolo et al. 2025).

State regulation in Uruguay focuses on accessibility, aiming to ensure safe, regulated access to cannabis for registered users (Queirolo et al. 2025). However, implementation through pharmacies has faced obstacles, with only a limited number of pharmacies participating (Alvarez et al. 2023). Cannabis clubs, where members cultivate together, have proven to be a popular alternative, but they face regulatory challenges. (Boidi and Queirolo 2016; Pardal et al. 2020). Home cultivation is also an alternative, providing greater autonomy over one's cannabis supply and its users (Aguiar and Musto 2022). Thus, one of the main objectives of the law was to guarantee safe and controlled access to registered users, to weaken organized crime and the influence of drug traffickers (Queirolo et al. 2025).

This cannabis regulation generated controversy on the international stage, as it contradicted global drug control agreements (Barry 2023; Boister 2016). While some criticized the measure for violating international agreements, others defended countries' right to implement drug policies tailored to their own realities (Sadeghi and Asadi 2023). These issues reflect a moment of transformation in the global substance control system, which is undergoing a process of adjustment (Collins 2021).

Uruguay's pioneering experience in cannabis regulation has become a crucial case study for other countries evaluating the restructuring of their drug policies. Although each nation faces specific challenges in this process, the Uruguayan model offers important insights into the impacts—both positive and negative—of change (Alvarez et al. 2023). As more countries and states move towards decriminalization or legalization, Uruguay remains a model, where future studies should analyze the long-term effects of regulation in areas such as public health, crime, and the economy (Manthey et al. 2024).

Over time, the Uruguayan experience will continue to provide rich guidance on the challenges and opportunities in the policy, health, and economic aspects of innovative drugs, consolidating its role as a global experiment in this complex and growing debate.

3.4 Mexico and Colombia

Mexico and Colombia have faced significant legal advancements and social challenges in discussions surrounding cannabis, influenced by international drug policies and local sociocultural dynamics (Hapsari et al. 2021; Arias 2015). In Mexico, debates about the legalization of cannabis have been on the agenda in recent years, while in Colombia, the legalization of the drug has been marked for decades by armed conflicts and repressive policies (Clerici et al. 2020; Agoff et al. 2021).

In 2021, Mexico moved towards the decriminalization and regulation of cannabis use, partly spurred by a Supreme Court decision that deemed the total prohibition of recreational use unconstitutional (Tinajero and Rivera 2010). However, the implementation of a forceful and comprehensive legal structure has faced difficulties, including cultural stigmatization and conservative public opinion as well as discrepancies in law enforcement (Agoff et al. 2021; Tinajero and Rivera 2010).

Cultural stigmatization is a significant challenge in Mexico, influencing perceptions and experiences of cannabis use (Agoff et al. 2021). Qualitative interviews with users in Mexico City reveal gender differences, with young women reporting using the plant to cope with family problems and to improve socialization (Agoff et al. 2021). These findings highlight the importance of considering diverse social contexts when addressing marijuana policies, where discrepancies between liberalization and legalization reforms aim to undermine public trust and mitigate illicit activities (Agoff et al. 2021; Clerici et al. 2020).

Colombia adopts a more progressive approach regarding the use and advancements of medicinal cannabis, aiming to stimulate business interest in creating medicinal cannabis businesses, which is emerging as an urgent need (Agoff et al. 2021). It is worth noting that in 2012, Colombia had one of the highest rates of cannabis consumption among Peru, Ecuador, and Bolivia (Arias 2015). However, the challenges are complex, but the country has made progress in developing a rational policy to minimize the harms associated with unregulated use through control policies (Hall and Lynskey 2009). The bioeconomy in the cannabis sector has been growing rapidly through innovations and efficient resource use, with a focus on promoting sustainable development (Grilli et al. 2024).

However, it is crucial to formally analyze the criteria and strategic factors to avoid future negative consequences (Grilli et al. 2024). In short, these two countries have made significant progress in addressing the legislative and social issues surrounding cannabis use. Although both face their own challenges, such as cultural stigma, corruption, and drug trafficking, they are innovating with groundbreaking approaches to regulating the use of the species and reducing harm. Scientific research, sociocultural dynamics, and the experiences of other countries can continue to support and strengthen the development of public policies for marijuana, defending public health and promoting social justice.

3.5 Brazil

In Brazil, the use of cannabis has been a topic of growing interest and discussion, traversing political stagnation, judicial advances, and medicinal regulation. The difficulty of the situation lies in the intersection between existing legislation, ongoing discussions, and emerging social practices (Feitosa et al. 2024; Silva et al. 2023; Jesus 2024).

The political stagnation surrounding cannabis in Brazil reflects the tension between different viewpoints and interests. We have Bill No. 399, which aims to legalize the medicinal use of cannabis; it has been under debate since 2015, demonstrating the slow pace of the legislative process (Feitosa et al. 2024; De Souza et al. 2022). The Drug Law (Law No. 11.343/2006) criminalizes the use, cultivation, and illegal acquisition of cannabis, but allows it for medicinal and scientific purposes (Feitosa et al. 2024). An ambiguity arises from the lack of a forceful and broad regulatory framework that addresses the cultivation, processing, and medicinal production of marijuana, as it requires specific technical standards from ANVISA (Brazilian Health Regulatory Agency) and its authorization (Feitosa et al. 2024; Gallassi et al. 2025).

Judicial authorizations for the cultivation of marijuana and the artisanal preparation of extracts have been granted in Brazil as advancements reflecting awareness of the medicinal benefits of cannabis and a demand for access to alternative treatments (Carvalho et al. 2023; Laranjeira and Martin 2019). However, the lack of clear regulation hinders access for the population for medicinal purposes. (Oliveira et al. 2025). The medicinal regulation of cannabis in Brazil faces significant challenges but also presents promising opportunities. The legalization of cannabis for medicinal purposes is a topic debated worldwide (Jesus 2024). Cannabis contains several chemical components, including THC (tetrahydrocannabinol) and CBD (cannabidiol), which are the main compounds responsible for its medicinal effects (Jesus 2024).

Many countries have already established regulations for the therapeutic use of cannabis, but there are still many barriers to overcome (Jesus 2024). Despite the challenges, the regulation of medical cannabis in Brazil could bring significant benefits to public health and the economy. The growing awareness of the medicinal benefits of cannabis, along with judicial advances and ongoing discussions in Congress, indicates a possible path towards regulation and access to cannabis-based treatments in Brazil (Câmara dos Deputados 2025).

4. European Countries

4.1 Netherlands

The Netherlands is often cited as one of the first countries to deviate from strict cannabis prohibition, adopting a model of pragmatic tolerance dating back to the 1970s. This system, known as the "closed-door policy," allows the sale and consumption of small amounts of cannabis in licensed establishments, known as coffee shops, without constituting a direct violation of criminal law (Ministry of Justice and Security n.d.). The rationale behind this approach is to separate the markets for soft and hard drugs, seeking to prevent cannabis users from meeting organized crime associated with more dangerous substances (Korf 2002).

Although the Netherlands is known for its tolerant approach, the situation regarding the production and supply of cannabis to coffee shops has remained ambiguous for decades. Large-scale cannabis cultivation is still largely illegal, creating an interesting paradox: sale is permitted, but the origin of the merchandise is often illicit (Blickman and Jelsma 2009). This paradox has led to challenges related to quality control, crime associated with cultivation and transportation, and tensions with municipalities seeking greater local control. Currently, the Netherlands is experimenting with pilot projects to establish a legally regulated cannabis supply chain, aiming to address this inconsistency and increase public safety and health (Knottnerus et al. 2023).

The Netherlands has a policy of tolerance, where the possession, sale, and production of drugs are technically illegal, but the sale of small amounts of "soft drugs" in "coffee shops" is tolerated under strict conditions. The rules for coffee shops include:

(1) Do not cause a nuisance.
(2) Do not sell hard drugs.
(3) Do not sell to minors.
(4) Do not advertise drugs.
(5) Do not sell large quantities (over 5 grams) in a single transaction.

Personal possession of up to 5 grams of cannabis and the cultivation of up to 5 plants for personal consumption are generally not prosecuted. The main objective of this policy is to safeguard public health, reduce harm, and combat drug-related crime by separating the cannabis market from the market for other illicit drugs. More recently, experiments with a controlled cannabis supply chain are being implemented in some municipalities to combat illicit exports and ensure quality control.

4.2 Portugal

In 2001, Portugal implemented a radical reform of its drug policy, decriminalizing the use and possession of all drugs, including cannabis, for personal consumption. This change was a response to a heroin addiction crisis that ravaged the country in the 1990s (Hughes and Stevens 2010). Instead of criminal sanctions, individuals found with small amounts of drugs are referred to Commissions for the Dissuasion of Drug Addiction (CDT), which are multidisciplinary panels focused on education, treatment, and social reintegration (Portugal 2000).

The Portuguese model is widely recognized internationally for its positive results. Studies indicate that decriminalization has led to a decrease in HIV/AIDS rates, fatal overdoses, and drug-related crime, without a significant increase in overall drug use (Mendes et al. 2019). The policy emphasizes public health and harm reduction, treating drug use as a health issue rather than a criminal justice issue. Although sale and trafficking remain illegal, the focus on decriminalizing the user represents a humanitarian and pragmatic approach that differs significantly from the Dutch model (European Monitoring Centre for Drugs and Drug Addiction 2011).

4.3 Germany

Germany represents one of the most recent and significant advances in the European cannabis policy landscape. After years of debate, the country moved forward with the legalization of cannabis consumption and cultivation for adults, with legislation coming into force in 2024 (Germany 2024). This new approach marks a fundamental shift from a system of prohibition with some tolerance for small quantities to a framework of legalization and state regulation.

German law allows limited cultivation of cannabis for personal use (up to three plants per adult) and possession of specific amounts in public and private places (Bundesgesundheitsministerium 2024). The initial distribution model provides for the creation of "cannabis social clubs" (Cannabis Social Clubs), non-profit associations that will grow and distribute cannabis to their members under strict regulation (Deutscher Hanfverband n.d.) The stated goal is to combat the black market, protect public health through quality control, and educate the population about the risks of consumption. Germany seeks to learn from other countries' experiences and implement a system that prioritizes safety and responsibility (Deutscher Bundestag 2025). Future phases may include regulated sales in specialized stores, after assessing the initial impact of social clubs (Thomasius 2024)

Germany passed the Cannabis Act (*Cannabisgesetz*) in February 2024, legalizing the use of cannabis by adults, as well as personal possession and cultivation of limited quantities, effective April 1, 2024. Adults (aged 18 and over) may possess up to 25 grams of cannabis in public and up to 50 grams of dried cannabis at home. The cultivation of up to three cannabis plants at home is also permitted. From July 1, 2024, adults will be able to join non-profit cannabis social clubs (cultivation associations) with a maximum of 500 members to collectively cultivate and distribute cannabis, with purchase limits of 25 grams per day and 50 grams per month (30 grams for those under 21). Public consumption is prohibited in certain areas, such as near schools and sports facilities, and in pedestrian zones before 8 p.m. The law aims to promote a rational, science-based drug policy and has already resulted in a significant decrease in cannabis-related criminal prosecutions (Germany 2024).

4.4 Other European Countries in Transition

In addition to the examples of the Netherlands, Portugal, and Germany, several other European countries are in different stages of reviewing and reforming their cannabis policies, reflecting a growing trend toward relaxation and the search for more effective approaches.

- **Malta** was the first country in the European Union to legalize the cultivation and possession of cannabis for personal use in 2021, also allowing the creation of non-profit cannabis clubs, in a model similar to that adopted by Germany under the Responsible Use of Cannabis Act (Malta 2021).

- **Luxembourg** has also legalized limited domestic cultivation and consumption of cannabis, seeking a balance between individual freedom and control (Luxembourg 2023).
- **Switzerland** is exploring pilot projects for the legal and regulated distribution of cannabis for non-medical purposes, seeking evidence for a future national policy (Switzerland 2020).

Other countries, such as the Czech Republic and Belgium, already have more lenient policies regarding possession of small amounts, and the debate on broader legalization remains active in their political and social spheres (European Monitoring Centre for Drugs and Drug Addiction 2024).

These examples demonstrate a diversity of approaches and the continuing evolution of cannabis policies in Europe, driven by different interests, including public health, crime reduction, individual freedom, and, in some cases, the potential for tax revenue.

5. Africa and Oceania

5.1 *South Africa*

South Africa has made the personal use and possession of *cannabis* a crime, as is the case in several countries around the world. In South Africa, the chemical substance is popularly known as dagga; however, in other parts of the world, it is called marijuana (National Prosecuting Authority of South Africa 2015). The criminalization of cannabis use in the country was established based on provisions in two Parliament laws: section 4(b) of the Drugs and Drug Trafficking Act No. 140 of 1992 (known as the Drugs Act) and section 22A(10) of the Medicines and Related Substances Control Act No. 101 of 1965 (Medicines Act) (Lubaale and Mavundla 2019). According to these laws, cannabis is considered a prohibited substance for personal use. According to international drug treaties, which will be discussed in the following sections of this article, there is a general belief that countries should criminalize both the possession and cultivation of the substance for personal use (Lubaale and Mavundla 2019).

However, this scenario underwent a significant change in September 2018, when the Constitutional Court of South Africa (ConCourt) upheld the Western Cape High Court's judgment. The Constitutional Court's decision in the case Minister of Justice and Constitutional Development and Others vs. Prince (2018) ruled that the criminalization of the use and cultivation of cannabis by adults in private settings is unconstitutional, although the prohibition on trade and use in public places remains in force. Supreme Court Deputy President Zondo explained that the use or possession of cannabis by adults in private places is no longer considered a crime; however, quantity limits must be defined by Parliament (Minister of Justice and Constitutional Development and Others vs. Prince, 2018). This decision reflects a more rational approach from a legal standpoint, while highlighting the inefficiency of criminal penalties in reducing consumption, revealing the waste of public resources in maintaining such punishments (Room and Reuter 2012).

According to Prohibition Partners' "The African Cannabis Report" (2019), South Africa is the first and only country in Africa to allow personal use of cannabis in private places, also known as recreational use. Despite this, the use of cannabis, for both medicinal and recreational purposes, remains illegal in most African countries, including Algeria, Angola, Benin, Botswana, Burkina Faso, Burundi, Cameroon, and the Central African Republic, among others.

5.2 *Oceania*

5.2.1 *Australia*

The vast majority of countries created laws prohibiting the use of cannabis and THC during the early and mid-20th century. An example of this occurred in 1928, when the state of Victoria became the first in Australia to ban cannabis, followed by South Australia in 1934 and New South Wales in 1935 (De Souza and Henriques 2022; Penington Institute 2022). However, over the past ten years, there has been a significant relaxation of cannabis regulations, increasing the legal availability of the substance around the world. Some countries, such as Uruguay and Canada, have decided to fully legalize cannabis use, while others have made more limited reforms (De Souza and Henriques 2022). In Australia, this change led to a major regulatory shift in 2016, when a law was passed allowing the medical prescription of cannabis-based medicines and the operation of companies that produce the substance (Therapeutic Goods Administration 2019).

Since this 2016 regulation, the medical cannabis landscape in the country has undergone a significant transformation. Before that, Australian patients who wanted to use the substance for therapeutic purposes had to resort to the illegal market, with no guarantee of quality or medical supervision (Lintzeris et al. 2018; Suraev et al. 2018). By 2024, the system had more than 800 different authorized medical cannabis products (Hewett 2023), accessible through Special Access Schemes (SAS) and the Authorized Prescriber (AP) system, both regulated by the Therapeutic Goods Administration (TGA), the federal agency responsible for drug oversight (Brook and Sambul 2023; MacPhail et al. 2022; Therapeutic Goods Administration 2023a; Therapeutic Goods Administration 2023b).

Following the November 1, 2016, amendment to the Narcotics Act of 1967, the TGA reclassified certain cannabis products from Schedule 9 (S9) to Schedule 8 (S8), paving the way for access via AP or SAS (Bawa et al. 2022). In the following years, however, patients reported difficulties obtaining these medications due to a complex regulatory system and the plant's classification as an "unapproved product" (O'Brien 2019). Only more recently has the number of prescriptions and authorized prescribers increased (Bawa et al. 2022). Still, factors such as high costs, public drug testing laws, and the limited training of many doctors mean that most of those seeking therapeutic relief resort to the illicit market (Lintzeris et al. 2022).

However, despite the diversity of studies on the use and representation of cannabis in different places, there is still a scarcity of research focusing on Australia. The exception is Lewis and Flood (2021), who analyzed how medical cannabis is framed in Australian professional medical publications, identifying it as a legitimate therapeutic alternative, but one with complex prescription and access, with evidence that is still not very robust, and safety issues that cannot be ignored. These findings serve as a starting point for future investigations into the integration of medical cannabis, especially from communicative and sociological perspectives, as little is known about its construction and legitimization in the Australian media.

5.2.2 New Zealand

In 2020, New Zealand put to a popular vote a proposal that could profoundly change its policy on the use and supply of cannabis for non-medical purposes. The referendum sought to gauge public support for adopting a "regulated legalization" model to replace the decades-long prohibitionist policy. Although many aspects of the proposed regime were still under development or undefined, the initiative followed the trend of other nations, especially in the Americas, that had already legalized cannabis, even though the issue remained controversial (Fischer and Bullen 2020; Manhire 2019).

The approaches to legalization adopted in different regions have their own characteristics, and neither their formats nor their results are directly transferable to other political realities. Therefore, the lessons learned from both the impacts of prohibition and the reforms already implemented elsewhere should serve as a basis, but the formulation of proposals for the New Zealand referendum requires support from data across various areas of knowledge and the consideration of fundamental value principles (Fischer et al. 2020).

The proposal to reform cannabis prohibition policy—especially in the New Zealand context, with emphasis on the arguments presented by leaders involved in the referendum—is based on the idea that prohibition represents an outdated and ineffective strategy, inherited from an international anti-drug campaign conducted decades ago. Three main arguments support this criticism: first, the disproportionate nature of the measure, considering that legal substances such as alcohol and tobacco, known to be more harmful to public health, remain widely available; second, its low effectiveness in preventing consumption, especially among young people; and, finally, the negative effects resulting from criminalization itself, such as the maintenance of illicit markets, the increase in the potency of products, and selective repression of vulnerable groups (Blumenson and Nilsen 2009; Crepault et al. 2016). In this scenario, advocates of reform have argued that policies grounded in public health, equity, and scientific evidence would be more appropriate for addressing the issue and have gained momentum in different countries throughout the 21st century (Fischer and Bullen 2020).

However, New Zealand still takes a prohibitive approach to cannabis control. Although authorities have the freedom to choose not to press charges when a health-oriented response would be more appropriate, this possibility is rarely used. If the 2020 referendum had resulted in a favorable majority, the country would have become the first outside the Americas to legalize the non-medicinal use of cannabis through legislation, after Uruguay, Canada, and several US states. Surveys conducted during the period indicated that the population was divided on the issue, and the negative result suggests that cannabis legalization is unlikely in the short term. Nevertheless, the process and its developments offer relevant insights for broader reflections on possible reforms in drug policy (Decorte et al. 2020; Fischer and Hall 2021).

6. Asia

6.1 Israel

Israel has had a medical cannabis program since the end of the 20th century, run by the country's Ministry of Health, which is responsible for regulating and licensing patients, producers, and suppliers. In 2017, the agency recorded an increase in the number of licenses for cannabis use, from approximately 28,000 in 2017 to 70,000 patients in 2020, according to data from the Israeli Ministry of Health (Zarhin et al. 2018; I.M.C.U. 2020).

The Israeli government, based on resolutions 1050 and 1587, recognizes the medicinal effects of cannabis. However, Israeli law follows the UN's single convention on narcotics (UN 1961), classifying cannabis as an illicit drug. Thus, cannabis remains a threshold substance, characterized as both a legitimate medicinal alternative and a dangerous drug (Zarhin et al. 2018).

Government Resolution No. 1050 initiated the process of opening up access to medical cannabis, establishing the functioning of the Israeli system for this issue by presenting five main points:

1) Respect for international conventions on drugs and narcotics.
2) Cannabis continues to be classified as a dangerous drug.
3) A government agency (Israeli Medical Cannabis Agency) is responsible for supervising and regulating its use for medicinal purposes.
4) Equality between treatment with cannabis and other medical products.
5) Prevention of abuse and crimes related to cannabis (Araújo et al. 2024).

Government Resolution No. 1587 reformulated the guidelines for the sale and distribution of medical cannabis, establishing rules for product standardization. It transferred the sale and distribution of medical cannabis from growers to pharmaceutical companies, allowing more doctors to prescribe medical cannabis for treatment (Lewis et al. 2024).

Another policy change involving cannabis was the "Non-Assault of Liability" bill passed by the Knesset (Israel's unicameral parliament and supreme authority of the state) in 2019, which decriminalized personal use of cannabis for recreational purposes. Thus, individuals caught using cannabis received a fine instead of being arrested and prosecuted; however, on the fourth offense, criminal proceedings may be initiated (Lewis et al. 2024).

6.2 India

Cannabis is the third most commonly used substance in India, alongside alcohol and tobacco, making it the most widely used illicit substance in the country. In 2018, 31 million people reported using cannabis (2.8% of the total population) and 2.5 million showed signs of dependence (Karki and Rangaswamy 2023).

Traditionally, India has used cannabis for religious purposes. The oldest reference to the preparation of cannabis (Bhanga) is from the Atharva Veda (2000 bC to 1400 bC), in which it is shown as a sacred herb. In the Sushruta Samhita (600 AD), cannabis-derived products were reported as valuable medicines in the treatment of certain diseases. Currently, cannabis consumption is common at Hindu festivals, as well as being an important part of religiosity (Russo 1998; Dasgupta 2013).

The habitual consumption of cannabis in India, linked to global influence for the decriminalization of its use, has promoted an increase in support for legalization in the country for medicinal and recreational purposes with the 2016 proposal of legislation for medicinal and commercial use, leading two Indian states, Uttarakhand and Madhya Pradesh, to allow cultivation for industrial and medicinal purposes in 2019 (Karki and Rangaswamy 2023).

In 2017, the Indian government's Union Minister for Women and Child Development again suggested the legalization of cannabis for medicinal purposes, citing a decrease in uncontrolled use and the assistance it provides to cancer patients, and her request was successful (Raza 2018).

The Indian government formed a council to research the use of *Cannabis* for various diseases. However, the research did not provide key information to inform regulations on the release of cannabis in the country (Karki and Rangaswamy 2023). Currently, the medicinal use of cannabis is prohibited under the Narcotics and Psychotropic Substances Act, which prohibits doctors from prescribing cannabis and blocks research focusing on possible medicinal uses (Verma 2021).

6.3 China

In China, cannabis is highly controlled as a narcotic drug and classified as a psychotropic drug, with strict legislation governing its use and opposition to any kind of revision aimed at relaxing its use. The Chinese administration's 2005 punishment law provides for 10 days' detention plus a fine for illegal possession, supply, or coercing a medical worker to prescribe the psychotropic substance or even deceiving the worker into purchasing it.

The country uses a licensing system for producers of industrial hemp leaves and flowers, standing out as a world leader in the production of cannabis seeds. The regulation on the administration of narcotic and psychotropic drugs is the main one in the management of industrial cannabis in China, with an extremely prohibitionist aspect. Industrial use is permitted at a low level of tetrahydrocannabinol in the manufacture of textiles, paper, oils, among others (Sun 2023).

6.4 Thailand

In Thailand, a public forum was held in 2016, organized by the agriculture council, focusing on the decriminalization of cannabis from anti-drug legislation. This led to the decriminalization of hemp in 15 districts and 6 provinces across the country (Bewley-Taylor et al. 2020).

In 2018, the use of medical cannabis was legalized as a way to improve the quality of life of communities located in the highlands. In the process of opening up legislation involving cannabis, a law was enacted to pardon patients and those convicted of cannabis possession (Jelsma and Bewley-Taylor 2019). Thus, over the years, the Thai government has adopted measures to regulate the cultivation of cannabis for medicinal and recreational purposes for adults, promoting the decriminalization of cannabis in 2022 (Putri 2020; Gómez 2024).

Table 1 shows the policy on recreational and medicinal use of *Cannabis sativa* in some countries.

Table 1: Regulations on the use of *Cannabis sativa* in some countries.

Country	Recreational Use	Medical Use	Observations
Canada	Adults may possess up to 30 grams of dried marijuana or equivalent in public.	The Access to Cannabis for Medical Purposes Regulations (ACMPR) allow patients with a medical prescription to grow it or purchase it from licensed producers.	One of the first countries to legalize both uses at the national level. It has a well-established recreational market. First country in the world to legalize the entire *Cannabis* chain. The model aims to control the market and combat trafficking.
Uruguay	Legalized nationally since 2013. State-controlled sale in pharmacies to registered citizens. Home cultivation and cultivation clubs permitted.	Legalized as part of the general legalization law. Access via the same mechanisms as recreational use for registered patients.	Uruguay was a pioneer in legalizing and regulating the entire *cannabis* chain (cultivation, production, distribution, and sale for medicinal and recreational use).
United States	Illegal at the federal level. Legalized for recreational use in several states (e.g., Colorado, California, Washington). Laws vary significantly between states.	Legalized for medicinal use in an even greater number of states (including some where recreational use is illegal). Medicinal programs vary in terms of eligible conditions and forms of access.	Complex legal landscape with federal laws conflicting with state laws. The medical market is broader than the recreational market in terms of the number of states.
Germany	Legalized for recreational use in April 2024, with rules for personal possession and cultivation. Commercial sale has not yet been implemented.	Legalized since 2017. Covered by health insurance in certain cases. Access via medical prescription and purchase at pharmacies.	The future marketing model is still under development. A strong medical access system is already established.
Netherlands	One of the largest economies to legalize recreational use. The future commercialization model is still under development. A strong medical access system is already established.	Legal for medicinal purposes since 2003. Accessible through medical prescription and purchase at pharmacies.	he tolerance model for recreational use is unique. The medicinal program is separate and more restrictive.
Brazil	Illegal	Legalized for medicinal use through the importation of products registered by Anvisa and controlled sale in pharmacies under medical prescription (RDC 327/2019). Cultivation for medicinal and scientific purposes is permitted under judicial or Anvisa authorization (RDC 327/2019).	The medicinal market is developing, with a focus on imported products and a few domestically produced ones. Ongoing debate about regulating cultivation for medicinal use. Recreational use is strictly prohibited.
Portugal	Decriminalization Law in 2001.	In 2018, the medicinal use of cannabis was legalized, allowing it to be sold in pharmacies and opening up opportunities for medicines based on the plant species.	There is still debate regarding the legalization of the plant in the country, with arguments that its free sale increases overall drug consumption in the country.
China	Prohibition of recreational use	Medicinal use is focused on cultural practices with severe restrictions and regulations.	The current policy is one of zero tolerance for recreational drug use and drug trafficking, in order to protect public health and order.
India	Depending on the part of the plant, the seeds and leaves are used as a basis for food and drinks, and as part of religious celebrations.	The medicinal use of *cannabis* is prohibited under the Narcotics and Psychotropic Substances Act, which prohibits doctors from prescribing cannabis and blocks research focusing on possible medicinal uses.	In 2017, the Indian government's Union Minister for Women and Child Development again suggested the legalization of cannabis for medicinal purposes, citing a decrease in uncontrolled use and the assistance it provides to cancer patients, and her request was successful.

7. Conclusion and Future Perspectives

The regulation of cannabis over the years in various countries still faces obstacles to its effective implementation. However, the advent of new medications and commercial opportunities has contributed to the loss of negative stigma and opened the wayfor less restrictive policies that integrate public health, safety, and education.

The state must position itself to assess the social and health impacts, while ensuring social participation in the formulation of these policies. The consolidation of regulatory frameworks will depend not only on the state's commitment but also on the population's commitment.

References

Agoff, C., Fondevila, G., and Sandberg, S. (2021). Cultural stigmatization and police corruption: cannabis, gender, and legalization in Mexico. *Drugs: Education, Prevention and Policy*, 29: 373–381.

Aguiar, S., and Musto, C. (2022). The regulation backyard: home growing cannabis in Uruguay. *Contemporary Drug Problems*, 49: 478–490.

Alvarez, E., Queirolo, R., and Sotto, B. (2023). Conflicting forces in the implementation of medicinal cannabis regulation in Uruguay. *Journal of Cannabis Research*, 5: 26.

Araújo, C. E., Messetti, P. A. S., and de Mendonça Cruz, C. A. (2024). A regulação da cannabis de grau medicinal em Israel e possíveis contribuições para o processo de regulação da cannabis medicinal no Brasil. Anais do Encontro Internacional e Nacional de Política Social 1.

Arias, J. M. C. (2015). Cannabis: challenges between legislation and cognitive competence. *International Journal of Psychological Research*, 8: 8–9.

Auguskani, L. J. (2025). Public health preparedness and response: lessons learned from recent global health crises. *Journal of Neonatal Surgery*, 14: 279–292.

Barry, R. A. (2023). 'We never thought this would be considered drug trafficking': international finance rules, policy space and Uruguay's regulation of recreational cannabis. *Global Public Health*, 18: 2283042.

Bawa, Z., McCartney, D., Manocha, R., and McGregor, I. S. (2022). Knowledge, experiences, and attitudes of Australian general practitioners towards medicinal cannabis: A 2021–2022 survey. *BMC Primary Care*, 23: 1–11.

Berk, R. (2025). Demystifying AI in criminal justice (Version 1). arXiv.

Bewley-Taylor, D., Jelsma, M., and Kay, S. (2020). Regulación del cannabis y desarrollo: alternativas comerciales (más) justas para mercados legales emergentes. International Development Policy| Revue internationale de politique de développement.

Boister, N. (2016). Waltzing on the Vienna consensus on drug control? Tensions in the international system for the control of drugs. *Leiden Journal of International Law*, 29: 389–409.

Blickman, T., and Jelsma, M. (2009). La reforma de las políticas de drogas: Experiencias alternativas en Europa y Estados Unidos (y II).

Blumenson, E., and Nilsen, E. (2009). No rational basis: The pragmatic case for marijuana law reform. Virginia *Journal of Social Policy and the Law*, 17: 43–82.

Boidi, M. F., Queirolo, R., and Cruz, J. M. (2016). Cannabis consumption patterns among frequent consumers in Uruguay. *International Journal of Drug Policy*, 34: 34–40.

Brasil, (2006). Lei n° 11.343, de 23 de agosto de 2006. Institui o Sistema Nacional de Políticas Públicas sobre Drogas. https://www.planalto.gov.br/ccivil_03/_ato2004-2006/2006/lei/l11343.html.

Brill, A., Miller, B. J., and Veuger, S. (2024). Implications of cannabis legalization for the US federal budget. *Public Budgeting and Finance*, 44: 22–43.

Brook, S., and Sambul, N. (2023). 'More acceptable now': Medicinal cannabis use rising, passes 1 million prescriptions. The Sydney Morning Herald. https://www.smh.com.au/healthcare/more-acceptable-now-medicinal-cannabis-use-rising-passes-1-million-prescriptions-20230511-p5d7oe.html.

Bruzelius, E., and Martins, S.S. (2024). Recreational cannabis legalization and immigration enforcement: a state-level analysis of arrests and deportations in the United States, 2009–2020. BMC Public Health 24.

Bundesgesundheitsministerium. (2024). Fragen und Antworten zum Cannabisgesetz (CanG). Bundesministerium für Gesundheit. https://www.bundesgesundheitsministerium.de/themen/cannabis/faq-cannabisgesetz

Câmara dos Deputados. (2025). Ficha de tramitação da Proposição n° 947642. https://www.camara.leg.br/proposicoesWeb/fichadetramitacao?idProposicao=947642

Carvalho, J. C. (2014). A emergência da política mundial de drogas: O Brasil e as primeiras Conferências Internacionais do Ópio. *Oficina do Historiador*, 7: 153–176.

Carvalho, V. M., Santos Carmo, J., Santos, L. M. G., Almeida, F.G., Rocha, E. D., Macêdo Vieira, A. C. et al. (2023). Pharmaceutical evaluation of medical cannabis extracts prepared by artisanal and laboratory techniques. *Revista Brasileira de Farmacognosia*, 33: 724–735.

Clerici, N., Armenteras, D., Kareiva, P., Botero, R., Ramírez-Delgado, J. P., Forero-Medina, G. et al. (2020). Deforestation in Colombian protected areas increased during post-conflict periods. Scientific Reports 10.

Collins, J. (2021). Evaluating trends and stakeholders in the international drug control regime complex. *International Journal of Drug Policy*, 90: 103060.

Crepault, J. F., Rehm, J., and Fischer, B. (2016). The cannabis policy framework by the Centre for Addiction and Mental Health: A proposal for a public health approach to cannabis policy in Canada. *International Journal of Drug Policy*, 34: 1–4.

Coggon, J., and Kamunge-Kpodo, B (2022). The legal determinants of health (in)justice. *Medical Law Review*, 30: 705–722.

Dasgupta, S. (2013). Legalization of Marijuana in India. Available at SSRN 2261316.

Decorte, T., Lenton, S., and Wilkins, C. (2020). Legalizing cannabis: Experiences, lessons and scenarios. Routledge.

De Faria, L., Mezey, L., and Winkler, A (2021). Cannabis Legalization and College Mental Health. *Current Psychiatry Reports*, 23: 17.

De Souza, M. R., Henriques, A. T., and Limberger, R. P. (2022). Medical *cannabis* regulation: An overview of models around the world with emphasis on the Brazilian scenario. *Journal of Cannabis Research*, 4: 33.

Deutscher Hanfverband (n.d.). Cannabis Social Clubs (CSC). Deutscher Hanfverband. https://hanfverband.de/nachricht/cannabis-social-clubs-csc

ElSohly, M. A., and Slade, D. (2005). Chemical constituents of marijuana: The complex mixture of natural cannabinoids. *Life Sciences*, 78: 539–548.

European Monitoring Centre for Drugs and Drug Addiction (2011). Drug policy profiles: Portugal. Publications Office of the European Union. https://op.europa.eu/en/publication-detail/-/publication/6ace2e2c-de64-4239-9c14-acb91ead097f/language-en

European Monitoring Centre for Drugs and Drug Addiction. (2024). European drug report 2024: Trends and developments. Publications Office of the European Union. https://www.euda.europa.eu/publications/european-drug-report/2024_en

Feitosa, C. M., Moura, A. S. M., Diniz, R. M. C. S. de C, Do Lago, L. C., Silva, M. A., Costa, J. V. et al. (2024). A legalização da *Cannabis sativa* L. (maconha) no Brasil como uso medicinal. *Revista Contemporânea*, 4: 831–853.

Fischer, B., Robinson, T., Bullen, C., Curran, V., Jutras-Aswad, D., Medina-Mora, M. E. et al. (2022). Lower-Risk Cannabis Use Guidelines (LRCUG) for reducing health harms from non-medical cannabis use: A comprehensive evidence and recommendations update. *International Journal of Drug Policy*, 99: 103381.

Fraga, P., and Brandão, M. (2025) Drogas, sociedades e a questão da saúde: Da proibição à regulação da cannabis para fins terapêuticos. Saúde e Sociedade, 34: 1–9.

Fischer, B., and Bullen, C. (2020). Emerging prospects for non-medical cannabis legalisation in New Zealand: An initial view and contextualization. *International Journal of Drug Policy*, 76: 102632.

Fischer, B., Daldegan Fischer, B., Daldegan-Bueno, D., and Boden, J. M. (2020). Facing the option for the legalisation of cannabis use and supply in New Zealand: An overview of relevant evidence, concepts and considerations. *Drug and Alcohol Review*, 39: 555–567.

Fischer, B., and Hall, W. (2021). New Zealand's failed cannabis legalization referendum – I mplications for cannabis policy reform. The Lancet Regional Health – Western Pacific 7: 100080.

Gallassi, A. D., De Oliveira, A. W. C., Mendes, N. S., Filev, R., and Nakano, E. Y. (2025). Evaluation of cannabidiol-based products in Brazil: How can current regulations influence their labeling quality? *Journal of Cannabis Research*, 7: 12.

Germany. (2024). Gesetz zum kontrollierten Umgang mit Cannabis und zur Änderung weiterer Vorschriften (Cannabisgesetz – CanG): Approved by the Bundestag on February 23, 2024. Federal Law Gazette, Part I 109.

Gómez, N. P. (2024). Influencia de la ideología en las actitudes hacia la legalización del cannabis en España. RIPS: Revista de Investigaciones Políticas y sociológicas 23.

Grilli, G., Cantillo, T., Turner, K., Erazo, J., Murcia López, M. A., Valle Parra, J. S. et al. (2024). A decision support procedure for the bioeconomy transition: a Colombian case study. *Journal of Environmental Management*, 352: 120042.

Hall, W. (2020). The costs and benefits of cannabis control policies. *Dialogues in Clinical Neuroscience*, 22: 281–287.

Hall, W., and Lynskey, M. (2009). The challenges in developing a rational *cannabis* policy. *Current Opinion in Psychiatry*, 22: 258–262.

Hall, W., Stjepanović, D., Dawson, D., and Leung, J. (2023). The implementation and public health impacts of cannabis legalization in Canada: a systematic review. *Addiction*, 118: 2062–2072.

Hapsari, R. D., Ramadhanti, H. N., and Putri, K. M. (2021). Comparative analysis of the United States' war on drugs policy in Mexico and Colombia: failure and success factors. *WIMAYA*, 2: 39–50.

Hasin, D. S., Sarvet, A. L., Cerdá, M., Keyes, K. M., Stohl, M., Galea, S. et al. (2017). US adult illicit cannabis use, cannabis use disorder, and medical marijuana laws. *JAMA Psychiatry*, 74: 579.

Hewett, A. (2023). Cannabis in Australia 2023. Policy Commons. https://policycommons.net/artifacts/11338802/cannabis-in-australia-2023/12227818/

Hong, G., Sideris, A., Waldman, S., Stauffer, J., and Wu, C. L. (2023). Legal and regulatory aspects of medical cannabis in the United States. *Anesthesia and Analgesia*, 138: 31–41.

Hussain, T., Jeena, G., Pitakbut, T., Vasilev, N., and Kayser, O. (2021) *Cannabis* sativa research trends, challenges, and new-age perspectives. *iScience*, 24: 103391.

Hughes, C. E., and Stevens, A. (2010). What Can We Learn from The Portuguese Decriminalization of Illicit Drugs? *British Journal of Criminology*, 50: 999–1022.

Israeli Ministry of Health - I.M.C.U. (2020). Current information on medical *cannabis* licenses in Israel.

Jelsma, M., Kay, S., and Bewley-Taylor, D. (2019). Opciones de comercio (más) justo para el mercado de cannabis. Informe de Políticas 1.

Jesus, J. V. S. M. D. (2024). Cannabis: uso terapêutico e desafios para sua aplicabilidade medicinal no Brasil. Revista Ft 28: 48–49.

Kamyab, H., SaberiKamarposhti, M., Hashim, H., and Yusuf, M. (2023). Carbon dynamics in agricultural greenhouse gas emissions and removals: a comprehensive review. *Carbon Letters*, 34: 265–289. https://doi.org/10.1007/s42823-023-00647-4.

Karki, P., and Rangaswamy, M. (2023). A review of historical context and current research on cannabis use in India. *Indian Journal of Psychological Medicine*, 45: 105–116.

Knottnerus, J. A., Blom, T., Van Eerden, S., Mans, J. H. H., Mheen, D. V. D., De Neeling, J. N. D. et al. (2023). Cannabis policy in The Netherlands: Rationale and design of an experiment with a controlled legal ('closed') cannabis supply chain. *Health Policy*, 129: 104699.

Korf, D. J. (2002). Dutch coffee shops and trends in cannabis use. *Addictive Behaviors*, 27: 851–866.

Laranjeira, R., and Martin, D. (2019). Traps in cannabis policies in Brazil. *Brazilian Journal of Psychiatry*, 41: 475–476.

Lewis, M., and Flood, J. (2021). The transition of cannabis into the mainstream of Australian healthcare: Framings in professional medical publications. *Journal of Cannabis Research*, 3: 1–48.

Lewis, N., Eliash-Fizik, H., Har-Even, A., and Sznitman, S. R. (2024). Media framing of causes, risks, and policy solutions for cannabis-impaired driving: does medical vs. non-medical cannabis context matter? *Health communication*, 39: 828-837.

Lintzeris, N., Driels, J., Elias, N., Arnold, J. C., McGregor, I. S., and Allsop, D. J. (2018). Medicinal cannabis in Australia, 2016: The Cannabis as Medicine Survey (CAMS-16). *Medical Journal of Australia*, 209: 211–216.

Lintzeris, N., Mills, L., Abelev, S. V., Suraev, A., Arnold, J. C., and McGregor, I. S. (2022). Medical cannabis use in Australia: Consumer experiences from the online cannabis as medicine survey 2020 (CAMS-20). *Harm Reduction Journal*, 19: 88.

Lubaale, E. C., and Mavundla, S. D. (2019). Descriminalização da cannabis para uso pessoal na África do Sul. *African Human Rights Law Journal*, 19: 819–842.

Luxembourg. (2023). Law amending various provisions relating to the fight against drug addiction. https://police.public.lu/en/reglementation/stupefiants/cannabis.html

MacPhail, S. L., Bedoya-Perez, M. A., Cohen, R., Kotsirilos, V., McGregor, I. S., and Cairns, E.A. (2022). Medicinal cannabis prescribing in Australia: An analysis of trends over the first five years. *Frontiers in Pharmacology*, 13: 885655.

Mallinson, D., Hannah, L., and Cunningham, G. (2020). The consequences of fickle federal policy: administrative hurdles for state cannabis policies. Cambridge University Press.

Malta. (2021). Act No. LXVI of 2021 – Authority on the Responsible Use of Cannabis Act, of 14 December 2021: Act on the Authority for the Responsible Use of Cannabis. Government Gazette of Malta 20.757.

Manhire, T. (2019). Cheat sheet: NZ cannabis legalisation bill, and the referendum question, revealed. The Spinoff. https://thespinoff.co.nz/politics/03-12-2019/cheat-sheet-nz-cannabis-legalisation-bill-and-the-referendum-question-revealed

Manthey, J. (2025). Treatment demand for *cannabis* use problems: analyses of routine data from 30 European countries. *European Archives of Psychiatry and Clinical Neuroscience*, 275: 355–363.

Martins, D. A., and Posso, I. P. (2023). Legislação atual sobre cannabis medicinal: Histórico, movimentos, tendências e contratendências no território brasileiro. *Brazilian Journal of Pain*, 6: S75–S79.

Mekonen Yimer, T., Hoch, E., Fischer, B., Dawson, D., and Hall, W. (2025). The adverse public health effects of non-medical cannabis legalisation in Canada and the USA. *The Lancet Public Health*, 10: e148–e159.

Mendes, R. D. O., Pacheco, P. G., Nunes, J. P. C. O. V., Crespo, P. S., and Cruz MS (2019). Literature review on the implications for drug user care of decriminalization in Portugal and Brazil. *Ciência e Saúde Coletiva*, 24: 3395–3406.

Menezes, S. M., Kumar, A., and Dutta, S. (2024). Navigating in turbulent times: using social media to examine small and family-owned business topics and sentiments during the COVID-19 crisis. *Information Systems Frontiers*, 1–21.

Miller, N. S., and Saad, Z. A. (2017). Comparative analyses of "medical marijuana" laws in the United States. *Journal of Addiction Research and Therapy*, S11.

Minister of Justice and Constitutional Development and Others vs. Prince (2018), National Director of Public Prosecutions and Others v. Rubin, National Director of Public Prosecutions and Others v. Acton and Others, ZACC 30.

Ministry of Justice and Security (Netherlands). (n.d.). Toleration policy regarding soft drugs and coffee shops. Government of the Netherlands. https://www.government.nl/topics/drugs/toleration-policy-regarding-soft-drugs-and-coffee-shops

Nargis, N., Westmaas, J. L., Orr, E., Alqahtani, M. M., Choudhury, P. P., Islami, F. et al. (2025). Cancer risk and legalisation of access to cannabis in the USA: Overview of the evidence. *The Lancet Public Health*, 10: e160–e164.

National Prosecuting Authority of South Africa. (2015). Annual report 2014/2015. https://www.ahrlj.up.ac.za/lubaale-em-mavundla-sd

Ng, J. Y., Homayouni, P., Usman, S., and Gomes, Z. (2022). The medical *cannabis* regulatory framework in Canada: a narrative review. *European Journal of Integrative Medicine*, 50: 102104.

O'Brien, K (2019). Medicinal cannabis: Issues of evidence. European Journal of Integrative Medicine 28: 114–120.

Oliveira, D. L., Amaral, A. C. F., and de Souza Ramos, A (2025). Factors for implementing medical *cannabis* cultivation in Brazil. *The Natural Products Journal*, 15.

Ortega-Bolaños, R., Bernal-Salcedo, J., Germán Ortiz, M., Galeano Sarmiento, J., Ruz, G. A., and Tabares-Soto, R. (2024). Applying the ethics of AI: a systematic review of tools for developing and assessing AI-based systems. *Artificial Intelligence Review*, 57: 110.

Pardal, M., Bone, M., Decorte, T., Queirolo, R., Parés, Ò., Johansson, J. et al. (2020). Hidden and uninterested populations: methodological insights and unresolved issues from the study of Cannabis Social Clubs. *Methodological Innovations*, 13.

Perlman, A. I., McLeod, H. M., Ventresca, E. C., Salinas, M. G., Post, P. J., Schuh, M. J. et al. (2021). Medical cannabis state and federal regulations. *Mayo Clinic Proceedings*, 96: 2671–2681.

Penington Institute. (2022). Cannabis in Australia: 2022. https://www.penington.org.au/wp-content/uploads/2022/12/Cannabis-in-Australia-2022.pdf

Pierro Neto, P. A., Pierro, L. M. C., and Fernandes, S. T. (2023) Cannabis: 12.000 anos de experiências e preconceitos. *Brazilian Journal of Pain*, 6: S80–S84.

Portugal. (2000). Law No. 30/2000, of November 29: Defines the legal regime applicable to the consumption of narcotics and psychotropic substances, as well as the health and social protection of people who consume such substances without a medical prescription. Diário da República, Series I-A, 277: 7531–7533.

Prohibition Partners (2019). The African cannabis report. https://pt.scribd.com/document/459275703/2019%E5%B9%B4%E9%9D%9E%E6%B4%B2%E5%A4%A7%E9%BA%BB%E6%8A%A5%E5%91%8A-P110-The-African-Cannabis-Report

Public Security Administration Punishment Law of the People's Republic of China, Art. 72. (2005). The Central People's Government of the People's Republic of China. https://www.cecc.gov/resources/legal-provisions/public-security-administration-punishment-law-chinese-text

Putri, D. (2020). Reclasificación del cannabis: Una introducción global. Londres: IDPC.

Queirolo, R., Repetto, L., Alonso, J., Álvarez, E., Sotto, B., Pardal, M. et al. (2025). Intended and unintended effects of cannabis regulation in Uruguay. *Policy and Politics*, 53: 553–570.

Raza, M. R. (2018). Should be Marijuana Legalized in India? Journal of Emerging Technologies and Innovative Research 5.

Room, R., and Reuter, P. (2012). How well do international drug conventions protect public health? *The Lancet*, 379: 84–91.

Rubin-Kahana, D. S., Crépault, J. F., Matheson, J., and Le Foll, B. (2022). The impact of *cannabis* legalization for recreational purposes on youth: a narrative review of the Canadian experience. *Frontiers in Psychiatry*, 13: 984485.

Russo, E. (1998). Cannabis for migraine treatment: the once and future prescription? An historical and scientific review. *Pain*, 76: 3–8.

Russo, E. B. (2016). Current therapeutic cannabis controversies and clinical trial design issues. *Frontiers in Pharmacology*, 7: 309.

Sadeghi, A., and Arab Asadi, S. (2023). Reevaluation of the international narcotics-control system in light of cannabis legalizations. *Public Law Studies Quarterly*, 53: 1911–1939.

Sandler, L. N., Beckerman, J. L., Whitford, F., and Gibson, K. A. (2019). *Cannabis* as conundrum. Crop Protection 117: 37–44.

Schauer, G. L. (2021). Cannabis policy in the United States: implications for public health. *JNCI Monographs*, 2021: 39–52.

Silva, G. C., Botelho, D. G., and Resgala Júnior, R. M. (2023). Cannabis e direito penal: implicações jurídicas do uso medicinal da planta, desafios e perspectivas da regulamentação jurídica da *cannabis* medicinal no Brasil. *Revista Ibero-Americana de Humanidades, Ciências e Educação*, 9: 6080–6100.

Shankar, R., and Gupta, L. (2024). Modelling risks in transition from Industry 4.0 to Industry 5.0. *Annals of Operations Research*, 342: 275–1320.

Sun, X. (2023). Research progress on Cannabinoids in *Cannabis* (*Cannabis sativa* L.) in China. *Molecules*, 28: 3806.

Suraev A, Lintzeris N, Stuart J, Blackburn R, Richards E, Arnold JC, McGregor IS (2018). Composition and use of cannabis extracts for childhood epilepsy in the Australian community. *Scientific Reports*, 8: 1–14.

Svrakic, D. M., Lustman, P. J., Mallya, A., Lynn, T. A., Finney, R., and Svrakic, N. M. (2012). Legalization, decriminalization and medicinal use of cannabis: A scientific and public health perspective. *Missouri Medicine*, 109: 90–98.

Switzerland. Federal Office of Public Health (2020). Swiss national drug strategy 2020–2030. Bern: Federal Office of Public Health. https://www.bag.admin.ch/bag/en/home/strategie-und-politik/nationale-gesundheitsstrategien/drogenstrategie.html

Tesalonika, N. S., and Kusumawardani, N. (2019). International law non-compliance: assessing Uruguay's decision to legalize *cannabis* under Jose Mujica regime. *AEGIS: Journal of International Relations*, 3.

Tinajero, J. H., and Rivera, L. (2010). IDPC Briefing Paper – *Cannabis* in Mexico: An open debate. SSRN.

Tobey, M. B., Binder, R. B., Chang, S., Yoshida, T., Yamagata, Y., and Yang, P. P. J. (2019). Urban systems design: a conceptual framework for planning smart communities. *Smart Cities*, 2: 522–537.

Therapeutic Goods Administration. (2019). Introduction to medicinal *cannabis* regulation in Australia. https://www.tga.gov.au/news/blog/introduction-medicinal-cannabis-regulation-australia

Therapeutic Goods Administration. (2023a). Medicinal *cannabis*: Access pathways and patient access data. Australian Government Department of Health and Aged Care. https://www.tga.gov.au/products/unapproved-therapeutic-goods/medicinal-cannabis-hub/medicinal-cannabis-access-pathways-and-patient-access-data

Therapeutic Goods Administration. (2023b). Medicinal cannabis products by active ingredients. Australian Government Department of Health and Aged Care. https://www.tga.gov.au/medicinal-cannabis-products-active-ingredients

Thomasius, R. (2024). Zur Diskussion / Up for Discussion. Gefährdet die Cannabislegalisierung Kinder und Jugendliche? / Does Cannabis Legalization Endanger Children and Adolescents? Praxis der Kinderpsychologie und Kinderpsychiatrie, 73: 652–664.

UN (1961). Single Convention on Narcotic Drugs.

Verma, C. (2021). Decriminalisation of *Cannabis*. Journal of Innovation and Social Science Research 8: 48-51.

Zarhin, D., Negev, M., Vulfsons, S., and Sznitman, S. R. (2018). Rhetorical and regulatory boundary-work: The case of medical cannabis policy-making in Israel. *Social Science and Medicine*, 217: 1-9.

Zuardi, A. W. (2006). História da cannabis como medicamento: uma revisão. *Revista Brasileira de Psiquiatria*, 28: 153–157.

Chapter 17

Cannabis in the Socio-Economic Context of the Southern Mid-Himalayas

Bijay Raj Subedee[1] and *Shandesh Bhattarai*[2,*]

1. Introduction

Cannabis sativa belongs to the Cannabaceae. It is distributed in Nepal at elevations of 100–2,800 m above mean sea level. It is native to East Asia, widely cultivated and naturalized in temperate and tropical regions worldwide (Shrestha et al. 2022). Its long cultivation makes it difficult to know its exact original distribution, although Eurasia is generally considered its primary region of origin (Clarke and Merlin 2013). Many studies have stated that cannabis originated in the Himalayan region of Asia and was traditionally cultivated as a source of durable fiber and highly nutritious oil seeds (Lambert 2024; Malabadi et al. 2023). Narcotic Drugs Control Act 1976 of Nepal prohibits the cultivation, production, manufacture, sales, and distribution of narcotic drugs, which also include various forms of cannabis (Pathak et al. 2024).

An estimated 4% of the world's population has used cannabis in the last year (World Drug Report 2022). In Asia, it is estimated that 2% of the population uses cannabis annually, which accounts for about one-third (approximately 54 million people) of the total number of cannabis users worldwide (Areesantichai et al. 2022). Cannabis utilization represents an eco-friendly option for diverse applications, including energy, food, pharmaceuticals, and textiles manufacturing (Lambert 2024). Various agricultural techniques have been continuously developed to enhance the yield and quality of cannabis for fiber, food, medicine, and mind-altering compounds (Clarke and Merlin 2016). Long-term cultivation and human selection for different desirable characteristics have led to significant biological variation in cannabis; however, classifying it into distinct species or the various varieties is probably not justified beyond the level of cultivated forms (Wu et al. 2003).

Cannabaceae comprises 170 species grouped in 11 genera globally (Rull 2022), about three genera (*Cannabis, Celtis,* and *Trema*) and eight species (*C. sativa, C. australis, C. tetrandra, C. timorensis, T. cannabina, T. orientalis, T. politoria,* and *T. tomentosum*) in Nepal (Shrestha et al. 2022. It is commonly called Bhang or Ganja in Nepali and Hemp or Marijuna in English (Shrestha et al. 2022; Rajbhandari et al. 2012; Rajbhandari and Rai 2019). Cannabis has been illegal in Nepal

[1] Research Centre for Applied Science and Technology, Tribhuvan University, Kirtipur, Kathmandu, Nepal.
[2] Faculty of Science, Nepal Academy of Science and Technology, Khumaltar, Lalitpur, Nepal.
* Corresponding author: shandeshbhattarai@gmail.com

DOI: 10.1201/9781003668190-21

since 1976, but the country has a long history of use of cannabis for Ayurvedic medicine, as an intoxicant, and as a holy offering for the Hindu God Shiva (Gairola et al. 2022). However, despite its high versatility, the prohibition against it persists. The statistics of the narcotics control bureau show cannabis as a consistently and most-seized substance in Nepal (Dahal 2019).

The production and use of cannabis products in India and Nepal were well documented during the 19th century (Clark 2007). The Nepali people have a long tradition of harvesting food, fiber, and drugs from a single field (Hodgson 1855), but such a tradition has not been reported from other regions (Clark 2007). The traditional Asian hemp farmers grow separate cannabis crops either for fiber production or for seed, and the illicit marijuana and hashish farmers target the resin (Clark 2007).

Cannabis sativa is an important plant that functions as a phytochemical factory (Shakil et al. 2021), contains over 500 chemical entities (Radwan et al. 2009), including over 100 phytocannabinoids and 120 terpenes (Calvi et al. 2018), of which less than 30 biosyntheses have been characterized (Booth and Bohlmann 2019). Terpenes represent the largest group of phytochemicals, with more than 100 compounds identified in cannabis. Terpenes are responsible for the aroma and taste of *Cannabis* spp. (Fukumoto et al. 2006). They exhibit a wide range of pharmacological properties, which have been documented in several reviews (Breitmaier 2006; Cox-Georgian et al. 2022; Perveen and Al-Taweel 2018). Under specific physiological conditions, phenolic compounds in *C. sativa* may act as antioxidants, protecting plants from oxidative damage (Andre et al. 2016). The flavones and flavonols present in cannabis exert a vast array of biological effects, including features shared by terpenes and cannabinoids (Pollastro et al. 2018). They are anti-inflammatory, anticancer, and neuroprotective (Soto-Hernández et al. 2017).

Cannabis sativa has been utilized across the globe for thousands of years due to its inherent biological activity, and there is no reported evidence suggesting that it is more toxic than several medicines currently used in clinical practice (Shakil et al. 2021). Recently, cannabis has been the hub of many scientific research studies, but the main focus is on chemical composition and medicinal values (Balant et al. 2021).

The utilization of cannabis is influenced by the percentage of cannabidiol (CBD) and *tetrahydrocannabinol* (THC) present in the plant. For medicinal purposes, priority is given to higher concentrations of THC and CBD, while cannabis with less than 0.3% THC content is referred to as "Industrial hemp" or "hemp," which is cultivated for natural fiber production (Fike 2016).

In Canada, a 0.3% THC threshold is used as an arbitrary threshold to distinguish hemp from marijuana based on cannabinoid content (Cherney and Small 2016; Small and Cronquist 1976). The European Union initially set the THC threshold at 0.8%, later reducing it to 0.3%, and eventually lowering it to 0.2%. The reduction to 0.2% was reportedly made for safety reasons, though the 0.3% threshold is commonly considered adequate (Cherney and Small 2016).

Socioeconomic context (SEC) refers to the relative wealth and living standards of an individual's community. It is associated with the environmental conditions in which the individual resides. The term socioeconomic refers to the interaction between a group's social and economic habits. Socioeconomic status was represented by educational attainment, employment status, and annual household income (Jeffers et al. 2021). In this chapter, socioeconomic links financial and social issues together in connection with cannabis and its use.

2. Methodology

Published papers for this review were obtained by searching the PubMed and Google Scholar databases. We reviewed published articles and included primarily research reported in English, along with a few studies published in Nepali. Some articles were also obtained from the reference lists of existing papers and reviews. The main aim of this search is to provide readers with information on cannabis research studies and to highlight important areas for future research in the Southern Mid-Himalayas to upgrade our understanding of cannabis use. Also, in this review, we discuss the linkage between cannabis and its direct socioeconomic relationship with the group of people, along with its social and economic perspectives. We also searched the relevant grey literature for the latest information on cannabis use incidence and legal status internationally. Additionally, some information was gathered from the author's field visits and is also included.

3. Botanical Description

Cannabis exhibits high genetic, morphological, and chemical diversity, and this variability has hindered taxonomic determination within the genus (Clarke and Merlin 2013). The genus is composed of either three species: *C. sativa, C. indica,* and *C. ruderalis* (Hillig 2005; Clarke and Merlin 2013; Sawler et al. 2015); two species: *C. indica* and *C. sativa* (Clarke and Merlin 2016); or one species: *C. sativa* (Small and Cronquist 1976; Small 2015; McPartland 2018; Zhang et al. 2018). Two hundred years of attempts have produced numerous interpretations, but it is widely accepted that the genus consists of a single species, *C. sativa*, with several subspecies and varieties (Balant et al. 2021).

Based on chemical composition, it is mostly divided into fibre-type (hemp or industrial hemp; < 0.3% Δ9-tetrahydrocannabinol (THC)) or drug-type (marijuana or medicinal cannabis; > 0.3% THC) plants (Farinon et al. 2020, Hurgobin et al. 2021). Drug-type plants are known in the vernacular nomenclature as "*sativa*" and "*indica*" plants based on their CBD/THC ratio (Balant et al. 2021). According to Clarke and Merlin (2016), in South Asia, *Cannabis indica* spp. *Indica* is found, which belongs to the narrow-leaf drug biotype group. Traditional drug landraces produce 5.0–20.0% THC (Small and Marcus 2003; Clarke and Merlin 2016). Traditional Nepali landraces are utilized for the production of drugs, fiber, and seeds (Clarke 2007). However, this does not always align with the taxonomic nomenclature of *C. sativa* and *C. indica*, nor does it necessarily reflect the common genetic ancestry (McPartland and Small 2020; Small 2015).

Cannabis L.

The taxonomic classification within the genus is not conclusively resolved, and this paper considers cannabis at the genus level. The botanical description of *Cannabis sativa* is based on (Wu et al. 2003), with slight modifications.

Cannabis sativa L., Sp. Pl. 2:1027. 1753

Cannabis sativa L. subsp. *indica* (Lam.) E.Small and Cronquist, Taxon **25**(4): 426. 1976; *Cannabis sativa* var. *kafiristanica* (Vavilov) E.Small and Cronquist, Taxon **25**(4): 429. 1976.

It is an annual herb, 1–3 m tall. Branchlets are densely white pubescent. Stipules linear. Leaves alternate; petiole 2–7 cm; leaf blade abaxially whitish green, strigose, and with scattered brownish resinous dots, adaxially dark green and with cystolith hairs; leaflets usually lanceolate to linear, 3–15 X 0.2–2 cm, with the longest in the middle, margin coarsely serrate, apex acuminate. Male inflorescences ca. 25 cm. Male flowers: yellowish green, nodding; pedicel 2–4 mm, thin; sepals ovate to lanceolate, 2.5–4 mm, membranous, with sparse prostrate hairs; petals absent; filament 0.5–1 mm; anthers oblong. Female inflorescences are crowded in apical leaf axils among leaflike bracts and bracteoles. Female flowers: green, sessile; calyx sparsely pubescent; ovary globose, ± enclosed by appressed calyx, surrounded closely by bract and bracteoles. Persistent bracts are yellow. Achenes flattened ovoid, 2–5 mm; pericarp crustaceous, finely reticulate.

The flowering months are May to June, and the fruiting month is July. It is found in open places (Wu et al. 2003).

4. Cannabis Applications

Cannabis is a highly versatile plant in Nepal, traditionally utilized for various purposes. Cannabis has been mostly used as medicine (whole plant), food (seeds), fibre (stem, bark), essential oil (leaves), narcotic (Shrestha et al. 2022), and for other purposes. The benefits and uses of cannabis were likely well known in many regions of Asia long before the advent of agriculture; however, cultivation was necessary to produce suitable crops for high-quality yarn. The use of a single *Cannabis* crop to produce seeds, fiber, and resin is presently limited to the mountainous regions of western Nepal (Clark 2007).

Balant et al. (2021) reported the traditional uses of cannabis from 41 countries worldwide. Cannabis use varied significantly by age, gender, race, marital status, education, employment, and income (Jeffers et al. 2021). These diverse applications, along with their deep-rooted cultural significance, suggest that Nepal, particularly the mid-Himalayan region, may represent one of the plant's historical centres of origin and utilization.

Medicinal Value

The leaves, flowers, and fruit are used medicinally (Wu et al. 2003). Cannabis has been used for treating diarrhoea, constipation, and snake bites in remote communities (Bhatt et al. 2021). The juice of the leaf, about six teaspoons twice a day, is given in cases of diarrhoea and dysentery. For cough, measles, and headache, 50 g of crushed leaves with onion paste was used as a medicine (Mustafa et al. 2021). For diarrhoea and dysentery in animals, powdered leaves are mixed with feed. A paste of the leaves is applied to cuts and wounds. A powder of dried leaves is fed to animals with coughs and colds. Powdered seeds in doses of about four teaspoons are given as an anthelmintic (Manandhar 2002).

Cannabis is considered an important medicinal plant in classical Indian Ayurvedic and medicinal texts (Tavhare and Acharya 2016). Traditional medicine systems such as Ayurveda use cannabis to treat ailments like food poisoning, gout, digestive issues, rheumatism, and as a pain relief. It is also used to stimulate appetite and treat sleep problems (Chopra and Smith 1974). Plant paste is taken for stomach problems (Gaire and Subedi 2011). Leaves, resin, buds, and seeds are used as an intoxicant (Manandhar 2002).

The severe effects of cannabis were mentioned as madness, weight loss, and decreased semen (Fisher 2011) and induced psychosis, schizophrenia precipitation, and association with depression (Acharya et al. 2014). A pinch of seed powder and flower is taken with a cup of boiled water for constipation, stomachache, and urinary tract infection. An overdose of this tea can cause vertigo/dizziness and headache (Bhattarai et al. 2006). The powder of seeds and leaves is smoked with tobacco to cure gastritis and constipation and is considered psychoactive (Bhattarai et al. 2010). The plant has diuretic, antiemetic, antiepileptic, painkilling, antiinflammatory, and antipyretic properties (Lozano 2001).

Cannabis is also utilized in the treatment of various ailments in domestic animals. People use it to treat food poisoning, digestive problems, diarrhoea, rheumatism, gout, to reduce pain and the exhaustion, to increase appetite and reduce insomnia, and to protect and heal illness related to evil spirits (Kuddus et al. 2013; Peetham 2013; Touw 1981; Robertson et al. 1996), used for cancer pain and chronic pain management (Blake et al. 2017; Lynch and Ware 2015), spasticity and pain management associated with multiple sclerosis (Mecha et al. 2020), inflammation reduction (Perisetti et al. 2020).

While cannabis has medicinal applications, such as treating anxiety disorders, its regular consumption has been associated with adverse effects, including lower birth weight, increased health risks in children, long-term respiratory complications, and a potential contribution to the development of lung malignancies (Lalsare 2022).

Food Value

Throughout Asia, cannabis seeds have been an important part of the human diet and are still consumed in several ways (e.g., raw, roasted, pickled, ground, parched, or pressed for oil) (Clarke and Merlin 2013). Cannabis seeds have long been used in culinary practices, such as pickle preparation. People of western Nepal chew roasted seeds and pickled vegetables. Hemp seeds are the key ingredient of popular Nepali and Indian pickles. A basic cannabis pickle is made by combining hemp seeds with many other ingredients (Bhattarai et al. 2010). Bhang is also eaten mixed with sweets or desserts (Manandhar 2002). Hemp seeds are a nutritionally valuable source of protein and essential fatty acids, and they are either consumed raw, roasted, or ground into flour and incorporated into cooked dishes. A nutritious trail snack is prepared by mixing roasted hemp seeds and honey with a majority of popped Amaranth grains.

Traditional drinks containing cannabis, which had healing, psychoactive, or spiritual benefits, were automatically added to the nutrient usage class (Balant et al. 2021). Cannabis-derived products are increasingly recognized as nutritious foods. Seeds are rich in lipids, magnesium, polyunsaturated fatty acids, carbohydrates, insoluble fiber, and protein, making them a popular health food (Shah 2004). They can be used in smoothies, salads, and dairy-free milk alternatives (Shah 2004). Oil can be extracted from cannabis and can be utilized to make paints, soaps, and cooking oil. Hemp seed oil and its byproducts are used in nutritional supplements, food processing, and animal feed. Furthermore, its nutritional value has improved health outcomes, such as decreased cholesterol and blood pressure (Crini and Lichtfouse 2020; Conrad 1997; John 1995).

Use as a Source of Fibre

Cannabis fiber has been utilized for thousands of years in the production of textiles, fabrics, yarns, ropes, canvas, and rugs. Unlike other natural fibers such as cotton, nettle, and flax, hemp fiber is very durable (Chaachouay et al. 2023). The plant's bark has been historically used for weaving textiles. The fibers of cannabis are hand-spun, often with the aid of a wheel spindle. Once spun into thread, the fibers are prepared for weaving by creating a warp, enabling the production of various items such as mats, bags, and fabrics. Many districts of Nepal, including Rukum, Rolpa, Bajhang, Darchula, Bajura, etc., still produce cloth and fiber from the cannabis plant (Clark 2007).

As part of this study, a field visit was conducted in the Bajura District of Western Nepal, where cannabis has a long-standing historical presence. Some of the items documented during the field study are presented here.

Cannabis sativa yields durable, robust fibers, locally known as "Septa," which are used to craft various items. The residents of Bajura District craft porter straps referred to as "Namlo," fishing nets, clothing materials known as "Ballyo," and robust ropes called "Guwadori" from the plant's fiber. These ropes are used for various purposes, such as tying a thick stick with turbines at one end, locally known as "Madani," to extract ghee from milk.

According to a local resource person, the community engaged in the extraction of hemp bark is commonly referred to as "Khsya." The Khsya are known for their expertise in weaving and embellishing hemp fabric.

Communities identified as Khsya actively participate in the cultivation, processing, and use of hemp-based clothing, such as the distinctive hemp cloth known as Bollya. It is essential to recognize the cultural significance embedded in these traditions and skills, emphasizing the need to protect traditional skills, cultures, and customs.

In Nepal, the stem and its bark provide good fiber for cordage, sacks, and rough clothes (see Figure 1 and Figure 2) and are widely used as fiber in the hills (Fisher 2011; Manandhar 2002). In Thailand, the fibre from the stems of male plants is used for rope making and textiles, especially by hill Tribes in northern Thailand (Phengklai 1981). In China, the long, strong fibers are used in the paper-making industry and for weaving cloth (Wu et al. 2003). The automobile industry also uses hemp in composites and plastics as a fiberglass substitute. Hemp fiber was cultivated largely for

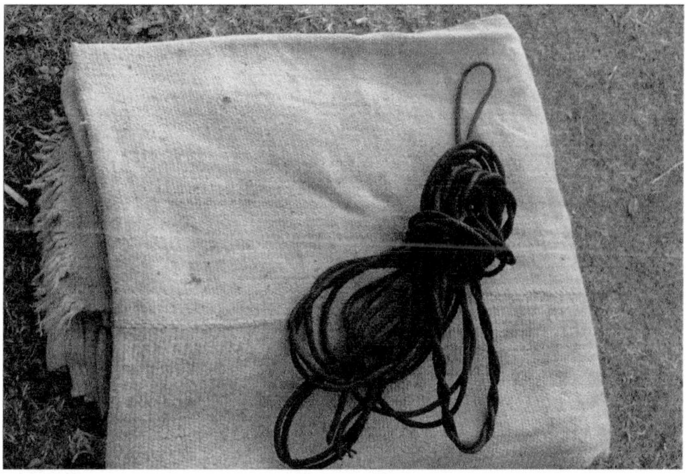

Figure 1: Locally crafted "Ballyo" cloth and "Guwadori" rope showcase the versatile applications of cannabis fiber in the community of Bajura District, Nepal.

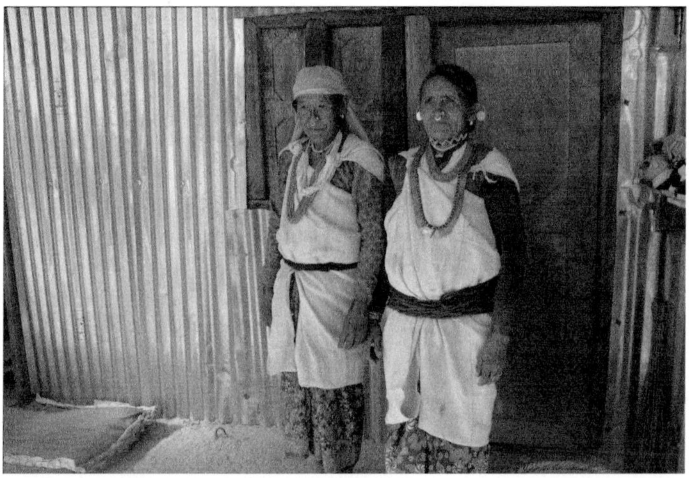

Figure 2: Women adorned in traditional attire crafted from *Cannabis sativa*, in a remote region of Nepal.

paper scrolls in ancient China (Robinson 1996). Hemp fibers are used for insulation and composites in the automotive, fashion, and furniture sectors, where synthetic fibers are substituted with hemp fiber (Chaachouay et al. 2023).

Hemp fiber is either spun into twine and rope, coarse yarn for weaving commercial-market cloth and rough sacking, or finer yarn for weaving their traditional cloth used domestically for blankets, sash belts, and grain storage sacks (Clark 2003). Smaller diameter stalks are preferred for spinning finer yarn for weaving. Very large, branched stalks can be used only for making rough cordage and are often simply stripped of their bark when still fresh and green. The retted stalks are dried and then beaten with wooden flails to break the woody pith into small pieces and release the fiber (Clark 2007).

In the Kailash Sacred Landscape (KSL) region of Nepal, species such as *Cannabis sativa* are traditionally used to extract natural fiber. Bajhang District of Western Nepal was once renowned for producing handwoven textiles from natural fiber. For fibre extraction, the stem and branches were first dried and then submerged in stagnant water for 5 to 7 days. The bark was then carefully peeled to extract the fiber. The fibre is sun-dried, then piled and stored (Chaudhary et al. 2017). Local communities still practice this traditional method of fiber extraction across Nepal.

Used to Extract Essential Oils and Resins

The seeds and leaves are used to extract essential oils and resins. The seeds are pressed to produce cooking or lighting oil (Wu et al. 2003; Clark 2007). Cannabis resin remains especially important to the local economy because farmers can produce and sell for cash (Clark 2007).

Narcotic Drugs

Hemp is a rich source of various narcotics. Cannabis was used by a few people as psychotropic agents (Fisher 2011). Seeds, Charas, and Ganja are extracted in many regions of Nepal where cannabis grows (Clark 2007). Rubbing and making charas represents considerably less labour and earns as much or more revenue than textiles or seeds (Clark 2007). A leaf from the female plant has been used as an euphoric drug for smoking (Phengklai 1981; Wu et al. 2003). In contrast, in Southern Asia, higher THC levels were cultivated for spiritual and recreational use (Cherney and Small 2016). Ganja and Bhang are smoked like tobacco, but charas is mixed with *Nicotiana tabaccum* or other smoking materials (Manandhar 2002). The plant's flowers and resin have been associated with recreational uses. People smoke cannabis at festivals and gatherings to feel relaxed, to reduce anxiety and stress, and to aid concentration.

The least potent form among different potencies in the Indian subcontinent is marijuana and bhang (Shakya et al. 2021). Marijuana is mixed and consumed in the form of cigarettes (joints). It is primarily ingested as bhang, a traditional edible preparation during the Holi festival. The leaves and flowering parts of female plants are crushed and inhaled through pipes. Similarly, the highly potent form of charas, obtained from the pure resin of the flowering tops and leaves of the female plant, is most often smoked in a conical clay pipe called a *chillum*, but may also be infused into hot milk and drunk as bhang (Chopra and Smith 1974). The majority of charas is produced by first drying the female plants, crushing the seeded flowers, and then using sieves to isolate the resin glands globally (Clarke 1998; Hamayun and Shinwari 2004). The flowers are aggressively rubbed between the hands so that the psychoactive resin, including extraneous dust, plant juice, leaf fragments, and insect parts, adheres to the palms and fingers (Kaplan 1969).

Cultural and Religious Values

Cannabis holds significant cultural and religious importance in its association with Lord Shiva. The plant is a figure of worship among the Rai people (Manandhar 2002), treated as a sacred plant used for meditation, showing their devotion towards Lord Shiva (Shakya et al. 2021). In Nepal, its use is largely tolerated without permission in the Shivaratri festival. People use the ground leaves and flowers of the female plants for smoking and drinking (Chopra and Smith 1974), at gatherings, festivals, and mourning time to reduce anxiety and stress (Chopra and Smith 1974).

Other Usage

The bark-removed stems are sun-dried for use as fuel (Clarke 2007). The peeled stalks are burned as torches (Clarke 2007). Cannabis was widely used as cattle fodder in the hills (Fisher 2011).

5. The Context of Psychoactive Compounds and Anti-Psychoactive Compounds

Cannabis produces approximately 80–100 naturally occurring compounds, among which the two main components are delta-9-tetrahydrocannabinol (Δ9-THC), a psychoactive compound, and cannabidiol (CBD), an anti-psychoactive compound, which are predominantly found in fiber and oilseed varieties (Barik 2023). Many parts of the world permit cannabis cultivation only when the THC content is equal to or less than 0.3%. In India, the Government of Uttarakhand enacted the Uttarakhand Hemp Policy 2016, which also permitted the cultivation of industrial hemp for non-narcotic purposes, such as in the production of medicine, textiles, and paper (Barik 2023).

6. Legal Aspects of Cannabis in Nepal

The legalization of cannabis refers to a system where cannabis production and sales are no longer considered a crime (Svrakic et al. 2012). For a country like Nepal, cannabis could be a potential means of generating economic benefits. Legalization could reduce the government's costs associated with enforcing anti-cannabis laws and the number of incarcerations for cannabis-related offences (Hall 2020), reduce the violence and illicit drug trafficking, thus reducing the power and wealth of drug traffickers and cartels, too (Review 2020). But the government of Nepal has yet to take any concrete steps towards the legalization of cannabis.

The use of cannabis in Nepal and India during the 19th century was well documented (Hodgson 1855; Clarke 2007). Hindu saints are observed smoking cannabis around the Pashupatinath Temple, the auspicious occasion of Shivaratri, a festival dedicated to the Hindu God Shiva. They consume a traditional drink, Bhang, prepared by grinding the female flowers and leaves of cannabis (Acharya et al. 2014). Between the 1960s and 1970s, the use of cannabis in Nepal was unrestricted (Dhital et al. 2001). The products (ganja and charas) made from cannabis were openly sold in the market. Its use was prevalent among hippies visiting Nepal (Shakya et al. 2021). However, under the influence of the US Government's campaign to control narcotic drugs, Nepal enacted the Narcotic Drugs (Control) Act of 1976. This legislation imposed strict prohibitions on the cultivation, production, consumption, distribution, import, and export of cannabis (Nepal 1976). As proponents of cannabis legalization increase across the country, it is equally crucial to analyze the contexts and practices in countries that have already adopted legalization (Pathak et al. 2024).

Under the Narcotic Drugs and Psychotropic Substances Act (1985), the Indian Government prohibited the cultivation, manufacture, and sale of cannabis: charas, hashis, and ganja, except for leaves or seeds (bhang), but a license from state governments in India will be provided for the cultivation of cannabis only for research and medical purposes. The medicinal use of cannabis in India is restricted to traditional systems of medicine (Ayurveda and Homeopathy) (Sharma 1985; National Policy on Narcotic Drugs and Psychotropic Substances 2017). Industrial cannabis can be cultivated and produced, but the medicinal, recreational use, and possession of cannabis are illegal in China (Sensi Seeds 2020). The leaves and roots of industrial cannabis can be used without processing in Chinese traditional medicine (World Law Group 2020).

7. Legal Frameworks for Cannabis in Nepal

Delta-9-Tetrahydrocannabinol (THC) is a main phytoactive ingredient found in cannabis. The THC less than 0.3% is also known as industrial hemp or hemp (Malabadi et al. 2023; Visković et al. 2023). Some countries that have adopted 0.1 to 0.3% THC include Austria, Canada, the Netherlands, and Uruguay (Kusi et al. 2080 (B.S.); Rathi et al. 2022). In 1961, the United Nations adopted the Single Convention on Narcotic Drugs, globally regulating the production and usage of narcotic substances, including cannabis labelled as a narcotic drug. Nepal, a UN member, adhered to this convention, leading to a 1973 (2030 B.S.) political declaration that banned cannabis cultivation, use, and trade in alignment with the international stance. Subsequently, Nepal implemented the Narcotics Control Act of 1976 (2033 B.S.). In a pivotal move, the 1993 (2049 B.S.) third amendment clarified cannabis as a non-drug status, and clarified the cannabis should be exempted from the drug to non-drug status controlled medicinal purpose (Kusi et al. 2080 B.S.). Despite this, producers and users have not been able to utilize this amendment made to the Narcotic Control Act, 1976 (2033 B.S.).

Due to the lack of infrastructure, governing body, and management regulations, even this treaty will not hinder the production of seeds and fibers (Kusi et al. 2080 B.S.). Overcoming these challenges requires a thoughtful approach to the legal framework and robust administrative measures. Cannabis cultivation and business currently face legal restrictions, leading traders to export hemp fibre products under alternative labels such as Allo (*Girardinia diversifolia*) fiber or other fiber-based goods; many products carry a symbolic hemp logo. Business claims indicate that approximately 70% of industrial products containing hemp fibers are exported to India, 20% to Europe, 5% to America, and the remaining 5% to various other countries (Kusi et al. 2080 B.S.).

The absence of formal revenue collection from this industry is a significant issue. Businessmen argue that both local people are adversely affected by these legal constraints. Research conducted by the Policy Research Institute suggests that legalizing hemp cultivation and business could yield substantial revenue and create additional economic opportunities (Kusi et al. 2080 B.S.). Nepal may learn from the USA, Spain, and Portugal about re-legalizing cannabis, by spreading awareness on controlled use, and creating a proper market. Following these countries' examples could help Nepal benefit from cannabis (Khanal et al. 2021).

In 2020, a private bill entitled "Marijuana Cultivation Regulation and Management in Nepal" was registered with the Parliament Secretariat of the House of Representatives. The bill proposed legalizing cannabis cultivation to generate economic benefits, primarily through export. However, it did not advocate for the legalization of public consumption of cannabis, although there were discussions regarding its use for medical purposes by patients. In the budget speech for the fiscal year 2081/82 (Nepali calendar), the Government of Nepal also mentioned developing acts and policies to commercialize cannabis, aiming to promote its medical use.

8. Conclusion and Future Perspectives

The taxonomic classification of cannabis exhibits significant variability. Three distinct species (*C. sativa*, *C. indica*, and *C. ruderalis*) are recognized (Hillig 2005; Clarke and Merlin 2013; Sawler et al. 2015), while others classify it into two species (*C. sativa* and *C. indica*) (Clarke and Merlin 2016). Additionally, a widely accepted perception holds that cannabis is a single species (*C. sativa*) with multiple subspecies and varieties (Small and Cronquist 1976; Small 2015; McPartland 2018; Zhang et al. 2018). The plant has been categorized into four distinct types based on percentage of THC and CBD (Clarke et al. 2016). Molecular analysis of *Cannabis* samples has not been extensively studied across Nepal's various regions. Therefore, there is a significant need for molecular studies that could contribute to resolving classification issues to some extent.

The cannabis grown in India, Nepal, and China is generally twice as potent as that grown in America (Chopra 1969). It is reported that cannabis in South Asian contains 5–20% THC (Small and Marcus 2003; Clarke and Merlin 2016; Joshi 2017). However, since many countries prohibit the cultivation of industrial hemp containing THC levels exceeding 0.3%, it is imperative to conduct comprehensive research on the THC content in cannabis found in Nepal.

According to the Uttarakhand Hemp Policy (2016), in India, the cultivation licenses for cannabis were issued with the requirement that the THC level must be equal to or less than 0.3%. However, farmers who have traditionally cultivated cannabis continued to use seeds preserved from their earlier practices. According to the policy, the responsibility for THC testing rests with the license holders themselves. Furthermore, it has been observed that many farmers are cultivating cannabis without obtaining the required licenses. As a result, implementing and enforcing the threshold of 0.3% or less THC has been demonstrated to be challenging (Barik 2023). The study on the legalization of cannabis as frontier capitalism concluded that the cannabis for medical purposes is justified. However, its distribution or sharing remains legally prohibited (Lagalisse 2018).

Presently, many cultivars of cannabis are being developed, and hybrid seeds are being produced to maximize economic benefits. As a result, these cultivars are becoming geographically and functionally isolated, with little to no gene exchange (Clarke and Merlin 2016). This isolation poses a threat to traditional landraces, as they risk contamination and loss. Nepal is also contributing to the preservation of these traditional landraces. Traditional practices related to cannabis in Nepal are gradually diminishing. Therefore, it is imperative to develop policies that emphasize the sustainable utilization and conservation of this highly versatile plant. More research is needed to determine the potential domestication area of cannabis in Nepal.

It is urgent to initiate a collaborative research program and allocate a budget at the Government level on cannabis use and associated policies in Nepal (Ransing et al. 2022). The cultivation of the cannabis crop creates jobs and may initiate industrialization. Thus, detailed research is necessary to understand the therapeutic benefits and risks of CBD and THC. If legalization is to be considered, the government must prioritize strict policies on trade, adulteration, smuggling, and illegal export to address concerns about an open border between Nepal and India (Pulami 2023). Policymakers need a robust plan to capture the economic benefits brought by legalization.

The Government of Nepal and national policymakers may examine both the positive and negative impacts and experiences from countries that have legalized cannabis. Policymakers may carefully consider the potential outcomes of the relegalization process, with particular emphasis on harm reduction and effective public health responses. To support this, socio-economic research is essential to identify the potential benefits and risks associated with legalization.

This chapter summarizes an ephemeral overview of the socio-economic aspects of cannabis use across the southern Himalayas, as well as general background, taxonomy, and traditional use of cannabis. Cannabis may be one of the least stigmatized of illegal drugs globally. It is the right time to understand cannabis use to guide and update national and global policies. There is noteworthy scientific evidence that supports the usage of cannabis as a traditional phytomedicine. The plant has been used for thousands of years worldwide for its biological activity, and thus, further biological evaluation to strengthen the pharmacological perspective of cannabis use is necessary in the future. The detailed toxicological analysis is necessary to conclude the safety of this plant.

References

Acharya, S. L., Howard, J., Panta, S. B., Mahatma, S. S., and Copeland, J. (2014). Cannabis, Lord Shiva and Holy Men: Cannabis Use among Sadhus in Nepal. *Journal of Psychiatrists' Association of Nepal*, 3(2): 9–14.

Andre, C. M., Hausman, J. F., and Guerriero, G. (2016). *Cannabis sativa*: the plant of the thousand and one molecules. *Front Plant Sci.*, 7: 19.

Areesantichai, C., Perngparn, U., and Pilley C. (2020). Current cannabis-related situation in the Asia-Pacific region. *Curr Opin Psychiatry*, 33(4): 352–359.

Balant, M., Gras, A., Ruz, M., Vall`es, J., Vitales, D., and Garnatje, T. (2021). Traditional uses of *Cannabis*: An analysis of the CANNUSE database. *Journal of Ethnopharmacology*, 279: 114362.

Barik, M. (2023). Political Ecology of Hemp in Uttarakhand: From Theory to Policy and Practice. *Research Journal of Berhampur University*, 75.

Bhatt, M., Adhikari, Y. P., and Kunwar, R. (2021). Ethnomedicinal values of weeds in Kanchanpur District, Far-Western Nepal. *Ethnobotany Research and Applications*, 21: 1–19.

Bhattarai, S., Chaudhary, R. P., and Taylor, R. S. L. (2006). Ethnomedicinal plants used by the people of Manang district, central Nepal. *Journal of Ethnobiology and Ethnomedicine*, 2: 41.

Bhattarai, S., Chaudhary, R. P., Quave, C. L., and Taylor, R. S. L. (2010). The use of medicinal plants in the trans-himalayan arid zone of Mustang district, Nepal. *Journal of Ethnobiology and Ethnomedicine*, 6: 14.

Blake, A., Wan, B. A., Malek, L., DeAngelis, C., Diaz, P., Lao, N. et al. (2017). A selective review of medical *Cannabis* in cancer pain management. *Ann. Palliat. Med.*, 6 (Suppl. 2): S215–S222.

Booth, J. K., and Bohlmann, J. (2019). Terpenes in *Cannabis sativa* - from plant genome to humans. *Plant Sci.*, 284: 67–72.

Breitmaier, E. (2006). *Terpenes: Flavors, Fragrances, Pharmaca, Pheromones*. John Wiley & Sons. p. 242.

Calvi, L., Pavlović, R., Panseri, S., Giupponi, L., Leoni, V., and Giorgi, A. (2018). Quality traits of medical *Cannabis sativa* L. inflorescences and derived products based on comprehensive mass-spectrometry analytical investigation. Recent Advances in Cannabinoid Research. London: IntechOpen; https://doi.org/10.5772/intechopen.79539.

Chaachouay, N., Azerouall, A., Bencharkil, B., Douira, A., and Zidane, L. (2023). *Cannabis sativa* L.: A Review on Traditional Uses, Botany, Phytochemistry, and Pharmacological Aspects. *Trad. Integr. Med.*, 8(1): 97–116.

Chaudhary, R. P., Bhattarai, S. H., Basnet, G., Bhatta, K. P., Uprety, Y., Bhatta, L. D. et al. (2017). *Traditional practice and knowledge of indigenous and local communities in Kailash Sacred Landscape, Nepal.* ICIMOD Working Paper 2017/1. Kathmandu: ICIMOD.

Cherney, J. H., and Small, E. (2016). Industrial hemp in North America: Production, politics and potential. *Agronomy*, 6(4): 58. doi.org/10.3390/agronomy6040058.

Chopra, G. S., and Smith, J. W. 1974. Psychotic reactions following cannabis use in East Indians. *Archives of General Psychiatry*, 30(1): 24–27.

Chopra, G. S. (1969). Man and Marijuana. *International journal of the addictions*, 4(2): 215–247.

Clark, R. C. (2007). Traditional *Cannabis* Cultivation in Darchula District, Nepal–Seed, Resin and Textiles. *Journal of Industrial Hemp*, 12(2): 19–42.

Clarke, R., and Merlin, M. (2013). *Cannabis: Evolution and Ethnobotany.* First edition, University of California Press, Berkley, Los Angeles, London.

Clarke, R. C., and Merlin, M. D. (2016). Cannabis domestication, breeding history, present-day genetic diversity, and future prospects. *Critical Reviews in Plant Sciences*, 35(5-6): 293–327.

Clarke, R. C. (1998). *Hashish*!. Red Eye Press, Los Angeles, California, USA: 387 pages.

Conrad, C. (1997). *Hemp for health: The medicinal and nutritional uses of Cannabis sativa.* Inner Traditions/Bear & Co.

Cox-Georgian, D., Ramadoss, N., Dona, C., and Basu, C. (2022). *Therapeutic and Medicinal Uses of Terpenes.* pp. 333–359. *In*: Joshee, N., Dhekney, S. A., and Parajuli, P. (Eds.). Medicinal Plants: From Farm to Pharmacy [Internet]. Cham: Springer International Publishing.

Crini, G., and Lichtfouse, E. (2020). *Sustainable Agriculture Reviews 42: Hemp Production and Applications.* Vol. 42. Springer Nature.

Dahal, L. (2019). From mellow to high: How the movement to legalize marijuana is lighting up Nepal. The Kathmandu Post.

Dhital, R., Subedi, G., Gurung, Y. B., and Hamal, P. (2001). *Alcohol and drug use in Nepal.* Kathmandu: Child Workers in Nepal Concerned Centre (CWIN).

Farinon, B., Molinari, R., Costantini, L., and Merendino, N. (2020). The seed of industrial hemp (*Cannabis sativa* L.): Nutritional quality and potential functionality for human health and nutrition. *Nutrients*, 12(7): 1935. doi.org/10.3390/nu12071935

Fike, J. (2016). Industrial hemp: renewed opportunities for an ancient crop. *Critical Reviews in Plant Sciences*, 35(5-6): 406–424.

Fisher, J. (2011). *Cannabis in Nepal: an overview.* pp: 247–256. *In*: Cannabis and Culture.

Fukumoto, S., Sawasaki, E., Okuyama, S., Miyake, Y., and Yokogoshi, H. (2006). Flavour components of monoterpenes in citrus essential oils enhance the release of monoamines from rat brain slices. *Nutr Neurosci.*, 9: 7380.

Gaire, B. P., and Subedi, L. (2011). Medicinal Plant Diversity and their Pharmacological Aspects of Nepal Himalayas. *Pharmacognosy Journal*, 3(25): 6–17.

Gairola, S., Singh, K., and Sharma, J. (2022). Plants used for Socio-Magico-Religious purposes by the indigenous communities of Sub-Himalayan Tract, Uttarakhand. *Ethnobotany Research and Applications*, 23: 1–19.

Hall, W. (2020). The costs and benefits of cannabis control policies. *Dialogues Clin Neurosci.*, 22(3): 281–287.

Hamayun, M., and Shinwari, Z. K. (2004). Folk Methodology of *Charas* (Hashish) Production and Its Marketing at Afridi Tirah, Federally Administered Tribal Areas (FATA), Pakistan. *Journal of Industrial Hemp*, 9(2): 41–50.

Hillig, K. W. (2005). Genetic evidence for speciation in *Cannabis* (Cannabaceae). *Genet. Resour. Crop Evol.*, 52: 161–180.

Hodgson, H. B. (1855). Hemp Cultivation in Nepal. pp. 314–340. *In*: Royle, J. F. (Ed.). The fibrous plants of India fitted for cordage, clothing, and paper. With an account of the cultivation and preparation of flax, hemp, and their substitutes. Smith, Elder and Co., London, England.

Hurgobin, B., Tamiru-Oli, M., Welling, M. T., Doblin, M. S., Bacic, A., Whelan, J. et al. (2021). Recent advances in *Cannabis sativa* genomics research. *New Phytol.*, 230: 73–89. doi: 10.1111/nph.17140.

Jeffers, A. B., Glantz, S., Byers, A., and Keyhani, S. (2021). Sociodemographic characteristics associated with and prevalence and frequency of *Cannabis* use among adults in the US. *JAMA Netw Open.*, 30; 4(11): e2136571.

Jones, K. 1995. *Nutritional and medicinal guide to hemp seed.* Rainforest Botanical Laboratory.

Joshi, D. R. (2020). Legalize Cannabis in Nepal to improve Health and Economy. *Journal of Drug Delivery and Therapeutics.*, 10(1-S): 185–186.

Joshi, M. P. (2017). The hemp cultivators of Uttarakhand and social complexity (with a special reference to the Rathis of Garhwal*). Acta Orientalia*, 78: 173–221.

Kaplan, J. (Ed.). (1969). *Marijuana: Report of the Indian Hemp Drugs Commission 1893–1894* (8 Vols.). Thomas Jefferson Press, Silver Springs, Maryland, USA: 15–84.

Khanal, S., and Christian, S. (2021). Cannabis legalization and potential impacts on Nepali economy and public health. *Global Journal of Agricultural and Allied Sciences*, 3(1): 25–28.

Kuddus, M., Ginawi, I., and Al-Hazimi, A. (2013). *Cannabis sativa*: an ancient wild edible plant of India. *Emirates Journal of Food and Agriculture*, 25(10): 736–745. doi: 10.9755/ejfa.v25i10.16400.

Kusi, M., Neupane, H. S., Kattel, M. R., Mainali, H. P., Gyawali, R., Regmi, P. et al. (2080). B.S. *Nepal ma ganga kheti ko baidanikaran: sambawana ra chunati* Kathmandu: Institute of Policy Research.

Lagalisse, E. (2018). The dangers of health and safety: marijuana legalization as frontier capitalism. *Journal of Ethnobiology*, 38(4): 473–488.

Lalsare, S. S. (2022). Cannabinoids: legal aspects, pharmacology, phytochemistry, probable targets from the biological system, and therapeutic potential. *Asian Journal of Pharmaceutical Research and Health Care*, 14(3): 127–141.

Lambert, C. F. C., Filho, E. A. B., Coronado, K. V. C., and Malabadi, RB. (2024). Exploring the potentialities of industrial hemp for sustainable rural development. *World Journal of Biology Pharmacy and Health Sciences*, 18(01): 305–320.

Lozano, I. (2001). The therapeutic use of *Cannabis sativa* (L.) in Arabic medicine. *J. Cannabis Ther.*; 1: 63–70.

Lynch, M. E., and Ware, M. A. (2015). Cannabinoids for the treatment of chronic non-cancer pain: an updated systematic review of randomized controlled trials. *J. Neuroimmune Pharmacol.*, 10: 293–301.

Malabadi, R. B., Kolkar, K. P., and Chalannavar, R. K. (2023). *Cannabis sativa*: Industrial hemp (fiber type)-An Ayurvedic Traditional Herbal Medicine. *International Journal of Innovation Scientific Research and Review*, 5(2): 4040–4046.

Malabadi, R. B., Kolkar, K. P., and Chalannavar, R. K. (2023). *Cannabis sativa*: Ethnobotany and phytochemistry. *International Journal of Innovation Scientific Research and Review*, 5(2): 3990–3998.

Manandhar, N. P. (2002). *Plants and People of Nepal*. Timber Press, Oregon, USA.

McPartland, J. M., and Small, E. (2020). A classification of endangered high-THC *cannabis* (*Cannabis sativa* subsp. *indica*) domesticates and their wild relatives. *PhytoKeyes*, 144: 81–112.

McPartland, J. M. (2018). *Cannabis* systematics at the levels of family, genus, and species. *Cannabis Cannabinoid Res.*, 3: 203–212.

Mecha, M., Carrillo-Salinas, F. J., Feliú, A., Mestre, L., and Guaza, C. (2020). Perspectives on cannabis-based therapy of multiple sclerosis: a mini-review. *Front. Cell. Neurosci.*, 14: 35.

Mustafa, A., Ahmad, K. S., Mehmood, A., Nawaz, F., Ahmed, H., Hamid, A. et al. (2021). Ethnobotany of Mountain Region of the Himalaya, District Poonch, Azad Kashmir. *Ethnobiology of Mountain Communities in Asia*, 245–267.

National Policy on Narcotic Drugs and Psychotropic Substances; 2017). Available from: https://taxguru.in/corporate-law/national-policy-on-narcotic-drugs-and-psychotropic-substances.html. Accessed March 11, 2023.

Nepal Law Commission. 1976. *Narcotic Drugs (Control) Act, 2033 (1976)*. Accessed from www.dda.gov.np on March 2025.

Pathak, N., Dhungana, S., Basyal, B., Jha, P. K., Shrestha, S., Thapa, P., and Paudyal, V. (2024). Current Status of *Cannabis* Legalization and Decriminalization Efforts in Nepal. *Substance Abuse and Rehabilitation*, 15: 163–171.

Peetham, S.-B. S. (2013). Ayurvedic View of Marijuana. Website: Retrieved December 10, 2014. http://www.somamatha.org/ayurvedic-view-of-marijuana.html.

Perisetti, A., Rimu, A. H., Khan, S. A., Bansal, P., and Goyal, H. (2020). Role of *Cannabis* in inflammatory bowel diseases. *Ann. Gastroenterol.*, 33: 134–144.

Perveen, S., and Al-Taweel, A. (2018). *Terpenes and Terpenoids*. BoD – Books on Demand. p. 154.

Phengklai, C. (1981). *Cannabidaceae.* E-Flora of Thailand. Volume 2 Part 4. Page 392 394.

Pollastro, F., Minassi, A., and Fresu, L. G. (2018). *Cannabis* Phenolics and their Bioactivities. *Current medicinal chemistry*, **25(10):** 1160-1185. doi.org/10.2174/0929867324666170810164636.

Pulami, M. J. (2023). Introducing the idea of border governance for Nepal-India open border. *J Polit Sci.*,77–97. doi:10.3126/jps.v23i1.52285.

Radwan, M. M., Elsohly, M. A., Slade, D, Ahmed SA, Khan IA, Ross SA. (2009. Biologically active cannabinoids from high-potency *Cannabis sativa. J. Nat. Prod.*, 72(5): 906–911.

Rajbhandari, K. R., and Rai, S. K. (2019). *A Handbook of the flowering plants of Nepal Volume 2*. Government of Nepal, Ministry of Forests and Environments, Department of Plant Resources.

Rajbhandari, K. R., Bhattarai, K. R., and Baral, S. R. (2012). *Catalogue of Nepalese Flowering Plants –III: Dicotyledons (Compositae to Salicaceae)*. Government of Nepal, Ministry of Forests and Environments, Department of Plant Resources, National Herbarium and Plant Laboratories, Godawari, Lalitpur, Nepal.

Ransing, R., Rosa, P. A. de la, Pereira-Sanchez, V., Handuleh, J. I. M., Jerotic, S., Gupta, A. K. et al. (2022). Current state of cannabis use, policies, and research across sixteen countries: cross-country comparisons and international perspectives. *Trends Psychiatry Psychother*. 44(Suppl 1). doi:10.47626/2237-6089-2021-0263.

Rathi, V. K., Singh, G., Kumar, P., Chaudhary, M., Singh, P., and Mishra, M. (2022). Legality of worldwide cannabis use and associated economic benefits. pp. 27–68. *In*: Belwal, T., and Belwal, N. C. (eds.). *Revolutionizing the Potential of Hemp and Its Products in Changing the Global Economy*. Cham: Springer International Publishing.

Review, T. B. (2020). How marijuana legalization would benefit the criminal justice system. The Blue Review; Available from: https://www.boisestate.edu/bluereview/how-marijuana-legalization-would-benefit-The-criminal-justice-system/(open in a new window). Accessed March 16, 2023.

Robertson, J., Miller, P., and Anderson, R. (1996). *Cannabis* Use in the Community. *British Journal of General Practice*, 46: 671–674.

Robinson, R. (1996). *The great book of hemp: the complete guide to the environmental, commercial, and medicinal uses of the world's most extraordinary plant*. Inner Traditions/Bear & Co.

Rull, V. (2022) Origin, early expansion, domestication and anthropogenic diffusion of Cannabis, with emphasis on Europe and the Iberian Peninsula. *Perspectives in Plant Ecology, Evolution and Systematics*, 55: 125670 .

Sawler, J., Stout, J. M., Gardner, K. M., Hudson, D., Vidmar, J., Butler, L. et al. (2015). The genetic structure of marijuana and hemp. *PloS One*, 10: 9.

Sensi Seeds. (2020). *Cannabis* Use in China - laws, history, uses and more info. Available from: https://sensiseeds.com/en/blog/countries/cannabis-in-china-laws-use-history. Accessed March 11, 2023.

Shah, N. C. (2004). Indigenous uses and ethnobotany of *Cannabis sativa* L. (*Hemp*) in Uttaranchal (India). *J. Ind. Hemp*., 9: 69–77.

Shakil, S. S. M., Gowan, M., Hughes, K., Azam, M. N. K., and Ahmed, M. N. (2021). A narrative review of the ethnomedicinal usage of *Cannabis sativa* Linnaeus as traditional phytomedicine by folk medicine practitioners of Bangladesh. *J. Cannabis Res*., 3(1): 8.

Shakya, D. R., Upadhaya, S. R., and Thapa, M. (2021). *Cannabis* Use and Abuse in Nepal: A Review of Studies. *J Nepal. Med. Assoc*., 59(241): 954–956.

Sharma, S. (2017). An overview on narcotic drugs and psychotropic substances act, 1985. *J Forensic Sci Crim Investig*., 4(4). doi:10.19080/JFSCI.2017.04.555644

Shrestha, K. K., Bhandari, P., and Bhattarai, S. (2022). *Plants of Nepal (Gymnosperms and Angiosperms)*. Heritage Publishers and Distributors, Bhotahity, Kathmandu, Nepal.

Small, E., and Marcus, D. (2003). Tetrahydrocannabinol levels in hemp (*Cannabis sativa*) germplasm resources. *Economic Botany*, 57(4): 545–558.

Small, E., and Cronquist, A. (1976). A practical and natural taxonomy for *cannabis*. *Taxon*, 25: 405–435.

Small, E. (2015). Evolution and classification of *Cannabis sativa* (marijuana, hemp) in relation to human utilization. *Bot. Rev*., 81: 189–294.

Soto-Hernández, M., Tenango, M. P., and García-Mateos, R. (Eds.). (2017). *Phenolic Compounds: Biological Activity*. BoD – Books on Demand, p. 238.

Svrakic, D. M., Lustman, P. J., Mallya, A., Lynn, T. A., Finney, R., and Svrakic, N. M. (2012). Legalization, decriminalization & medicinal use of cannabis: a scientific and public health perspective. *Mo Med*., 109(2): 90–98.

Tavhare, S., and Acharya, R. (2016). Bhanga (*Cannabis sativa* L.) as an activity potentiator in Ayurvedic classics and Indian alchemy (Rasashastra): A critical review. *Int. J. Ayurvedic. Med*., 7(3): 136–152.

Touw, M. (1981). The religious and medicinal uses of Cannabis in China, India, and Tibet. *Journal of Psychoactive Drugs*, 13(1): 23–34.

U.N.O.D.C. World Drug Report 2022). (2022). Available from: www. unodc. org/ unodc/ en/ data- and- analy sis/ world- drug- report-2022). Html.

Visković, J., Zheljazkov, V. D., Sikora, V., Noller, J., Latković, D., Ocamb, C. M. et al. (2023). Industrial hemp (*Cannabis sativa* L.) agronomy and utilization: a review. *Agronomy*, 13(3): 931.

World Law Group. (2020). Global Cannabis Guide- China. Available from: https://www.theworldlawgroup.com/news/2020-global-cannabis-guide-china. Accessed March 16, 2023.

Wu, Z. Y., Raven, P. H., and Hong, D. Y. (eds.). (2003). *Flora of China. Vol. 5 (Ulmaceae through Basellaceae)*. Science Press, Beijing, and Missouri Botanical Garden Press, St. Louis.

Zhang, Q., Chen, X., Guo, H., Trindade, L. M., Salentijn, E. M. J., Guo, R. et al. (2018). Latitudinal adaptation and genetic insights into the origins of *Cannabis sativa* L. *Front. Plant Sci*., 9 https://doi.org/10.3389/fpls.2018.01876.

Index

S

T

V

Editors Biography

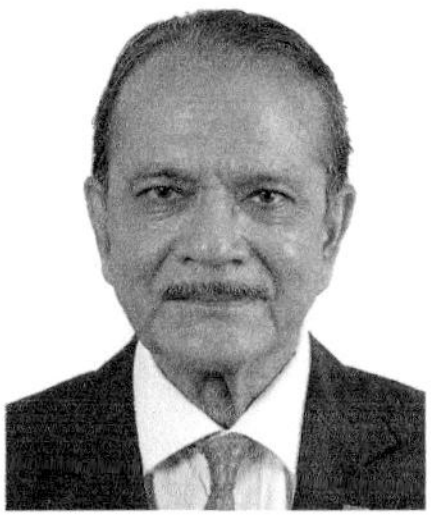

Dr. Mahendra Rai is presently a senior visiting Professor at the Department of Chemistry, Federal University of Piaui (UFPI), Teresina, Brazil. Formerly, he was a Professor and Head of the Department of Biotechnology at SGB Amravati University in Maharashtra, India. He has also held positions as a visiting scientist at several prestigious institutions, including the University of Geneva, Debrecen University in Hungary, the University of Campinas in Brazil, VSB Technical University of Ostrava in the Czech Republic, the National University of Rosario in Argentina, and the University of São Paulo. Dr. Rai has an impressive publication record, with over 450 research papers published in national and international journals with 95 h-index. In addition, he has edited/authored more than 70 books and holds six patents. Notably, he has recently been featured in Stanford's list of the top 2% of scientists in nanoscience and nanotechnology, and ranks 7th nationally in biology and biochemistry, according to Research.com.

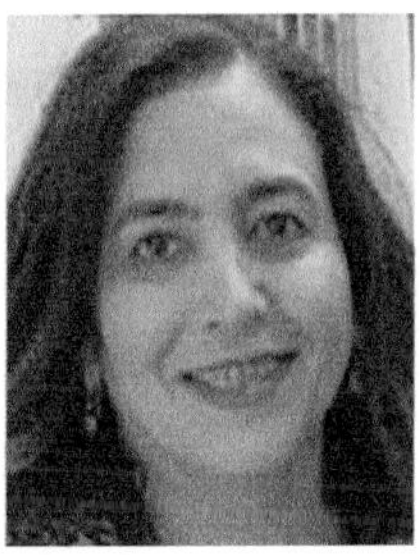

Dr. Chistiane M. Feitosa is a Professor of Chemistry at the Federal University of Piauí (UFPI), Teresina, Brazil. She specializes in Natural Products Chemistry, with research interests in acetylcholinesterase enzyme bioassays, antioxidants, medicinal plants (extracts, secondary metabolites, and essential oils), and Alzheimer's disease.

She was awarded the CNPq Technological Productivity Scholarship (2012–2015) for her scientific contributions. At UFPI's Teresina campus, Dr. Feitosa teaches in the Chemistry Master's program and in Pharmaceutical Sciences, with a focus on the production and quality control of medicines.

She has published more than 75 scientific articles and over 10 books in English and Portuguese. In addition, she serves as an active peer reviewer for several international journals, including the Brazilian Journal of Pharmacognosy, Pharmaceutical Biology, and the Journal of Medicinal Plants Research.

For Product Safety Concerns and Information please contact our
EU representative GPSR@taylorandfrancis.com Taylor & Francis
Verlag GmbH, Kaufingerstraße 24, 80331 München, Germany